D1586661

Icers

For Elsevier:

Commissioning Editor: Mairi McCubbin
Development Editor: Claire Wilson
Project Manager: David Fleming, Andrew Palfreyman
Design Direction: Erik Bigland
Illustration Manager: Bruce Hogarth
Illustrator: Cactus

Leg Ulcers

A problem-based learning approach

Edited by

Moya J Morison BA BSc(Hons) MSc PhD PGCE RGN

Emeritus Professor of Health and Nursing,
School of Social and Health Sciences, University of Abertay, Dundee, UK

Christine J Moffatt RGN NDN MA PhD CBE

Professor of Nursing & Co-director, The Centre for Research & Implementation of Clinical Practice,
Faculty of Health & Human Sciences, Thames Valley University, London, UK

Peter J Franks BSc Grad. Stat MSc PhD.

Professor of Health Sciences & Co-director,
The Centre for Research & Implementation of Clinical Practice,
Faculty of Health & Human Sciences, Thames Valley University, London, UK

Foreword by

Keith Harding

Head of Department of Surgery and Professor of Rehabilitation Medicine (Wound Healing),
University of Wales College of Medicine, Cardiff, UK

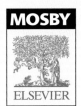

MOSBY

ELSEVIER

EDINBURGH LONDON NEW YORK OXFORD PHILADELPHIA ST LOUIS SYDNEY TORONTO 2007

MOSBY
ELSEVIER

First published 2007

ISBN 10: 07234 33119
ISBN 13: 9780 7234 33118

British Library Cataloguing in Publication Data
A catalogue record for this book is available from the British Library

Library of Congress Cataloging in Publication Data
A catalog record for this book is available from the Library of Congress

Notice

Knowledge and best practice in this field are constantly changing. As new research and experience broaden our knowledge, changes in practice, treatment and drug therapy may become necessary or appropriate. Readers are advised to check the most current information provided (i) on procedures featured or (ii) by the manufacturer of each product to be administered, to verify the recommended dose or formula, the method and duration of administration, and contraindications. It is the responsibility of the practitioner, relying on their own experience and knowledge of the patient, to make diagnoses, to determine dosages and the best treatment for each individual patient, and to take all appropriate safety precautions. To the fullest extent of the law, neither the Publisher nor the Editors assume any liability for any injury and/or damage to persons or property arising out or related to any use of the material contained in this book.

The Publisher

The publisher's policy is to use **paper manufactured from sustainable forest**

Printed in China

CONTENTS

CONTRIBUTORS

Magnus S Ågren DMSci
Associate Professor, Department of Surgery K, Bispebjerg Hospital, Copenhagen University Hospital, Copenhagen, Denmark

Elizabeth N Anionwu RN PhD
Professor of Nursing, Mary SeaCole Centre for Nursing Practice Thames Valley University and Honorary Professor, London School of Hygiene and Tropical Medicine

Baldur T Baldursson MD PhD
Consultant Dermatologist, University Hospital, Reykjavik, Iceland

Janice M Beitz RN PhD CS CNOR CWOCN
Associate Professor of Nursing, La Salle University School of Nursing and Health Sciences, Philadelphia, USA

Nick Bosanquet BA MSC
Professor of Health Policy, Imperial College, London, UK

Michael Clarke MD
Wound Healing Research Unit, Cardiff UK

Patricia M Coutts RN
Wound Care Specialist and Clinical Trials Coordinator, Ontario, Canada

Mary Dyson BSc PhD FCSP (Hon) FAIUM (Hon) LDH (Hon)
Retired Emeritus Reader in Tissue Repair Biology, Kings College London, London, UK

Mike Edmonds MD
Diabetic Foot Clinic, Kings College Hospital, London, UK

Vincent Falanga MD
Professor of Dermatology and Biochemistry, Boston University, School of Medicine, Boston, USA

Peter J Franks BSc Grad. Stat MSc PhD
Professor of Health Sciences & Co-director, The Centre for Research & Implementation of Clinical Practice,

Faculty of Health & Human Sciences, Thames Valley University, London, UK

Katia Furtado
Community Nurse, Centro de Saude de Penha de Franca, Lisbon, Portugal

Finn Gottrup MD DMSci
Professor of Surgery, University of Southern Denmark, Head of University Center of Wound Healing, Department of Plastic Surgery, Odense University Hospital, Odense, Denmark

Marwali Harahap MD PhD
Professor of Dermatology, Indonesia

Andrew B Jull RN MA
Research Fellow, Clinical Trials Research Unit, University of Auckland, Auckland, New Zealand

Jonathan Kantor MD MSCE MA
Resident Physician, Department of Dermatology, University of Pennsylvania School of Medicine, Philadelphia, USA

Alison Kite BSC (Hons) RGN
Vascular Nurse Specialist, UHCW, Walsgrave Hospital, Coventry, UK

Theo D Kwansa PhD Med MTD Dip Nurs (CT) RM RN
Lecturer Advisor of Studies, School of Social and Health Sciences, University of Abertay, Dundee, UK

Susan M McLaren BSc (Hons) PhD RGN
Professor of Nursing, Faculty of Health and Social Care Sciences, Kingston University and St George's Hospital Medical School, Kingston upon Thames, UK

David J Margolis MD PhD
Associate Professor of Dermatology and Epidemiology, Center for Clinical Epidemiology and Biostatistics, University of Pennsylvania School of Medicine, Pennsylvania, USA

William A Marston MD
Associate Professor, Division of Vascular Surgery Medical Director, Wound Healing Limb Salvage Center, University of North Carolina, School of Medicine, Chapel Hill, NC, USA

Christine J Moffatt RGN NDN MA PhD CBE
Professor of Nursing & Co-director, The Centre for Research & Implementation of Clinical Practice, Faculty of Health & Human Sciences, Thames Valley University, London, UK

Philip A Morgan RGN RCNT DipN DipNEd RNT BSc(Hons) MA EdD
Post-Doctoral Research Fellow, Centre for Research and Implementation of Clinical Practice, Faculty of Health and Human Sciences, Thames Valley University, London, UK

Moya J Morison BA BSC(Hons) MSc PhD PGCE RGN
Emeritus Professor of Health and Nursing, School of Social and Health Sciences, University of Abertay, Dundee, UK

Peter Mortimer MD FRCP
Professor of Dermatological Medicine to the University of London at the Royal Marsden Hospitals, London

Olle P Nelzen MD PhD
Consultant Vascular Surgeon, Vascular Surgery Unit, Skaraborg Hospital, Skovde, Sweden

Adebayo Olujohungbe Dip Haem MD MRCP MRCPath
Consultant Haematologist, Department of Haematology, University Hospital Aintree NHS Trust, Liverpool, UK

Hugo Partsch MD
Professor, Emeritus Head, Dermatological Department, Wilhelminen Hospital, Vienna

Elaine Pina MD
Clinical Microbiologist, Former Co-ordinator of the National Infection Control Programme, Portugal

Janet T Powell PhD MD FRCPath
Medical Director, University Hospitals Coventry and Warwickshire NHS Trust, Coventry, UK

Patricia Price BA (Hons) PhD CHPsychol AFBPsS
Director, Wound Healing Research Unit, Cardiff University, Cardiff, UK

Marco Romanelli MD PhD
Consultant Dermatologist, Department of Dermatology, University of Pisa, Pisa, Italy

Paolo Romanelli MD
Department of Dermatology and Cutaneous Surgery, University of Miami, Florida

Siobhan Ryan MD FRCPC
Staff Dermatologist, Women's College Ambulatory Care Center, Dermatology Day Care and Wound Healing Clinic, Toronto, Canada

Gary Sibbald MD, BSc, FRCPC (Med. Derm), ABIM DABD, M. Ed
Department of Medicine, University of Toronto, Director of Continuing Education Professor of Medicine, Departments of Medicine and Public Health Sciences

Luc Teot
Associate Professor Plastic Surgery, Hospital Lapeyronie, Montpellier, France

Kathryn Vowden MSc BSc (Hons) RGN
Consultant Nurse Acute and Chronic Wounds, Bradford Royal Infirmary, Bradford, UK

Peter Vowden MD FRCS
Professor Wound Healing Research, University of Bradford and Consultant Vascular Surgeon, Department of Vascular Surgery, Bradford Royal Infirmary, Bradford UK

Anne F Williams RGN DN DipNEd
Research Fellow and Specialist Lymphoedemo Practitioner, Napier University and NHS Lothian, Edinburgh, UK

FOREWORD

Not another textbook on leg ulcers! You may believe that there have been enough books published on this subject in recent years but no-one, in my opinion, has yet managed to produce a comprehensive and practical book on this subject. This book, however, seems to achieve the impossible. It provides individuals from diverse backgrounds with information on all of the key aspects of this disease and for clinicians it will enable them to improve the standards of care they can provide to their patients.

The book is edited by three individuals who are all internationally renowned for their work in this area and can truly call themselves experts in the field. A problem based learning approach is used not because it is flavour of the month in educational circles but rather because it lends itself as a relevant method of providing practical assistance to individuals dealing with patients who have leg ulcers.

The case studies in Section 2 of the book provide clinicians with scenarios that they are likely to meet in practice and inform others of the real challenge of caring for patients with leg ulceration. They also provide individuals with an opportunity to test themselves to see if they would offer good care if they were treating such patients.

32 chapters deal with a wide variety of subjects written by experts in this field from across the globe. The subjects include traditional topics found in textbooks on leg ulceration but also information on epidemiology, models of care delivery, frameworks for assessing patients, nutrition, pain, health related quality of life and patient education that are all novel and often neglected aspects of providing care for patients with leg ulceration. The chapters discussing the various aetiologies of leg ulceration are comprehensive, practical and provide readers with a single source of information to enable them to increase their knowledge and understanding of each subject. The chapters on adjunctive therapy and wound bed preparation reflect how up to date this work is and provide individuals new to the area with an opportunity to identify new directions in this clinical area.

The book is over 500 pages long and has extensive references throughout with good illustrations and tables used to highlight key issues, has achieved a remarkable feat. It is able to provide detailed information in a readable format that is relevant to current practice. Its styles allow readers to dip into sections to obtain specific pieces of information as well as enabling students to have a comprehensive review of each subject. The book is essential, in my opinion, for all those interested in this important, neglected and challenging clinical problem. The editors, authors and publishers should be congratulated. To those who access this book – read, digest and enjoy!

Keith Harding
Cardiff 2006

PREFACE

Leg ulcers are a major health problem affecting people throughout the world and consuming considerable healthcare resources. They can impact on many aspects of a patient's life, physically, psychologically and socially. In spite of a burgeoning of knowledge in this field over the last twenty years the practical reality is that many leg ulcers become chronic and fail to heal.

Written by internationally acknowledged experts in the field, this book has a tremendous breadth as well as depth of coverage, and as such it is a high quality resource. The most common pathologies are explored in detail, as are those less commonly encountered in routine practice such as tropical ulcers, and ulcers associated with malignancy or haematological disorders.

The educational philosophy underpinning this book is problem-based learning (PBL), which is particularly appropriate for such a practical subject. While it is now widely accepted that health care provision should be evidence-based, approaches to fostering high quality teaching and learning in wound care have tended to lag behind the evidence provided by educational research. The arguments for using a PBL approach in this context are now compelling. Appropriate case studies are an invaluable aid to teaching clinical problem solving and it is no accident that the case studies in Section 2 are brought to the fore and are regarded as a particularly important component of the present book. The case studies can be approached at many levels and from several viewpoints. Most present ethical and organisational as well as clinical challenges.

Knowledge in this field is far from static and a chapter is included on sources of knowledge and evidence-based practice. Other practice-related chapters include models of service provision and health economics. A framework for patient assessment and care planning is presented which encourages a holistic approach and presents new insights into patient and carer beliefs. Generic issues are addressed such as nutritional assessment and support, pain management and health promotion.

The present text can be used as a resource by health care professionals for independent study or it can be used as the basis of interactive small group work, in both higher education and practice settings. Its strength lies in drawing on knowledge from many different disciplines to enable the reader to solve complex clinical problems. It should therefore be regarded as a spring board to encouraging self-directed, lifelong learning in an ever changing and clinically challenging field.

It has been written by a multidisciplinary team and is meant for use by all members of the multidisciplinary team. As such it acknowledges the important contributions that each professional group make for the optimum management of patients with leg ulcers.

We hope that you find this volume useful, both as a reference guide and as a stimulus for further student learning and research.

Moya Morison, Christine Moffatt and Peter Franks
2006

ACKNOWLEDGEMENTS

No endeavour such as this is undertaken without a personal cost to those involved, either directly or indirectly. It is a tribute to the authors that each has seen their chapter through to completion, despite many competing demands on their time. We would like to extend our warmest thanks to them for their outstanding contributions and for their commitment to this project. Special thanks are also extended to all the families and friends of those involved for their support and forbearance during the duration of this complex undertaking. We hope that you find this a useful book, and that your patients may benefit from the best practice identified within it, and the multidisciplinary approach to care adopted.

Moya Morison, Christine Moffatt and Peter Franks

Introduction

What is problem-based learning?

Moya J. Morison

INTRODUCTION

The responsibility for caring for patients with leg ulcers is commonly shared by general physicians, surgeons, nurses and specialists such as dermatologists. While a number of excellent teaching programmes have been developed by specialist centres, on the whole the care of patients with leg ulcers tends to be under-represented on the undergraduate medical and nursing curricula, and in many countries opportunities for continuing professional development and specialist practice development are fragmented. There are a number of possible explanations for this, which have not yet been fully researched. In many countries there is the lack of a recognized 'core curriculum' for leg ulcer care, lack of suitably qualified teachers and lack of suitable, high-quality learning resources. The development of nationally and internationally accredited programmes with explicit learning outcomes, underpinned by a sound competency framework, is the ideal.

What is less certain is the influence that the approach to teaching the subject might have on knowledge acquisition, problem-solving skills and clinical outcomes. There are concerns that many undergraduate and continuing professional development programmes rely too heavily on didactic teaching approaches, are insufficiently interactive, pay insufficient attention to fostering clinical reasoning skills and do not sufficiently mirror the situations that clinicians will encounter in real life. Problem-based learning (PBL) may be a valuable means for overcoming these deficiencies and is being adopted by medical schools worldwide to teach all or part of undergraduate and postgraduate programmes.

This chapter describes the emergence of PBL, its educational objectives and philosophy, some curriculum designs and the PBL process as it might be applied to wound care. The approach is suitable for both specialist practitioners and for generalists who encounter patients with leg ulcers during routine practice. It is suitable for novices, ideally under the supervision of a clinically-based mentor, and for experienced practitioners, who realize that learning is a lifelong process. PBL has the potential for enhancing interprofessional collaboration and shared learning in the workplace. PBL is not without its critics, and both the strengths and the limitations of this approach are acknowledged.

NEW APPROACHES TO TEACHING AND LEARNING

Over the millennia, learning through problem-solving has enabled the human species to evolve in a rapidly changing environment. Today, problems still drive the search for new knowledge and stimulate research questions and scientific inquiry (Margetson 1993). However, the traditional model of teaching and learning fails to capitalize on this approach to problem solving for, in a typical curriculum, knowledge is presented first, often by teaching staff from different disciplines and without integration (Harden 2000), and problem-solving exercises are generally used later with the aim of encouraging students to apply information (Glen & Wilkie 2000, Wilkie & Burns 2003). PBL is an approach in which the problem comes first and knowledge is then acquired during the process of studying real-life scenarios (Morrison 2004). It is now a well established approach in medical education and can provide a motivating, challenging and enjoyable approach to learning (Bligh 2000, Smits et al 2002).

THE EMERGENCE OF PROBLEM-BASED LEARNING

The impetus for PBL came from employers over 40 years ago who observed that students on placements and newly qualified graduates could not apply knowledge effectively in real-life situations. An unintended consequence of the traditional knowledge – problem – solution sequence is that it can foster superficial rather than deep learning, with many students memorizing facts and studying without reflection in order to pass examinations rather than seeking real understanding for themselves (Sadlo 1995). A PBL curriculum has a different philosophy, which puts the responsibility for learning squarely on to the student. It entails a problem – knowledge and understanding – solution structure. From the very beginning individuals work on scenarios that they will be expected to manage successfully in their professional lives. The scenarios trigger both a need and a desire for relevant knowledge, and many studies have shown that both students and their teachers find this method of learning more motivating, enjoyable and satisfying than traditional methods (Smits et al 2002). The recent history of PBL dates back to the setting up of a PBL course in medicine at McMaster University, Canada, in the mid 1960s. It has now spread from medical courses to other health professions, including nursing, dentistry and professions allied to medicine. A number of medical schools around the world now use PBL as the main teaching strategy (pure PBL). Many others use it for part of their curricula in specific clinical contexts, such as emergency medicine (Kelly 2000).

THE EDUCATIONAL OBJECTIVES AND PHILOSOPHY UNDERPINNING PROBLEM-BASED LEARNING

The practice of medicine has changed dramatically in the past decade with rapid advances in biomedical knowledge, the requirement for evidence-based practice and changes in the organization and delivery of care. Understanding how health professionals learn, select best practices and change their behaviour is very important if educators are to equip their students to cope with these demands (Bennett et al 2000, Grol & Jones 2000, Slotnick 2000).

PBL is based on cognitive learning theory and assumes that learners are active processors of information, rather than passive recipients of knowledge. The key educational objectives of PBL, as it applies to health care are:

- the acquisition of an integrated body of knowledge related to commonly encountered health problems
- the development and application of problem-solving skills
- the learning of clinical reasoning skills.

PBL is thought to facilitate these objectives by building on students' prior knowledge and helping them to assimilate new information, providing a context for applying knowledge to clinical problems (Morrison 2004).

PBL adopts a coherentist view of knowledge (Margetson 1993) which recognizes that knowledge is ever-changing. Subjects are learned and assigned importance in accordance with the needs of the problem situation. In vocational programmes this approach allows practice issues to be raised from the start of a programme. Self-motivated learning is more likely to endure, and is often referred to as deep learning (Wilkie 2004).

PBL is characterized by learning in context, student-centredness and an acknowledgement of individual learning styles.

Learning in context

Research has shown that knowledge is better recalled in the context in which it was originally learned (Norman & Schmidt 1992). Smits et al (2003) describe the complex nature of many medical problems where patients may present confusing, contradictory and inaccurate information and problems can be compounded by the interaction between other concurrent medical conditions. PBL encourages the handling of such complexity and as such mirrors real life.

Student-centredness

An oft quoted benefit of PBL is student-centredness. There is evidence that students prefer being actively involved in the learning process (Bligh et al 2000, Smits et al 2002, Wagenaar et al 2003). There is also evidence that the way doctors study and learn changes during their career as they progress from undergraduate student to practising professional (Slotnick 2001). PBL accommodates these changes and acknowledges the importance of individual learning styles.

Individual learning styles

The learning style inventory developed by Kolb (1976) is used widely in medical education. Kolb describes experiential learning as a cyclical process involving four stages:

1. The learner has a concrete experience
2. This experience is observed and reflected upon
3. The experience is then abstracted, conceptualized and generalized
4. The generalization is tested in new situations.

He differentiates between two distinct dimensions in the learning process: concrete experience versus abstract conceptualization, and active experimentation versus reflective observation. In a study of factors predictive of successful learning in postgraduate medical education Smits et al (2004) found that the 'accommodator' learning style (dominated by active experimentation and concrete experience) showed a relationship with knowledge increase but had no influence on clinical performance. In this study a PBL approach yielded a better clinical performance outcome than a lecture-based approach but had no influence on knowledge tests. However, Smits et al (2004) were unable to establish any interactive effects between learning style and the educational approach used (PBL or lecture-based learning) and could not draw any firm conclusions about which educational approach might best

match different individuals' learning styles. Differences in learning styles have actually been demonstrated between specialties, with more concrete specialties attracting more 'concrete' learners and vice versa. Applying this knowledge to curricula in different specialties is a challenge for the future.

DESIGNS FOR PROBLEM-BASED LEARNING CURRICULA

PBL was originally devised as a learning philosophy to be applied across the whole curriculum, structured around problem scenarios. Lectures were reduced to a minimum, often offered at student request on given topics. The McMaster undergraduate medical programme reduced lectures on anatomy and physiology from 1,000 hours to nil. Other resources were developed to support student learning. In addition to library facilities, and in later years computer databases and Internet access, resources included laboratories and contact numbers for expert practitioners. PBL is potentially a resource-intensive strategy. This attribute has led educational institutions to look at alternative ways of designing problem-based curricula where PBL is just one of several teaching strategies (Box 1.1). A single-strand PBL approach has been successfully used, for example, in the teaching of basic pharmacology (Antepohl & Herzig 1999). However, there are potential pitfalls. Where PBL is used in only part of a programme, students may be unfamiliar with the technique and this can lead to feelings of insecurity and anxiety.

The value of computer-supported problem-based learning

The place and value of computer-supported learning in medical education is still the subject of considerable debate (Devitt & Palmer 1999, Stromso et al 2004). Ryan et al (2004) have demonstrated the benefits of using an on-line *Clinical Reasoning Guide* to assist with the integration of PBL in the clinical setting and to promote further development of the students' clinical reasoning skills. On-line materials can be used as key resources to stimulate and support the integrated

> **Box 1.1 Some designs for problem-based curricula**
>
> - **Pure problem-based learning** – where PBL is the only approach employed
>
> - **Parallel track problem-based learning** – the PBL option is offered to part of the student intake and runs concurrently with the subject-based curriculum (often used for experimental purposes when attempting to evaluate the success of PBL in achieving specific outcomes, such as knowledge acquisition or clinical problem solving capabilities)
>
> - **Single strand problem-based learning** – PBL is used in specific parts of a programme, for example a single module
>
> - **Hybrid problem-based learning** – PBL is used in combination with other teaching strategies in the same module or programme

> **Box 1.2 Examples of problem-based learning trigger materials**
>
> - **Paper-based cases** – e.g. anonymized case notes, referral letters, charts, discharge summaries
>
> - **Clinical photographs** – which can include a sequence of clinical images over time
>
> - **Video clips**
>
> - **Simulated patients/carers** – who can be given 'histories' and simulated clinical conditions

learning that occurs around the PBL course. Materials can be generated 'in house' but this is time-consuming and expensive. Some high-quality materials are also available commercially (see, for example: www.elsevier.com).

THE PROBLEM-BASED LEARNING PROCESS

The PBL process consists of a series of stages: engaging with the material presented in the problem, identifying the issues, defining individual learning needs, undertaking the learning and applying the learning to the original problem to create a solution. Students work in small groups (ideally of five to eight) with a tutor who acts as a facilitator. The role of the facilitator is to assist students with identifying their learning needs, to keep the PBL process moving, to ensure that all students are involved and to probe students' understanding.

Examining the trigger material

The first step in the PBL process consists of examining the 'trigger'. 'Triggers' are material that is

intended to stimulate learning. They come in a variety of formats, as summarized in Box 1.2. Using case studies to teach clinical problem solving has a long history of success (Dowd & Davidhizar 1999). Some PBL scenarios include a PBL task such as the creation of a care pathway or compilation of a discharge plan.

Examples of two paper-based cases are illustrated in Boxes 1.3 and 1.4. The first case is a 'classic' presentation of a commonly encountered clinical problem – a venous leg ulcer. The second is a far less commonly encountered scenario and presents as a series of 'snapshots' over time, illustrating the possible course of an initially life-threatening problem and its psychosocial as well as clinical consequences. Students are encouraged to take time to consider the trigger material. When working in groups, they should ensure that they have a similar understanding of the trigger. Students using PBL in an open, distance or electronic setting may want to discuss the trigger with others on the programme or with colleagues to identify and prioritize the key issues.

Identifying learning needs and seeking out the evidence

When the situation has been discussed, students then clarify the issues to be explored. Prior learning is noted and applied at this point. Students have the opportunity to share any personal previous learning with the group and to relate it to the

Box 1.3   *An example of a problem-based learning scenario at one point in time*

Case study 1   *An elderly lady with a leg ulcer living at home*

Mrs Andrews, aged 68 years, lives at home with her husband in a ground floor flat and has a daughter living nearby. A year ago she underwent surgery for varicose veins. She had previously experienced a deep vein thrombosis (DVT) following a long air flight to visit her family living in Australia. Over the past few months Mrs Andrews has become increasingly aware of the brown staining in the gaiter area of her lower leg. Two months ago a leg ulcer developed following a minor injury (Fig. 1.1). It has failed to heal despite her own self-help measures, which have included the application of topical antiseptics that she has bought over the counter from the local pharmacist. The pharmacist recommended that Mrs Andrews seek medical help and she was commenced on a 5-day course of broad-spectrum oral antibiotics after a wound swab revealed the presence of a number of microorganisms in the wound bed. Mrs Andrews currently smokes 15–20 cigarettes a day and has done so ever since leaving school at the age of 16. She is complaining of pain at the wound site and increasing lethargy, and now leaves it to her husband to exercise their dog. She

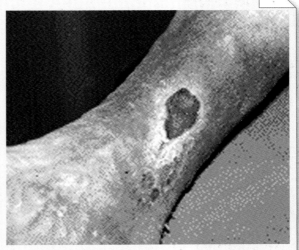

Figure 1.1   A leg ulcer in an elderly woman

feels socially isolated because her ulcer is malodorous. She also feels depressed and increasingly apathetic because, as a child, she had watched her grandmother suffer from a leg ulcer for many years before she died. In her grandmother's case the ulcer never healed and she was eventually bedridden by it. Mrs Andrews describes the situation as 'history repeating itself'.

---

problem under consideration. Following exploration of the problem, learning needs are identified (Wilkie 2004). An example of the learning needs that might be identified from the first case study (Box 1.3) by undergraduate students, or by clinicians with little experience of patients presenting with chronic leg ulcers, is given in Box 1.5. The needs are expressed as a series of questions. This example illustrates the depth and breadth of issues that may be identified, such as issues relating to pathology, the availability of properly validated assessment tools suitable for use in clinical practice, patient education and issues relating to multiprofessional working.

The resulting work is divided among the group members through a process of negotiation. Students then seek out the evidence to supply the necessary information, either individually or in small groups. They are encouraged to seek out highly reputable sources of evidence. In relation to Case study 1 (Boxes 1.3 and 1.5), these might include:

- Cochrane Collaboration, www.cochrane.org
  - *Compression for Venous Leg Ulcers* (Cochrane Review), at www.cochrane.org/cochrane/revabstr/ab000265.htm
  - *Compression for Preventing Recurrence of Venous Ulcers* (Cochrane Review), at www.cochrane.org/cochrane/revabstr/ab002303.htm
- European Wound Management Association, www.ewma.org – position papers:
  - *Understanding Compression Therapy* (2003)
  - *Pain at Wound Dressing Changes* (2002)
  - *Wound Bed Preparation in Practice* (2004).

Box 1.4 *An example of a four-stage problem-based learning scenario*

Case study 2   *A young woman presenting with lesions following a meningococcal infection*

This scenario presents a sequence of events for the same patient. Students are encouraged to use the PBL process to work through each stage of Sharon's history.

Stage 1
Sharon is an 18-year-old who developed septicaemia following meningococcal infection. Extensive purpuric lesions over her skin, particularly on the extremities and her face, have left her with tissue necrosis of varying degrees on all of her limbs (Fig. 1.2).

Stage 2
Three weeks later Sharon requires amputation of several fingers from both hands and of her right leg, below the knee.

Stage 3
Sharon spends 5 months in hospital for skin grafting and hand surgery to promote optimum function. She is discharged but has to spend time away from home to have her leg prosthesis fitted and to attend rehabilitation to encourage her to walk.

Stage 4
Sharon is re-admitted for a repeat skin graft to her right knee (Fig. 1.3) and to surrounding areas, using stored skin. She has numerous superficial wounds on her knees and elbows (Fig. 1.4). Many of these areas have been grafted – with varying degrees of success. On admission, Sharon is angry and depressed. Her mother admits that she is finding things difficult. Her second marriage has crumbled under the pressure of attending to Sharon's hygiene needs and daily wound dressing changes. Fearful of infection, she has limited visits from Sharon's friends. Angry, isolated and in pain, Sharon has subjected her mother to intense

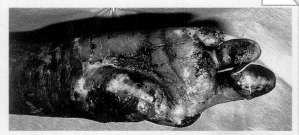
Figure 1.2   Extensive tissue necrosis following meningococcal infection

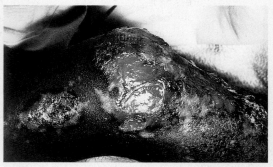
Figure 1.3   The previous graft to the knee has failed

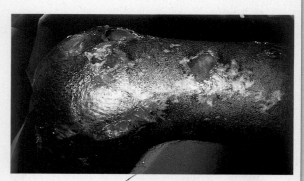
Figure 1.4   Numerous superficial wounds

psychological pressure and verbal abuse. Both Sharon and her mother complain that they are receiving conflicting information and advice from different professionals in the multidisciplinary team responsible for Sharon's care.

Box 1.5 *The learning needs that might be identified by students studying Case study 1: An elderly lady with a leg ulcer (Box 1.3)*

1. The leg ulcer
- What factors are likely to have led to the development of this leg ulcer?
- How should we assess the underlying pathology?
- In what circumstances should we consider a vascular specialist referral?
- If assessment confirms that the ulcer is of mixed venous and arterial aetiology, what are the main treatment options?
- How should we attempt to prevent recurrence of the leg ulcer in the future?

2. Local wound assessment and management
- What are the challenges relating to local wound assessment and management in this case?
  - How should we record the local problems at the wound site?
  - How should we evaluate whether the wound is in fact infected?
  - What dressing regimen should we choose at this point and why?
- Is there a role for adjuvant therapies such as ultrasound or low-level laser therapy?
- How should we assess and manage the skin surrounding the ulcer?
- How should we assess and manage the pain at the wound site?

3. Patient education, care planning and health promotion
- What self-help advice should we give to Mrs Andrews?
- We should encourage her to stop smoking. What methods should we use and what patient-centred information might we give her? Which methods are most effective and how has their effectiveness been demonstrated/tested?
- How could we involve Mrs Andrews and her husband in the care planning process and in treatment evaluation?

4. Liaison with other health-care professionals
- Are there any other healthcare professionals with whom we should liaise in this case?

Formulating a solution

Learning is brought back to the group, integrated and applied to the problem to create a solution (such as a care plan). During the discussion students are expected to challenge the materials brought to the group and to justify their findings.

THE STRENGTHS OF PROBLEM-BASED LEARNING

Advocates of PBL point out a number of educational advantages of this approach, including the currency of learning, the development of critical thinking skills and as a means of following complex cases as they develop over time. However, controversy rages about the benefits of this approach in relation to the individual's professional development.

While PBL students show little or no improvement in written examinations compared with students following traditional curricula, there is evidence that PBL students score better in clinical examinations (Albanese & Mitchell 1993) and small but significant effects have been demonstrated using measures of clinical reasoning and diagnostic ability (Doucet et al 1998, Norman & Schmidt 2000). PBL can be a useful strategy for gaining the support of health care professionals in the implementation of clinical practice guidelines (Benjamin et al 1999). While there is some evidence that PBL can change professional practice for the better there have been few well conducted trials (Davis et al 1999, Sanci et al 2000). There is evidence that PBL can provide a motivating, challenging and enjoyable approach to learning both for students (Bligh et al 2000, Smits et al 2002) and for faculty staff (Quinlan 2003). Albanese (2000) suggests that the positive effect that PBL has on the learning environment is a worthwhile gain in and of itself. Students' intrinsic interest in medicine and their self-directed learning skills may be enhanced, and may persist throughout their professional careers (Miflin et al 2000, Norman & Schmidt 2000). These benefits could be highly important, especially if they help to foster career satisfaction and a commitment to lifelong learning, but these longer-term benefits are difficult to measure.

THE LIMITATIONS AND CHALLENGES OF PROBLEM-BASED LEARNING

A number of concerns about the merits of PBL over more traditional curricula have been extensively aired, including resourcing issues, such as the training of tutors, and educational challenges, such as the development of suitable 'problems' and student assessment. There is evidence that some students feel insecure with PBL and come to rely on resources provided by their faculty rather than being truly self-directed in their learning (Lloyd-Jones & Hak 2004). The tutor/facilitator's skills are crucially important in overcoming such anxieties, as discussed by Wilkie & Burns (2003).

Following an extensive review of the literature from 1992 to 1998, Colliver (2000) questioned whether the magnitude of the effects of PBL in improving both knowledge acquisition and clinical performance justified the resources involved in running a PBL course. In the debate that followed the publication of this article Norman & Schmidt (2000) highlighted the limitations of relying on randomized controlled trials to demonstrate the effectiveness of PBL in the complex, multifaceted learning environment and pointed to the need for more sophisticated research methods and a wider range of research instruments and outcome measures. The validity of judging the effectiveness of PBL (compared with more traditional approaches to teaching and learning, such as lecture-based programmes) by comparing examination results is questionable, as written examinations may not be

the most appropriate means of assessing performance in practice (Dornan et al 2004). The 'limitation' of PBL in enhancing knowledge acquisition may be a red herring. Dornan et al (2004) argue that effective behaviour in authentic clinical situations should be the ultimate goal of medical education. PBL shows great promise in fulfilling this goal, as noted above in relation to its strengths.

REQUIREMENTS FOR SUCCESS

Henk Schmidt's research group in Maastricht has conducted a series of studies using structural equation modelling to clarify the complex relations among variables thought to be important in PBL. One such study was aimed at testing a theoretical model of PBL against data collected over six consecutive academic years in the PBL curriculum of Maastricht University. It involved 1350 undergraduate medical students enrolled on 120 courses over that period. For each course data were collected about:

- the prior knowledge of the students
- the quality of the problems presented
- tutor performance
- tutorial group functioning
- time spent by students on individual study
- students' interest in the subject matter
- academic achievement (Norman & Schmidt 2000).

The findings suggest that all these components are important. However, whether the tutors acting as process facilitators should be subject-matter experts or whether they can be non-specialists is still hotly debated (Schmidt & Moust 1995).

In a study in which fourth-year medical students were randomly allocated to the teaching of eating disorders by an expert or a non-expert tutor, Hay & Katsikitis (2001) found that students taught by subject experts scored more highly in the end-of-course test. Assuming that these results are transferable to other clinical situations, such studies suggest the benefits of employing subject experts as facilitators in wound care programmes. However, the number of clinically-based specialists in wound care is quite small. Subject experts could themselves benefit from being trained in group management and other facilitator skills (Haith-Cooper

2000) but high clinical case loads can make attending such courses difficult in practice.

Clearly, the clinical environment will influence the transfer of knowledge and changes to clinical practice. The role of the clinical facilitator and the service infrastructure may either enhance or prevent beneficial changes in practice. This is in line with research that demonstrates that education alone does not change practice.

ENCOURAGING INTER-PROFESSIONAL LEARNING

Policy documents relating to service innovation, education priorities and professional development exhort professions to learn together and to work collaboratively (Ross & Southgate 2000). The benefits of shared learning include improved communication and understanding of professional roles, enhanced interprofessional working and more efficient use of resources. PBL lends itself to this philosophy, especially in relation to the continuing professional development of clinically-based teams.

CONCLUSION

While it is now widely accepted that health care provision should be evidence-based, approaches to fostering high-quality teaching and learning in wound care have tended to lag behind the evidence provided by educational research. The theoretical arguments for using a PBL approach in this context are strong, especially in relation to fostering a commitment to team working, and collaborative life-long learning. However, the evidence base in this context is very limited. The present text can be used as the basis of interactive small-group work, in both higher education and practice settings, or it can be used by health-care professionals for independent learning. Its strengths lies in fostering skills that enable the reader to access knowledge from many sources and to solve complex clinical problems. It should therefore be regarded as a springboard to encouraging self-directed, lifelong learning in an ever changing and clinically challenging field. High-quality problem scenarios are important for effective learning, as is access to high-quality learning resources. This book aims to provide such scenarios and resources.

References

Albanese M 2000 Problem based learning: why curricula are likely to show little effect on knowledge and clinical skills. Medical Education 34: 729–738

Albanese M, Mitchell S 1993 Problem based learning: a review of literature on its outcomes and implementation issues. Academic Medicine 68: 52–81

Antepohl A, Herzig S 1999 Problem-based learning versus lecture-based learning in a course of basic pharmacology: a controlled, randomised study. Medical Education 33: 106–113

Benjamin E, Schneider M, Hinchey K 1999 Implementing practice guidelines for diabetes care using problem-based learning: a prospective controlled trial. Diabetes Care 22: 1672–1678

Bennett N, Davis D, Easterling W et al 2000 Continuing medical education: a new vision of the professional development of physicians. Academic Medicine 75: 1167–1172

Bligh J 2000 Problem-based learning: the story continues to unfold. Medical Education 34: 688–689

Bligh J, Lloyd-Jones G, Smith G 2000 Early effects of a new problem-based clinically oriented curriculum on students' perceptions of teaching. Medical Education 34: 487–489

Colliver J 2000 Effectiveness of problem-based learning curricula: research and theory. Academic Medicine 75: 259–266

Davis D, O'Brien M A, Freemantle N et al 1999 Impact of formal continuing medical education. Do conferences, workshops, rounds, and other traditional continuing education activities change physician behaviour or health outcomes? Journal of the American Medical Association 282: 867–874

Devitt P, Palmer E 1999 Computer-aided learning: an over-valued educational resource? Medical Education 33: 136–139

Dornan T, Boshuizen H, Cordingley L et al 2004 Evaluation of self-directed clinical education: validation of an instrument. Medical Education 38: 670–678

Doucet M, Purdy R, Kaufman D, Langille D 1998 Comparison of problem-based learning and lecture format in continuing medical education on headache diagnosis and management. Medical Education 32: 590–596

Dowd S B, Davidhizar R 1999 Using case studies to teach clinical problem solving. Nurse Educator 24(5): 42–46

Glen S, Wilkie K (eds) 2000 Problem-based learning in nursing: a new model for a new context? Macmillan, Basingstoke

Grol R, Jones R 2000 Twenty years of implementation research. Family Practitioner 17(Suppl): 32–35

Haith-Cooper M 2000 Problem-based learning within health profession education: what is the role of the lecturer? Nurse Education Today 20: 267–272

Harden R 2000 The integration ladder: a tool for curriculum planning and evaluation. Medical Education 34: 551–557

Hay P, Katsikitis M 2001 The 'expert' in problem-based and case-based learning: necessary or not? Medical Education 35: 22–26

Kelly A 2000 A problem-based learning resource in emergency medicine for medical students. Journal of Accident and Emergency Medicine 17: 320–323

Kolb D 1976 Learning style inventory. McBer, Boston

Lloyd-Jones G, Hak T 2004 Self-directed learning and student pragmatism. Advances in Health Sciences Education 9: 61–73

Margetson D 1993 Understanding problem-based learning. Educational Philosophy and Theory 25: 40–57

Miflin B, Campbell C, Price D 2000 A conceptual framework to guide the development of self-directed, lifelong learning in problem-based medical curricula. Medical Education 34: 299–306

Morrison J 2004 Where now for problem-based learning? Lancet 363: 174

Norman G, Schmidt H 1992 The psychological basis for problem-based learning: a review of the evidence. Academic Medicine 67: 557–565

Norman G, Schmidt H G 2000 Effectiveness of problem-based learning curricula: theory, practice and paper darts. Medical Education 34: 721–728

Quinlan K 2003 Effects of problem-based learning curricula on faculty learning: new lenses, new questions. Advances in Health Sciences Education 8: 249–259

Ross F, Southgate L 2000 Learning together in medical and nursing training: aspirations and activity. Medical Education 34: 739–743

Ryan G, Dolling T, Barnet S 2004 Supporting the problem-based learning process in the clinical years: evaluation of an online Clinical Reasoning Guide. Medical Education 38: 638–645

Sadlo G 1995 Problem-based learning. Tertiary Education News 5(6): 8–11

Sanci L A, Coffey C M, Veit F C M et al 2000 Evaluation of the effectiveness of an educational intervention for general practitioners in adolescent health care. British Medical Journal 320: 224–230

Schmidt H, Moust J 1995 What makes a tutor effective? A structural equation modelling approach to learning in problem-based curricula. Academic Medicine 70: 708–714

Slotnick H 2000 Physicians' learning strategies. Chest 118(Suppl): 18–23

Slotnick H 2001 How doctors learn: education and learning across the medical school to practice trajectory. Academic Medicine 76: 1013–1026

Smits P, Verbeek J, de Buisonje C 2002 Problem based learning in continuing medical education: a review of controlled evaluation studies. British Medical Journal 324: 153–156

Smits P, de Buisonje C, Verbeek J 2003 Problem-based learning versus lecture-based learning in postgraduate medical education. Scandinavian Journal of Work, Environment and Health 29: 280–287

Smits P, Verbeek J, Nauta et al 2004 Factors predictive of successful learning in postgraduate medical education. Medical Education 38: 758–766

Stromso H, Grottum P, Hofgaard Lycke K 2004 Changes in student approaches to learning with the introduction of computer-supported problem-based learning. Medical Education 38: 390–398

Wagenaar A, Scherpbier A, Boshuizen H, van der Vleuten C 2003 The importance of active involvement in learning. Advances in Health Sciences Education 8: 201–212

Wilkie K 2004 What is problem-based learning? In: Morison M, Ovington L, Wilkie K (eds) Chronic wound care: a problem-based learning approach. Mosby, Edinburgh, pp 12–23

Wilkie K, Burns I 2003 Problem-based learning: a handbook for nurses. Palgrave Macmillan, Basingstoke

CHAPTER 2

Sources of knowledge, evidence-based practice, and the development and effective use of reflective portfolios to enhance professional practice

Theo D. Kwansa, Moya J. Morison

INTRODUCTION

Kenkre et al (2000) noted that for many years traditionalism and intuitive knowing formed the basis of leg ulcer management. However, current health-care practice challenges this approach to care provision. Emerging concepts and scientific and technological advancements cannot be ignored. Therefore, practitioners involved in the care of patients with leg ulcers have a responsibility to pursue quality-assured care and clinical excellence, in terms of the rate and quality of healing, patient satisfaction and cost-effectiveness.

However, the nature and complexity of professional knowledge in this context reflects the complex sources and multiple dimensions from which this knowledge derives. Currently, the challenge for the individual and the health-care team is to take appropriate action when many practices in habitual use are untested and non-validated. Clinical guidelines can help in dealing with this situation, especially where they are adapted to meet local circumstances.

The following sections examine evidence-based practice and the role of tacit and implicit knowledge. An attempt is then made to demonstrate how these means of knowing can be realistically assimilated in a particular local clinical context. The roles of critical thinking and reflectivity are explored. The development and effective use of reflective portfolios is described as a means of enhancing professional practice and facilitating lifelong learning.

RESEARCH AND EVIDENCE-BASED PRACTICE

Evidence-based practice is based on the philosophy that sound theoretical knowledge is required for safe, effective and cost-effective clinical practice. The concept encompasses the processes of problem identification and extensive review and systematic critique of the related research literature. It also entails identification of examples of best practice in terms of the most effective interventional procedures, practices and policies. The information gained can then be utilized as the basis for decisions and actions in clinical and other aspects of health-care professional practice. The aim is to ensure that care and service provision reflect emerging new knowledge and technological advancements that have withstood the rigours of scientific research testing and validation. Effective problem solving is the ultimate goal.

In the context of nursing, Sisk's (2002) conceptualization of evidence-based practice indicates a process of making clinical decisions based on best available evidence. It could be argued, therefore, that in order to achieve this practitioners ought to give consideration to a wide range of sources of evidence including the following:

- Evidence from related published research (seminal work) in the field of professional practice
- The practitioner's own professional knowledge and expertise
- The expressed views, demands, expectations and preferences of the consumers, the patients/clients
- Evidence from clinical surveys conducted in the primary and acute sectors of health-care provision
- Guidelines, regulations and policies that have been developed by a team of experts in the field of professional practice
- The professional codes and regulations relating to the education and practice in terms of the curricular structure and content, as well as the stipulated codes of conduct and behaviours of practitioners within the context of professional practice
- The set governance available to guide care and service provision.

Key requirements

Evidence-based practice requires:

- An ongoing process of systematic literature search and critical appraisal
- Skills in problem identification, critical analysis and evaluation
- Establishment of an evidence-based culture that consistently and actively seeks to effect the following principles:
  - Fostering of the philosophy, professional values and beliefs, the principles and skills of evidence-based practice in the professional development of the novice and future practitioners (the newly qualified staff and students)
  - Role modelling, practice and non-traditional teaching, since these are modes of education and training that are frequently employed in the context of evidence-based practice
  - Recognition that evidence-based practice requires appropriate skills, commitment and conscientiousness on the part of both the

teacher or expert practitioner and the novice practitioner/student
- Continuous activity in the conduct and utilization of research, as well as quality assurance audits. Awareness of the need for high standards and quality in practice is crucial. Therefore, evidence-based practitioners must seek a clear insight and understanding of the principles of clinical governance and clinical effectiveness.

To adopt examples of best practice a sound understanding of the nature of the problem is crucial. Therefore, an extensive and systematic search of the literature must be conducted to select studies that directly relate to the identified clinical problem situation or specific topic.

The critical appraisal of the content of each of the selected studies allows the practitioner to examine what is known in practice and to judge validity, accuracy and reproducibility for future implementation. To achieve this, effective use could therefore be made of earlier, well documented case studies, which requires judicious selection and appraisal of similar critical incidents. The critique must follow clearly devised, well tested and generally accepted criteria.

An example of such set guidelines is provided later in this chapter.

The role of tacit and implicit knowledge

There is an abundance of published guidelines and criteria for critical review of the literature, research development and utilization.

Ideally, researchers in the health-care professions should also determine approaches that would be suitable for exploiting tacit and implicit knowledge as a means of solving particular practical problems. Rather than dismissing tacit and, indeed, cultural knowledge as unscientific and therefore unacceptable within the professional context, a general recognition and acceptance of different types of knowledge can lead to a richer professional knowledge base. However, as Gormley (1995) noted, the knowledge must be recognized as appropriate and valuable, and must withstand critical analysis and rigour.

Once expressed and documented into an explicit form the information can be integrated with personal experience in order to solve problems competently in professional practice. Within the team context, interpersonal contacts serve as a means of conveying knowledge among the experts at the advanced level of practice and to the inexperienced practitioner at the novice level.

This requires that working environments afford opportunities for practitioners to isolate and distinguish traditional and intuition-based practices.

Reflection and articulation of ideas must therefore feature as a regular pattern of practitioner behaviour in the context of leg ulcer management. This can only be achieved within a culture of evidence-based practice, as demonstrated in Box 2.1.

Box 2.2 outlines the stages of actions from the practitioner's personal recognition of the habitually used intuitive implicit knowledge through

---

Box 2.1   *A practical exemplar*

Context
Primary care setting (a health centre).

Procedure policy
All team members employ the technique of compression bandaging in the management of venous leg ulcers.

Observed outcomes
The healing rate and quality of final outcomes of venous leg ulcers managed by one colleague, Nurse Dean, remain consistently higher than those managed by other team members.

Practitioner responsibility within the team
Need for shared knowledge, the intuitive decisions employed in the assessment processes and criteria applied, the choice of specific material, the particular techniques employed and the nature of client education and supervision provided by Nurse Dean.

Reflection, articulation and rationalization
- An environment of mutual respect and support
- Opportunities for team reflection on the existing practices employed within the team – in this case the management of venous leg ulcers
- Nurse Dean encouraged to reflect on and articulate her intuitive ideas and her rationale for her decisions and actions
- Team discussions and clarifications and comparisons to isolate and distinguish the specific differences in their leg ulcer care provision
- Team collaboration in extensive and systematic exploration of the literature for: research evidence, new techniques, effective material and examples of best practice and the factors associated with the healing rates and the quality of outcomes

Audit, research and improvement of practice
- Team collaboration in carefully planned audit exercises and research activities – such exercises should incorporate critical review of existing audit tools designed for leg ulcer management
- Consensus agreement and team review of the existing procedures and protocols based on the scientific findings but, crucially importantly, underpinned by research evidence about leg ulcer management
- A period of testing and refinement prior to dissemination of the newly generated knowledge and techniques

– A team effort in which the originator, Nurse Dean, plays a key role

Box 2.2 *Tacit/implicit knowledge in professional practice: the stages of action from identification through exploration, testing and refinement*

Stage 1
- No active premeditation, reflectivity or rationalization in practitioners' use of inherent tacit and implicit knowledge
- Decisions and actions are intuitive/habitual

Stage 2
- Practitioner's awareness of professional responsibility to implement evidence-based practice
- Practitioner's awareness of the need for the inherent tacit and implicit knowledge to be articulated, tested, validated and confirmed for implementation
- Therefore, documentation of the events, critical incidents or clinical phenomena in which particular decisions and actions are taken intuitively
- Creation of supportive working environments with opportunities to encourage articulation of the identified tacit/implicit actions and behaviours – verbal and/or written explanation of the nature of decisions and actions
- Fostering of critical reflection in and on intuitive/habitual decisions and actions
- Practitioner's recognition of the existing body of professional knowledge, personal experiences, patient/client needs and demands, changes in society and societal expectations. Therefore:
  - Preliminary search of the literature appraisal and or meta-analysis of sound research on the particular phenomenon, the existing scientifically validated evidence-based interventions and the patient/client outcomes
  - Initial articulation and discussion with colleagues who have similar backgrounds of professional knowledge and expertise
    (*Intradisciplinary dialogue: Purpose* – Initial externalization, sharing of tacit knowledge, determination of dimensions and related concepts)
  - Collaborative critical examination of the identified clinical phenomenon or incident and the related decision and action taken by the practitioner
    (*Purpose* – Further externalization through sharing of ideas, brainstorming, exploring all the different dimensions for further creation and justification of other emerging concepts)

Stage 3
Team recognition of need for research for rigorous scientific validation of identified tacit/implicit knowledge into formal explicit knowledge. Therefore, identification and shared problem solving:
- Further more extensive literature search and critique of related published research by the group of colleagues (*advantage of intradisciplinary journal clubs*)
- Discussion with the multi-disciplinary team of carers (*inter- or multiprofessional dialogue*)
- More intensive literature review and discussion (*the seminar context*)
- Implementation of the research process (see Box 2.3)

Stage 4
Dissemination and importation of the newly validated knowledge into the existing body of professional knowledge with ongoing testing, refinement and expansion in the multidisciplinary context.

intradisciplinary and multiprofessional collaborative initiatives. Guidelines for research development and practice are also outlined in the subsequent examples.

The team research project

In the clinical team scenario of the primary care context outlined in Box 2.1 the team's research project may set out to explore the following speculative questions. These are questions that may arise in relation to Nurse Dean's relatively higher success rate for venous leg ulcer management.

- What factors form the basis of Dean's assessment of the patients and her categorization of the leg ulcers to determine the suitability of the patient and the type of ulcer for the chosen treatment method?
- What factors influence this practitioner's decisions in patient referrals for specialist care?
- What factors form the basis of Dean's decisions and criteria for selecting specific therapeutic materials for the management of venous leg ulcers?
- If compression therapy is identified as appropriate, what assessment criteria does this experienced colleague use in deciding between high compression techniques and lower compression techniques for particular presentations of venous leg ulcers?

These questions may lead the team to agree to explore the literature for research evidence. Additionally, the team may decide to conduct a randomized controlled phase IV clinical trial for sound scientific evidence that takes account of local policies, resources and procedures. The aim might be to compare the impact, e.g. the healing rates, and patient satisfaction and comfort, of two regimens for which there is already a sound evidence base but where a high-quality comparative clinical trial has not yet been carried out.

In their review of the literature these practitioners should attempt to critically evaluate the range of relevant published material, including clinical practice guidelines for the management of patients with venous leg ulcers as well as the relevant Cochrane Library and other reviews. Account would need to be taken of the characteristic profiles of the patients and potential variables that might influence the education, training and support systems designed to facilitate patient self-care as incorporated in the overall management strategy. The context of care is a crucially important variable. McGuckin et al (2000) set out to determine the variables associated with healing rates for patients with venous leg ulcers who were managed collaboratively by district nurses and general practitioners. In this study the practitioners took account of particular variables in their local practice to investigate the possible impact on the identified problem – the healing rates of the venous leg ulcers within their practice. The practitioners' aim was to review and modify their management protocols for venous leg ulcers.

Boxes 2.3–2.6 provide summaries of the processes that may be employed by individual researchers or by teams of practitioners.

As an example, Box 2.7 sets out the guidelines that we provide to students to guide them in the preliminary stages of a literature review.

STAGES OF A LITERATURE SEARCH STRATEGY

The literature search strategy involves a systematic process of exploring or seeking through various sources to find the most relevant and substantive information about a specific topic. The purpose is to identify all potentially useful reference sources and select works or published material that directly relate or have appreciable relevance to the topic.

It involves locating the required information and evaluating the relevance of the content (Oiler & Munhall 1993).

Commonly used databases for such a search include:

- MEDLINE
- Cochrane Database of Systematic Reviews
- ASSIA (Applied Social Science Index and Abstracts)
- CINAHL (Cumulative Index of Nursing and Allied Health Literature)
- ERIC (Education Resource Information Centre)
- DHSS-databases
- RCN ROM.

Box 2.3 *Implementation of the research process in development of the new explicit knowledge*

Formulation of the topic title

This is usually influenced by the source and incentive for the study. For example:

- Professional expertise – ideas emerging from the knowledge and skills acquired through formal education, training and practice, as well as through workshop situations, seminars, study days and conferences
- Practitioner awareness of policies, practices and procedures that lack sound scientific research evidence
- Identification of a gap in the existing professional knowledge
- Practitioner awareness of effective and high-standard routine practices based on the personal intuition of an advanced level/expert practitioner but without sound theoretical underpinnings – accumulated over a number of years these may have resulted in habitual/intuitive decisions and actions that could not be articulated or explained at the time
- An idea gained from exploration of the literature or other text
- An emerging phenomenon or critical incident occurring in patient/client care situations or the practitioner's own personal experience
- Observations by the consumers of the care/service provision through evaluative processes and complaints procedures
- Identified Health Service or national priorities based on observed demographic phenomena, changes in society or changes in health-care needs, demands and expectations.

Whatever the source or incentive the topic must be clearly formulated, realistic and researchable. A proposal must be developed outlining all the anticipated processes to be employed in the development of the research. Therefore, clear insight and understanding of the research processes is crucial.

The research aim, purpose and justification

Formulating an overarching aim of the research helps to focus and communicate the purpose and justification for the study in a concise statement. This often requires refinement following review of the literature and the gaining of greater insight and understanding of the research problem.

Many novice researchers and practitioners find it difficult to distinguish between the terms aim, purpose and justification and are inclined to use the terms interchangeably. The following simple explanation may be useful. For the

- *Aim*, consider the overall *goal*. For example: The aim of the proposed research is to:
  - ◆ develop or generate new knowledge about …
  - ◆ contribute to or fill an identified gap in the existing body of knowledge
  - ◆ bring about improvement or change in practice.
- *Purpose*, consider the *reason* for the proposed study. For example: The purpose of the study is to:
  - ◆ explore
  - ◆ describe
  - ◆ evaluate.
- *Justification*, consider the *rationale* or *need* for the study. This therefore requires a strong and convincing statement or argument in support of the proposed study based on the significance of the problem.

These processes help in guiding and explaining the direction of the study and in selecting the most appropriate research design.

Box 2.4   *Formulating a researchable question*

This requires careful thought. It is always useful to refer to and ensure that the main research question and subquestions directly relate to the identified problem and, therefore, the key element in the topic title.

The main research question, which conveys the nature of the problem, key variables and inter-relationships between them, may also convey predictions or infer speculations. For example:

- To what extent does ...?
- In what ways ...?
- How does X relate to Y?
- What are the interrelationships between ...?

The main question must be formulated at the stage of development of the proposal. Subquestions evolve when more insight is gained about the research problem from review of the literature to enable the practitioner to determine the different dimensions of the topic.

It is important to have a clear understanding of the typology of research questions in terms of the nature, levels and purpose of each type. These will influence the research design and methods of data collection, processing and analysis.

The question(s) must be clearly formulated, concise and investigable. Of equal importance, there must be a direct and consistent link to the aim and purpose of the study.

(Refer to published text on research processes for typology and formulation of research questions.)

Box 2.5   *Locating and selecting related published studies*

The literature review forms a major component of the research process. It is important to explore the existing knowledge and seminal work in the field. The review enables the practitioner to:

- Find out what is known about the research topic and the types of studies that have been carried out on the identified problem
- Determine whether the topic is realistic and feasible for exploring through the scientific processes of research
- Gain greater insight and understanding about the problem – this enables the practitioner to refine or reformulate more focused, clear and concise topic title, aim and research questions
- Find out what research approaches, designs and methods have been used by previous researchers, in exploring the different dimensions of the topic, how effective was each of these and what claims have been made by previous researchers.

Therefore, the following processes are required:

- Access to substantive academic and professional material
- Extensive systematic search and identification of material that specifically relates to the research topic
- Conscientious reading for critical analysis and evaluation of the content of the selected material
- Note writing to record key findings from the literature.

It is important to:

1. Have a clear statement of the full title of the topic.
2. Highlight the key words and concepts. Create a list of related terms and concepts. These can then be used for searching and selecting the required material. It may be useful to categorize the terms into two sets of criteria based on relevance – for inclusion and exclusion – and then to reject the irrelevant studies that show up in the search.
3. Commence the search by exploring the key, directly relating words, terms and concepts.

Box 2.6 *The search strategy*

This may require an information technology training session for the practitioner who lacks the necessary knowledge and skills.

The search should be extensive and methodical to obtain substantive information that is relevant to the research topic.

- The first stage is to determine the key words in the research problem and formulated topic title. Consider terms and concepts with similar meanings (synonyms).

- Explore different sources both primary and secondary. For example:
  - Printed documents such as:
    Textbooks
    Journals
    Conference Proceedings and Papers
    Abstracts including:
      Health Service Abstracts
      Nursing Abstracts
  - Indices for evidence-based healthcare, including:
    The Cochrane Library databases – a series of separate databases accessible by subscription on the Internet and CD-ROM; provides databases of abstracts of reviews of effectiveness (DARE) produced by the different Health Boards, e.g. the NHS Centre for Reviews and Dissemination
    CINAHL – Cumulative Index of Nursing and Allied Health Literature
    NHS electronic database
    MEDLINE
    ASSIA – Applied Social Science Index and Abstracts
  - Published and unpublished dissertations/research reports
  - Documented archival records
  - Electronic databases both on-line and off-line such as:
    The institutional intranet
    The Internet
    CD-ROMs
    Electronic journals

- Record the references of all the selected literature. For example:
  - Create an electronic database,
  - Enter references on index cards
  - Devise a simple spreadsheet
  For each article note and record the title correctly.

- For journal articles, record the surname and initials of the author, followed by:
  - Year of publication
  - Title of the article
  - Name of the journal in *italic* or underlined
  - Volume number
  - Part/issue number, month of publication if supplied
  - Page numbers

- For textbooks record the author's or editor's name correctly in a similar way, followed by:
  - Year of publication
  - Title in *italic* or underlined
  - Edition (if not the first), e.g. 2nd edition
  - Publisher
  - Place of publication

- For example:
  Book/journal:
  Author:
  Year:
  Title:
  Edition:
  Place:
  Publisher:
  Journal title:
  Volume/part/issue nos:
  Page nos:

Box 2.7 *Guidelines for planning, exploring and writing up the first draft of findings from the literature*

- The first stage involves identification of the topic of particular relevance to the given area of professional practice. It could be a topic of particular professional interest in the current practice of a specific discipline or clinical specialism.
- The next stage is to conduct a thorough and systematic review of the literature. Where specific material is not available or cannot be accessed in an institutional or NHS library, an interlibrary loan may need to be explored. This could take considerable time and therefore requires careful planning and organization to allow time for the required material to arrive.
- Careful and judicious selection is crucial, bearing in mind that it may not be possible to read through every single one of the articles collected. Nevertheless, aim to read extensively and conscientiously around the subject, allowing ample time for the full review.
- It is useful to start by developing a basic outline of concepts and ideas. Attempts should also be made to establish the possible relationships between all the emerging concepts. A consistent note must be kept of all the sources of reference of those concepts and the different contexts in which they occur. This avoids being overwhelmed by the abundance of ideas that have to be put together and losing track of some references.
- Conscientious and accurate note-keeping is invaluable in the review and appraisal of published studies.
- Note should be kept of the full reference of each piece of material read for this purpose. If any passages are selected to be quoted verbatim a detailed note must be made of the page number(s) where the quotation appears. This also avoids the frustration and harassment of having to search later for details of a reference source that has escaped the memory.
- Reflectivity is crucial. This enables the practitioner to think critically and to draw on personal and professional experiences and the experiences of senior colleagues to develop a convincing and progressive argument when writing up and discussing the findings.
- When planning the write-up of the literature findings it is important to sustain a clear focus, logical content organization and progression. The argument should be comprehensive, coherent and readable.
- There should be an introduction, which provides an overview about the topic, what it means and what it involves. In essence, the introduction signposts to the reader the logical sequence of the main ideas and how these are intended to be developed. A brief and convincing statement should also be provided that conveys the background to how the topic evolved and the underlying reasons for investigating it.
- A brief outline or summary could be presented to show the search strategy employed; this should indicate the search engines and keywords used.
- The main body of the review report should contain a critical evaluation of the identified studies, illustrating arguments with specific examples from existing theories and personal professional experiences where applicable.
- The final part of the review should provide a considered conclusion, which reflects and summarizes the key issues addressed in the main body of the text.
- Meticulous referencing is vital. All sources cited must be recorded and must conform to the requirements of an identified reference system both for the in-text referencing and for the reference list. Where necessary a bibliographical list could also be compiled of all the relevant books and articles that were read and used to generate the concepts and ideas but are not specifically cited in the text.
- After completion of this preliminary review, reread the draft constructively and critically checking, even at this early stage:
  - Clarity of expression
  - Sequencing of the key issues discussed
  - The coherence, progression and quality of the argument
  - The degree of accuracy of the reference citations in the text and the reference list compiled
  Proof-reading and spell-checking are crucial.

4. Organize the search plan in the format of a table showing the following details:

Database	Keywords	Directly-related words	Word combinations
e.g. CINAHL			
MEDLINE			
ASSIA			
ERIC			
RCN ROM			

COLLABORATIVE REVIEW FOR RESEARCH AND EVIDENCE-BASED PRACTICE: A CONSTRUCTIVE EXERCISE FOR SYSTEMATIC APPRAISAL

The following is designed for useful application by a team of professional colleagues who share the same motivation and interest in exploring current research findings and emerging new knowledge to advance their evidence-based practice.

Having identified a particular inherent tacit or implicit knowledge and having conducted an extensive search of the literature, the team of health-care practitioners would then be faced with further challenges. The next involves selecting and appraising a number of relevant published studies for meta-analysis. The following formula also developed for students by the current author outlines the key criteria and questions for conducting a critical appraisal of published research studies. This could effectively be employed as a collaborative team exercise by qualified staff. The purpose is to explore and gain more knowledge and insight about the different dimensions of an identified knowledge deficit, clinical problem or even intuitive action in practice based on tacit or implicit knowledge. The process provides another means of resourcing substantive, validated theories/knowledge for professional practice.

The collaborative review exercise is particularly applicable where the group of colleagues comprise a multiprofessional and multidisciplinary team of staff with varied backgrounds and specialties. Each member of the group committed to the development of the new explicit knowledge applies the formula to critically appraise selected studies focusing on a specific dimension or aspect of the topic from a different perspective. The application of set guidelines affords standardization and repeatability in the review exercise which could serve as the first part of the full and more extensive process of meta-analysis.

Formula of essential criteria for critical appraisal of published studies: a preliminary process in meta-analysis

The following criteria and questions serve as a useful guide for a collaborative appraisal exercise for the preliminary stage of systematic appraisal of studies for meta-analysis.

The study title
- How clearly formulated is the study title?
- Does it convey a clear focus and relevance?
- To what extent does the topic title relate to the identified area of professional practice, clinical problem or phenomenon explored in the study?

The abstract or summary
Evaluation of how informative this is. Does the content of the abstract:

- Provide an executive summary or clear overview of the research study?
- Serve as an adequate frame of reference stating what the study set out to explore?
- Present a concise information of the design, methods employed, the main results the researcher's claims and implications of the study for professional practice?

In essence the abstract should provide an informative summary of what the study was about.

The introduction
This should provide explanations about each of the following components in the research report.

- The research topic
  - How clearly is the research topic explained?
- Background to the study:
  - Does the researcher explain the context in which the problem occurs?

- ◆ How clear, concise and relevant are the aim(s) of the study?
- ◆ Do the aims raise practical questions in terms of how realistic and achievable?
- Overall purpose and justification for the study
  - ◆ How clearly does the researcher explain the rationale for the study?
  - ◆ In what way does the researcher explain the clinical significance and implications of the identified problem and what he/she envisaged to achieve from the study for the relevant target population, the patients/clients of the health service?
  - ◆ How convincing is the argument in showing the significance of the study for professional practice and how the findings might contribute to improvement of specific procedures and policies?
  - ◆ How convincing is the argument in relating the background and other issues addressed to the general topic area?
  - ◆ Does the researcher present a convincing argument to show what specific gaps in professional knowledge and practice the study attempts to fill?

The introduction should set the scene for the study and convey the concern, drive and enthusiasm of the researcher. It should also demonstrate the link between the research problem or question and possible implications for professional practice.

The literature review

The literature review of a published research report should contain a comprehensive appraisal of material from both the primary and secondary sources. Relevance is vital therefore: there should be a purpose for the review. The selected material should have particular relevance to the topic of the current study. The criteria and questions to bear in mind are:

- What are the range and sources of the selected studies?
  - ◆ From what perspectives of health-care practice do these address the research problem?
  - ◆ What specific dimension(s) of the topic has each study focused on?
- How is the structure and content of the review organized?

- ◆ Does the review show judicious selection of relevant material?
- ◆ What is the degree of emphasis on the main pertinent, classic and most recent studies?
- ◆ Where do these appear in the review in relation to the other selected studies?
- What is the standard and quality of the review?
  - ◆ To what extent does the researcher demonstrate appropriate skills in critical analysis and evaluation with critical examination of the main ideas, similarities and contradictions in the major studies reviewed?
  - ◆ How convincing is the researcher's argument in justifying the relevance of other related studies included in the review?
  - ◆ Is there a convincing argument to refocus and re-emphasize the identified gaps and is there evidence of an attempt to maintain consistency in the arguments presented?
- What are the types and quality of the research questions?
  - ◆ What are the levels of question asked and how clear, concise and researchable do they appear to be?
  - ◆ Does the researcher demonstrate how the research question(s) for the current study link to the key findings from the literature and the identified gaps?

The review should have direct relevance to the topic of interest. The standard and style of writing should convey a progressive and coherent argument in which the researcher demonstrates critical analytical and evaluative skills. There should be a clear focus and consistency in the arguments presented, with clear explanations.

The methodology

Appraisal of this section of the report is crucial. The researcher should provide a detailed explanation of each aspect of the methodological strategy, the processes employed and the underpinning rationales. The key criteria and related questions to bear in mind are:

- What research methodology was employed, how appropriate and how clearly explained?
  - ◆ Does the researcher provide a detailed description and sound rationale for the choice of research approach and study design?

- ◆ How relevant are these to the problem, topic title, aims and research questions?
- ◆ In what ways do these consistently interlink?
- What kind of research subjects were involved in the study?
  - ◆ What kind of information does the researcher provide about the subject selection or sampling technique? For example:
    - – Are explanations provided about identification of the target population and the source of subject selection?
    - – What criteria did the researcher use for inclusion and exclusion of subjects?
    - – How appropriate were these for the type of study and the information required?
    - – How appropriate is the sample size for the type of study conducted?
  - ◆ What kind of rationales does the researcher provide for the decisions and actions of the research strategy?
    - – How appropriate and convincing are these in relation to the research topic and aims of the study?
- Within what kind of setting was the study conducted?
  - ◆ Is the nature of the study setting, reason for choice and its impact on the study convincingly explained?
- What strategy did the researcher employ for the data collection?
  - ◆ Does the researcher provide a detailed description of the instrument for data collection, its development, rationales and underpinning theories?
  - ◆ What methods were employed for testing the validity and reliability of the instruments?
  - ◆ To what extent does the researcher provide a step-by-step description of the procedure employed to collect the data and how appropriate was this?
  - ◆ What explanations has the researcher provided about any problems encountered in the development of the instrument(s) and data collection and how these were addressed?

This section on methodology should address all issues relating to the study approach, design and methods employed. Additionally, the report should convey the reasons and justification for the decisions and actions taken in the processes with a convincing argument about the fit between the methodological strategies and the research questions.

Measures for ethical considerations

- To what extent and what does the researcher report about actions he/she took to deal with ethical considerations relating to:
  - ◆ Seeking access to the study setting and subjects and negotiating a means of respecting and providing privacy for the subjects during the data collection?
  - ◆ Obtaining informed consent from the subjects?
  - ◆ Confirming confidentiality and anonymity?
  - ◆ Respecting the data protection regulations?
  - ◆ Dealing with role conflict, if the subjects are professional colleagues?
  - ◆ Dealing with possible dilemmas involving subject abuse, victimization or criminal acts?

The strategy employed for the data analysis

- What strategy did the researcher employ to analyse the data?
- To what extent does the researcher provide a detailed description of the technique(s) employed in processing and analysing the data?
  - ◆ How appropriate is the selected system of data processing and analysis?
  - ◆ To what extent does the researcher provide detailed explanations and rationale for the ways in which the data were coded and categorized?
  - ◆ How clearly does the researcher explain the validity and reliability testing of the coding and categorization systems employed?
  - ◆ For qualitative and interpretive data analysis how clear are the researcher's explanations about how the emerging themes and theoretical constructs generated from the responses?
  - ◆ How effectively does the researcher make use of direct quotations from the responses to demonstrate the credibility of the emerging categories?
  - ◆ To what extent does the researcher make effective use of realistic examples from the responses to substantiate the themes and related interpretations?

- For quantitative data analysis, how clearly does the researcher explain the selected statistical package and the rationale for his/her choice?
- How sensitive is the actual technique in providing accurate information from the data?

This section of the report should provide explicit details of the trail of all decisions and actions taken in analysing the data.

Techniques employed for presentation of the results

- What is the standard and quality of the presentation of the results?
  - How substantive is the researcher's summary of the results?
  - What format does the researcher employ in presenting the results?
  - How clearly does he/she explain the diagrammatic illustrations, tables and graphs? (How simply presented, and how comprehensible to the reader?)
  - For narrative formats, how clear, relevant and comprehensive are the explanations provided about the data?

Clarity and comprehensibility are crucial in the presentation of the results.

The standard and quality of the discussion of the findings

- How effectively and comprehensively has the researcher discussed the findings from the study?
  - Where the interpretive and narrative stance was adopted for the data analysis, how effectively does the researcher make use of selected quotations from the responses in demonstrating how the results derived from the data?
  - How effectively does the researcher use such quotations to substantiate the arguments developed and the claims made from the study?
  - Does the discussion include an explanation of the limitations or any bias that emerged in the study?
  - Does it provide a reflective account of how the study could be improved, extended or further illuminated from another angle?

- To what extent do the findings directly relate to the results from the data analysis?

The nature of claims and conclusions drawn from the study

- How relevant and convincing are the conclusions drawn from the study?
  - Do the conclusions provide an adequate summary of the key results in context?
  - How directly related to the results are the conclusions re-emphasizing the key findings from the study?
  - Does the researcher demonstrate the links between the aims, research question(s), theoretical ideas and propositions that emerged from the study?
  - How convincing are the researcher's final arguments about the implications and recommendations of the findings for professional practice and future research?
- How accurately and consistently have the principles of the adopted system of referencing been applied?
  - How accurate are the reference citations throughout the text?
  - How correctly do the referencing technique and reference list conform to the recommended system?
  - Does the list include all the sources of reference cited in the text?
  - How comprehensive is the bibliographical list?
- Where applicable (e.g. in full research reports), how relevant is the material supplied as appendices?
  - How accessible are the following materials for the reader's scrutiny?
    - Copy of the instrument for data collection
    - Copy of field notes from Observational studies
    - Copies of the letters of ethical approval, access and relevant consent forms.

These should be organized in the order in which they appear and the exact locations in the research report.

For the purpose of meta-analysis the practitioner or researcher(s) would normally omit those components of this relatively comprehensive review that do not apply to that process. Box 2.8 provides

Box 2.8 *Critical reading and writing up the review findings*

Stage 1: Critical reading for appraisal

Effective reading is crucial to be able to grasp what the authors are conveying to the professional readers. It is useful to begin with a careful selection of the material that is most relevant and directly addresses the topic of interest.

Careful consideration should be given to:

- The title of the article chapter or text – how relevant to the identified research problem is the information conveyed in the title of the selected material?
- The name and professional background, if supplied, of the author(s)
- What perspective of the problem has the author addressed in this particular case? (It is usually helpful to read the abstract)
- What elements in that summary are applicable to the research topic and how can they be used to develop the discussion and arguments in the report of the review?
- The date, to determine how current and up-to-date the work is
- How readable, clear and comprehensible are the explanations, figures, charts and other illustrations provided?

Strategic reading yields greater insight and understanding about the topic:

- Read conscientiously with the primary objective of being able to identify and extract relevant information from the text
- Look at the way the content has been structured and organized, then concentrate on one particular section at a time
- Reflect on what you have read, interpret and write down the information gained and what sense you make of it; in particular, note what argument the author is trying to put across – what claims, what ideas, how convincing?
- If uncertain, re-read that section, reflect on it, review your interpretation and make refinements as necessary.

Stage 2: Writing up the findings from the literature

The literature review should show logical structure and organization. Careful planning with use of appropriate subheadings enables you, the author, to address the topic extensively and comprehensively from different perspectives with appropriate examination of all the relevant dimensions.

Structure of the review

The content structure could be organized in three key sections as follows:

The introduction

This section should provide a concise explanation of the nature of the problem.

The first part presents an outline of the author's intentions, indicating the key issues to be addressed, in what logical sequence, what approach will be employed and the rationale for that strategy. This signposts to the reader how the content is organized and the main objectives of the review. A strong and convincing argument must be presented to explain the purpose of and justification for the study.

The main body of the review

Using the notes compiled from the critical reading, develop a logically structured discussion, which should consist of a balanced critical appraisal of the findings from the literature.

Box 2.8 (cont'd)   *Critical reading and writing up the review findings*

The main studies, primary work directly relating to the identified problem, are critically examined and evaluated first, followed by appraisal of other secondary work. The appraisal should show:

- A critical examination of the topic
- The explanations provided about the dimensions, related concepts and inter-relationships
- The methods employed:
  - choice of study design and appropriateness for investigating the topic
  - the type of subjects and selection strategy, i.e. what inclusion and exclusion criteria were used in selecting the subjects?
  - the type of data collected and instruments used
  - the technique used for analysis of the data
  - the results obtained
  - the claims made and
  - to what extent those claims reflect the results presented.

What gaps are identifiable from these findings in relation to the existing professional knowledge and skills? Discuss which aspects of these have relevance to the current study and in what ways specific elements might feasibly be applicable to the current ideas and intended strategies.

Cross-referencing enables the writer to compare and contrast the strengths and limitations in the approaches, claims and conclusions drawn by the different researchers.

Apart from demonstrating the ability to extract and organize relevant information for the review, it is also important to demonstrate analytical and evaluative skills, which are vital for effective critique of published material. They also allow evaluation of the ways in which the researchers have addressed the topic from different perspectives. The style of writing should demonstrate the development of progressively strong and convincing arguments with a cohesive and lucid flow.

In-text referencing

In-text referencing and citations are crucial for the following reasons:

- They enable the writer to demonstrate the authenticity of the information used in developing the discussion in the review
- They indicate acknowledgement of indebtedness to the original authors' work, thus avoiding plagiarism
- They enable the writer to substantiate the key points addressed in the review.

Additionally, the references within the text serve the purpose of directing professional readers to the sources of the information or quotations cited.

The system of referencing used should be maintained throughout the text and should reflect the development of the reference list, for example the 'name and date' system demonstrated below. Both printed and electronic sources could be used, based on the following principles.

- Within the text the reference may be given in the form of the author's surname and the year of publication. For example, where the names of the authors occur naturally in the sentence the reference may appear as 'Matthews and Dean (2004) describe sepsis as …'. Where more than two authors are involved the reference may be cited as 'Eden *et al.* (2003) explain that …'.
- In a passing reference or paraphrase, the names and dates of the authors are cited at the end of the statement. For example: 'Concepts interrelate in explaining theory (Eden & Benns 2002)'.

Detailed instructions for the different systems of referencing can be found in most research books. Alternatively, the preferred system of referencing may be supplied in the guidelines issued by different higher academic institutions.

detailed guidelines for critical reading and writing up of the findings of an extensive and comprehensive review of the literature.

SYSTEMATIC APPRAISAL AND SEQUENTIAL STAGES OF META-ANALYSIS

One of the main objectives of this chapter is to consider the sources of knowledge for evidence-based practice. Research is seen not only as the fundamental component but as an ultimate and vital requirement for effective professional practice in evidence-based health care. Extensive and ongoing research activities and research utilization have increasingly become characteristic features in the multidisciplinary approach to evidence-based care and service provision.

Two ways of achieving high-standard evidence-based professional practice in health care are:

- Application of published findings from rigorous research studies identified through extensive review of the literature
- Through active engagement by conducting appropriate research studies.

The key processes of critical review of the literature are outlined in Boxes 2.5–2.7 above. However, as previously mentioned, another process of review and utilization of published studies that could be employed by practitioners involves meta-analysis of multiple studies, in cases where the different sources of the literature show that the topic has been extensively researched from different perspectives. This approach combines detailed systematic reviews with statistical calculations of the pooled and summarized results from a number of different studies that have explored or investigated similar factors on the same topic (Crookes & Davies 1998, Robson 2002). Specialized statistical techniques are used to pool the results of the selected studies to estimate overall effects and associations among attributes and specific findings from the selected studies (Crookes & Davies 1998). The process of systematic review is crucial in conducting meta-analysis but the fundamental components in this scientific research process are the two stages of statistical estimating. Precision is vital in these calculations, which therefore require sound statistical

knowledge and skill. Alternatively, practitioners may seek specialized guidance and support from expert statisticians. Since this level of statistical expertise and the detailed techniques necessary are beyond the scope of this chapter, only a broad outline of the key principles and sequential stages of meta-analysis are presented here. Full details can be found in a range of research and statistical books on health care, nursing and social science research.

The key stages of meta-analysis are presented in Box 2.9. This provides an overview of what meta-analysis involves. It is a useful exercise and a productive means of extensive exploration and systematic appraisal of published studies to discover emerging new knowledge and research for evidence-based practice. Although its application in nursing and allied health has been relatively minimal to date, meta-analysis is gaining increasing recognition among practitioners in these fields. Its most frequent application has been in relation to quantitative and, particularly, experimental studies. However, its use is extending to involve qualitative and other types of research design where numerous studies have been conducted to explore or test similar factors on a particular topic. The important thing to bear in mind is that the processes are applied with scientific rigour. The main advantage is that, conducted properly with accurate statistical calculations and effect estimates, meta-analysis is capable of yielding substantive information and greater scope of knowledge and understanding about specific clinical and other service related problems. Therefore, it is important that more consideration be given to this potentially rich source of knowledge.

CRITICAL THINKING AND CRITICAL REFLECTIVITY: THE REFLECTIVE PRACTITIONER

The common conception of critical reflection in health-care practice is that it involves in-depth review of events and experiences in practice. The process, therefore, involves critically examining, analysing and evaluating phenomena in order to enhance learning and improve professional knowledge, practice and personal development.

Box 2.9   *Sequential stages of meta-analysis*

Identification of the specific topic
- The title must be clearly focused, as it is vital that reliable sources of research are explored for selection of studies that directly relate to the particular topic of interest in professional practice
- Unfocused or broad and abstract titles result in ambiguous criteria and inconsistent selection of studies for the analysis

Extensive literature search
- This must be methodical, comprehensive and systematic using appropriate search engines and databases to:
  - select relevant material focusing on appropriate research studies
  - survey the titles to determine how closely related each study is to the focus of the problem and key element in the topic title (see Box 2.7 and apply the guidelines for critical search of the literature)
- Accurate recording of all references is crucial – this is important for providing correct in-text referencing in substantiating key issues addressed in the appraisal arguments
- Judicious selection and conscientious reading of abstracts enables practitioners to:
  - commence identification of variables and to continually add more newly emerging variables
  - develop an appropriate and sensitive coding system for the variables identified from each study, noting, in particular, the operational definitions provided in each of the research reports

Generation of eligibility criteria
- This is important for selecting studies that have explored the same topic and tested or examined similar factors (a vital requirement for meta-analysis)
- It is crucial to establish clear and unambiguous criteria for inclusion and exclusion. Exact quality standards must be defined for deciding which studies to include in the meta-analysis. The following may help to enhance the rigour of the study selection process:
  - An appropriate pro forma should be developed for assessing the eligibility status of each study
  - A scoring system must be developed and tested for validity and reliability
  - Additionally, it is necessary to devise a system for calculating the quality of each study (the use of a standardized system helps to ensure inclusion of important studies while rejecting studies with dubious and non-significant results)

Critical reading and critical appraisal of the selected studies
- The relevance, standard and quality of the selected studies is vital for a successful and productive meta-analysis.
- The study designs must be thoroughly scrutinised in terms of the scientific rigour in the processes employed and the validity and reliability of the instruments and methods employed.
- The sampling techniques must be critically examined for:
  - the statistical basis for arriving at the appropriate sample size
  - the process of implementation and conditions under which these were applied.
  - The strategies employed in dealing with systematic errors must be examined including:
    - the system of randomisation and allocation of subjects *(Selection Bias)*,
    - measures to avoid inconsistencies and for dealing with emerging errors in the experimental or other research interventions *(Performance Bias)*,
    - measures for dealing with subject losses *(Attrition Bias)*,
    - Measures to avoid differences in assessing the outcome measures and effectiveness of the research interventions *(Detection Bias)*.

(Changing Practice, 2000, Supplement I p. 4)

Box 2.9 (cont'd) *Sequential stages of meta-analysis*

- Appraisal of the Degree of Precision in the Statistical Techniques Employed for Synthesis of the Data
  - ◆ This stage is vital as it enables the researchers or practitioners engaged in the meta-analysis to determine a summary estimate of effects
  - ◆ An appropriate measure of effects must be applied. For example measure of the difference in the rates of occurrence of an identified condition among the experimental treatment group and that of the control group.
  - ◆ A fixed effects model is feasible where the aim is to determine if:
    - the experimental exposure or treatment did on average, produce the predicted outcome
    - the conclusions drawn from the meta-analysis of the selected studies were valid.
  - ◆ A random effects model is feasible where the studies in the meta-analysis have been randomly selected from a large sample of similar (homogenous) studies. This calculation is used to determine if:
    - an association will emerge between the experimental exposures or treatments and the predicted outcomes
  - ◆ A sensitivity analysis is important to substantiate the suitability of the model(s) applied

- Presentation of the results must be in a format that is informative and comprehensible:
  - ◆ The exact protocol devised for entering the results from the studies.
  - ◆ The technique for calculating the estimates of the results from the individual studies separately.
  - ◆ The method employed for combining, transforming and summarising the results from all the identified studies.
  - ◆ The statistical technique employed for calculating the pooled results to present the overall estimate effects should be clearly explained and substantiated

- Reporting of the findings from the meta-analysis should represent a logical format as for other scientific research studies. Therefore aspects to be reported should include:
  - ◆ A clear statement of the topic title indicating the exact focus
  - ◆ The search strategies employed
  - ◆ The methods of identification and selection of the studies
  - ◆ The procedure employed for the systematic appraisal of the studies and the method of recording the findings
  - ◆ The statistical techniques used for calculating and synthesising the combined results
  - ◆ The conclusions drawn from analysis and the recommendations based on the findings.

Halpern (1996) maintains that critical thinking is a purposeful, reasoned and goal-directed process that is applied in making decisions and solving problems. In leg ulcer management this should enable practitioners to gain more awareness, deep insight and understanding of the different patient/client care scenarios or critical incidents that they may encounter. The retrospective contemplation involved allows for re-examination and deeper exploration of the experience in its totality, related knowledge, rationales, perceptions and feelings. Figure 2.1 illustrates the processes of critical reflection in practice.

In this way reflective practitioners are able to identify deficits in their own knowledge, competencies and professional expertise. The aim is to improve practice in response to the clinical governance that emphasizes practitioners' accountability to continually improve quality and safeguard standards of care' (Royal College of Nursing 2003, p. 7).

Continual exposure to the rich resources of the environment of professional practice enables

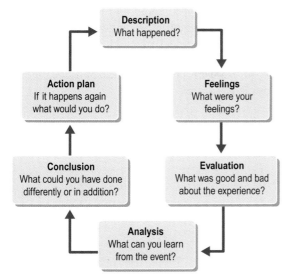

Fig. 2.1 Gibbs reflective cycle (Gibbs 1988) – the processes of critical reflection in practice

health-care professionals to constantly expand and deepen the scope and depth of their knowledge. Tumin (1976) described a fundamental characteristic of experiential learning as a sense of achievement associated with successful performance underpinned by the practitioner's knowledge and skills. The acquired knowledge from that exposure enables the practitioner to implement, rationalize and justify his/her professional decisions and actions.

Development of a reflective portfolio fosters an incentive for the practitioner to retrospectively re-examine specific events relating to the care and service provision.

Development and effective use of a reflective portfolio

Rationale
A reflective portfolio enables health-care professionals to compile a comprehensive evidence of their acquired knowledge, competencies, key professional achievements, personal contributions and aspirations. It also enables the practitioner to examine other personal attributes, strengths and weaknesses. Its purpose is to help the individual to engage in contemplative practice by freely exploring, analysing and evaluating personal professional and clinical issues.

Key characteristics
- Portfolios should be constructed over a period of time.
- It is useful to take advantage of the knowledge and expertise of a 'critical friend' such as the clinical supervisor mentor or preceptor to advise, provide guidance and facilitation in the reflective processes.
- The mutually beneficial relationship established between the two should enable the critical friend to listen, evaluate and reflect back to the practitioner the ideas, main points, concerns and aspirations expressed by the practitioner.
- The critical friend should be in a position to help the practitioner to relate relevant theoretical underpinnings to the practicalities of leg ulcer management.

In leg ulcer management the practitioner is faced with the challenges of the holistic dimensions of physical, psychological, cultural, socio-economic and environmental considerations. Key challenges in the care provision, therefore, require that:

- Optimal conditions be established aimed at achieving effective healing of the ulcer – this requires implementation of health promotion with appropriate client education and support
- Effective procedures be identified for dealing with such potential complications as infection and oedema
- Conscientious observation and assessment be provided to ensure early detection and referral of conditions that need specialist intervention
- Preventive measures be implemented to guard against recurrence of the ulcers (Royal College of Nursing 1998).

Framework of the leg ulcer management portfolio

The organization of the portfolio could comprise different types of leg ulcer, for example the practitioner's experience with management of:

- Venous leg ulcers
- Diabetic foot ulcers.

The detailed evidence compiled on each of these client-care situations should be clearly titled and fully addressed separately from any others. The boxed summaries and exemplars provide a useful guide to reflective leg ulcer practitioners for compiling evidence of their professional practice, personal progress and development.

Content

- A brief introductory section could be presented giving an overview of the purpose and justification for the development of the portfolio of leg ulcer management. This could be followed by an outline of the structure and logical organization of the content.

- Begin by formulating an *overarching aim* followed by clearly stated *objectives*.

Box 2.10 gives a framework for the treatment of one critical incident described in a leg ulcer care portfolio.

Box 2.10   *The main reflective processes*

Critical thinking

This process enables the practitioner to:

- Retrospectively contemplate and reflect on the critical incident or client care situation in its totality
- Examine the potential factors that may have influenced particular decisions and actions
- Examine the perspectives and motives of other parties involved or affected by the care situation
- Convey an intellectual consideration of alternative options that could have been employed.

A key aspect of critical reflectivity involves a description of the experience to a supervisor or senior colleague of appropriate level of expertise. The listener may pose challenges or highlight specific critical questions to encourage reflectivity.

Self-awareness

The self-awareness process enables practitioners to:

- Analyse personal characteristics and attributes, which entails self-assessment of personal values and beliefs, previous experiences and reactions to given situations
- Re-examine and reflect on what impact the particular experience has had on them
- Re-examine in what way their particular personal characteristics may have affected the client care situation.

Description

- This section of the reflective portfolio should portray the practitioner's ability to identify and organise the essential elements in the problem scenario
- The content should portray reflection on the specific event or critical incident
- Do not hesitate to articulate or express personal experience in terms of associated feelings, conflicts or uncertainties relating to the specific situation
- Colleagues may be approached in organising one's thoughts and recall; this helps in presenting the account comprehensively in a logical manner
- The aim of this section is to provide an informative background illustrating the nature of the problem(s) associated with the particular patient's leg ulcer

Critical analysis of the situation

This process enables the practitioner to:

- Demonstrate critical analytical skill and to identify and examine all the different aspects of the event, the related challenges that it posed and the personal assumptions made about these at the time
- Examine the degree of expertise in leg ulcer management and what prior knowledge the practitioner had when confronted with the situation

Box 2.10 (cont'd)   *The main reflective processes*

- Examine how these influenced the practitioner's reaction to the complexity, or otherwise, of the situation,
- Reflect on the decisions and actions that the practitioner might have taken in dealing with such venous leg ulcer management before acquiring the new research/evidence-based knowledge and competencies.

Thus the reflective account should include self-diagnosis of knowledge deficits and identified limitations in professional competence. Practitioners are then able to explore what additional knowledge and expertise they require to develop to enable them to deal more effectively with leg ulcer management.

Synthesis

Involves practitioners' ability to:

- Integrate and use previous and newly acquired knowledge, through assimilation, to deal with similar situations in future practice
- Articulate how significantly the nature and complexities of that event affects the standard and quality of the care provision in the identified area of clinical practice
- In relation to identified models of excellence in leg ulcer management, critically discuss what model or aspects of it relate to the policies, procedures, decisions and actions employed in care provision
- On reflection, explain and justify personal views about the appropriateness of the strategy used in dealing with that client problem/care situation
- Critically discuss the theoretical underpinnings of each of the identified models; your argument should show research/evidence-based reflective application of the models of excellence or aspects of the models referred to in this section
- Provide a reflective account of the new learning acquired to function more effectively in the management of venous leg ulcers
- Reflect on how they think the new knowledge will affect their future practice.

Although speculative, in essence this reflective process enables the practitioner to explore alternative courses of action and to demonstrate envisaged professional growth and development in the practitioner role.

Evaluation

- Overall what impact do you think the processes involved in this experiential reflective practice will have on the effectiveness of your future role in leg ulcer management?
- Which aspect(s) of your leg ulcer/nursing role could be further improved by research into a particular model of excellence if no such study exists in the current literature?

Presentation

The portfolio should comprise distinct sections with each section focusing on a different client scenario of leg ulcer management. For example:

Management of patients with venous leg ulcers

- *Assessment procedures employed* and special considerations taken into account such as: the patient's medical condition, assessment of the nature and extent of the ulcer, assessment of associated pain
- *Treatment decisions*: cleansing, debridement, selected dressings and contact sensitivity
- *Education and nature of support* required by the patient
- *Treatment outcome, referral and follow-up assessments.*

> **Box 2.10 (cont'd)** *The main reflective processes*
>
> This should convey a comprehensive account of the practitioner's reflection on their personal role and involvement in each aspect of the management, i.e. what decisions, what rationales, what impact on the patient, self and team interactions? Examine the identified education and training needs and related quality assurance issues.
>
> The content must be research/evidence-based with accurate in-text referencing and a comprehensively compiled reference list.

CONCLUSION

Among the varied interpretations and usage of the term 'knowledge' is the notion of an individual's ability to use the information they have acquired through formal or informal learning in making decisions, solving problems and taking particular actions. This use of the term refers to the state of 'knowing how' in terms of the practitioner's competence and capability to take actions and decisions based on acquired knowledge.

The current drive in health-care practice is to apply sound theoretical knowledge in describing, rationalizing, planning, implementing and evaluating care provision. To that end, the sources of knowledge are explored in relation to research and evidence-based practice in leg ulcer management.

To enable the practitioner to make effective and realistic application of the content of this chapter specific aspects have been structured and developed in a format that can be used to developing purposeful systems of creating, converting and constructing sound research and evidence-based professional knowledge. The notion of sharing of ideas from an individual's accumulated resources of knowledge is strongly encouraged as this is a useful and effective means of problem identification within the context of evidence-based practice. The team of colleagues in a given discipline must aim at implementing rigorous scientific processes. Appropriate designs and methodologies must be employed in converting intuitive and implicit knowledge that underpins traditionalism in practice into the desired empirical knowledge for evidence-based practice.

References

Crookes P, Davies S 1998 Research into practice: essential skills for reading and applying research in nursing and health care. Baillière Tindall, London

Gibbs G 1988 Learning by doing: a guide to teaching and learning methods. Further Education Unit, Oxford

Gormley K 1995 From theory to practice. In: Basford L, Slevin O (eds) Theory and practice of nursing: an integrated approach to patient care. Campion Press, Edinburgh

Halpern D F 1996 Thought and knowledge: an introduction to critical thinking, 3rd edn. Lawrence Erlbaum, Hillsdale, NJ

Kenkre J, Brette J, Burl G 2000 Undertaking leg ulcer research in primary care. Nursing Standard 14(40): 66–68

McGuckin M, Brooks J, Cherry G 2000 Venous leg ulcers: the role of the GP and district nurse. Nursing Standard 14(40): 46–48

Oiler B, Munhall P L 1993 Qualitative research proposals and reports. In: Munhall P L, Oiler B (eds) Nursing research: a qualitative perspective, 2nd edn. National League for Nursing Press, New York, pp 424–453

Robson C 2002 Real world research: a resource for social scientists and practitioner-researchers, 2nd edn. Blackwell, Oxford

Royal College of Nursing 2003 Clinical governance: an RCN resource guide. Royal College of Nursing, London

Royal College of Nursing Institute Centre for Evidence-Based Nursing 1998 Clinical practice guidelines: the management of patients with venous leg ulcers. RCN Publishing, University of Manchester, Manchester

Sisk B 2002 Evidence-based nursing. Clinical Nursing Resources Newsletter 1(13)

Tumin M 1976 Valid and invalid rationales. In: Keeton M T and associates (eds) Experiential learning rationale, characteristics and assessment. Jossey-Bass, San Francisco, CA

3

How to make the most of this book

Moya J. Morison, Peter J. Franks, Christine J. Moffatt

INTRODUCTION

Learning through problem-solving is an everyday process that has enabled the human species to survive and to evolve in an ever-changing world. Problems drive the search for new knowledge by stimulating research questions and scientific inquiry.

Problem-based learning is an attractive strategy for use in wound care programmes at all levels because learning is integrated and contextualized (Ch. 1). So far, however, most textbooks in this field have tended to take a somewhat didactic approach, even when case studies have been included and have been recognized as providing important opportunities for learning (e.g. Morison 2001). Appropriate case studies are an invaluable aid to teaching clinical problem-solving (Dowd & Davidhizar, 1999) and it is no accident that the case studies in Section II are brought to the fore and are regarded as a particularly important component of the present book.

This book can be a valuable resource whether the approach taken to teaching the subject is 'pure' problem-based learning, a hybrid approach, or more traditional. Its strengths lie in fostering skills that enable readers to access knowledge from many sources to solve the complex clinical problems that they are likely to encounter in practice.

Chapter 2 described means of selecting and evaluating the latest research evidence. It also explored the essential skills of critical thinking, reflectivity and the benefits of developing reflective portfolios to facilitate the exploration, analysis and evalua-tion of personal professional and clinical issues. Reflective portfolios are a potent means of enhancing current professional practice and facilitating life-long learning. The results of engaging with the case studies given in Section II can be incorporated into such a portfolio.

WHEN SHOULD THE BOOK BE USED AND WHO CAN BENEFIT?

This text can be used by health-care professionals for individual, independent learning. It can also be used by teachers as the basis of interactive small-group work in both higher education and practice settings, whether or not a problem-based learning approach has been adopted for the programme as a whole. It is suitable for both novices (ideally under the supervision of a clinically based mentor) and for experienced practitioners who realize that learning is a lifelong process.

By the individual based in clinical practice

Reflection is an important skill for enhancing and improving practice, as discussed in Chapter 2. The identification of learning needs is often triggered by challenging cases encountered in real life. Engagement with the case studies presented in Section II of this book can further stimulate the identification of learning needs, especially in relation to the less commonly encountered presentations of leg ulceration. It is fully recognized that everyone's learning needs will be different and the case studies presented in Section II can be undertaken at many levels.

Chapter 7 gives a coherent overview of issues relating to patient assessment and care planning, which is especially helpful for those who appreciate a structured approach. Chapters 23, 28 and 29 provide a useful overview of key issues, such as wound bed preparation nutrition, and pain management, and these chapters may, in themselves, trigger new questions and stimulate further enquiry.

Individuals with a special interest in a clinical topic may prefer to begin by reading the relevant chapters and then testing their understanding by applying the insights gained to the relevant case studies. This is a more traditional approach, but it can be a useful way of consolidating existing knowledge as well as identifying further learning needs.

In the classroom

Developing credible and appropriate teaching materials can be a very time-consuming activity (Wilkie & Burns 2003). The scenarios presented in Case Studies 1–15 (Section II) have been developed by Professor Christine Moffatt and have been inspired by her years of practical experience of caring for patients with leg ulcers, as well as the depth and breadth of her theoretical knowledge. Teachers can review the scenarios and match them to the learning needs of students at particular stages in their education and training. Once the basic principles of patient assessment and care planning have been established (Ch. 7) it can be useful to include more unusual cases and to explore ethical and management issues associated with care delivery. Case studies can be modified, and multistage case studies can be developed by teaching staff so that topics can be explored in more breadth and depth (see, for example, Case study 2 in Ch. 1). Following a patient's progress over time adds realism and can make students more aware of the consequences of the avoidable and unavoidable complications that may arise.

When a traditional problem-based learning approach is used, students work in small groups with a facilitator to gain knowledge and acquire problem-solving skills (Ch. 1). Problems are presented in the context in which they are most likely to be encountered and students are asked to:

1. Clarify terms and concepts not readily understood
2. Define the problems
3. Analyse them
4. Generate learning issues
5. Collect information outside the tutorial group
6. Report back to the group and synthesize the new information.

Chapters 4–32 are a valuable resource for students to tap into but they should merely be regarded as a helpful map of the territory and a starting point in

---

Box 3.1   Other sources of information and opportunities for networking

Cochrane Wounds Group
   Department of Health Sciences
   University of York
   York YO10 5DQ
   UK
   Website: www.cochranewounds.org

European Wound Management Association (EWMA)
   Membership, PO BOX 864
   London SE1 8TT
   UK
   Website: www.ewma.org

World Wide Wounds
   Website: www.worldwidewounds.com

Tissue Viability Society (TVS)
   Glanville Centre Salisbury District Hospital
   Salisbury SP2 8BE
   UK
   Website: www.tvs.org.uk

Wound Care Society
   PO Box 170
   Hartford
   Huntingdon PE29 1PL
   UK
   Website: www.woundcaresociety.org

World Union of Wound Healing Societies
   Website: www.wuwhs.org

the search for further information. Other sources of information and opportunities for networking are included in Box 3.1. The practicalities of finding further information are described by Anthony (2004).

CONCLUSION

While it is now widely accepted that health care provision should be evidence-based, approaches to fostering high quality teaching and learning in wound care have tended to lag behind the evidence provided by educational research. The arguments for using a problem-based learning approach in this context are now compelling.

The present text can be used as the basis of interactive small group work, in both higher education and practice settings, or it can be used by health-care professionals for independent learning. Its strength lies in fostering skills that enable the reader to access knowledge from many different sources to solve complex clinical problems. It should therefore be regarded as a springboard to encouraging self-directed, lifelong learning in an ever-changing and clinically challenging field.

References

Anthony D 2004 Finding information. In: Morison M, Ovington L G, Wilkie K (eds) Chronic wound care: a problem-based learning approach. Mosby, Edinburgh, pp. 30–45

Dowd S B, Davidhizar R 1999 Using case studies to teach clinical problem solving. Nurse Educator 24 (5): 42–46

Morison M (ed.) 2001 The prevention and treatment of pressure ulcers. Mosby, Edinburgh

Wilkie K, Burns I 2003 Problem-based learning: a handbook for nurses. Palgrave Macmillan, Basingstoke

Case Studies

Chris Moffatt and Moya Morison

CASE STUDY 1: *A SIMPLE VENOUS ULCER*

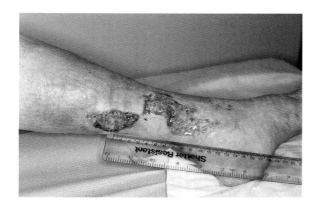

A 65-year-old lady presents with an ulcer on her right medial malleolus measuring 5 × 2 cm. On further discussion she reveals that the wound has resulted from a traumatic injury 4 months ago while she was gardening. She has no history of ulceration or any obvious reasons for delayed wound healing and there is no reported family history of ulceration. Her medical history reveals that she has mild hypertension for which she is monitored by her general practitioner but does not require medication. She underwent a hysterectomy 3 years ago for uterine cancer followed by chemotherapy. There is no evidence at present of recurrence and she reports that she feels generally well although she tires easily.

When questioned about the care of her ulcer she reports that she has been caring for the wound herself using antiseptic lotions and cream and a dry dressing. She only sought medical advice when her local pharmacist questioned her about the repeated purchase of dressing materials. It is clear that she expected the wound to heal and was unaware that she had significant venous disease. On examination she has palpable oedema extending to the calf region, which is generally soft and pitting although in some areas there is evidence of woody induration suggestive of lipodermatosclerosis. On standing, varicosities are evident on the inner aspect of both legs. She reports that her mother suffered from varicose veins and that she developed them in her early twenties but has never been bothered by them or sought medical opinion. When questioned about the development of staining in both legs she reported

that this began about two years ago as an insidious process and coincided with leg swelling, particularly if she had been standing or during hot weather. She states that she considered that these changes were to do with getting old and were best ignored.

Examination of the skin reveals varicose eczema around the gaiter region. Areas of atrophie blanche are present and ankle flare extends around both malleoli. Her general mobility is good and she walks to town daily with her dog and generally remains active. She reports that she is lonely since her husband died 6 years ago but that she does have friends that she visits locally. Her two children have moved away from the area but keep in contact regularly. When questioned about pain in the ulcer she reports that this is worse during the evening and that walking causes wound pain from the dressing. On a visual analogue scale of 1–10 she rates her pain at present at 4; however there are many variations in intensity during the day, depending on what she is doing. She gains relief from ibuprofen, which she takes periodically. She finds that the pain subsides during the night but is particularly severe when she first gets up. She describes the pain as bursting in nature.

The wound appears clean, with evidence of granulation tissue. There is no sign of clinical cellulitis or odour but localized maceration from exudate around the wound periphery. She reports having difficulty in finding appropriate footwear and the shoes she is using do not support the foot well. Examination of her ankle function shows that she still has good movement, although she finds that flexion and extension exercises exacerbate her pain. From the discussion it is evident that she is unaware of the underlying problem causing her ulcer and that, while she is pleasant and cooperative, she does not seem to want to become actively engaged in her care. During the assessment she has described using denial as a major coping strategy in a number of circumstances.

Investigations show that she has mild anaemia with a haemoglobin (Hb) of 11.2 g/dl. Further discussion reveals that her diet is poor since the loss of her husband. She relies on ready-made meals and does not enjoy vegetables or fruit. Her thyroid function is within normal limits, as are her other routine blood tests. Assessment of her circulation involves a careful clinical examination. Both feet are warm and well perfused with a rapid capillary refill time of 2 seconds. Her sensation, tested with a microfilament, is normal in both legs. She has palpable foot pulses and an ankle to brachial pressure index of more than 1 in both legs, suggesting normal peripheral perfusion. A duplex ultrasound scan, performed later, reveals bilateral long saphenous vein incompetence from the saphenofemoral junction and evidence of an old thrombosis in the right popliteal vein.

CASE STUDY 2: *NON-HEALING VENOUS ULCERATION*

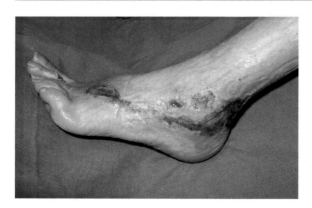

A 63-year-old lady is referred to a hospital ulcer clinic with an ulcer that has failed to heal for 38 years. During this period she has undergone numerous treatments, including episodes in hospital for bed rest and skin-grafting. Her ulcer improved while in hospital but rapidly deteriorated on discharge. Close questioning reveals that postoperative care following grafting did not include the use of compression therapy. She is accompanied to the clinic by her husband, who appears very supportive, and she is extremely knowledgeable about leg ulceration and the range of treatments that she has received. She seems anxious and clearly does not enjoy visiting hospital.

A careful history is taken, with particular attention to how she is coping with her leg ulcer and the impact that it is having on her life. Discussion with her reveals that the ulcer has dominated her life and she feels that it has significantly affected her role as wife and mother. With sadness she reflects that her ulcer began when her children were small, the same age as her grandchildren now are. Over the last 10 years she has dressed her own ulcer and her husband has applied the bandage. She is visited occasionally by the community nurse to check for progress. The nurse was reluctant to agree that the patient was capable of doing her own dressings but was persuaded by the argument that it gave her greater freedom and that she was quite capable of identifying if the ulcer was deteriorating.

The referral to the hospital has been made following a severe bout of cellulitis that extended into lymphangitis. The bacteria isolated were *Staphylococcus aureus* and anaerobes. During this episode of infection, she was hospitalized and received intravenous antibiotics. The infection has resolved but has left a new area of ulceration across the dorsum of the foot. It is thought that the infection gained entry through a fungal infection present between the toe webs. The clinical team are unsure whether infection remains a major cause of her slow-healing ulceration and discuss methods to stimulate the wound bed and promote healing. A number of alternative therapies are considered, including negative pressure and laser therapy.

A treatment plan is devised by the multidisciplinary team to address the various problems she is facing. Further vascular investigations are ordered to establish the extent of the venous pathology. A venous duplex scan shows that she has significant saphenous vein incompetence originating from the saphenofemoral junction, and segmental venous reflux in the popliteal vein. Attempts to undertake photoplethysmography to establish her calf muscle function are abandoned because of her lack of ankle movement. The surgical team are unwilling to perform surgery because her venous pump function is so poor and surgery could create further wounds that will not heal.

An orthopaedic surgeon is consulted about surgery to correct her equinus deformity. He is also unwilling to perform surgery because of the associated risk of infection. An orthotic assessment leads to her being made a pair of boots that greatly improve her ability to mobilize. During her hospital stay the wound granulates well with the (VAC) negative pressure applied. A split-skin graft is applied, which takes well. She remains on bed rest for one week and is then allowed to mobilize with compression bandaging applied. Infection was controlled by the use of antibiotics. The donor site was particularly painful but this was resolved by the application of a silicone-coated dressing rather than the conventional paraffin tulle dressing that was applied in theatre.

Staff on the ward note that her anxiety levels have dropped and she is now more optimistic about her future. A careful discharge plan is devised with the community nursing team. On discharge, her ulcer progresses well for the first few months but never completely heals. A bout of cellulitis and heavy colonization with *Pseudomonas aeruginosa* leads to rapid ulcer deterioration. Following this episode she becomes increasingly depressed and isolated. The community team refer her to a psychologist to begin work on helping her to adjust to living with her ulcer as a chronic illness. She develops new strategies to cope with her leg ulcer and takes control of her own dressings. Her pain is now well controlled with the addition of amitriptyline, a tricyclic antidepressant, which allows her to sleep well. These changes lead her to a more fulfilled lifestyle with less emphasis on the effects of having a leg ulcer.

CASE STUDY 3: *COMPLEX VENOUS/LYMPHATIC ULCERATION*

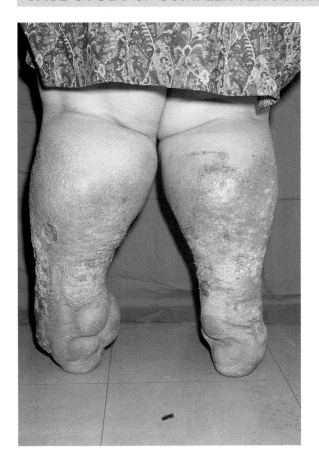

A 67-year-old lady presents with a 20 year history of recurrent leg ulceration and increasing lymphoedema. She reports that her leg swelling began in her late teens and has become progressively worse over the years, but particularly since she had a deep-vein thrombosis 10 years previously. Her mother and sister also suffer with leg swelling but it is less severe and not accompanied by ulceration. Because of the risk of deep-vein thrombosis, she is maintained on warfarin, for which she is closely monitored. Investigations for her venous disease have included a venogram performed 10 years ago that showed a deep-vein thrombosis in the right femoral vein with partial obstruction and some signs of recanalization. A recently performed venous duplex scan showed that the femoral vein remains partially obstructed and that she has developed superficial vein incompetence in the long and short saphenous vein of both limbs. Photoplethysmography revealed considerable functional disruption with a refill time of 5 seconds in her left leg and 6 seconds in her right. She found performing this procedure extremely difficult because of her reduced ankle mobility, which doubtless is a major factor exacerbating her venous disease. She has not undergone investigations for her lymphoedema although she and her family have been invited for genetic screening as it is likely that there is a familial component to her lymphoedema.

On clinical examination she is morbidly obese, weighing 20 stone (127 kg) and her mobility is significantly affected. She is only able to walk around at home and spends the majority of her time sitting in a chair. She reports that sometimes she does not go to bed because the effort is too great for her. Staff assessing her at this stage suspect that she has clinical depression, which is affecting her mood and desire to move. She is tearful about her condition and feels helpless. Previous treatment experiences have not been positive and she believes that little can be done to improve her situation. It is clear that her situation causes her considerable embarrassment and this contributes to her social isolation since she fears that people stare at her in public, a situation she has experienced since her teens when the lymphoedema developed. Family support consists of her mother, who is 93 and lives in a sheltered housing complex 20 miles away, and her sister, who lives locally. She sees her sister about once a week but states that they are not close. Her circle of friends is now depleted since her immobility prevents her going out with them, but they visit her at home occasionally. Her legs are dressed and bandaged by the community nurses, who have referred her for specialist advice as her condition is deteriorating.

On examination of her legs there are gross signs of venous disease and lymphoedema. She has extensive hard, indurated, sclerotic tissue extending around the gaiter region and extending towards the knees. The oedema cannot be pitted below the knee and the oedema extends to the mid thigh but does not involve the genital area, buttocks or abdomen. The oedema in the thigh area can still be pitted and the tissue in this area has only early signs of induration. Stemmer's sign is positive on both feet and there are deep skin folds around the ankle. There is considerable loss of limb shape, and foot deformities are developing, causing a change in gait.

There are multiple areas of ulceration on both legs, at varying stages of healing. These produce copious exudate and require dressing every day. Lymphorrhoea leaks from numerous areas on the leg. There are large areas of thick hyperkeratosis extending over both legs. Signs of localized infection are present. Mycosis is visible between the toes and in the skin folds. The right leg feels particularly warm to the touch, with erythema around the largest ulcer. She reports that she has experienced numerous infections, some requiring hospitalization and intravenous antibiotics. She does not take prophylactic antibiotics and states that the oedema seems to worsen after each episode.

A comprehensive treatment plan is developed and discussed with her. This involves a period of intensive therapy involving isotonic exercises, a skin care regime, manual lymphatic drainage and multilayer inelastic bandaging over a period of weeks. In addition she commences treatment with penicillin and is advised that she will need to continue with this long-term.

The team begin to try to involve her in all aspects of her care. Her depression is treated with paroxetine, a selective serotonin re-uptake inhibitor. It is clear that she has very little understanding of her condition. A patient support group is contacted and asked to visit her. She finds being able to talk to other people in a similar situation to herself an enormous help.

CASE STUDY 4: *AN ARTERIAL ULCER PROGRESSING TO BELOW KNEE AMPUTATION*

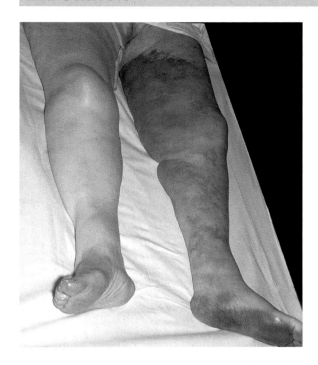

A 70-year-old lady is admitted to a surgical ward with an acute arterial embolism that requires a femoropopliteal bypass operation. Prior to admission she developed severe pain in her right leg, which became pale and cold, and on admission no pedal pulses were present. She was developing paraesthesia and had little movement in her foot or leg. She had a history of atrial fibrillation and reported that she had been experiencing pain on walking. She had reduced her walking distance to compensate for this and reported that she smoked 10 cigarettes a day and had smoked continuously from the age of 13.

On admission she is accompanied by her anxious daughter. The daughter demands to see a doctor and paces up and down the ward using her mobile phone, to the annoyance of patients and staff. This clearly upsets her mother, who pleads with her to sit quietly. The doctor is delayed in theatre, which aggravates the situation further.

A duplex scan is performed, followed by an emergency angiogram that confirms that surgery is urgently required. Prior to surgery an area of necrosis develops over the dorsum of the foot that, after surgery, develops into a deep ulcer extending to reveal tendon.

Postoperatively, her daughter remains demanding and insists that the area of tissue loss is due to negligence. Ward staff are intimidated by her and this leads to the patient being ignored or avoided by certain members of staff. She appears withdrawn and depressed and has little interest in her condition. Although she has many visitors, she seems relieved when they leave. When her family visit the staff note that there are frequent arguments about plans for her discharge and where she should live. Her daughter insists that she should come to live with her but is extremely anxious about how she will cope with the situation given her very demanding career. She contacts a number of home care agencies and is appalled at the cost of providing care at home.

Staff talk to the patient about where she would like to live and it becomes clear that she wishes to return to her own home rather than live with her daughter. Before her admission to hospital she saw little of her daughter and the staff suspect that some of the daughter's demanding behaviour is associated with feelings of guilt. Staff are requested to intervene in planning the patient's discharge.

The initial results from her surgery are successful, although she has extreme swelling immediately after surgery. Her ankle to brachial pressure index improves and she has an absolute systolic ankle pressure of 95 at the posterior tibial artery, although the signal is of poor quality. Her foot is warm and perfused. However, 4 days after surgery the pulses become impalpable and a duplex scan reveals an extensive thrombosis within the vein graft. Her general condition also deteriorates and she develops a chest infection. Over the following 2 weeks it becomes clear that her femoropopliteal graft has failed and she develops increasing sepsis and signs of spreading gangrene in her foot. A case conference involving the family is held and a decision is made to perform a below-knee amputation. During this time the patient continues to show little interest in her condition and appears to use denial as a method of coping with the situation. The family dynamics continue to be problematic for both patient and staff. The family are anxious to encourage the patient to address the reality of the situation and are frustrated by her unwillingness to do so.

Below-knee amputation is performed and a rehabilitation programme is commenced. She makes good clinical progress over the weeks but continues to manifest signs of depression and is reluctant to actively engage in her rehabilitation programme. A psychologist is asked to assess her and to begin helping her to grieve the loss of her limb and come to terms with her altered life.

CASE STUDY 5: *MIXED VENOUS/ARTERIAL ULCER*

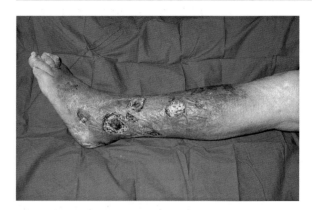

An 80-year-old man has been treated for recurrent bouts of ulceration over the last 10 years by his general practitioner. His ulceration was treated with simple non-adherent dressings and multilayer bandaging and each episode healed within a few months and he was discharged with compression hosiery. Over the last year his general health has deteriorated: he suffered from a myocardial infarction and was hospitalized for a week. He complains of episodes of dizziness and on one occasion had numbness and loss of power in his right arm for a short period, which spontaneously recovered. He is hypertensive, with a blood pressure of 190/100.

He presents with an ulcer that has developed over 3 weeks in the gaiter region. This has deteriorated and enlarged, with new areas of ulceration developing. These are sloughy, with no signs of granulation, and are causing him extreme pain. While his previous ulceration was painful, he reports that the pain is much more severe with this episode and keeps him awake at night. He finds elevating his leg particularly painful and this is

exacerbated at night when, in addition to severe pain in his feet, he also complains of pins and needles. He often stays up and sleeps in a chair, and finds this more comfortable. He has been a fairly active man who took a walk to town daily. On close questioning it is found that over the last 6 months he has become less active and reports that he develops cramp if he walks long distances. Before this episode of ulceration he could only walk a short distance without resting. He has smoked for over 40 years and still enjoys a pipe, which he feels is much healthier than cigarettes.

On clinical examination there is evidence of severe venous disease with extensive lipodermatosclerosis over both limbs. He has ankle flare and atrophie blanche around the gaiter region. He has reduced ankle function, with loss of rotation and limited extension and flexion.

When assessed, the pedal pulses are impalpable and it is only possible to record an ankle to brachial pressure index using the posterior tibial artery. Having little knowledge of vascular assessment it does not concern the practitioner that only one pedal pulse can be found to record an ankle to brachial pressure index. The pulse is difficult to locate and he describes the sound as 'sluggish'; however, the systolic pressure in this vessel appears to be very high – 200 mmHg – and treatment with compression bandaging is commenced. A diagnosis of recurrent venous ulceration is made.

The following morning, having worn high-compression therapy overnight, the patient contacts the practitioner and complains of severe pain during the night for which he was tempted to call an ambulance. When the patient is reassessed it is found that he has multiple new areas of ulceration and that his affected leg is cooler than the other. Somewhat bemused, the practitioner decides to send the patient to hospital for a vascular assessment.

On arrival at hospital he is given morphine to help control the pain he is now experiencing in his leg. Careful examination reveals that he has severe peripheral vascular disease, which the practitioner had not recognized. The Doppler studies are repeated and it is found that the reason the other pulses could not be palpated was because there is occlusion in these vessels. The remaining patent vessel, which was used to record the systolic pressure, is so calcified that no reliable reading can be obtained and the signal is monophasic, confirming severe peripheral vascular disease.

An arterial colour duplex ultrasound confirms multiple short occlusions in a number of vessels, and an angiogram supports these finding.

Treatment involves angioplasty to the occluded vessels and following this his arterial perfusion improves considerably, with an ankle to brachial pressure index of 0.7. He is persuaded to stop smoking and change to a healthier diet. He continues to suffer with oedema and ulceration. Under strict supervision he begins inelastic multilayer bandaging with a sub-bandage pressure of less than 25 mmHg. His ulceration takes 6 months to heal. He is regularly monitored for his peripheral vascular disease and has entered an intermittent claudication programme.

CASE STUDY 6: *ARTERIAL ULCERATION IN A PATIENT WITH RHEUMATOID*

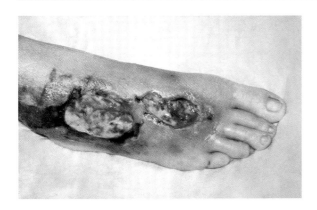

A 65-year-old lady presents with severe rheumatoid arthritis, which she has had for 40 years, and ulceration of her right leg and foot. She complains of excruciating pain, particularly in the ulcer, which lies on the dorsum of her foot and is deep, punched out and sloughy.

Clinical examination reveals evidence of peripheral arterial disease. Her pedal pulses are impalpable and her capillary refill time is very slow (>5 s). Her foot is cold and dusky red and she is only able to hold her limb in a dependent position. She reports that she is extremely sensitive to changes in temperature and touch, however light. Because of the pain she is unable to tolerate the recording of an ankle to brachial pressure index.

The signals from her vessels when the probe is placed on them are extremely difficult to hear and appear muffled (monophasic flow). There are other areas of ulceration on her leg and toes. An ulcer lies behind the lateral malleolus and small ulcerated areas appear at the base of the great toe and between the third and fourth toes. She has considerable foot deformity, with claw toes and hallux valgus. Her other leg also appears to have reduced perfusion, although it is warmer to the touch and an ankle to brachial pressure index of 0.65 can be recorded.

This lady is severely crippled with rheumatoid arthritis and tells staff that she feels she cannot cope with her condition and that the ulceration is yet another problem she must deal with. She has had bilateral hip and knee replacements and surgery on both hands. Involvement of her spine means that she finds sitting in one position for long periods of time extremely painful, and she wears a soft collar when sitting in her wheelchair. For the last 5 years she has been unable to care for herself and now has a residential carer who lives at home with her. She can no longer transfer herself from bed to chair but is moved using a hoist.

She is increasingly finding that she spends long periods thinking about her illness and wondering what catastrophe will happen if different events occur. She has lost interest in television and reading of late and states that she is aware that she is hard to live with and intolerant of those around her. When asked what is her most important problem she replies that the unremitting pain is the worse problem and that it intrudes on every aspect of her life and prevents her having any quality of life. There are times when she has been suicidal and felt that life is not worth living.

It is clear from her history that until recently she was a positive person who managed to continue working with her condition until she was 50 years of age. Her current problems centre around the loss 4 years previously of her husband, who was her main care-giver, and have been exacerbated by her daughters leaving home. She describes her condition and her symptoms as imploding on her and says that she is not able to see a way forward.

Medical management of this lady proves a major challenge. Investigations confirm that she has severe peripheral vascular disease with microcirculatory involvement. Surgical revascularization is not considered appropriate, because her potential for wound healing is so poor and because of the diffuse nature of her arterial disease. A regional nerve block brings enormous relief of pain, which results in a significant improvement in her depression, which was already responding to antidepressant therapy. As her mental state improves, she takes a greater interest in her surroundings and becomes more positively engaged with her condition. She wants to understand the true extent of her condition. It is decided that, if the condition of her leg deteriorates, she will have an elective amputation and that she will be involved in this decision. Her main concern is to remain pain-free and she feels that if this can be achieved that she will be able to manage at home with her carer and the district nurses for the foreseeable future.

She returns home with extensive community support and undergoes a below-knee amputation 9 months later. Although her rehabilitation has been very slow she states that she now has a future worth looking forward to.

CASE STUDY 7: *A NEUROPATHIC DIABETIC FOOT ULCER*

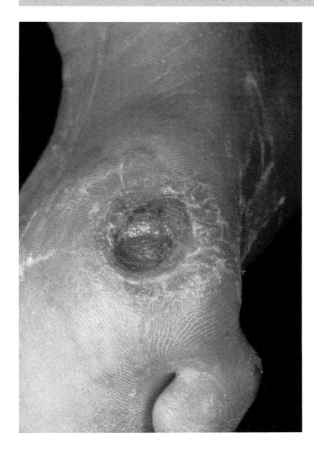

A 55-year-old gentleman presents with painless ulceration over the plantar area of his foot. On examination his foot is warm and well perfused with distended dorsal foot veins. The skin is dry with no evidence of sweating and small fissures appear over the calloused area of the heel. The arch of the foot is raised and the toes are clawed.

There are signs that his shoes are too small and causing pressure damage. He reports that he has been wearing smaller shoes of late as his shoes have felt loose. He has whitish yellow discoloration of the toenails of both feet due to onychomycosis and a small subungual haematoma on the second toe of his right foot.

His investigations reveal that his blood glucose level is 18 mmol/l. On further questioning it appears that his diabetic control is erratic with periods of very high blood sugar. He attends his diabetic

appointments regularly but frequently misses podiatry appointments despite rapid build up of callus on both feet. On inspection he has loss of mobility of the metatarsophalangeal joints. His medical history states that he has suffered from retinopathy, for which he has received laser therapy, and he is hypertensive.

On vascular examination his ankle to brachial pressure index is 1.3 and a wave form analysis shows him to have good triphasic flow in all pedal vessels. Because of the risk of calcification obscuring these findings his toe pressures are also recorded and are found to be normal. Examination of the plantar surface of his feet reveals extensive callus formation over the entire surface with a perforating ulcer which is discharging foul-smelling exudate. Probing of the ulcer reveals considerable tracking down to the joint with the drainage of viscous, bubbly synovial fluid during this procedure. There are signs of erythema (>3 cm) developing around the ulcer, suggestive of severe clinical cellulitis. During the deep probing, tissue samples are sent for culture and sensitivity and blood cultures are also collected. The tissue samples reveal that a number of organisms are causing the infection: *Staphylococcus aureus*; *Enterococcus*, *Klebsiella* and *Bacteroides* spp. X-ray of his foot suggests that osteomyelitis is already present with some loss of bone density and cortical outline of the metatarsal heads. His routine observations show him to be apyrexial and he reports feeling well, although tired.

Assessment highlights that he has severe neuropathy which he was unaware of. A 10 g monofilament is used over the plantar aspect of the first toe, the first, third and fifth metatarsal heads, the plantar surface of the heel and the dorsum of the foot. Reduced sensation is present at all sites, suggesting that he has severe neuropathy and that the protective pain sensation has been lost.

Given the severity of his condition admission to hospital is arranged. During this time he appears frightened and bemused by the interest that is being taken in his foot. When he is questioned about his condition it becomes evident that he has failed to understand the potential seriousness of his condition. Facing this crisis is causing him much anxiety and over time he begins to respond to attempts to educate him and encourage him to become involved in his condition. His wife is also engaged in this process of adjustment over his protracted hospital stay.

CASE STUDY 8: *AN ISCHAEMIC DIABETIC FOOT*

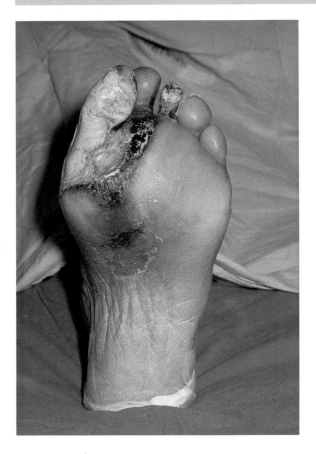

A 52-year-old lady arrives at an accident and emergency unit complaining of pain in both feet and foot ulceration. She has an unkempt appearance and is clutching an assortment of carrier bags. Further investigation reveals that she has been found sleeping in an alley and was brought to hospital by ambulance suspected of suffering from hyperthermia. She is agitated and aggressive towards the staff and it is obvious that she has recently consumed a large amount of alcohol. She is persuaded to allow staff to examine her. From her appearance she has been sleeping rough as she is extremely dirty with evidence of scabies between her fingers and around her wrists. She tells staff that she has been sleeping in a hostel but because of her alcohol consumption was asked to leave. She appears distrustful of staff but begins to respond when given a warm drink and a meal.

Her social history suggests that her problems began 10 years ago when her husband and only daughter were killed in a car crash. She began to drink after this and lost her job around this time. She lived in a council flat which she was evicted from a year ago because she was behind with payments on her rent. There is no evidence that she has sought professional help to address her problems.

She developed diabetes at the age of 40 and her previous medical notes show that at this time she was very compliant with her medication of glibenclamide and regularly attended follow-up appointments. These ceased when she lost her family and no follow-up care has been provided over the last 10 years.

On clinical examination she is underweight and hypertensive with a BP of 180/110. She reports smoking up to 60 cigarettes a day and has smoked regularly from the age of 15. Eye examination reveals bilateral advanced retinopathy. There is no history of transient ischaemic attacks, cerebrovascular accidents or myocardial infarction and she does not complain of chest pain.

Examination of her feet is extremely painful and she is given morphine prior to this. Her feet are cool and a dusky red colour with a very sluggish capillary refill time (>6 s), with an area of partially dry gangrene over the hallux (great toe) and signs of offensive discharge. Her pedal pulses are impalpable and the ankle to brachial pressure index cannot be calculated because of severe calcification. Obliteration of the systolic reading cannot be achieved although the monophasic signal is suggestive of severe peripheral vascular disease. Her toe pressure is 34 mmHg, confirming significant disease. She finds these procedures extremely painful. Examination of her sensation with a monofilament reveals a degree of neuropathy in both feet and she reports changes in sensation with burning pain in her feet and lower limbs at night.

Further examination of her feet reveals claw toes and the presence of tinea pedis between them. Surrounding the area of gangrene are clear signs of extending sepsis. Blood culture revealed infection with group A *Streptococcus*, *Bacteroides* and *Clostridium*. Because of the severity of her condition she is immediately commenced on intravenous antibiotic therapy. Later investigations reveal occlusion of the lower superficial femoral artery. There is considerable debate about her management. Because of her refusal to stop smoking, staff are divided about whether she should undergo a popliteal bypass. Severe conflict occurs within the multidisciplinary team over this ethical dilemma. A magnetic resonance imaging scan confirms that the underlying infection is spreading rapidly and an emergency femoropopliteal bypass and ray amputation are performed.

Postoperatively she improves, with good perfusion through the new graft. Control of pain proves problematic and dressing procedures and debridement are a particularly difficult time. This is managed by giving pain relief prior to the procedure in order to eliminate background pain. Entonox is used during each dressing change. Of particular help is the involvement of the patient in each stage of the procedure, including allowing her to remove her own dressings. She finds listening to music relaxing and benefits from the ability to stop the procedure and have time out when ever she requires. Attention is also placed on having a calm, quiet, undisturbed environment and avoiding delays that mean the wound is exposed. She finds touching the wound and the surrounding skin extremely painful. Her pain level is monitored by a pain diary and her medication is adjusted accordingly.

During her stay she has cut down her smoking to less than ten a day. As she begins to build up a therapeutic relationship with staff she begins to talk of how she has got to the point she has. This involves a great deal of grieving over her lost family and a psychologist is asked to work with her on these issues. A long-term discharge plan is developed and housing in sheltered accommodation is organized. After a 3-month period she is discharged to the community team to begin rebuilding her life.

CASE STUDY 9: *AN ULCER DUE TO WALDENSTRÖM'S CRYOGLOBULINAEMIA*

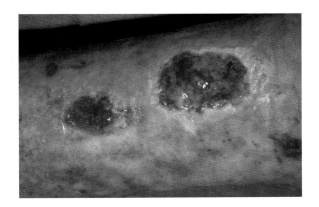

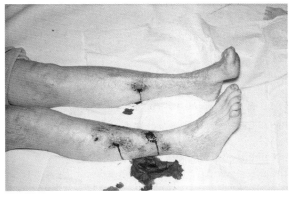

A 77-year-old lady is referred to a vascular department with suspected venous ulceration that has been treated with compression bandaging for the previous 9 months. A vascular assessment reveals mild peripheral vascular disease with an ankle to brachial pressure index of 0.8 in the right leg and 0.85 in the left. A venous colour duplex ultrasound reveals that she has superficial incompetence of the long saphenous vein originating from mid-thigh in the right leg and from the saphenofemoral junction of the left leg. Reflux is minimal, and all deep vessels are patent and competent.

She is a frail lady who is thin and immobile and has difficulty transferring from the chair to the couch. She is accompanied by her elderly sister, who expresses great concern over her deteriorating health. Until just over a year ago she was fit and mobile and both sisters enjoyed an active social life. Her condition was insidious in its development, beginning with fatigue and a general cachexia with loss of appetite. Over the year she has lost 20 kg in weight. She also reports having repeated nose periods over the last few months and eye examination reveals extended retinal veins and small areas of haemorrhage.

Her leg ulceration appeared spontaneously and began as small blisters that coalesced into areas of ulceration. Lesions at varying stages of development and healing are present. These range from blisters and bullae to deep, punched-out ulceration with a necrotic base. The ulceration extends up the limbs and over both knees, with more extensive areas of ulceration over these exposed areas. Greater healing is evident in those lesions that were covered with wool padding and compression bandaging, which presents a dilemma. There is evidence of diffuse staining over the gaiter region, although there is little induration. Her legs are thin with little calf muscle or natural limb contour. There are signs of slight pressure damage from the bandaging over the prominent tibial crest. During removal of the dressings she experiences severe pain. She reports that the pain is most severe as new lesions develop and that the pain lessens considerably when granulation tissue begins to form. The referral letter from the community nurse highlights that as new areas of ulceration began others spontaneously occurred and that when she commenced bandaging the community staff felt that the ulcers would heal and are surprised by her lack of progress. Numerous different dressings have been tried over the previous months, including products containing iodine and silver.

A dermatologist is asked to review her case and suggests that she has vasculitis, although the cause is not yet clear. He notes that, in addition to the skin changes already observed, there are also raised areas of purpura and Raynaud's phenomenon in her hands and feet. Routine observations reveal that she has a low-grade fever with a temperature of 37.3°C. Investigation of her reduced mobility reveals that she has a generalized arthralgia, with minimal signs of osteoarthritis on X-ray. Urinalysis reveals proteinuria and haematuria, although she does not complain of renal symptoms. A urine Bence–Jones protein test reveals the presence of partial immunoglobulins and she is found to be suffering from advanced renal failure. A magnetic resonance imaging scan showed a tumour around the right kidney with secondary deposits in the peritoneal area and extensive lymph node involvement in the inguinal and axillary regions.

Blood tests reveal an increased sedimentation rate, elevation of total proteins (particularly gammaglobulins), positive antinuclear factor, reduction of the total complement of the C3 fraction, circulating immunocomplexes, positive latex test and the presence of mixed cryoglobulin IgG–IgM type kappa. A biopsy is taken from an ulcer site. Histology and direct immunofluorescence reveal dilation of capillaries, luminal obstruction and large deposits of IgM in the vessels and deposition of C3 in the vessel wall. A diagnosis of Waldenström's cryoglobulinaemia with multiple myeloma is confirmed. This syndrome frequently involves multiple myeloma, polycythaemia vera, lymphoma, collagen vascular disease and cirrhosis.

Treatment of her ulceration includes several courses of plasmaphaeresis to help reduce the hyperviscosity of the blood and stimulate ulcer healing. This results in short periods of improved healing with reduction in pain, but these improvements are not maintained over time and after three transfusions the treatment is discontinued.

Treatment of the myeloma includes a combination of chlorambucil and prednisolone, which has been reported to be effective in 57% of cases. Sadly, chemotherapy is unable to inhibit the rapid metastasis of the tumour and the patient dies within 4 months.

CASE STUDY 10: *MALIGNANCY IN A LONG-STANDING VENOUS ULCER*

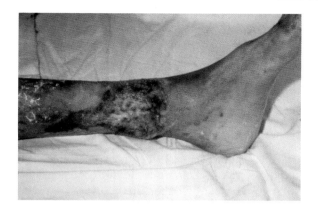

A 93-year-old gentleman living in a residential home is referred to a hospital dermatology department for assessment of a non-healing ulcer. He has a long history of venous ulceration, which has been treated with a wide range of products over the years. He has been a resident in a nursing home for 8 years and has an extensive medical history. The reason for admission to the home was his increasing frailty and a number of falls. He was found to be suffering with atherosclerotic dementia and has become increasingly confused over the past year. During his hospital visit he becomes very confused and distressed. His medical history indicates that, 20 years ago, he suffered a severe fractured tibia and fibula in the affected limb, which required surgery. It is thought that he suffered an acute deep vein thrombosis during this time as the episodes of ulceration began some years afterwards. He has diverticulitis and staff report that they have great difficulty persuading him to eat and drink. He appears thin and his skin is dry, suggesting dehydration. During the assessment it is noted that he has urinary incontinence.

His niece arrives during his visit to the hospital and is clearly upset to see her uncle's deterioration since she saw him a few months ago; she becomes very demanding with staff. Clinical examination of his ulcer reveals signs of malignant change. The base of the wound is filled with necrotic tissue and the edges of the ulcer are raised. There are signs that the tumour within the base of the wound is beginning to fungate and produce foul-smelling exudate. When the wound is cleaned it bleeds profusely, suggesting the tissue is very vascular beneath the necrotic layer. There are signs of previous venous ulcer scars and it is difficult to determine how long the current changes have gone unrecognized. Because of the patient's distress it is decided to undertake a biopsy while he is at the clinic and this is rushed to histology to allow for a diagnosis to be made. The patient finds the procedure extremely difficult to tolerate. The histology confirms that he has a well-differentiated squamous cell carcinoma (Marjolin's ulcer) with some local invasion of tissue.

Discussion takes place with his niece, who is his next of kin, concerning the treatment plan. The medical team are unwilling to perform surgery or radiotherapy on this gentleman because of his confused mental state and advanced age. His niece strongly disagrees with their decision, accusing them of refusing treatment on the grounds of age. Attempts are made to explain how traumatic surgery would be for him. There is no evidence of metastatic spread and it is recommended that he is managed conservatively with dressings and bandaging and, if necessary, local curettage to remove the bulk of tumour under a local anaesthetic. Despite the medical position, agreement over his treatment plan cannot be reached and the niece threatens the medical team with legal action. The patient returns to the nursing home unaware of the conflict that surrounded him and settles into familiar territory. The case remains under discussion.

CASE STUDY 11: *AN ULCER ASSOCIATED WITH PYODERMA GANGRENOSUM*

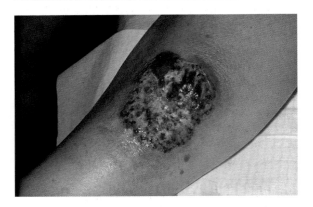

A 30-year-old man presents with spontaneous ulceration and discoloration of his lower leg. The ulcer is surrounded by a deep purple edge and an area of erythema. The ulceration is rapidly increasing in size. His previous medical history reveals that he has suffered with Crohn's disease in the past for which he had a partial colon resection. This episode of ulceration coincides with a recurrence of bowel symptoms over the last month. A diagnosis of pyoderma gangrenosum is suspected and he is admitted to hospital. A full range of investigations are undertaken and a magnetic resonance imaging (MRI) scan confirms active bowel disease. An infective cause of the ulceration is ruled out by the microbiologists, who find only normal skin flora in the wound and blood cultures are negative. A biopsy taken from the wound edge confirms the diagnosis of pyoderma gangrenosum and high-dose steroid therapy is commenced.

Because of the virulence of this condition the wound area is examined every few hours and the area of demarcation of normal skin marked with a pen. The MRI scan reveals that the lesion is partially extending into the dermis and the plastic surgeons are asked to consider excision and skin grafting.

After one week his condition is stable and the area of ulceration no longer extending. There are early signs of dehiscence of the central area of dead tissue and the patient still complains of severe pain requiring morphine, particularly during dressing changes. Discussion takes place at this stage concerning whether the wound should be surgically debrided and left to heal by secondary intention or whether a skin graft should be applied. Concern is expressed that surgical intervention may activate the lesion, as has previously been reported. It is decided that a skin graft should be performed because of the age of the patient and the relative stability of the Crohn's disease since admission to hospital.

The wound is surgically debrided and a split-thickness graft is taken from the thigh and applied to the ulcer bed. The donor site is covered with an alginate dressing and a secondary dressing to prevent slippage. The patient experiences a great deal of pain from the donor site, particularly when the wound begins to dry out. On examination it is found that the alginate is deeply adherent to the donor site and difficult to remove. A soft silicone dressing that does not require regular removal is applied, along with a secondary dressing that can be changed when ever necessary. This rapidly reduces the pain he is experiencing and healing proceeds uneventfully.

The ulcer site was dressed with a non adherent dressing in theatre. The wound is left undisturbed for 5 days and the patient is kept on bed rest and high elevation. The surgeon is concerned that, if a haematoma developed beneath the graft, this would lead to graft failure. Antibiotics were given to the patient prior to surgery and are continued for a number of weeks.

On first examination it is apparent that the graft has taken well. There is slight shrinkage of the graft, leaving a small area of the wound margins still exposed; however, these are granulating well. There is no evidence that the pyoderma gangrenosum is returning and the patient is now experiencing very little pain since the skin graft has been applied. 10 days after the graft he is discharged from the hospital and within 2 months has returned to work. Throughout this episode of illness he remains positive and cheerful, despite bouts of severe pain. He has numerous visitors and is visited daily by his wife and small son. He is warned to be aware that this condition may return and that, if he has surgery or an injury in the future, he should inform the medical team of his history.

CASE STUDY 12: *AN ULCER ASSOCIATED WITH TUBERCULOSIS*

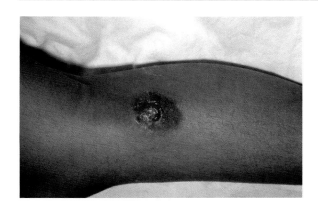

A 40-year-old man presents at a hospital accident and emergency unit complaining of feeling generally unwell and with a leg ulcer that has been present for a few months. He is extremely vague about his previous medical history and who has treated him in the past. He is not registered with a local general practitioner.

On examination he appears tired and thin. He stated that he has been feeling unwell and tired for several months and that this is associated with a loss of appetite. He has a low-grade fever and reports night sweats.

His ulcer began as an indurated, circumscribed red-brown nodule that has now ulcerated. The ulcer is irregular in shape with a sloughy base and a low level of exudate. Crust formations are present when the dressing is removed. The surrounding skin appears normal. The patient reports that the ulcer causes discomfort but is not acutely painful.

His social history reveals severe deprivation. He is living with his partner and three children under the age of 5 in bed-and-breakfast accommodation. When asked if he has applied for rehousing he becomes very agitated and says that he does not want the authorities involved. He states that he works long hours in a shop and this means that he has little time for rest. The entire family are living in one room and sharing a bathroom and kitchen with five other families. Staff wonder if his reluctance to seek help is because he is either an asylum seeker or an illegal immigrant.

A biopsy of the lesion is performed, which reveals an infiltrate of epithelioid cells, Langhans cells and various inflammatory cells, including lymphocytes, plasma cells and polymorphonuclear leukocytes. Tuberculoid structures with a moderate amount of necrosis are seen, in addition to a few tubercle bacilli.

His ulcer is dressed with an occlusive dressing and bandage to help reduce the risk of cross-infection. Staff discuss the importance of continuing with his multidrug therapy and talk to him about the high risk that other members of his family are also infected, particularly his children. While he is waiting to be seen he is given a meal and a drink. While waiting to be seen again he leaves the hospital without informing staff. Later on it is discovered that the address he has given is not correct and that he does not have a national insurance number. Staff feel frustrated and deeply concerned that he did not trust them enough to allow them to treat him.

CASE STUDY 13: *AN ULCER ASSOCIATED WITH SICKLE CELL DISEASE*

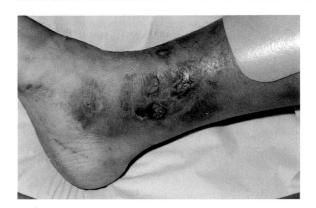

A young lady of 18 years of age presents with an ulcer on the medial malleoli of 6 months duration. She suffers with sickle cell disease, which manifested at the age of 2, and experienced her first leg ulcer at 7 years of age. On presentation her main complaint is of excruciating pain and she is contemplating suicide because of its severity. Because of her sickle cell disease and multiple allergies she is unable to tolerate many of the traditional pain medications. The immediate priority is to ensure her safety and she is admitted to hospital for assessment and pain management.

On admission opiates are used to control her pain, with the addition of amitriptyline, a tricyclic antidepressant. Her pain is quickly controlled and attention can now be focused on the wider issues surrounding her leg ulcer. She proves to be an engaging girl who is determined not to let her condition prevent her from achieving her ambition of becoming a dress designer, for which she has great talent. Despite her ill health and frequent episodes in hospital for treatment of sickle-cell-related crisis she has managed to obtain a place at university with a scholarship to travel to Europe for a year. Her priority is to be able to manage the ulcer while it heals and to reduce the severity of the pain she is experiencing. She has cared for her own ulcer for the past 3 years and is expert in what worked for her. Sadly, she reports that professionals are often far from caring and have

little insight into the expertise that a patient develops from living with a condition.

Clinical examination of her leg reveals a deep, punched-out ulcer with a dark, discoloured base and well-defined margins, positioned behind the malleoli. The surrounding area of skin is thin and fragile, with evidence of previous scars from ulceration. On palpation the area is indurated and pigmented, with small areas of atrophie blanche. A biopsy is taken to ensure that the aetiology is correctly defined. The histology reveals atrophic epithelial margins, cellular infiltration and intimal proliferation in the arterioles from the base of the ulcer. These findings are consistent with those previously reported in patients with sickle cell ulceration. A colour duplex ultrasound scan shows normal venous and arterial vessels. Photoplethysmography, however, shows that the refill time is very rapid despite the absence of gross venous pathology. Bacteriology fails to identify organisms requiring treatment and there is no sign of clinical cellulitis.

Her medical history is complex. Her sickle cell crises frequently involve her joints and she complains of chronic joint pain, although her mobility is surprisingly good. During one crisis she required a splenectomy and she has had two bouts of pneumonia. During the progress of the disease she has undergone two courses of blood transfusions, which were associated with her leg ulcer healing, and she reports feeling generally better after these treatments. Her haemoglobin level remains constant at 8 g/dl.

During her hospital admission she talks more about the difficulties of living with her condition and the fears she has for the future. Of particular concern is whether she should have a further course of blood transfusions, which have helped her previously. During her stay she has a skin graft to the ulcer, which takes well. Her university is contacted, asked to ensure that she is well-supported and advised of her special needs.

CASE STUDY 14: *A TROPICAL ULCER (YAWS)*

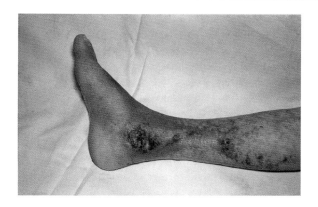

A 49-year-old gentleman is referred to a hospital ulcer clinic with a 41-year history of having a non-healing ulcer on his leg. He reports that numerous different treatments have been used in an attempt to heal his ulcer, including topical antimicrobial and antibiotic therapy, compression bandaging and two failed pinch skin grafts. The ulcer is small, with indurated edges, and is relatively painless. There is some evidence of hyperpigmentation around the ulcer and the area feels indurated.

His history reveals that a diagnosis of venous ulceration was made many years ago and since then the focus of treatment has been to provide compression therapy. This diagnosis appears to have been made on the basis of excluding peripheral vascular disease or diabetes. His previous notes reveal that the pigmentation and position of the ulcer were major factors used to define his ulcer as venous in origin. Initially the wound made some improvement when compression therapy was commenced. This coincided with a reduction of oedema around the wound area; however, the wound failed to heal completely. He states that he can hardly remember a time when he did not have an ulcer and that in the tropics, where he was born and lived for many years, leg ulcers were endemic

and people had little expectation of them healing. He is unable to remember whether the development of the ulcer followed a period of illness but does remember the ulcer becoming infected as a child and requiring antibiotics.

Investigations reveal that he has normal peripheral arterial circulation with an ankle to brachial pressure index of more than one in both legs. A venous colour duplex scan confirms normal deep and superficial veins and no evidence of previous thrombosis. A biopsy is taken from the wound and shows marked acanthosis and papillomatosis. The epidermis is oedematous, with neutrophils migrating into the area. Serology tests are positive and confirm infection with *Treponema pertenue*, a rigid spirochaete morphologically and serologically indistinguishable from the causative agent of syphilis. It is transmitted non-venereally and is generally a disease of childhood, occurring before puberty. It passes through four stages: primary; latent; secondary (non-destructive) and late (destructive) lesions. The patient's current ulcer is in the latent stage and the ulcer extends deeply through the subcutaneous tissues. A bone scan confirms that there is no secondary osteomyelitis or underlying involvement of the bone.

When the diagnosis and treatment are presented to the patient he expresses amazement and pleasure that healing is a possibility. He states that his ulcer has become part of his life and that it will be exciting to consider what he will now be able to do. He is prescribed a single intramuscular injection of 1.2 megaunits of benzathine penicillin. His ulcer is dressed with a non-adherent dressing and a support bandage to avoid the formation of oedema, which might impair healing. He returns to the community, where he continues to care for his ulcer. At a follow-up appointment 2 months later the ulcer has completely healed.

CASE STUDY 15: *A SELF INFLICTED ULCER*

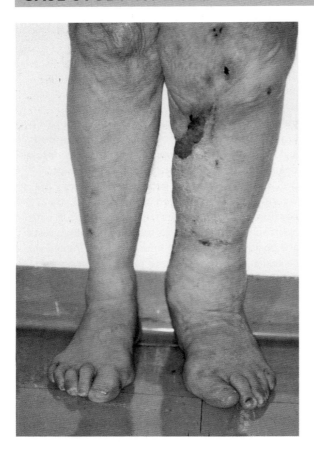

A 40-year-old gentleman presents with ulceration of the left leg that involves the lower limb and extends into the inner side of the thigh. There is gross unilateral oedema extending to the groin, with evidence of sclerotic skin changes throughout the entire limb. Examination of the contralateral limb reveals normal skin, shape and colour.

Assessment of this gentleman proves difficult as he seems unwilling to describe his previous history, preferring to concentrate on the current state of his wound and his demands for treatment. He reports that he has only recently moved into the area and that his notes may not yet have reached his new general practitioner. The professionals involved in his current care are unable to contact his previous carers using the information he gives them. During the assessment it is obvious that he is

very anxious. He has sweaty palms and becomes agitated during some of the questioning.

While he is elusive about the history of his wounds he does talk about his social situation. He lives alone, having separated from his partner, who retains custody of his children. He is unable to work because of his ulceration and generally states that his life is grim. His medical history reveals that in his early twenties he had a major traffic accident, during which time he sustained a fractured femur and broken pelvis. He spent over 3 months in hospital and described his care as excellent. There is no evidence that he experienced a deep vein thrombosis during this time, despite the risk of this occurring. A colour duplex scan shows that he has dilated veins, which remain competent, and no evidence of a thrombosis. He does not report any abdominal or genitourinary problems such as cancer, a frequent cause of unilateral swelling of the lower limbs, although he has not been investigated for this.

His knowledge of the wound treatments available is considerable and he reports being allergic to a number of unrelated dressings. Attempts to use compression in the past have been unsuccessful because he complained of extreme pain. He reports that he has previously required morphine to control the pain and that he feels that he needs it at present. He is vague about changes in pain during the day but describes his pain as excruciating. During dressing removal he complains of severe pain but during consultation, when distracted, the pain seems less of an issue.

Because of the lack of information, assessment has to be carried out over a number of episodes. None of his previous records can be traced and staff begin to wonder if he has changed his name recently. Staff report that he is using manipulative behaviour. In particular, he appears to favour certain staff over others and complains about the care he receives from those he dislikes.

Closer examination of his limb reveals evidence that a tourniquet is being applied to the top of his limb, which is creating swelling (Secrétan's syndrome). When questioned about this he becomes upset and denies the accusation. The wounds are angular in shape and during dressing procedures he frequently scratches the wound and skin. It is noted that he is right-handed and that all wounds are easily accessible to him. There is also evidence that the full-leg compression bandaging he is receiving is being tampered with. He reports having to reapply the bandage because of slippage. Although this may in part be true, a cohesive bandage is used over the entire bandage system to help prevent slippage. There is also evidence that he is applying the bandages himself, as there is localized trauma over the lower third of his leg from excessive bandage pressure. Over a period of many months he fails to make progress. Any small improvements in wound healing are not maintained the following week. Despite this he seems surprisingly unconcerned about his lack of progress. Suggestions of admission to hospital are greeted with enthusiasm.

Following extensive medical examination, including magnetic resonance imaging scan, arterial and venous duplex scan and lymphoscintigraphy, no reasonable cause for his ulcer, other than induced swelling from the tourniquet, can be established. The increasing diameter in the veins and lymphatics that are noted during examination are thought to be due to the enforced congestion in the limb from the tourniquet.

A diagnosis of self-inflicted wounding is concluded by the multidisciplinary team, which includes a psychiatrist. On being faced with this conclusion he discharges himself from the care of the team and is thought to have left the area.

Leg ulcer management: principles and resources

CHAPTER

4

Epidemiology

Jonathan Kantor, David J. Margolis

INTRODUCTION

Epidemiology, broadly speaking, is the study of the distribution and determinants of disease in populations. It is the basic science underlying essentially all clinical research. Appreciating the epidemiology of leg ulcers is important for researchers and clinicians alike. Researchers must understand the trends in the illnesses they study, while clinicians may tailor therapy based on an understanding of the risk factors for disease, likelihood of healing with standard care and potential consequences of failure to heal. Understanding the characteristics of an illness, the definition of an illness and the expected outcomes of an illness are all essential components of the design of a clinical trial. Broadly speaking, all these descriptions of an illness can be thought of as falling under the general rubric of epidemiology. Furthermore, from a policy standpoint, appreciating the prevalence of a disorder can help to determine the appropriate funding (whether from government in the form of grants or from industry in the form of targeted drug design) and assessing the burden of disease. Unfortunately, however, there is only a relatively small body of literature that addresses the epidemiology of lower extremity ulceration. We will describe that literature by first focusing on 'traditional' epidemiology such as incidence and prevalence and then focusing on more analytical use of epidemiologic principles such as determining those likely to do well with a therapy.

PREVALENCE OF LEG ULCERS: BURDEN OF DISEASE

Many investigators have attempted to estimate the prevalence of lower extremity ulcers. These esti-mates vary broadly as regards the prevalence of such ulcers. The difficulties in determining a good population-based estimate are many and these studies are generally limited by insufficient sample size, lack of generalizability and bias. Despite the importance of this question, and despite the large number of separate studies that have been performed in order to address this issue, further research in this area is still needed. Unfortunately, prevalence studies in particular are sensitive to methodological limitations, since the population of interest in a study may or may not reflect the population of interest for the clinician attempting to synthesize the information included in the study. For example, looking only at the prevalence of lower extremity ulcers in the broad group of patients over the age of 45 will probably dilute the burden of disease if one is really interested in the prevalence in an *elderly* population (i.e. >65) because the risk of developing a wound increases with age; alternatively, it may overestimate the risk if one is actually interested in the impact of lower extremity ulcers on the whole population. As always, the central issue for both the researcher and the consumer of research remains the formulation of a clinically meaningful question of interest.

Venous ulcers

Recently, a systematic review of the prevalence of lower extremity ulcers was published. This article comprehensively reviewed the extant literature through 2002 (Graham et al 2003). The authors reviewed 22 separate prevalence studies, including 15 population-based studies and six population-segment-based studies. One of the major conclusions of this systematic review was the realization of the need for further rigorous research in this area, since the actual prevalence estimates from the included studies varied wildly. A minority of these studies used validated measures of ulcer diagnosis and there was no uniformity in reporting of other important issues that have implications for generalizability.

Clearly, lower extremity ulcers are major problems in developed nations. A recent study using the General Practice Research Database found the incidence of venous ulcers in people in the UK over the age of 65 to be 0.76 (95% confidence interval (CI), 0.71, 0.83) per 100 person-years for men and 1.42 (95% CI 1.35–1.48) per 100 person-years for women (Margolis et al 2002). The prevalence of venous ulcers in this population was 1.69% (95% CI 1.65–1.74). Information from this study cannot be extrapolated to those under 65 years of age.

A Swedish questionnaire-based community study of more than 5000 individuals over the age of 65 suggested a prevalence of all lower extremity ulcers – including venous, arterial, and diabetic foot ulcers – to be 1.02% (±0.29% standard deviation (SD)), although their raw data suggested a higher prevalence at 2.15% (±0.45% SD; Andersson et al 1993).

Another Swedish study that included 12 000 patients found a prevalence of lower extremity ulceration of 1.8%. When the question was limited to active, open ulcers, the prevalence dropped to 0.63%. This study also showed a trend of increasing prevalence of ulceration in patients of increasing age: the prevalence in patients aged 50–59 was 0.9%, and this climbed to 3.2% in those aged 80–89 (Nelzen et al 1996a).

In long-term care facilities, it is possible that the prevalence of venous leg ulcers is higher than in the general population because in general these patients are older and sicker. One study of more than 30 000 nursing home patients in Missouri found the point prevalence of venous leg ulcers to be 2.5% at the time of admission to a nursing home, with an annual incidence in the first year of institutionalization of 2.2% (Wipke-Tevis et al 2000).

The effect of age on the prevalence of lower extremity ulcer was noted in several Swedish studies. First, a Swedish population-based study that used nurses to assess ulceration found a prevalence of 0.305% in the overall population. Examining older subsets of patients predictably revealed higher prevalences of lower extremity ulceration. For example, the prevalence in men over the age of 85 was 3.3% (Nelzen et al 1991). Using a subset of this population, the authors found a prevalence of 0.16% (95% CI 0.15–0.18) for venous leg ulcers. A similar trend was seen reflecting an increasing prevalence of lower extremity ulcers in older patients: women aged 10–19 had a prevalence of 0.01% while those aged 90–99 had a prevalence of 2.65% (Nelzen et al 1994). This finding was confirmed in yet another Swedish study, which found a prevalence of 0.12%. The prevalence was highest, at 1.0%, for patients over the age of 80 (Lindholm et al 1992). Additionally, other studies in Sweden also found a prevalence of 0.12% (0.08–0.16%) in all patients over the age of 34 (Ebbeskog et al 1996); the prevalence of lower extremity ulcers in factory workers was 1.9% in those aged 30–65, although these estimates included both healed and active ulcers (Nelzen et al 1996b). Finally, another study found a prevalence of 0.32% (0.2–4.0), although it is unclear what age group was evaluated (Andersson et al 1994).

A British survey of general practitioners and long-term-care facilities found a prevalence of 0.18% for lower extremity ulceration (Cornwall et al 1986). Of note, this population included all individuals aged 40 or more. Another British study found a crude prevalence of 0.19% for all patients over the age of 45 (Lees & Lambert 1992). A British study of hospital inpatients found a prevalence of 1.8% (Deeley 1999).

A Scottish study found the prevalence to be 0.148%, rising to 1.9% for women over the age of 85 (Callam et al 1985). Another Scottish study of patients over the age of 65 found a prevalence of 0.8% (Dale et al 1983).

An American study found the prevalence of all ulcers, both active and healed, to be 0.2%. This included all patients aged 10 or more. The prevalences in this study increased with age until the age of 70, at which point the prevalence of lower extremity ulcers dropped off (Coon et al 1973). The prevalence of venous ulcers has been estimated at 0.3%, with 1% of the population having either a history of a venous ulcer or active ulceration (Fowkes et al 2001).

An Australian study of non-institutionalized individuals found numbers similar to those in the above studies, suggesting a prevalence of approximately 1.1% in patients over the age of 60 (Baker & Stacey 1994).

A survey-based British study found the prevalence of lower extremity ulcers to be 0.12% (Franks et al 1997). The prevalence increased to 2.1% in women over the age of 85.

A British study of patients under age 45 found a prevalence of 1.97%. Importantly, this population included hospital inpatients and must therefore be interpreted with caution (Barclay et al 1998).

An Irish study found a prevalence of 1.03% for lower extremity ulcers in patients over the age of 70 (O'Brien et al 2000). The overall prevalence (crude prevalence rate) was 0.12%, however, highlighting the need to carefully define the population at risk for ulceration so that results of different studies can be compared in a meaningful way. In their population, venous disease represented 81% of all ulcers, arterial disease was responsible for 16.3% of ulcers, and diabetic ulcers and ulcers of other aetiologies were responsible for the remaining few lesions.

A separate Irish study found a prevalence of 1.5% in all patients over the age of 25. Here again, a strong trend to increasing prevalence in older patients was evident, as those over the age of 65 had a prevalence of 5.69% (Henry 1986).

A Swiss study found the prevalence of active and healed ulcers to be 1.3% in a group of factory workers (Widmer et al 1977).

Clearly, age is an important factor that needs to be taken into account when discussing the prevalence of lower extremity ulceration. For example, a study by Marklund et al (2000) performed in Sweden found a prevalence of 8.5% for lower extremity ulceration; these findings must be qualified by appreciating that this study included only patients over the age of 70.

Recently, a study in the *American Journal of Epidemiology* addressed the prevalence of and risk factors for venous ulcers. While this study did not address ulceration per se, and instead focused on trophic changes and functional disease, it does suggest that – as is clear from numerous other studies – lower extremity ulcers are a common problem and their prevalence probably increases with age (Criqui et al 2003). This study also showed that the prevalence of venous disease differs according to whether one relies on clinical judgement or on making the diagnosis using duplex ultrasonography.

Finally, chronic wounds are often thought of as a disease of industrialized nations; however, a study of patients in rural Brazil suggests that the prevalence of venous ulcers in non-Western nations may be as high as – or higher than – that seen in North America and Europe (Maffei et al 1986). The prevalence of chronic venous insufficiency with either an active or healed lower-extremity ulcer was 3.6%, higher than most estimates from Western populations. This study may have been limited by selection bias, which may have led to an inflated estimate of prevalence, but it nevertheless highlights the need for further research in this area. In summary, the prevalence of leg ulcers ranges from 0.12% to 1.1% in the whole population. The prevalence increases with age and in the elderly may be as high as 8.5%. Future studies need to try to define their population of interest uniformly and will need to define diagnostic criteria carefully.

Diabetic foot ulcers

Several studies have separately addressed the prevalence of diabetic foot ulcers. As with the studies that addressed all lower extremity ulcers and venous leg ulcers alone, these studies are subject to a number of limitations. A Swedish study of 395 patients with diabetes between the ages of 15 and 50 found the prevalence of foot ulcers to be approximately 3% (Borssen et al 1990). Another study on a US population with diabetes found that the incidence of foot ulcers over a 4-year period was 9.5–10.5%, depending on the population being studied (Moss et al 1992).

Several studies in the UK have found similar rates of foot ulcers in diabetics. A British study of diabetic patients found a prevalence of 7.4% (95% CI 5.8–9.0) for past or present foot ulcers (Walters et al 1992). Interestingly, they found the prevalence of past or present foot ulcers in the non-diabetic group of patients that they examined to be as high as 2.5%. Another British study limited to 811 patients with type 2 diabetes found the prevalence of current or previous ulceration to be 5.3%

(95% CI 3.8–6.8; Kumar et al 1994). Finally, a large 3-year retrospective cohort study of patients with diabetes was conducted between 1993 and 1995. The authors found a cumulative incidence over a 3-year period of 5.8% for lower extremity ulceration in this group of diabetic patients (Ramsey et al 1999).

Very recently, an issue of the US Centers for Disease Control *Morbidity and Mortality Weekly Reports* addressed the prevalence of foot ulcers in patients with diabetes in the US (Aguiar et al 2003). Data from the Behavioral Risk Factor Surveillance System (BRFSS) was reviewed. The BRFSS is a random sample of the non-institutionalized US population over the age of 17. The median response rate to this survey was 48.9% in 2000, 51.1% in 2001 and 58.6% in 2002. Patients were classified as having diabetes based on self-report that they had been told by a physician that they had diabetes. During the period from 2000–2002 approximately 11.8% of those questioned reported a history of a foot ulcer. Secondary analyses demonstrated a significantly lower prevalence of foot ulcer history among respondents who were black, married, non-obese and non-insulin-users. The prevalence was higher among current smokers (15.8%) than in former smokers (11.9%) and never-smokers (10.3%). Of the many factors examined in this study, those that were associated most strongly with a history of a foot ulcer were duration of disease of more than 20 years (odds ratio (OR) 2.3), insulin use (OR 1.6) and current smoking (OR 1.6).

In summary, diabetic foot ulcers are a major problem for individuals with diabetes. Their prevalence varies depending on the population being evaluated and ranges from 3% to more than 15%. As with other lower extremity ulcers, future studies must focus on carefully defining both a population of interest (all patients with diabetes, those with only type 2 diabetes, etc.) and an outcome of clinical relevance (active ulcer versus history of ulceration, etc.).

LIMITATIONS OF PREVALENCE AND INCIDENCE RATES

Unfortunately, it may be very difficult to draw comparisons or a conclusion from the studies presented above because all the studies did not evaluate the same population. For example, some prevalence estimates examine patients over the age of 60, some look at patients over the age of 65 and some restrict their population to those over the age of 70. These differences can lead to dramatic changes in the observed prevalence of lower extremity ulceration. Studies that do not include age ranges – including some noted above – are of questionable value when interpreting the literature, since it is not clear to the consumer of medical information what to do with the findings. A prevalence rate of 5% that is not qualified by an age range is essentially meaningless, since it could reflect a marked elevation in a population-based estimate or a less-than-surprising finding in a clinic composed of elderly patients with venous disease.

Another important limitation, and one that can make the difference between meaningful, clinically-relevant research and misinformation, relates to diagnosis. Most of the studies discussed in this section did not adequately address the diagnosis of the underlying ulceration; instead, they simply documented the presence or absence of an ulcer. Again, if we are to use this information for meaningful research, we need to be able to delineate whether the ulcers in question are diabetic neuropathic ulcers, venous ulcers or ulcers as a result of arterial disease. Only in this way can we better tailor therapies, as well as channelling funding, to the appropriate clinical entity. This also touches on another issue that can represent a problem in survey-type studies: misclassification. We have to assume that those coded as having an ulcer do indeed have one and that those coded as being ulcer-free are indeed ulcer-free. Unfortunately, this is sometimes not the case, and the problem of differential misclassification – and the ensuing introduction of bias – must certainly be addressed in any such research study.

What is clear from a brief overview of the research, however, are several trends in prevalence. First, most studies support the belief that the prevalence of lower extremity ulceration increases with age. For those caring for patients with these ulcers, this point is also abundantly clear, as elderly patients represent by far the largest subset seen in the clinic setting. Second, venous ulcers appear to be more common in women, something that is also borne out of clinical experience. Importantly, however, when examining the point prevalence of disease – as was done in all the studies reviewed – we are able to assess only a snapshot in time. Therefore, for example, if a subset of the population has ulcers that last for longer than others (whether unhealed or not amputated), or who clinically fare better than their contemporaries, it is possible that this group could effectively be over-represented in a prevalence study.

Epidemiology, however, is not simply the study of the prevalence of disease. Important ongoing research in areas such as risk factors, surrogate markers, cost-effectiveness and prognostic modelling must also be addressed in order to better understand the world of chronic wound management.

RISK FACTORS AND SURROGATE MARKERS

Being able to predict whether or not an ulcer will heal has important implications both for clinical management of patients with these wounds and for the design of further studies to assess the efficacy of leg ulcer therapy. At the core of this research area is the appreciation that, while a proportion of all wounds – say, 30% – will heal, the chance of any individual wound healing is not necessarily equal to 30%. This is because the overall number reflects variations in the population in question: just as an 85-year-old woman's chance of having a leg ulcer is higher than a population estimate for all women aged 18–90, so too an individual's chance of healing may not be equal to the crude population estimate.

Why bother with risk factors? In medicine in general – and chronic wound care in particular – there is a myriad of choices available to the clinician. Certain treatments have been broadly accepted as 'standard care'. This is in part a function of the therapies employed in the control arm of clinical studies, although of course these choices themselves are guided by the standard of care accepted by most healthcare practitioners. For diabetic foot ulcers, standard care includes offloading of the affected limb, debridement and good wound care. For venous ulcers, standard care includes adequate limb compression and good wound care. Other therapies, are available for patients with chronic wounds, but many of these treatments are both

cost- and labour-intensive. Therefore, clinicians, patients and payers need tools to help choose which patients would most benefit from these adjunctive therapies. If an individual is likely to heal within a few weeks with standard care alone, it may not be a wise use of existing limited resources to treat this person with expensive growth-factor-based therapies. Similarly, if patients are known to have multiple risk factors for not healing with standard care within a defined period of time, then perhaps they should be started on these adjunctive therapies immediately on presentation to the clinician.

Understanding risk factors can also help design better – and less costly – clinical trials. If a study can selectively enrol patients who are unlikely to heal with standard care, this can lead to significant benefits in terms of required sample size and resulting power. Finally, for many patients with chronic wounds, the wounds are not likely to heal in a few weeks, which is a time frame that they have come to expect from a lifetime of acute wounds. Clinically, being able to reassure a patient that they are indeed going to heal can be critically important. Epidemiologic prognostic models, properly explained, can be very helpful in consoling such a patient. In the following paragraphs we have reviewed several epidemiologic studies of risk factors. The available literature on this topic has grown significantly in the past few years. As a result, this review is not meant to be comprehensive but is meant to give the reader a general understanding of the topics that can be and have been addressed.

Diabetic foot ulcers

Several studies have addressed risk factors both for developing lower extremity ulcers and for having ulcers that fail to heal with standard care. A meta-analysis, which is a pooled analysis of many patients with diabetic foot ulcers from several trials, was performed in 2000 (Margolis et al 2000). This study pooled data from five separate clinical trials in order to assess what clinical features were associated with the failure of an ulcer to heal after 20 weeks of standard care. Several clinical characteristics were associated with an increased likelihood of healing: smaller wound size (OR 0.67, 95% CI 0.55–0.81), shorter wound duration (OR 0.73, 95% CI 0.61–0.87) and being non-white (OR 0.64,

95% CI 0.43–0.96) were all baseline features that were associated with an increased chance of healing within 20 weeks of standard care. Interestingly, age and glycosylated haemoglobin level at the time of the entry into the study were not significantly associated with an increased risk of not healing within 20 weeks of care. By pooling data from the control arms of five separate clinical trials, this study was able to include data on a large number of patients – over 500.

More formally, a retrospective cohort study was conducted using a wound care database covering more than 27 000 person (Margolis et al 2003a). This study showed that several baseline factors are associated with a diabetic foot ulcer failing to heal after 20 weeks of care. Factors that were associated with an increased likelihood of not healing included: male sex (OR 1.17, 95% CI 1.10–1.23), age (OR per 5 years 1.02, 95% CI 1.01–1.02), wound grade (e.g. grade 6 versus grade 1 OR 18, 95% CI 12–27), duration (log months OR 1.26, 95% CI 1.24–1.28), size (log mm^2 OR 1.34, 95% CI 1.32–1.37) and the presence of multiple wounds (e.g. four or more wounds versus single wound OR 2.01, 95% CI 1.86–2.18). Finally, using this same database the authors demonstrated their ability to predict who would heal. A simple prognostic model was created in which 1 point was assigned each for a wound older than 2 months, larger than 2 cm^2 or with a grade of 3 or more. Using this system, they found that the likelihood that a wound would not heal was 0.35 for a count of 0, 0.47 for a count of 1, 0.66 for a count of 2 and 0.81 for a count of 3.

Venous ulcers

A single-centre retrospective cohort study was performed in 1999 to assess risk factors for venous leg ulcers failing to heal within 24 weeks of care (Margolis et al 1999). This study included data on 260 patients with venous leg ulcers, and baseline characteristics were recorded at the initial office visit. Several factors were associated with the failure of a venous ulcer to heal within 24 weeks of standard care (Vaseline gauze and compression stockings). These included larger wound size, longer wound duration, history of venous ligation or stripping, history of knee or hip replacement surgery, an ankle to brachial index of less than 0.8

and the presence of fibrin on more than 50% of the wound surface.

A British study of 200 patients with a venous ulcer larger than 2 cm^2 was performed more than a decade ago (Skene et al 1992). The authors found that smaller wounds (RR 1.92, 95% CI 1.58, 2.33), those of shorter duration (halving duration RR 1.35, 95% CI 1.17–1.56), younger patients (for a 10 year decrease, RR 1.34, 95% CI 1.12–1.59) and those with no deep venous involvement (RR 1.8, 95% CI 1.19–2.78) were more likely to heal quickly. Several other studies have found similar findings (Skene et al 1992, Franks et al 1995, Phillips et al 2000).

Endpoints

For all these wound care studies, the ultimate result is a healed wound. Of note, however, is that different endpoints are often used in chronic wound studies. For example, in most of the earliest studies a 20 week endpoint was used for diabetic foot ulcers and 24-week endpoint was used for venous ulcers. The choice of these different endpoints and the endpoints used in our current studies is not based on any a priori reasoning or basic science principles that would explain the meaningfulness of these differing endpoints for patients with lower extremity ulcers. Instead, they are guided by the existing literature: since many studies of diabetic foot ulcers include 20- or 12-week outcome data, a patient-level meta-analysis must rely on existing studies and existing endpoints. Similarly, the venous ulcer retrospective cohort study used a 24-week endpoint because most venous ulcer studies have used a 24-week endpoint. In order to keep the findings meaningful in the context of the existing literature, these different endpoints were adopted by the authors. Determining the appropriate endpoint for a study is not a trivial question; for example, if a therapy is theorized to have an effect on the acute phase of wound healing, then using an earlier endpoint (4 weeks in lieu of 40 weeks) may help to minimize type II error. Conversely, using an early endpoint when studying a therapy that may take weeks or longer to lead to a benefit (such as a topically-applied growth factor) may also lead to excess type II error. Therefore, a thorough clinical understanding, as well as an appreciation of the extant literature, is needed to guide the establishment of appropriate clinical endpoints.

One potential solution would be to use a surrogate endpoint for a healed wound. When an outcome is delayed in time – such as wound healing – it can be more efficient from the perspective of both clinical management and clinical trial design to use an endpoint that occurs earlier in the course of treatment and that would predict the outcome of interest. In some ways, the use of surrogate markers represents a more advanced form of risk factor analysis.

Several studies have addressed the use of surrogate markers for predicting healing of venous ulcers. One study found that percentage change in ulcer area after the first 4 weeks of care could be used as a prognostic index of healing after 24 weeks (Kantor & Margolis 2000). A more recent study that included data on more than 20 000 patients explored surrogate endpoints for healing for venous leg ulcers (Gelfand et al 2002). This study found that several features could be used to discriminate between wounds that would and would not heal, including percentage change in ulcer area, log rate and log area ratio.

More recently, one study has evaluated the use of surrogate endpoints in the treatment of diabetic foot ulcers (Margolis et al 2003b). As with venous ulcers, the authors found that percentage change in area, log healing rate and log area ratio all discriminated between wounds that did and did not heal at 12 and 20 weeks of care. These findings are most useful in the design of future clinical trials, by not only allowing for smaller sample sizes but also permitting the use of short exploratory studies to assess whether novel therapies might be effective while using only a fraction of the resources – and time – that would be required for a traditional study.

COST AND COST-EFFECTIVENESS

Venous and diabetic foot ulcers are very expensive to treat and several attempts have been made to study this important health policy issue. One study has suggested that between 25% and 50% of costs related to inpatient diabetes care may be directly attributable to the diabetic foot (Apelqvist 1998). Moreover, a separate study of almost 9000 patients looked at costs associated with the development of a diabetic foot ulcer (Ramsey et al 1999). In men between 40 and 65 years old, the attributable cost of a new foot ulcer was just under US$28 000 for the first 2 years after diagnosis. Even patients with less complicated wounds often see their healthcare provider on at least a monthly basis and may miss days of work, meaning that the economic cost – both of direct care and of lost productivity – may be substantial indeed.

Despite the availability of treatments such as becaplermin for diabetic neuropathic foot ulcers and allograft skin substitutes for venous ulcers and diabetic neuropathic foot ulcers, most patients do not receive these therapies for their wounds. We performed a cost-effectiveness study several years ago to evaluate the cost-effectiveness of different therapies available for the treatment of diabetic neuropathic foot ulcers (Kantor & Margolis 2001). We used data from a meta-analysis, multicentre randomized controlled trials and a large database to assess the effectiveness of the most widely used treatments for neuropathic diabetic foot ulcers. Commercially available adjunctive growth-factor therapies did indeed cost more than standard care, but they also resulted in modestly improved healing rates. Ultimately, the patient or insurance provider needs to decide whether the modest improvement is worth the increased cost. To date we are not aware of any studies indicating what the level of the willingness of a patient is to pay for these new therapies. Overall, these findings highlight the need for better studies of risk factors and prognosis so that these expensive therapies can be selectively used in the groups of patients who are likely to benefit from them most.

CONCLUSIONS

Chronic wounds are a major problem and affect a significant proportion of the population. Further studies are needed to more clearly delineate the prevalence of these wounds. Still, most studies agree that, among elderly individuals, venous ulcers affect at least 1% of the population. The rate of diabetic foot ulcers is not as clearly defined and probably varies according to the patient's lower limb arterial status, the type of diabetes and the length of time that they have had diabetes. An overall estimate of 5% of patients with diabetes, however, is probably realistic. New data on risk factors for both ulceration and failure to heal may help to better guide therapy and tailor treatments so that patients who are most likely to benefit from more expensive and intensive therapies are also more likely to receive them. Risk factors such as sex, wound size and wound duration may be used to help predict which wounds are likely to heal after 20–24 weeks of therapy. Moreover, these data will help guide clinical trial design and may make new drug development less costly and allow for more aggressive research in this area. Further research in the area of chronic wound epidemiology will focus both on improving prevalence estimates and on better understanding risk factors and surrogate markers to help care for patients with these debilitating and frustrating ulcers.

References

Aguiar M E, Burrows N R, Wang J et al 2003 History of foot ulcer among persons with diabetes – United States, 2000–2002. Morbidity and Mortality Weekly Reports 52: 1098–1102

Andersson E, Hansson C, Swanbeck G 1993 Leg and foot ulcer prevalence and investigation of the peripheral arterial and venous circulation in a randomised elderly population. An epidemiological survey and clinical investigation. Acta Dermato-Venereologica 73: 57–61

Andersson E, Hansson C, Swanbeck G 1984 Leg and foot ulcers. An epidemiological survey. Acta Dermato-Venereologica 64: 227–232

Apelqvist J 1998 Wound healing in diabetes. Outcome and costs. Clinics in Podiatric Medicine and Surgery 15: 21–39

Baker S R, Stacey M C 1994 Epidemiology of chronic leg ulcers in Australia. Australian and New Zealand Journal of Surgery 64: 258–261

Barclay K M, Granby T, Elton P J 1998 The prevalence of leg ulcers in hospitals. Hospital Medicine 59: 850

Borssen B, Bergenheim T, Lithner F 1990 The epidemiology of foot lesions in diabetic patients aged 15–50 years. Diabetic Medicine 7: 438–444

Callam M J, Ruckley C V, Harper D R, Dale J J 1985 Chronic ulceration of the leg: extent of the problem and provision of care. British Medical Journal (Clinical Research Edition) 290: 1855–1856

Coon W W, Willis P W III, Keller J B 1973 Venous thromboembolism and other venous disease in the Tecumseh community health study. Circulation 48: 839–846

Cornwall J V, Dore C J, Lewis J D 1986 Leg ulcers: epidemiology and aetiology. British Journal of Surgery 73: 693–696

Criqui M H, Jamosmos M, Fronek A et al 2003 Chronic venous disease in an ethnically diverse population: the San Diego Population Study. American Journal of Epidemiology 158:448–456

Dale J J, Callam M J, Ruckley C V et al 1983 Chronic ulcers of the leg: a study of prevalence in a Scottish community. Health Bulletin 41: 310–314

Dealey C 1999 Measuring the size of the leg ulcer problem in an acute trust. British Journal of Nursing 8: 850–852, 854, 856

Ebbeskog B, Lindholm C, Ohman S 1996 Leg and foot ulcer patients. Epidemiology and nursing care in an urban population in south Stockholm, Sweden. Scandinavian Journal of Primary Health Care 14: 238–243

Fowkes F G, Evans C J, Lee A J 2001 Prevalence and risk factors of chronic venous insufficiency. Angiology 52(suppl 1):S5–S15

Franks P J, Bosanquet N, Connolly M et al 1995 Venous ulcer healing: effect of socioeconomic factors in London. Journal of Epidemiology and Community Health 49: 385–388

Franks P J, Morton N, Campbell A, Moffatt C J 1997 Leg ulceration and ethnicity: a study in west London. Public Health 111: 327–329

Gelfand J M, Hoffstad O, Margolis D J 2002 Surrogate endpoints for the treatment of venous leg ulcers. Journal of Investigative Dermatology 119: 1420–1425

Graham I D, Harrison M B, Nelson E A et al 2003 Prevalence of lower-limb ulceration: a systematic review of prevalence studies. Advances in Skin and Wound Care 16: 305–316

Henry M 1986 Incidence of varicose ulcers in Ireland. Irish Medical Journal 79: 65–67

Kantor J, Margolis D J 2000 A multicentre study of percentage change in venous leg ulcer area as a prognostic index of healing at 24 weeks. British Journal of Dermatology 142: 960–964

Kantor J, Margolis D J 2001 Treatment options for diabetic neuropathic foot ulcers: a cost-effectiveness analysis. Dermatologic Surgery 27: 347–351

Kumar S, Ashe H A, Parnell L N et al 1994 The prevalence of foot ulceration and its correlates in type 2 diabetic patients: a population-based study. Diabetic Medicine 11: 480–484

Lees T A, Lambert D 1992 Prevalence of lower limb ulceration in an urban health district. British Journal of Surgery 79: 1032–1034

Lindholm C, Bjellerup M, Christensen O B, Zederfeldt B 1992 A demographic survey of leg and foot ulcer patients in a defined population. Acta Dermato-Venereologica 72: 227–230

Maffei F H, Magaldi C, Pinho S Z et al 1986 Varicose veins and chronic venous insufficiency in Brazil: prevalence among 1755 inhabitants of a country town. International Journal of Epidemiology 15: 210–217

Margolis D J, Berlin J A, Strom B L 1999 Risk factors associated with the failure of a venous leg ulcer to heal. Archives of Dermatology 135: 920–926

Margolis D J, Kantor J, Santanna J et al 2000 Risk factors for delayed healing of neuropathic diabetic foot ulcers: a pooled analysis. Archives of Dermatology 136: 1531–1535

Margolis D J, Bilker W, Santanna J, Baumgarten M 2002 Venous leg ulcer: incidence and prevalence in the elderly. Journal of the American Academy of Dermatology 46: 381–386

Margolis D J, Allen-Taylor L, Hoffstad O, Berlin J A 2003a Diabetic neuropathic foot ulcers: predicting which ones will not heal. American Journal of Medicine 115: 627–631

Margolis D J, Gelfand J M, Hoffstad O, Berlin J A 2003b Surrogate end points for the treatment of diabetic neuropathic foot ulcers. Diabetes Care 26: 1696–1700

Marklund B, Sulau T, Lindholm C 2000 Prevalence of non-healed and healed chronic leg ulcers in an elderly rural population. Scandinavian Journal of Primary Health Care 18:58–60

Moss S E, Klein R, Klein B E 1992 The prevalence and incidence of lower extremity amputation in a diabetic population. Archives of Internal Medicine 152: 610–616

Nelzen O, Bergqvist D, Lindhagen A, Hallbook T 1991 Chronic leg ulcers: an underestimated problem in primary health care among elderly patients. Journal of Epidemiology and Community Health 45: 184–187

Nelzen O, Bergqvist D, Lindhagen A 1994 Venous and non-venous leg ulcers: clinical history and appearance in a population study. British Journal of Surgery 81: 182–187

Nelzen O, Bergqvist D, Lindhagen A 1996a The prevalence of chronic lower-limb ulceration has been underestimated: results of a validated population questionnaire. British Journal of Surgery 83: 255–258

Nelzen O, Bergqvist D, Fransson I, Lindhagen A 1996b Prevalence and aetiology of leg ulcers in a defined population of industrial workers. Phlebology 11: 50–54

O'Brien J F, Grace P A, Perry I J, Burke P E 2000 Prevalence and aetiology of leg ulcers in Ireland. Irish Journal of Medical Science 169: 110–112

Phillips T J, Machado F, Trout R et al 2000 Prognostic indicators in venous ulcers. Journal of the American Academy of Dermatology 43: 627–630

Ramsey S D, Newton K, Blough D et al 1999 Incidence, outcomes, and cost of foot ulcers in patients with diabetes. Diabetes Care 22: 382–387

Skene A I, Smith J M, Dore C J et al 1992 Venous leg ulcers: a prognostic index to predict time to healing. British Medical Journal 305: 1119–1121

Walters D P, Gatling W, Mullee M A, Hill R D 1992 The distribution and severity of diabetic foot disease: a community study with comparison to a non-diabetic group. Diabetic Medicine 9: 354–358

Widmer L K, Mall T H, Martin H 1977 Treatment of venous disorders. In: Hobbs J T (ed.) The treatment of venous disorders. MTP Press, Lancaster, pp 4–12

Wipke-Tevis D D, Rantz M J, Mehr D R et al 2000 Prevalence, incidence, management, and predictors of venous ulcers in the long-term-care population using the MDS. Advances in Skin and Wound Care 13: 218–224

Health economics

Peter J. Franks, Nick Bosanquet

INTRODUCTION

While it is known that wound care treatment and prevention consume large quantities of resources in terms of disposables, equipment and nursing time, there is still little objective evaluation of the economic burden of wound care on the health services. Moreover, the health service costs may inadequately describe the total cost of care, as this burden falls increasingly outside the formal health services and on to patients and their families. In addition, the assessment of cost burden of disease does not describe the complete evaluation. Cost information alone is limited and needs to be assessed in relation to some measure of health outcome. Cost-effectiveness is therefore a balance between input (resources) and output (effectiveness). The best treatments are low cost per unit of health gain, but it is important to appreciate that the cheapest option is not necessarily the most cost-effective.

Measuring the cost burden of leg ulceration

When we think of the economic burden of a disease it is tempting to examine the costs of providing health services to patients suffering from the disease in question. However, this may be a very limited view of cost. Social appraisal requires that not only should costs related to the health service be considered but also costs to the patient and their family and the cost of the disease to society. Costs may be divided into the 'direct' costs of treating the patient and the 'indirect' cost to society. Typically, direct costs would include health service costs as well as the cost of drugs and travel associated with the health care. Conversely, indirect costs would be derived from estimates of lost production by the patient or family members caused by the disease, losses to society caused by the patient being unable to function to their potential, and quality of life issues, particularly problems associated with pain, poor mobility, discomfort and distress.

Assessing cost burden

In its simplest form cost burden can be estimated by determining the number of patients suffering from the condition and the mean (average) cost of treating patients on an annual basis. This approach is highly dependent on the exact prevalence of ulceration. A number of studies have been undertaken to evaluate prevalence in different westernized populations (Graham et al 2003), most of which give estimates around 1.2–3.2 per 1000 population. Selecting a prevalence in this range would potentially increase costs nearly threefold. This indicates the need for a systematic approach to the evaluation of prevalence from within the population studied.

While prevalence is clearly an essential part of the equation, the average cost of treating patients is also highly variable. Notwithstanding the problems associated with which costs to include (direct versus indirect, etc.), care must also be undertaken when using the available literature. Frequently, the mean cost of treatment is given over a short period of time and will therefore also include patients who heal. In a steady state, the numbers of patients who heal will be equal to the number of patients who either recur or develop their first ulcer. Thus the average cost required must be that 'on treatment'. Using mean costs in a situation where patients are being healed but where patients newly presenting for treatment are not accounted for will seriously underestimate the cost of care.

Clearly, this is the simplest model of cost burden. More complex models may be needed to identify particular patient groups whose cost of care is greater or less than the average. These differences can then be factored into the crude prevalence estimates to give a more realistic cost estimate. This method has been used successfully in developing models for the diabetic foot, where the cost consequences of conservative treatment, arterial reconstruction and amputation have been evaluated (Ragnarson Tennvall & Apelqvist 1997).

Which measure of effectiveness?

In studies of acute life-threatening disease survival would be the most widespread measure of effectiveness. However, when dealing with chronic, (generally) non-life-threatening diseases we must consider what our best outcome measure will be. In general, clinical measures of effectiveness are preferred since these are of direct relevance to the clinician. In wound management one might consider the following outcomes:

- Change in wound area
- Change in the severity of the wound
- Subjective improvement in wound
- Wound-free days
- Complete wound healing (clinical cure).

The last of these is the most commonly used outcome, since most clinicians believe that it provides a hard (irrefutable) endpoint for clinical studies. However, it does have its limitations, since it assumes that complete ulcer healing is the only outcome of value to the patient. Thus, an ulcer that reduces dramatically in size or causes less perceived pain, but does not heal, is still considered a treatment failure. In addition, clinical cure may be poorly correlated with the patient's perceived health. This has led researchers to investigate the role of health related quality of life (HRQoL) in determining outcomes of treatment (see Ch. 30).

METHODS OF COST ANALYSIS

Because of the need to balance cost with effectiveness, different types of economic appraisal have been proposed. The choice of method will depend on the expectations of the treatment outcome and the level of funds available. In the following sections we will outline the major cost evaluation methods.

Cost minimization

This term is used to describe studies where the outcomes of treatment are expected to be the same but the costs are likely to differ. This type of analysis becomes more important when assessing the introduction of new therapies when the current treatment is already highly effective. An example might be a comparison of hernia repair performed laparoscopically or by the conventional open procedure. In this analysis the outcome is the same (hernia repaired) but the costs of treatment may vary considerably.

Cost-effectiveness

While cost minimization may be useful in situations where the outcome is expected to be identical, frequently there is a balance between the effectiveness of a treatment and the cost of each procedure. There are four possible outcomes when introducing a new procedure into medical practice:

- *Outcome is better, cost is lower.* This is the ideal situation, since implementing the new procedure both improves the outcome and reduces cost. This new technique should be adopted
- *Outcome is poorer, cost is higher.* This situation is the worst possible, since not only is the new technique more expensive but it produces a poorer outcome. The new technique should be discarded immediately
- *Outcome is better, cost is higher.* This is a complicated problem, since the patients have improved but at extra cost
- *Outcome is poorer, cost is lower.* As with the previous outcome, a decision has to be made about the relative reduction in outcome and the appropriate level of spending reduction.

Cost-effectiveness studies are designed to evaluate the latter two models of care. In these analyses it is important that the outcome is the same for both treatment groups.

Cost-benefit

While cost-effectiveness studies rely on common outcomes of treatment, there may be multiple outcomes of interest, some of which may show benefit while others may not. Clearly, to evaluate the overall relative benefits of each treatment one must relate all outcomes to one common value. The common value most frequently used is a monetary unit. All outcomes, be they wound-free years, medical complications avoided or improvements in social functioning, are converted into a monetary equivalent. The analysis that uses both the costs and consequences (outcomes) of treatment in monetary terms is called a cost-benefit study. Most studies referred to as cost-benefit studies are actually cost-effectiveness studies.

Cost-utility analysis

Early evaluation of treatment effectiveness revolved around the survival of patients from life-threatening diseases. However, the shift in focus from infectious to chronic diseases required a re-evaluation of the appropriate outcomes of treatment. While quantity of life was the key outcome measure, quality of life has also become a key outcome indicator, leading to the development of quality of life tools. Utilities are values placed on health states that include zero (death) and 1 (perfect health). The principle depends on the trade-off between quality of life and survival. It makes the assumption that years of perfect health can be traded off for longer periods of poorer health. Thus, 1 year of perfect health is equivalent to a health utility of 0.5 over 2 years. Utilities can have negative values, reflecting health states that are considered to be worse than death. An example of this may be intractable pain unrelieved by medication. The values of these utilities are derived from population studies in which participants are asked to rate certain disease states to evaluate their potential worth on this scale. The utilities derived at different stages in a patient's life (or disease) may then be multiplied by the years of life within each state to derive a single index that incorporates both quality and quantity of life (the so-called QALY, or quality-adjusted life year). This has the advantage of producing a single outcome measure that can be used in economic assessment.

The use of QALYs has many advantages in health economics since it allows for comparisons not only across different medical interventions for the same disease but also between diseases. However, their use remains controversial and emotive, particularly with respect to the evaluation of the relative benefits of high-cost, life-saving surgery and low-cost interventions that may help many people. There may also be issues in relation to the assumption that all life has the same value. Thus, 1 QALY in a child is equivalent to 1 QALY in someone aged over 85 years. However, this is a popular method of analysis for health economists, policy decisions on health being made with the use of QALYs.

REVIEW OF THE LITERATURE ON COST-EFFECTIVENESS

Method

The review of articles discussing cost-effectiveness was undertaken following a literature search. For this chapter the medical databases of MEDLINE and EMBASE were combined with the nursing database CINAHL. Searching was undertaken using the terms 'cost effectiveness' and 'cost utility' and combined with the terms 'leg ulcer', 'venous ulcer' and 'diabetic foot'. Articles were included provided they gave comparative evidence of both outcomes and costs of treatment in at least two groups. Individual case studies, non-comparative series and descriptions of disease burden without outcome measures were not included. Following the search and fulfilment of the inclusion criteria, papers were categorized into either leg/venous ulcers or diabetic foot ulcers. The leg ulcer/venous ulcer papers were then subdivided into:

- Cost-effectiveness studies of dressing materials
- Studies of other treatment products (bandages, pharmaceuticals and other therapies)
- Studies of care delivery.

Cost-effectiveness of dressing materials in chronic leg/venous ulcers

In total, eight studies were identified that fitted this criterion (Table 5.1). Of these, four were from the UK and one each from the USA, France, Sweden

Table 5.1 Cost-effectiveness studies on dressings used in leg and/or venous ulceration

Reference	Aim	Study design	Participants	Methods	Results	Conclusions
Ohlsson et al 1994 Sweden	To compare clinical and cost-effectiveness of two wound dressings in the primary care setting	RCT comparing saline gauze (SG) soaks with use of hydrocolloid (HCD; DuoDerm). All patients treated using short-stretch bandaging (Comprilan)	30 patients with venous or mixed venous/arterial ulceration	Patients followed up for 6 weeks, with healing as primary endpoint. Costs included use of wound care products, nurse time and travel costs	Mean cost of wound care products were SEK608 with gauze and SEK653 with HCD. Mean overall cost of care SEK4126 with SG and SEK1565 with HCD. 2/15 healed with SG compared with 7/15 with HCD	Results showed both reductions in overall cost of care and improvements in healing. HCD more cost-effective than SG dressings
Armstrong & Ruckley 1997 UK and France	To compare clinical and cost-effectiveness of two wound dressings in three specialist centres	RCT comparing a hydrofibre dressing (HFD; Aquacel) with an alginate dressing (AGD; Kaltostat)	44 patients with moderately or heavily exuding leg ulcers (diameter <7.5 cm). Aetiology 36 venous, 6 mixed, 2 others	Dressing changed if leakage, pain or wear time of 7 days. Secondary dressing of HCD (DuoDerm Extra Thin), orthopaedic padding and class 3c compression bandage (Tensopress). Followed for up to 6 weeks. Direct and indirect costs calculated	21 randomized to HFD, 23 to AGD. 6 healed on HFD compared with 2 on AGD. Similar total costs – £1424 with HFD compared with £1375 with AGD	More cost-effective with HFD than with AGD because of greater effectiveness
Bale et al 1998 UK	To compare the dressing costs of treating different wound types in the community	RCT comparing the use of hydrocellular dressing (HCE; Allevyn) with HCD (Granuflex)	100 patients (32 pressure ulcers, 30 leg ulcers, 34 others)	Dressings changed if leakage or imminent leakage, clinical reason such as pain. Total cost of materials calculated for patients. Patients who withdrew had costs scaled up to 8 weeks. Followed for up to 8 weeks	At study end of the 30 leg ulcers, 2/16 (12.5%) had healed with HCE compared with 1/14 (7%) on HCD. Cost of dressings was £1290 with HCE compared with £932 with HCD. Cost per patient higher on HCE (£81 vs £67) but greater cost-effectiveness with HCE (£645 vs £932 per healed ulcer)	Need for full costing including nursing time and cost of complications

Table 5.1 Cost-effectiveness studies on dressings used in leg and/or venous ulceration, cont'd

Reference	Aim	Study design	Participants	Methods	Results	Conclusions
Harding et al 2000 UK	To evaluate cost-effectiveness of HCD (Granuflex) and skin replacement (SR; Apligraf) with SG within UK practice	Information derived from published data was pooled to develop cost-effectiveness models	Literature search of MEDLINE undertaken to identify trials where clinical effectiveness and cost-effectiveness evaluated. Only studies with >100 patients included	Expert panel used to supplement published information. Results fitted into a probability-based cost-effectiveness model. Costs based on UK published data for wound products and other health-care costs	Most cost-effective model was use of HCD, since it gave lowest cost per healed ulcer (£342). SG had highest nursing costs because of short wear time (£541). Use of SR highest overall cost per healed ulcer because of high dressing costs (£674).	Cost-effectiveness using published results may offer a valuable adjunct to published clinical evidence
Schonfeld et al 2000 US	To assess use of Apligraf for hard-to-heal venous leg ulcers	Semi-Markov model	Based on available literature	Direct costs of health services only evaluated	Annual cost of hard to heal ulcers was $20 041 with Apligraf compared with $27 493 treated with Unna boot. Apligraf led to 3 more months healed per year	Lower overall cost of care together with greater cost-effectiveness when using Apligraf compared with Unna boot
Harding et al 2001 UK	To evaluate cost-effectiveness of HFD with AGD in leg ulceration	Open, prospective RCT of HFD (Aquacel) compared with AGD (Sorbsan) in four centres in the UK	131 patients with moderate or heavy exudate. 103 venous, 15 mixed, 11 arterial and 2 diabetic ulcers	Dressing change according to clinical need (up to 7 days). Absorbent pad and class 3c bandage used over orthopaedic padding in those clinically indicated. Costs included wound material costs, and cost of nurse time evaluated for up to 12 weeks of treatment	17/66 patients healed on HFD compared with 17/65 on AGD. Costs per healed ulcer were £1184 with HFD compared with £1201 with HCD. Average cost per cm² reduction in area was £59.22 with HFD and £92.27 with HCD	Authors concluded that HFD was more cost-effective than HCD despite no difference in cost per healed ulcer

table continued on following page

Table 5.1 Cost-effectiveness studies on dressings used in leg and/or venous ulceration, cont'd

Reference	Aim	Study design	Participants	Methods	Results	Conclusions
Sibbald et al 2001 Canada	To explore cost-effectiveness of adding tissue engineered skin (TES; Apligraf) to the care of patients with venous ulcers treated by outpatient services	Decision analysis model using published data and expert panel	Expert panel of 5 dermatologists and 2 family practitioners. Models based on 4LB (Profore) alone and 4LB with TES	All costs of health care plus time lost from work (societal costs). Assumed one application of Apligraf per patient	Healing rates assumed to be 60% with 4LB alone and 67.5% with 4LB + TES. Healing time 56 days with 4LB and 26.1 days with 4LB + TES. 3-month costs $1454 versus $1758 respectively. Ulcer days averted with TES = 22. Cost per day averted $14	TES more costly but more effective than 4LB alone. TES more cost-effective over longer follow-up and in ulcers of longer duration. However, key assumptions made by panel, not clinical evidence
Kerstein et al 2001 US	To explore costs, outcomes and effects of outcomes on costs of wound care protocols	Model development using published data supplemented by expert panel. Comparisons made between SG, HCD and TES	Searches of MEDLINE and CINAHL revealed 18 studies that fitted inclusion criteria	Costs for dressings, bandages, debridement and infection. Staffing costs for nursing and physicians over 12 weeks of treatment.	Healing assumed to be 39% with SG, 51% with HCD and 45% with TES. Costs per healed patient were lowest for HCD at $1873, then SG $2939 and $15 053 for TES	Authors conclude that cost analysis should not only include cost of products, as purchase price is not an indication of cost-effectiveness.
Meaume & Gemmen 2002 France*	To evaluate cost-effectiveness of HCD (Granuflex) and SR (Apligraf) with SG within France	Information derived from published data was pooled to develop cost-effectiveness models	A literature search of MEDLINE and CINAHL was undertaken to identify trials where clinical effectiveness and cost-effectiveness were evaluated. Only studies with >100 patients included	Expert panel used to supplement published information. Results fitted into a probability-based cost-effectiveness model. Costs based on French published data for wound products and other health-care costs	Most cost-effective model was use of HCD, since this gave the lowest cost per healed ulcer (€1436). SG had the next highest cost (€2763). Use of SR highest overall cost per healed ulcer because of high dressing costs (€11 396).	Need to move away from SG as treatment

*This paper is based on the same literature as Harding et al 2000
RCT, randomized controlled trial

and Canada. Four presented data from original randomized controlled trials (RCTs), with the remainder pooling information from previously published literature to develop cost models.

The first identified study was published in Sweden (Ohlsson et al 1994), and was a randomized trial to compare the cost-effectiveness of a hydrocolloid (HCD; DuoDerm) with saline gauze (SG) soaks. A total of 30 patients with venous or mixed arterial/venous ulcers were randomized, with the nurse in charge of the patient recording all treatments given over a 6 week period. All patients were treated using Comprilan short-stretch compression bandaging. Dressing changes occurred twice daily in patients randomized to SG and weekly (more frequently if clinically indicated) in the HCD group. Nine patients healed over the study (seven on HCD, two on SG). The mean cost of dressings, cleansers and bandages was £47 (SEK608) with SG compared with £50 (SEK653) with HCD. However, the cost of nursing time and travel more than cancelled this difference out. Mean costs of this were £271 (SEK3518) with SG and £70 (SEK912) with HCD. The mean direct cost of care was therefore £318 (SEK4125) with SG compared with £120 (SEK1565) with HCD. It is worthy of note that the trial protocol dictated the frequency of dressing changes and may therefore have influenced the final cost-effectiveness analysis. However, this study did indicate that, while the cost of the dressing could be cheaper using saline gauze, the total cost of care might be substantially higher using this product because of the increased frequency of dressing changes required.

Later studies using published clinical data have since found similar results. Harding et al (2000) used published literature to compare the cost-effectiveness of saline gauze with Granuflex (UK name for DuoDerm), and tissue engineered skin (TES; Apligraf) over a 12-week follow up. They identified 12 studies involving 843 ulcers, of which 205 were treated with SG, 509 with HCD and 278 with TES. A multinational panel of four wound care experts was used to supplement the clinical information where areas of doubt existed. Cost-effectiveness was evaluated as the total cost of care of the cohort divided by the number of healed ulcers to give a cost per healed ulcer of £342 for HCD, £541 for SG and £6741 for TES. Few details

were given in the paper about how these costs were calculated and their precise composition. The results of this study were also adapted to give a French perspective on the relative cost-effectiveness of the three treatment regimens (Meaume & Gemmen 2002). The expert panel in this study consisted of five French wound care experts. While the system of care is different between the UK and France the pattern of cost-effectiveness was consistent, with HCD being most cost-effective at £1974 (€2763) per healed ulcer, £1026 (€1436) with SG and £8140 (€11,396) with TES.

A similar study was undertaken in the US by Kerstein et al (2001). They undertook a broader literature review, which included the CINAHL database, to evaluate the cost-effectiveness from a US perspective of SG, HCD and TES in patients with venous ulceration. They identified 18 studies that fitted their search criteria and identified 223 patients on SG, 530 on HCD and 130 on TES. This paper used a similar methodology to that adopted by Harding et al (2000), but gave more details of how the model was developed and analysed. The average cost of dressings was lowest with SG at £62 ($112), followed by HCD at £124 ($223) and then TES at £3406 ($6130) over 12 weeks. However, the difference in SG and HCD was reversed when considering nursing costs, at £311 versus £126 ($559 versus $227). The cost per healed patient was estimated at £1633 ($2939) for SG, £1041 ($1873) for HCD and £8363 ($15 053) for TES.

Other studies have made similar efforts to evaluate the relative cost-effectiveness of other dressing types. Bale et al (1998) evaluated the relative performance of a hydrocellular dressing (HCE; Allevyn) with a HCD (Granuflex) in a trial of 100 patients (32 pressure ulcers, 30 leg ulcers, 34 others) over 8 weeks. Dressing changes were made according to need, particularly for leakage, imminent leakage or another clinical reason such as wound pain. There was no indication in this trial of the protocol adopted for compression therapy in the two groups, although Tensopress compression bandage was clearly used in some instances. Cost analysis was undertaken for dressing and other material costs only. The total material costs of treatment were £1290 in the 16 leg ulcer patients randomized to HCE compared with £932 in the 14 patients randomized to HCD, with 2/16 (12.5%)

healing on HCE and 1/14 (7.1%) healing on HCD. In this limited analysis the mean dressing costs were higher in the HCE group (£81 versus £67), but a cost-effectiveness analysis (per healed ulcer) would favour HCE because of its greater effectiveness (£645 versus £932). Clearly a more detailed analysis would be required to investigate the wear time, nursing and medical costs associated with these two dressing types. While the results from this trial must be treated with caution because of the limited data collected, this study does have a major advantage in that patients underwent dressing changes according to need, not according to the trial protocol. This may therefore better reflect the real clinical situation than other studies of this type.

Armstrong & Ruckley (1997) compared the clinical and cost-effectiveness of a hydrofibre dressing (HFD; Aquacel) with an alginate (AGD; Kaltostat) in an RCT. Forty-four patients with moderately or heavily exuding leg ulcers were randomized to one of the two dressings in combination with a secondary dressing (DuoDerm Extra Thin), orthopaedic padding and a class 3c compression bandage (Tensopress). Changes of dressing were dictated by clinical need (leakage or pain) to a minimum of once per 7 days for up to 6 weeks. The wound types included in this trial were venous (36), mixed arterial/venous (six) and two others. In this trial direct costs of care were evaluated, which included costs of dressing materials and nurse time. Over the 6 weeks 6/21 (29%) healed on HFD compared with 2/23 (9%) on AGD. There were similar total costs of treatment, at £1424 and £1375 in the two groups. The cost per healed ulcer as given by the data in the paper was £237 for HFD compared with £688 with AGD. Here the overall costs of care were similar, but with greater effectiveness the HFD was shown to be more cost-effective.

A similar study was undertaken by Harding et al (2001) using the same HFD but a different AGD (Sorbsan replacing Kaltostat). This was an open RCT undertaken in four centres in the UK. A total of 131 patients (103 venous, 15 mixed, 11 arterial and two diabetic) were randomized to one of the two dressings. An absorbent pad was used as a secondary dressing, with orthopaedic wool and class 3c compression bandage used in those in whom it was clinically indicated, for up to 12 weeks. Again, dressing changes were undertaken according

to clinical need to a minimum of once per 7 days. Costs were calculated according to information collected on materials used at dressing change, with a notional cost of £15 added for the cost of nursing time per visit. After 12 weeks 17 patients had healed in both groups. Cost-effectiveness was determined in three ways, as the cost per healed ulcer, the cost per 1 cm^2 reduction in ulcer area and the cost per 10% reduction in area. While the cost per healed ulcer was similar between groups (£1184 in HFD versus £1201 with AGD), there was greater cost-effectiveness when examining cost per 1 cm^2 reduction (£59 versus £92) and per 10% reduction in area (£80 versus £105). The authors stated in their conclusions that this showed that the HFD was more cost-effective than AGD. While reductions in ulcer area may have clinical importance, this is unlikely to have a major impact in cost-effectiveness studies. While the area may be reduced, the patient still has an ulcer present and therefore will require a similar level of care. The difference in reductions in area might be explained by different median areas between the groups, but these data were not presented in the paper.

Finally, two papers have evaluated the potential cost-effectiveness of the use of tissue engineered skin (TES; Apligraf) in the management of patients with venous ulceration. The first of these used data derived from the RCT of Apligraf to develop a semi-Markov model of care (Schonfeld et al 2000). Clinical trial data were supplemented with information provided by a panel of physicians. The patients for the trial had an ulcer present for a minimum of 1 month and had failed to respond to standard treatments. Direct costs were estimated from the cost of products, physician visits, inpatient stays and home visits over a 1-year period. Overall healing rates were 48.1% with TES compared with 25.2% without after 1 year, with a mean ulcer-free period of 4.6 months with TES and 1.75 months without. The total annual cost of care was £11 134 ($20 041) with TES compared with £15 274 ($27 493) without. While the results do show a cost advantage in using TES, there was little information in the paper about how many TES applications were assumed to be used in the model.

Sibbald et al (2001) explored the use of TES as an adjunct to four-layer bandage (4LB) high-compression therapy using a similar decision model approach. They used information derived from the literature supplemented with expert opinion. In addition to the direct costs of care this study also attempted to evaluate the indirect costs of care through the impact of the ulceration and its treatment time lost from work. Costs were assessed using two models, one at 3 months and one for a 6-month follow up. The results showed that the mean cost of care was higher for patients treated with TES + 4LB at £977 ($1758) compared with £808 ($1454) using 4LB alone. However, the mean number of ulcer days per patient was considered to be lower with TES + 4LB at 45 days compared with 67, giving an average number of ulcer days averted at 22. The cost per ulcer-free day was estimated to be £7.78 ($14). With the 6-month model this cost per day healed was reduced to less than £2.78 ($5). While this was an interesting take on the method of cost-effectiveness analysis, a number of caveats must be considered. The cost models are highly dependent on the assumptions made about costs and outcomes. In this model, with no clinical evidence of the use of TES under 4LB compression, the panel decided on their best guess estimate of healing based on the only RCT available. They decided that 4LB alone would provide a 60% healing rate compared with 67.5% when combined with TES. Related to this, the mean days to heal was lower at 26.1 with TES + 4LB compared with 56 with 4LB alone. A further assumption was that one piece of TES was required per patient at a cost of £528 ($950). While this may be the case in most situations, any lower relative healing or additional use of TES would have a marked impact on the relative cost of providing care within this group.

Cost-effectiveness of bandages, pharmaceuticals and other treatments

While the cost-effectiveness of wound dressings has been the subject of a number of studies, evidence of this nature has been less common with respect to other areas of care (Table 5.2). The use of compression bandaging is considered to be the cornerstone of care, with the Cochrane Review considering high compression to be the best available treatment. Despite this, there is little evidence on the relative cost-effectiveness of high compression

against no compression and a dearth of studies undertaken to compare the relative costs of different compression systems.

In 1999 Carr et al published the results of a Markov decision model to evaluate the potential cost-effectiveness of using high compression in venous ulceration. Two comparisons were made: the cost-effectiveness of high compression versus usual care, and the comparative cost-effectiveness of two four-layer bandage systems (Profore versus the original Charing Cross system). While the authors wished to test the impact of high compression on care, they were hampered by the fact that little evidence was available on the care of patients without compression. It was assumed that the evidence of pre-implementation studies would provide similar results to no compression, since compression bandages were not routinely available when these studies were undertaken. The follow-up for the model was 1 year, with analysis also including the costs of recurrence. The assumed healing over 52 weeks was 71% with 4LB compared with 60% with usual care, with median time to ulcer healing of 19.5 weeks with 4LB and 35.5 weeks with usual care. Different models were used to test the robustness of the results (sensitivity analysis). Assessed total cost of care averaged £1404 with usual care compared with £631 with 4LB, with a mean cost per healed ulcer of £2200 and £815 respectively. The difference was largely due to improved healing rates, shorter healing times and reduced frequency of visits when using 4LB. A comparison of the use of Profore with the original 4LB system revealed greater cost-effectiveness with Profore, due to the shorter healing times given by a previous RCT. More recently, O'Brien et al (2003) published the results of an RCT comparing the use of 4LB with the usual care of patients treated in the community by nurses or general practitioners. Two hundred patients were randomly assigned to receive 4LB or continue with their usual care within the community. After 12 weeks of treatment 52% of patients had healed on 4LB compared with 34% with usual care. The mean cost per patient was £150 (€209.7) on 4LB compared with £168 (€234.6) with usual care. The study indicated a better outcome of treatment using 4LB at no extra cost. Therefore, it was concluded that the 4LB was a cost-effective method of the care of patients with venous ulceration in the community.

Table 5.2 Cost-effectiveness studies of bandages, pharmaceuticals and other leg ulcer treatments

Reference	Aim	Study design	Participants	Methods	Results	Conclusions
Carr et al 1999 UK	To investigate the potential cost-effectiveness of four-layer bandaging (4LB)	Markov model using published literature. Comparison of four-layer bandaging with usual care and Profore with Charing Cross (CX)4LB	Information from the published literature. Model developed to examine the effects within 100 patient cohorts run for 52 weeks of follow-up	Transition probabilities determined from healing curves within the literature. Costs determined from cost of treatments (products and nursing). Tested for robustness using different assumptions	Model predicted slightly better cost-effectiveness with Profore compared with CX4LB, due to shorter median time to heal (£412 vs £494 per healed ulcer). Substantially more cost-effective than usual care (£1932 vs £980) per healed ulcer	Systematic use of 4LB compression reduces time to healing and increases proportion who heal. This leads to both cost reduction and improved outcomes. Can treat 162–222 with compression for the same cost as 100 patients treated with usual care
Iglesias et al 2004 UK	Investigate the cost-effectiveness of 4LB versus short-stretch compression bandaging (SSB) in venous ulcers	Information collected in parallel with an RCT of therapy	387 adults with venous ulcers	Analysis based on cost of NHS and personal social service, followed for 1 year. Health benefit determined as QALYs and ulcer-free days	Small difference in QALYs between groups (−0.02), although 4LB took 10.9 fewer days to heal compared with SSB. Costs were £227 less per patient per year with 4LB compared with SSB	4LB produced greater health benefits and lower costs than SSB
Korn et al 2002 USA	To examine the cost-effectiveness of compression hosiery (CS) in leg ulcer prevention.	Markov model comparing a prophylactic programme with reimbursed hosiery and patient education versus no programme	Theoretic model based on a cohort of patients aged 55 years	Transition probabilities determined for states of health including ulcer recurrence, no ulcer, cellulitis, amputation and death. Probabilities based on published results. Included utility measures based on states of health	Cost of stockings $300/year. Average cost of recurrence $1621. Use of CS and education was cost-saving ($5904) and increased QALYs by 0.37 compared with alternative strategy. Lifetime saving of $17 080	The use of CS and education are cost-saving and lead to improved outcomes, even with most conservative outcomes. Insurers should reimburse CS for ulcer recurrence prevention

Table 5.2 Cost-effectiveness studies of bandages, pharmaceuticals and other leg ulcer treatments, cont'd

Reference	Aim	Study design	Participants	Methods	Results	Conclusions
Glinski et al 1999 Poland	To determine increase in healing with micronized purified flavinoid fraction (MPFF) compared with usual care alone	RCT	140 patients with venous ulcer >3 months, 2–10 cm diameter	Patients randomized to MPFF in an open trial over 6 months. Patients bandaged own legs with Setopress elastic bandage. Direct medical costs determined including treatments, nursing, physician and hospital costs	Total costs were lower with MPFF (€476 vs €515) and more effective (healing 46.5% vs 27.5%). Cost per healed ulcer was €1026 vs €1871 respectively	Authors conclude that MPFF has good therapeutic effect and is cost-effective in patients with venous ulcers
Oien et al 2001 Sweden	To compare the relative cost-effectiveness of pinch skin grafting in hospital versus community	Patients in community compared with a historical group of patients treated in hospital	29 patients in community compared with 29 patients in hospital service	Direct costs estimated for hospital stay and care within the community following discharge. Primary care group assessed for community costs only	9/29 healed in both groups over 12 weeks. Costs were £6738 for hospital group vs £1806	Treatment costs for hospital patients were 3.3 times that of patients in the community
Wayman et al 2000 UK	To examine cost-effectiveness of larval therapy (LDT) compared with hydrogel in debridement	RCT of debridement for sloughy ulcers	12 patients diagnosed with sloughy venous ulcers	Dressings changed every 72 hours. Covered with secondary dressing alone. Costs based on 1 month follow-up	Debridement occurred more rapidly in the LDT group. Mean cost of nursing time greater in hydrogel group (£54 vs £11). Mean cost of dressings greater in hydrogel group (£90 vs £10). Overall medina costs £136 vs £79, p <0.05)	Larval debridement more cost-effective than standard hydrogel for sloughy venous ulcers. Need for a larger study to confirm results

table continued on following page

Table 5.2 Cost-effectiveness studies of bandages, pharmaceuticals and other leg ulcer treatments, cont'd

Reference	Aim	Study design	Participants	Methods	Results	Conclusions
O'Brien et al 2003 Ireland	Compare cost-effectiveness of 4LB with usual care in venous ulceration	RCT comparing the introduction of 4LB with the usual care provided by community nurses and physicians	200 patients (100 in each group) randomized	Patients followed for up to 12 weeks. Standard care not controlled, but determined by nurse or GP treating the patient. Costs included GP and nurses time and travel costs	After 12 weeks 52% healed with 4LB compared with 34% in control group. Mean costs were €209.7 with 4LB and €234.6 in the control group	Costs were lower and outcomes better in the patients treated with 4LB. The 4LB provides increased health benefits at no added cost

RCT, randomized controlled trial

Moffatt et al (2003) reported an RCT comparing the use of 4LB (Profore) with a two-layer system (2LB; Surepress) in 109 patients, which included a cost-effectiveness analysis. While there was a marginal improvement in healing over 24 weeks of follow-up in the 4LB group (88% vs 77%), the largest impact on costs was the dressing frequency, which occurred on average 1.1 times per week with 4LB compared with 1.5 times/week with 2LB. The mean weekly costs on treatment were therefore higher with 2LB (£83.56) compared with 4LB (£79.91), despite 4LB being a more costly product. The average total costs per patient over the 24 weeks were £876 on 4LB compared with £916 on 2LB. A recent economic analysis based on a trial comparing four-layer versus short-stretch compression (SSB) in venous ulceration (Iglesias et al 2004) demonstrated that the 4LB system cost on average £227 less per patient per year than the SSB system, because of improved healing and 10.9 fewer days on treatment. The authors stated that this indicated greater health benefits and lower costs then the SSB system, confirming cost-effectiveness.

While compression therapy has been advocated for the treatment of venous ulceration it may also play an important role in the prevention of ulcer recurrence following healing. Korn et al (2002) used a Markov decision model approach to examine the potential cost-effectiveness of compression hosiery to health insurers. Included within this was an educational component to provide training for the patient to improve compliance. The base case model used direct costs only, although sensitivity analysis included an assessment for time off work (indirect costs). The assumptions made included that patients with stockings would be compliant while those who received no stockings would be non compliant. Recurrence rates were assumed to be 1.8% per month with stockings and 5.3% per month without, with mean time to recurrence 53 months and 18.7 months respectively. The provision of hosiery led to a mean lifetime cost saving of £3280 ($5904) and an additional 0.37 QALY gained. Again, the biggest criticism for this paper comes from the use of the reference data used. Information on studies that categorized patients as compliant or non-compliant was used as the major determinant of recurrence. Patients who are non-compliant for whatever reason have a higher inci-

dence of recurrence, but they are not representative of the general healed ulcer population. This does not mean that similar recurrence rates would occur in a population of patients not supplied with hosiery, and as such the results must be treated with caution.

Few pharmaceuticals have been advocated in the management of venous ulceration, and of these fewer still have been adequately evaluated in RCTs. The literature search undertaken for this chapter revealed just one study on cost-effectiveness, in relation to the use of micronized purified flavonoid fraction (MPFF) on venous ulcer healing. The cost-effectiveness study was part of an open RCT of MPFF undertaken in Poland (Glinski et al 1999). One hundred and forty patients with venous ulceration were randomized to either receive the drug or not. All patients were taught how to manage their own ulcers, including the application of a class 2 bandage (Setopress), which was reapplied on a daily basis. Nine clinical assessments were made over the 24-week follow-up period. Direct costs included costs of materials, physician and nursing costs. Hospitalization occurred frequently, with 19% in the control group and 14% on MPFF receiving in-patient care for an average of 45 and 34 days respectively. The average total costs of care were £368 (€515) in the control group and £340 (€476) with MPFF. The cost per healed ulcer was £1339 (€1874) in the control group and £731 (€1024) with MPFF. While this is an interesting study, there are a number of issues around the trial that need to be explored. The leg ulcer practice undertaken in Poland is quite different from that used in Western populations, particularly with respect to patients treating their own ulcers. While it is not stated in the paper, it is assumed that the bandages were re-used. Moreover, there was a high reliance on inpatient services, which is comparatively rare in western Europe and north America. It is likely that the cost-effectiveness in other countries is somewhat different from that experienced in this study.

While pharmaceuticals have rarely been evaluated in clinical trials of venous ulceration, other alternative therapies are used, some of which have been evaluated in cost-effectiveness studies. Wayman et al (2000) undertook a small study ($n = 12$) to examine the relative cost-effectiveness of larval therapy compared with a standard hydrogel in the debridement of sloughy venous ulcers. The outcome for this trial was resolution of slough rather than time to complete healing, patients being followed to 30 days. Direct costs included cost of materials and nursing time, the larvae costing £58 per treatment. The total cost in the larval group was £492 compared with £1054 using a hydrogel, the differences being largely due to the higher number of visits required using the hydrogel and the corresponding nursing and materials costs associated with them. While this trial may show the cost-effectiveness using larvae there are a number of difficulties in determining their true value. In the paper it was assumed that all patients received one dose of larvae, yet in the text it indicated that dosage may have been more frequent. Moreover, the endpoint of this trial (slough resolution) is probably more difficult to determine, particularly since evidence of the value of debridement on ulcer healing is still lacking. Despite this, the study was of interest and may indicate a potential benefit of using larval therapy in patients with sloughy wounds.

Cost-effectiveness in development and evaluation of leg ulcer services

While the literature so far reviewed has examined particular products, cost-effectiveness arguments can equally be applied to systems of care that provide services to patients. Care delivery is a complex, multidimensional process that rarely relies on one product. It is as important to try to evaluate the system that offers care as to evaluate the components that make it up (Table 5.3).

The focus of cost-effectiveness evaluation of systems has been in the UK, with the introduction of community leg ulcer clinics run by community nurses in collaboration with specialist nurses from the hospital and direct links to specialist physicians and surgeons (Moffatt et al 1992). While this is not the only potential model of care, to date it is the only one that has evaluated costs together with outcomes of treatment. The concept of community clinics was developed in the Riverside Leg Ulcer project undertaken during the late 1980s and early 1990s. At that time leg ulcer care was largely undertaken in patients' homes by community nurses, with little medical input. The study aimed to implement a system of care that included assessment using Doppler, treatment using high-compression 4LB and appropriate referral to specialists within the hospital. Cost-effectiveness was determined by combining the clinical results prior to and following implementation with the costs of services from questionnaire and audit data provided by patients and professionals (Bosanquet et al 1993). The study indicated that the cost of care in Riverside was £433 600 prior to the new service compared with just £169 000 in the new service. This was also associated with improvements in outcome from a 12-week healing rate of 22% prior to the new service to 80% in the new clinics. In this study outcomes improved together with reductions in cost made the new service clearly cost-effective. Despite this success, there was concern over the use of a historical control group in this analysis. A further implementation study was undertaken by Simon et al (1996) in two neighbouring health authorities (Stockport and Trafford) in the UK. To minimize the temporal effects on the data, one authority (Stockport) implemented a new service based on the Riverside model while the other (Trafford) maintained their service using existing practices. In Stockport the 12-week healing rates improved from a baseline of 26% during 1993 to 42% in 1994, while in Trafford they remained static at 23% in 1993 and 20% in 1994. Annual expenditure reduced in Stockport from £409 991 to £253 371, while in Trafford it rose from £556 039 to £673 318. Again the evidence showed improvements in outcome combined with reduction in cost, a powerful cost-effectiveness argument. This work has since been extended by implementing a similar service in the control (Trafford) authority (Ellison et al 2002). The Stockport service was able to maintain healing rates at 40%, while those in Trafford rose from 20% to 42% following implementation. The cost of the service increased in Stockport from £65 545 to £83 344, while in Trafford it reduced from £151 375 to £53 176 in 1999. Again, an improved outcome was demonstrated at a lower cost.

Despite these studies showing demonstrable improvements of care and lower cost it has been argued that the use of historical control groups may exaggerate the differences, while comparisons

Table 5.3 Cost-effectiveness studies of services for the management of leg ulceration

Reference	Aim	Study design	Participants	Methods	Results	Conclusions
Bosanquet et al 1993 UK	To investigate the cost-effectiveness of community leg ulcer clinics in one UK health authority	Pre- and postimplementation evaluation.	Patients attending new community leg ulcer service compared with patients treated by community nurses in their homes prior to implementation	Pre- versus postimplementation analysis. Information collected prospectively from nurses and retrospectively from patients. Follow up to 12 weeks	Healing rates were substantially greater in the clinics compared with home prior to service (80% versus 22%) Total cost of care for the provider was £433 000 prior to service compared with £169 000 postimplementation	Community leg ulcer clinics providing high-compression bandaging lead to both cost reduction and more cost-effective care than in the standard care offered by community nurses without high compression
Simon et al 1996 UK	To determine outcome and cost-effectiveness for community leg ulcer clinics within two health authorities	Pre- and postimplementation in one area (Stockport), compared with control area (Trafford)	All patients attending for leg ulcer treatment within the two districts audited in 1993 and 1994	Pre (1993) versus (1994) audit in Stockport compared with control audits in Trafford in the same years, followed for 12 weeks	Healing rates in Stockport increased from 26% to 42%, whereas in Trafford they stayed static at 23% and 20% respectively. Annual expenditure reduced in Stockport from £409 991 to £253 371. Expenditure increased in Trafford from £556 039 to £673 318	In the first year of a leg ulcer clinic based service healing increased, and costs reduced

table continued on following page

Table 5.3 Cost-effectiveness studies of services for the management of leg ulceration, cont'd

Reference	Aim	Study design	Participants	Methods	Results	Conclusions
Morrell et al 1998 UK	To establish the relative cost-effectiveness of community leg ulcer clinics using 4LB versus usual care provided by district (community) nurses	RCT with 1 year of follow up	233 patients with venous ulcers randomized to community clinics (120) and usual care (113)	Weekly treatment of patients either in clinics or at home. Direct costs evaluated for staff time, materials, transport and overheads	Patients in clinic had higher healing rates than those treated at home (34% vs 24% at 12 weeks). Mean costs were £878 vs £859 respectively	A small additional cost of using 4LB by trained nurses in community leg ulcer clinics improves patient outcomes
Kerstein et al 2000 US	To explore the outcomes and costs of managing patients with venous ulceration in a physician's office or in the patient's home	Non randomized prospective longitudinal study	81 patients with acquired venous disease with ulceration, followed up at least 6-monthly	Use of Unna's boot, wet-to-dry dressings, HCD dressings and compression hosiery in both facilities. Costs based on health-care charges	Outcomes did not differ between the home care and physician's office. Patients preferred home care but costs were higher than for physician's office ($159 vs $55 per visit respectively)	Authors concluded that HCD dressings more cost-effective than Unna's boot or saline gauze. Need RCTs to examine cost-effectiveness in different settings, treatments and care systems
Ellison et al 2002 UK	Follow up of the Simon 1996 study	Comparison of two health districts, the latter audit (1999) following implementation in control site	All patients with active leg ulcers cared for in the two health authorities	Community clinic held in both areas providing multilayer high compression bandaging	Healing rates in Stockport maintained at 40%, those in from 20% to 42% following new clinics. Costs rose in Stockport to £83 344 but reduced in Trafford from £151 375 to £53 176	Costs and outcomes can be sustained in mature community leg ulcer clinics staffed by specialist leg ulcer nurses

of authorities may be limited because of differences in patients, populations and other health-care factors. To overcome this, Morrell and co-workers (1998) undertook an RCT comparing patients treated in clinics with high compression bandaging with those being cared for in their homes by nurses providing usual care over a 12-month period. In total, 233 patients were randomized. The annual cost for patients randomized to clinics was £878, compared with £859 in usual home care setting. 12-week healing rates were 34% in the clinic compared with 24% in the home care. Thus, outcomes were improved at a similar cost within the community clinics. While this result cannot prove that community clinics are more cost-effective per se, since the treatments offered were different, it does show that the system of care offered within the clinics was superior to the system of care offered in the home by community nurses.

While most studies have come from the UK, one study from the USA has examined the cost-effectiveness of patients being cared for by physicians or home care nurses. Kerstein & Gahtan (2000) identified 81 patients cared for either by a physician or by home care nurses and followed them for at least 6 months. Patients were given similar treatments, including Unna's boot, wet-to-dry and hydrocolloid dressings and compression hosiery. Costs were based on health-care charges rather than true costs of care. The outcomes of treatment were similar between treatment systems. While patients preferred to be cared for in their own homes, this was at a higher cost of £88 versus £31 ($159 versus $55) per visit. The authors concluded that an RCT would be required to examine the costs in different health-care settings.

Pinch skin grafting was introduced to allow for the rapid coverage of ulcerated areas using a technique that could be carried out in the community. Oien et al (2001) evaluated the relative cost-effectiveness of undertaking this procedure either in hospital or within community services. This was a non randomized study using historical data from the hospital service compared with patients from primary care receiving the same grafting technique undertaken by physicians in the hospital and one general practitioner in the community. Patients in hospital were restricted to bed for 1 week following surgery and cared for using Vaseline gauze or silicone dressing and compression. Patients in the community were treated using hydrocolloid dressings and compression. Direct costs included the inpatient stay, home care nursing and GP visits and all related travel costs. In both groups 9/29 (31%) were healed after 12 weeks of care. The total mean costs of treatment were £6738 in hospital and £1806 in primary care. The majority of this difference could be explained by the time spent as an inpatient (mean 31 days) in the hospital group, with the corresponding cost accounting for 98.7% of the total cost. While this is an evaluation of one treatment within two systems of care, it does illustrate that the same procedures can have different costs associated with them depending on where care is being delivered and precisely which protocol is being used.

Cost-effectiveness of products in diabetic foot ulcers

The evaluation of cost-effectiveness of wound care products for the diabetic foot is presented in Table 5.4. While a number of studies have been undertaken to examine the role of antibiotics in the prevention of amputation, there are relatively few studies that have evaluated particular products in the treatment of diabetic foot ulceration. The majority of evaluations have been undertaken in the comparison of standard care with the addition of high cost tissue engineered skin equivalents.

The first of these was undertaken by Allenet et al (2000). They used a Markov model to simulate the healing of diabetic foot ulcers over a 1 year period, drawing on the results of a RCT and the application of information from a modified Delphi panel. Only direct costs were evaluated, with the assumption from the trial of an average seven pieces of Dermagraft. The healing was assumed to be 76% using TES and 69% in control group. Total costs per patient were higher in the TES group (FF54 384 vs FF47 418). However, when considering the effectiveness of treatment, the cost per healed ulcer was FF53 522 with TES and FF56 687 with standard care. The additional cost of healing one ulcer was estimated at FF38 784. A similar study was undertaken in the US using Apligraf using information from a randomized trial of 198 patients (Steinberg et al 2002). On average 3.9 applications of TES

Table 5.4 Cost-effectiveness studies of dressings, pharmaceuticals and other diabetic foot ulcer treatments

Reference	Aim	Study design	Participants	Methods	Results	Conclusions
Allenet et al 2000 France	Assess CE of Dermagraft (TES) in the treatment of diabetic foot ulcer	Markov model simulation over a 1 year period	Information from RCT of TES. Modified Delphi process used clinicians from centres of excellence in France	Used published data to estimate unit costs using DRGs standard costs. Assumed average seven pieces of TES per course. Direct costs only measured	Healing estimated as 76% TES and 69% control. Cost per patient FF54 384 with TES vs FF47 418 standard care. Cost per healed ulcer FF53 522 TES vs FF56 687 standard care. Cost to heal one additional ulcer FF38 784	Addition of TES important contribution when used in optimal setting
Ghatnekar et al 2001 Sweden	CE of treating diabetic foot ulcers with Regranex (becaplermin) + good wound care (GWC) versus GWC alone	Markov simulation model examining CE in 4 European countries	Information from study of 183 patients, and meta-analysis of 449 patients	Country specific data collected and combined with disease model to estimate incremental cost per ulcer-free month gained. Analysis run over 1 year	Patients on becaplermin predicted to spend 0.81 months free of ulcers, and 9% lower risk of amputation. Net saving in Sweden, Switzerland and UK. In France, increase in cost $19 for each ulcer-free month gained	Use of becaplermin is cost-effective in a variety of European countries, with different costs of services, and management systems. Use of becaplermin may be cost-saving in some countries and at low cost per ulcer-free period in others

Table 5.4 Cost-effectiveness studies of dressings, pharmaceuticals and other diabetic foot ulcer treatments, cont'd

Reference	Aim	Study design	Participants	Methods	Results	Conclusions
Steinberg et al 2002 USA	Evaluate the economic outcomes of TES (Apligraf) versus standard care for DFUs	Cost-effectiveness analysis from an RCT	112 patients randomized to TES and 96 controls on standard care. 3.9 applications of Apligraf per patient at a mean cost of $5598	Costs assigned for all non protocol driven clinical events. Patients followed for 6 months. Total cost of care derived for all patients using Medicare reimbursement rates. CE analysis for the incremental cost per amputation/resection avoided and cost per ulcer-free month	22 patients (15 control, 7 TES) underwent amputation or resection. Mean costs were higher in the TES group ($7366 vs $2020). Cost per amputation/resection avoided $86 226. Cost per ulcer-free month gained $6683	May be beneficial with low application rate (1.5 per patient) giving cost per ulcer free month gained of $2356. May have best cost-effectiveness in ulcers <2months duration
Sibbald et al 2003 Canada	To evaluate the cost-effectiveness of adding Regranex (becaplermin) to best clinical care	Markov model using a clinical trial of becaplermin supplemented with an Expert panel	Delphi panel of 6 nurses, 2 chiropodists, 2 dermatologists, 2 infectious disease specialists, 1 endocrinologist, 1 GP	Questionnaire on care of patients to Delphi panel. Cost per day calculated and multiplied by days on treatment. Reported over 1 year of treatment. Recurrence factored into decision tree	Assumed 35% healed by 20 weeks on best care and 49% using becaplermin. Ulcer days per patient 237 on standard care versus 211 days with becaplermin. Mean cost per patient $16 513 on best care versus $16 680 with becaplermin. 26 ulcer days averted at a cost per day of $6	Clinical benefits of becaplermin deserve further investigation
Abidia et al 2003	Evaluate the role of hyperbaric oxygen in the management of ischaemic diabetic ulcers	Double-blind RCT of 100% oxygen or air at 2.4 atmospheres	18 patients with ischaemic non-healing diabetic ulcers. 2 patients dropped out of the study	Patients given treatments for 90 minutes/ day for 5 days/week. For 6 weeks	Complete healing occurred in 5/8 with hyperbaric oxygen compared with 1/8 in control group. After 1 year, 5/8 still healed compared with 0/8 in control group	Limited CE analysis. Reduced frequency of visits led to a mean reduction in treatment cost of £2960 over 1 year

were made at an average cost of $5598 per patient. Costs were assigned for all non-protocol-driven clinical events, with follow-up for 6 months. After 6 months 22 patients (7 TES vs 15 controls) had undergone amputation or resection. Mean costs were higher in the TES group ($7366 vs $2020). Cost per amputation/resection avoided was $86 226, with cost per ulcer-free month gained $6683. The conclusions of this study were that a lower application rate of 1.5 experienced in routine clinical practice would offer a much greater cost-effectiveness at $2356 per ulcer-free month gained. It would appear that cost-effectiveness was greatest in patients whose ulcers had been present for less than 2 months.

The other major area of investigation has been with the addition of becaplermin gel (Regranex) to the routine wound care in the diabetic foot. Becaplermin is a biotechnology product that contains a platelet-derived growth factor (rhPDGF-BB) that stimulates the healing process in neuropathic ulcers. Ghatnekar et al (2001) developed a Markov model using information from a study of 183 patients and a meta-analysis of 449 trial patients to estimate costs in four European countries. They used country-specific cost data which they combined with the clinical data to determine the cost per ulcer-free month gained over a 12-month follow up. Patients on becaplermin were predicted to spend an additional 0.81 months ulcer-free, with a 9% lower risk of amputation. There were net savings in cost within the Swedish, UK and Swiss systems. In France the addition of becaplermin led to a slight increase in cost, although the cost per ulcer-free month gained was just $19. From this the authors concluded that the addition of becaplermin could provide cost savings in some health systems, or at a low cost per ulcer-free month in others. A similar model was developed for the Canadian health-care system. Sibbald et al (2003) used a Delphi panel of a variety of health-care professionals involved in the management of patients with diabetic foot ulceration. The lower healing in the standard care group (35% at 20 weeks) compared with those on becaplermin (49%) led to fewer days with ulceration in the becaplermin (211 vs 237). Mean costs per patient were similar between groups at $16 513 on standard care versus $16 680 with becaplermin. On average 26 ulcer days were averted using the product at an estimated additional cost of $6 per day. The authors concluded that the clinical benefits of becaplermin deserved further investigation.

Finally, one study has evaluated the role of hyperbaric oxygen in the healing of ischaemic diabetic foot ulcers (Abidia et al 2003). Eighteen patients were randomized double-blind to either 100% oxygen or air, both at 2.4 atmospheres. Patients were given treatment for 90 minutes per day, five days per week, for 6 weeks. Complete healing occurred in 5/8 on hyperbaric oxygen compared with just 1/8 on air (two patients withdrew from the trial). After 1 year the five ulcers had remained healed in the oxygen group, while the patient who had healed in air had recurred. In this limited cost-effectiveness analysis the reduced frequency of visits led to a mean reduction in treatment cost of £2960 over the 1-year period.

Cost-effectiveness studies of services for the management of diabetic foot ulceration

There has been much interest in the development of services to prevent the development of diabetic foot ulceration and its consequences such as infection and amputation. However, few of these studies have examined in detail the potential cost-effectiveness of intensive foot management programmes. McCabe et al (1998) evaluated the potential cost-effectiveness of a foot screening programme in a RCT of 2001 patients attending their diabetic clinics (Table 5.5). Patients were randomized to either continue with standard care, or to enter a foot screening programme (FSP) to identify high risk of foot damage and to then enter these patients into a foot protection programme. In all, 128/1001 randomized to screening were considered to be at high risk of foot problems and entered the programme. After 2 years of follow-up, there were 11 fewer ulcers in the FSP group. Amputations were lower in this group at seven (one major) compared with the standard care group of 23 (12 major). While formal cost-effectiveness analysis was not undertaken, the total cost of the programme was estimated at £100 372, while the cost of the 11 major amputations averted were £132 000. With lower incidence of other outcomes (ulcer development

Table 5.5 Cost-effectiveness studies of services for the management of diabetic foot ulceration

Reference	Aim	Study design	Participants	Methods	Results	Conclusions
McCabe et al 1998 UK	Evaluate a clinical foot screening programme to reduce the incidence of ulceration and lower limb amputation	RCT of foot screening programme (FSP) versus usual care	2001 patients randomized to intervention vs control. 128 high risk patients identified in FSP group, entered into foot protection programme	Primary and secondary screening for high risk of foot problems in FSP patients. Follow up for 2 years to examine incidence of foot ulcers and amputations	11 fewer ulcers in FSP group. 7 (1 major) amputations in FSP compared with 23 (12 major) in control. Total cost of programme £100 372 (mean cost per patient £100). Cost of major amputation was £12 000, therefore CE system. Cost of £3000 per amputation averted	Foot-screening programme is effective in reducing major amputations and foot ulcers. Cost of new service lower than cost of amputations averted. However, limited CE evaluation
Ragnarson Tennvall & Apelqvist 1999 Sweden	Evaluate CE of intensified prevention strategy for foot ulceration and amputations	Markov model of current vs optimal prevention strategies	Clinical data on 1677 diabetic patients used in model. Four risk groups	5-year model, with eight health states. Transition probabilities based on published literature. Outcomes were incidences of foot ulcers, amputations and deaths, costs, cost-effectiveness and QALYs	For high-risk patients, intensive prevention strategy is cost saving, with a reduced incidence of foot ulcers and amputation of 25%. In the low-risk group not cost-effective	Costs of patient education, foot care and footwear are small. Prevention must be provided for a large number of patients over many years to observe the benefit

and minor amputations) it is likely that the magnitude of this difference would be greater. The estimated cost per amputation averted was £3000.

Finally, a major study to evaluate the cost-effectiveness of a prevention programme to prevent amputations and ulceration used data from 1677 diabetic patients with the results given for four categories of risk (Ragnarson Tennvall & Apelqvist 1999). The developed Markov model was run over a 5-year period, with eight health states. Transition probabilities were based on the literature. Outcomes included incidence of foot ulceration, amputation, death and costs/cost-effectiveness. The results indicated that for medium- and high-risk patients the strategy was not only cost-effective but also led to cost savings. The strategy was not cost-effective in the lowest risk group where no specific risk factors for foot ulceration were identified. The con-clusion was that, since the cost of education, foot care and footwear was small, the overall benefits of an appropriate prevention programme were shown. However, the provision had to be for large numbers of patients who require long-term follow-up for these benefits to become apparent.

DISCUSSION

In this chapter we have reviewed the evidence on the cost-effectiveness of products and services to patients with leg ulceration. While much attention has been placed on the examination of clinical effec-tiveness of these, relatively little emphasis has been placed on the relative cost of different interventions. With ever increasing cost consciousness within health services, and greater demand for 'value for money', these types of study are expected to increase their quality and quantity in leg ulceration.

References

Abidia A, Laden G, Kuhan G et al 2003 The role of hyperbaric oxygen therapy in ischaemic diabetic lower extremity ulcers: a double blind randomised controlled trial. European Journal of Vascular and Endovascular Surgery 25: 513–518

Allenet B, Paree F, Lebrun T et al 2000 Cost effectiveness modelling of Dermagraft for the treatment of diabetic foot ulcers in the French context. Diabetes and Metabolism 26: 125–132

Armstrong S H, Ruckley C V 1997 Use of a fibrous dressing in exuding leg ulcers. Journal of Wound Care 6: 322–324

Bale S, Hagelstein S, Banks V, Harding K G 1998 Costs of dressings in the community. Journal of Wound Care 7: 327–330

Bosanquet N, Franks P, Moffatt C et al. 1993 Community leg ulcer clinics: cost effectiveness. Health Trends 25: 146–148

Carr L, Phillips Z, Posnett J 1999 Comparative cost-effectiveness of four-layer bandaging in the treatment of venous ulceration. Journal of Wound Care 8: 243–248

Ellison D A, Hayes L, Lane C et al 2002 Evaluating the cost and efficacy of leg ulcer care provided in two large UK health authorities. Journal of Wound Care 11: 47–51

Ghatnekar O, Persson U, Willis M, Odegaard K 2001. Cost effectiveness of becaplermin in the treatment of diabetic foot ulcers in four European countries. Pharmacoeconomics 19: 767–778

Glinski W, Chodynicka B, Roszkiewicz J et al 1999 The beneficial augmentative effect of micronised purified flavinoid fraction (MPFF) on the healing of leg ulcers: an open, multicentre, controlled, randomised study. Phlebology 14: 151–157

Graham I D, Harrison M B, Nelson E A et al 2003 Prevalence of lower-limb ulceration: a systematic review of prevalence studies. Advances in Skin and Wound Care 16: 305–316

Harding K, Cutting K, Price P 2000 The cost effectiveness of wound management protocols. British Journal of Nursing (Supplement) 9: S6–S24

Harding K G, Price P, Robinson B et al 2001 Cost and dressing evaluation of hydrofiber and alginate dressings in the management of community based patients with chronic leg ulceration. Wounds 13: 229–236

Iglesias C P, Nelson E A, Cullum N, Torgerson D J 2004 Economic analysis of VenUS 1, a randomised trial of two bandages for treating venous leg ulcers. British Journal of Surgery 91: 1300–1306

Kerstein M D, Gahtan V 2000 Outcomes of venous ulcer care: results of a longitudinal study. Ostomy/Wound Management 46: 22–29

Kerstein M D, Gemmen E, van Rijswick L et al 2001 Cost and cost effectiveness of venous and pressure ulcer protocols of care. Disease Management and Health Outcomes 9: 651–663

Korn P, Patel S T, Heller J A et al 2002 Why insurers should reimburse for compression stockings in patients with chronic venous statis ulcers. Journal of Vascular Surgery 35: 950–957

McCabe C J, Stevenson R C, Dolan A M 1998. Evaluation of a diabetic foot screening and protection programme. Diabetic Medicine 15: 80–84

Meaume S, Gemmen E 2002 Cost-effectiveness of wound management in France: pressure ulcers and venous leg ulcers. Journal of Wound Care 11: 219–224

Moffatt C J, Franks P J, Oldroyd M et al 1992 Community leg ulcer clinics and impact on ulcer healing. British Medical Journal 305: 1389–1392

Moffatt C J, McCullagh L, O'Connor T et al 2003 Randomized trial of four layer and two-layer bandage systems in the management of chronic venous ulceration. Wound Repair and Regeneration 11: 166–171

Morrell C J, Walters S J, Dixon S et al 1998 Cost effectiveness of community leg ulcer clinics: randomised controlled trial. British Medical Journal 316: 1487–1491

O'Brien J F, Grace P A, Perry I J et al 2003 Randomised clinical trial and economic analysis of four layer compression bandaging for venous ulcers. British Journal of Surgery 90: 794–798

Ohlsson P, Larsson K, Lindholm C, Moller M 1994 A cost-effectiveness study of leg ulcer treatment in primary care. Comparison of saline-gauze and hydrocolloid treatment in a prospective, randomised study. Scandinavian Journal of Health Care 12: 295–299

Oien R F, Hakansson A, Ahnlide I et al 2001 Pinch skin grafting in hospital and primary care: a cost analysis. Journal of Wound Care 10: 164–169

Ragnarson Tennvall G, Apelqvist J 1997 Cost effective management of diabetic foot ulcers. Pharmacoeconomics 12: 42–53

Ragnarson Tennvall G, Apelqvist J 1999 Prevention of diabetes related foot ulcers and amputations: a cost utility analysis based on Markov model simulations. Diabetologia 44: 2077–2087

Schonfeld W H, Villa K F, Fastenau J M et al 2000 An economic assessment of Apligraf (Graftskin) for the treatment of hard-to-heal venous leg ulcers. Wound Repair and Regeneration 8: 251–257

Sibbald R G, Torrance G W, Walker V et al 2001 Cost-effectiveness of Apligraf in the treatment of venous leg ulcers. Ostomy/Wound Management 47: 36–46

Sibbald R G, Torrance G, Hux M et al 2003 Cost effectiveness of becaplermin for non healing neuropathic diabetic foot ulcers. Ostomy/Wound Management 49: 76–84

Simon D A, Freak L, Kinsella A et al 1996 Community leg ulcer clinics: comparative study in two health authorities. British Medical Journal 312: 1648–1651

Steinberg J, Beusterien K, Plante K et al 2002 A cost analysis of a living skin equivalent in the treatment of diabetic foot ulcers. Wounds 14: 142–149

Wayman J, Nirojogi V, Walker A et al 2000 The cost effectiveness of larval therapy in venous ulcers. Journal of Tissue Viability 10: 91–94

Models of service provision

*Christine J Moffatt, Peter J Franks,
Moya J. Morison*

INTRODUCTION

There has been great investment in the development and evaluation of wound care products for the treatment of leg ulceration, but relatively little attention to how these products are integrated into clinical practice. This chapter will draw on the organizational and change management literature as well as experience in developing leg ulcer services in different organizations and cultures. It will address some of the key issues in service planning and development and examine some of the approaches to care offered by different health-care systems. It will not consider the delivery of care for the diabetic foot, which will be dealt with in Chapter 18.

ASSESSMENT OF NEED

To evaluate the level of service required it is important to understand the needs of the patient population for whom care is being delivered (Thomas 1996). In many situations this stage is inadequately addressed, with service planners frequently relying on published literature to estimate the need within their population (Gooch et al 2000). Major epidemiology studies were undertaken in the UK in the 1980s and the evidence from these is still being used to make assumptions about the current patient populations (Callam et al 1985, Cornwall et al 1986). While these studies have been of great importance in stimulating the development of the field of leg ulcer management, changes in the population as well as general improvements in practice

may have altered the patient profile considerably (Moffatt et al 2004). All studies of prevalence have been undertaken in Western populations, particularly, the UK, Scandinavia and Australia (Baker et al 1991, Nelzen et al 1991a, Lees & Lambert 1992, Andersson et al 1993). There is little evidence from other countries and anecdotal reports from Asia imply that there are few patients with this condition in these countries. The complexities of the US system also make evaluations of this nature problematic. Studies that purport to evaluate need often rely on patients already in the clinical areas. Thus, a true prevalence including unmet need is rarely undertaken (Nelzen et al 1991a).

In epidemiological terms, need can be defined as: 'indicators of disease that require intervention because their level is above that generally accepted in society.... Needs always reflect prevailing value judgements as well as the existing ability to control a public health problem.' Perceived need may be felt by the person or community concerned, but may not be perceived by health professionals (Last 1995).

The description of the needs of these patients has been framed by the medical model of care. Very little attention has been given to the psychological or social issues facing patients or their families (Callam et al 1988). Relatively little is known about the realities of living with a leg ulcer, although one aspect, the quality of life of patients, has been examined in more depth (Ch. 30). Scant attention has been given to the examination of patients' choice of leg ulcer strategies and how patients might wish to engage in their care delivery.

While an understanding of the number of patients who may wish to access a service is crucial, it is also important to understand the geographical location of patients, as this will have an impact on service design (Moffatt et al 1992). The needs of a rural population will be different from those of an urban population and it is important to factor this into a service plan (Thomson et al 1996). This may also have an impact on which professional group will care for the patient. Educational strategies need to be planned on the basis of this information to ensure that the professionals have the appropriate skills and knowledge to deliver the care required for all patients in their care (Moffatt & Karn 1994). The geographical spread of patients will also help to inform the model of service delivery that is required and can reasonably be delivered within the constraints of funding and staffing levels.

There has been a great emphasis on the role of the multi-professional team in the care of patients with leg ulceration (Gottrup et al 2001). However, research has not been undertaken to show the ideal contribution that individual professional groups can make. Pragmatically, it is important for areas to draw on the expertise they have in their area and to identify the key stakeholders who can develop an effective service (Leathard 1994).

While a population-based service is the ideal, it is acknowledged that many professionals work in areas where there are multiple agencies serving a geographical population (Graham et al 2001). This makes evaluation of need more complex and may lead to patients failing to access adequate care. Even in population-based services, many challenges may be faced in ensuring that acute and community services are working effectively in partnership (Moffatt & Franks 2004).

Little is known of the experience of patients with leg ulceration from ethnic minority groups. One study in west London (UK) identified fewer patients from a south Asian background than would be predicted based upon the demographic details of the resident population (Franks et al 1997). The reasons for this remain obscure but it may be due to poorer uptake of leg ulcer services or a lower prevalence in this ethnic group. This observation has been confirmed in a second study in another part of London (Moffatt 2001, Franks et al 2002). Moreover, the latter study also showed an increased

prevalence of African–Caribbean patients. This may imply a greater risk of leg ulceration in this group or a higher incidence of different aetiologies such as sickle-cell disease. While there has been some research examining ethnic differences, there is little evidence on cultural differences in attitudes to care (Menzies Lyth 1989). Service planners may have to engage in dialogue with community leaders to ensure that these patients receive an appropriate level of service. Similarly, to access marginalized groups such as drug users and the homeless may require collaboration with other agencies. As an example of this, the Riverside Community Leg Ulcer Project found that approximately 25% of the patients identified, many of whom were homeless, were unknown to clinical services (Moffatt et al 1992).

One of the reasons why services have not been developed using a co-ordinated national approach relates to its profile in the health-care agenda (Bosanquet 1992). Priority areas are often associated with mortality or excessive use of hospital resources, and are often emotive issues that capture the public's attention. Leg ulcer patients are predominantly elderly, cared for by community staff and often viewed as unpopular by hospital staff, who find them time-consuming and unrewarding (Callam et al 1985, Browse et al 1988, Moffatt et al 1992). It is only over the past decade that there has been an appreciation of the morbidity associated with leg ulceration and its impact on the patient. Many health initiatives attempt to tackle the major health problems of our age, such as heart disease and cancer. This can have a negative affect on the provision of other services that are considered low priority. As an example of this, the UK government has established National Service Frameworks for these high-priority areas, which have to be delivered to meet agreed targets. The resources have become focused on delivery of these services, as financial penalties will be levied should the targets not be met. It is very difficult in this type of climate to attract funds for areas considered to be low-priority.

DEVELOPING A STRATEGIC ORGANIZATIONAL APPROACH TO SERVICE PROVISION

The sense of need is the greatest driver for change in any system (Lewin 1951). However, developing this may entail engaging key stakeholders in the organization in the provision of evidence to support the argument for service development. Part of this must include the needs assessment. Policy changes seek to place patients in a more central position in health care. The availability of information on the World Wide Web means that patients are becoming more informed and more vocal about demanding effective care (Chambers 2000). As an example of this, the Multiple Sclerosis Society was instrumental in overturning the recommendation by the National Institute for Clinical Effectiveness that beta-interferon was not cost-effective and should not be used in patients with multiple sclerosis (Dobson 2000).

With greater demands on health services, there is a need for the efficient use of financial resources. The collection of cost data can be a driver for change when the scale of investment is known and the potential benefits of adopting an evidence-based approach to care are understood. There is an increasing need for this within evaluation, yet the quality of these studies is generally poor, making interpretation problematic (Ch. 5).

A systematic review of the effectiveness of implementing guidelines has shown the paucity of research that is available at present to guide service development (Bero et al 1998). However, it has shown the importance of using multiple strategies in implementation. Because of the dynamic nature of organizations, it may be very difficult to determine the most effective strategies to be used, as these will always have to be tailored to the complex needs of the organization (Senge 1990).

Implementation does not rely on the presence of research evidence alone but requires the organization to develop a realistic vision for the new service. Successful service development requires a systems approach to implementing change (Leathard 1994). A service plan should be developed that will include both short-term and long-term goals, and should consider how the integration of the different parts of the service will be achieved (Evans & Haines 2000). An example of this is how community and acute (hospital) services will work together to achieve seamless care. This may well require issues of funding to be addressed as patients move from one setting to another. For the development of this plan, key stakeholders within the organization must be involved and committed to the change process, although this can be very difficult if the individuals have a vested interest in maintaining the status quo (Hinshelwood 1987).

Managing the change process requires effective leadership (Covey 1989, Georgiades & Macdonell 1998). The person responsible for leading the service development should have clinical credibility and sufficient authority within the organization to bring about the changes. Much has been written on managing change, but a major factor is an appreciation of how people react to the requirement to adopt new practices. The literature suggests that responses will range from early adopters to late laggards, who delay in adopting change or fail to adopt at all. Successful change will require sensitivity in understanding where people are on this continuum and the pressures they face in their daily work.

LEADERSHIP AND QUALITY ASSURANCE

There has been a burgeoning of the literature relating to effective leadership principles and practices, and their application in health-care organizations. Quality assurance, quality improvement and effective leadership are interconnected, as this literature reflects.

An excellent organization is characterized by:

- Technical excellence in its core services – in this case the clinical care of patients with leg ulcers
- High levels of customer satisfaction
- Excellence in managing its staff – indicated, for example, by high levels of employee motivation and high retention rates
- Cost-effectiveness, and keeping costs under control.

Excellent results in these domains are achieved through leadership driving policy and strategy, people, partnerships and resources, and processes (European Foundation for Quality Management 2003).

Excellent leaders:

- Develop the mission, vision, values and ethics of their organization and are role models of a culture of excellence – this includes prioritizing improvement activities and stimulating and encouraging collaboration within the organization

- Are personally involved in ensuring that the organization's management system is developed, implemented and continuously improved
- Interact with customers, partners and representatives of society (e.g. by being involved in lay and professional working groups and organizations seeking to improve the situation strategically and more globally, and presenting at conferences and seminars)
- Reinforcing a culture of excellence within and outwith the organization (e.g. by being accessible, actively listening, inspiring, uniting and responding to people)
- Identifying and championing organizational change (European Foundation for Quality Management 2003).

Kouzes & Posner (2002) summarize the five practices of exemplary leadership as: modelling the way, inspiring a shared vision, challenging the process, enabling others to act and encouraging the heart. The importance of rewarding and recognizing others is also stressed by Kouzes & Posner (1998).

BARRIERS TO CHANGE

The literature would suggest that it is important to identify the barriers that exist to the planned change in order to overcome them (Bero et al 1998). In leg ulceration there are a number of common areas that have been highlighted, although there will be individual issues in each practice setting.

Developing new services require a major commitment both in time and effort. Health services are frequently overburdened, with staff shortages common. While those leading an innovation may appreciate the vision for change, staff in the clinical area may have a different view and may perceive this to be an additional burden of which they question the value. These difficulties can often be overcome by effective communication strategies that, as well as informing them, engage them in the dialogue of the new service development (Leathard 1994). It is important that clinicians feel that their views are valued and that these are used to inform service development.

The development of leg ulcer services requires the adoption of new practices in assessment and treatment. Staff may find evaluation of their practice threatening and may fear that management will view the findings negatively and treat them punitively as a result (Argyris 1990). The development of new skills requires a sound educational programme to help overcome the anxiety associated with adopting new practices. It is essential that practitioners are supported in the clinical environment where they are required to make these changes rather than in a purely academic setting. Many implementation projects are hampered by the lack of educational programmes and resources for staff in the early stages of new service provision.

The role of the nurse in leg ulcer care has been extended in many services. They have an increasing diagnostic role with the use of non-invasive vascular equipment, and in some models are able to refer directly to hospital consultants (Moffatt et al 1992). Nurses have taken on pinch skin grafting and punch biopsy, which was previously the domain of surgeons. There are large international variations in the academic preparation of nurses and in their position within the multidisciplinary team. Approaches that seek to challenge the traditional divide between medical and nursing practice may create conflict.

A major barrier to the implementation of new services is access to modern wound care products and compression bandages (Moffatt 2003). The reimbursement of these products varies between countries and the mechanisms required to get products reimbursed are complex (Franks & Posnett 2003). There is no international agreement on which products should be reimbursed, nor what the patient's financial contribution (if any) should be towards the cost of products and care.

EVALUATION METHODS

Evaluating service development is a complex process, with competing demands from the different groups involved in the change process. Clinicians may require evidence of clinical improvements in their patients and seek to reduce their workload, whereas health-care managers may prioritize a reduction in the cost of service provision. There has been little evaluation of what the priorities are for patients with leg ulceration, although it is likely that quality of life issues may dominate, with healing an important goal. The priorities for policy-makers are likely to include the estimate of need, and the potential for reduced prevalence and use of health-care resources while improving the health of the population (Korn et al 2002).

Time to healing as an outcome measure

To date, the majority of evaluations have examined the healing potential with different systems of care, occasionally supplemented with cost arguments and quality of life evaluations (Moffatt et al 1992, Simon et al 1996, Vowden et al 1997, Morrell et al 1998). This approach has been as a response to the need for real clinical data that reflects the clinical challenges of the patient population. These analyses have focused on the clinical outcomes of care, particularly time to complete healing. The literature frequently refers to 12- and 24-week healing rates; however, these time points are arbitrary and are not necessarily the most valuable in assessing true change. If the time frame is too short it is possible that there may be insufficient difference between groups, whereas with a longer evaluation period the percentage healed may also fail to reflect real differences in performance. As an example of this, a trial of two bandage systems achieved a similar percentage healed after 24 weeks but the rate of healing was substantially greater in one group (Moffatt et al 2003). The time on treatment was therefore less in this group, which had an impact on the use of resources and cost effectiveness.

Examining the patient population

Evaluation should include patients who cannot tolerate standard treatments, and the reasons for this, and also identify and continue to follow up patients who withdraw, for whatever reason. This will remove the bias experienced in the clinical trial situation, where patients are only followed up while they are receiving the trial treatment, and give a more realistic view of the impact of changes in care. The literature would suggest that there is little attention paid to the longitudinal follow-up of patients, which would provide more evidence of changes in prevalence, but might also provide evidence on the incidence of leg ulceration (Lambourne et al 1996). Cross-sectional studies are often compared, but there may be fundamental differences in the methodologies and the maturity of the services. There is anecdotal evidence from services that have been established for a number of years that the patient population may be changing (Moffatt et al 2004). These changes include a lower prevalence, and a higher proportion of patients with complex ulceration. The difficulties are further compounded by the lack of standardization in evaluation methods, particularly the method of patient ascertainment, and the non-invasive diagnostics and clinical descriptors used in classifying the patient groups.

Challenges in outcome measurement

The emphasis on outcomes has revolved around healing, with little attention to other outcomes. However, with the changes in patient profile, there is a growing awareness of the challenges involved in evaluating success in patients who do not heal, where the priorities of care may be very different (Moffatt & Franks 2004). Healing is still a key outcome of care, since it has a major impact on resource usage; however, reduction in the size of the wound or improvements in symptom management may have profound benefits to patients that cannot be captured by measuring healing alone. However, these unhealed patients still represent a major resource burden, which may not be valued by health-service managers in the same way. It remains to be seen where outcomes other than complete healing are placed in the hierarchy of evaluation.

Professionals and the change process

Little is known about professional attitudes to the implementation of leg ulcer services. There has been some evaluation of changes in professional practice such as the use of Doppler ultrasound, but little of the impact that the changes have had on professional practice and how these are viewed (Flanagan et al 2001). It is assumed that the professionals view complete healing as a positive outcome; however, in some cases professionals may miss the relationship that they have established with long-term patients. Evaluation of leg ulcer services requires commitment on the part of the staff, and the evaluation process may require additional time to be spent with this patient group. This may be a significant burden, which leads to resentment if the benefits to them as individuals are not immediate. Implementation is always likely to require additional time, whether it is due to additional training, increases in patient numbers or time spent with patients, or the burden of the evaluation process. The attitude of professionals to these changes will be highly dependent on how they value the new service in relation to their other work commitments. This attitude may be influenced and modified by their perception of the management's commitment to the new service. The leadership role will have a major influence on the motivation of staff to work towards the proposed changes (Georgiades & Macdonell, 1998).

Organizational responses

Research has not focused on evaluating the organizational challenges in developing leg ulcer services. This will be influenced by the culture of the organization and the turbulence within health care that requires continual adaptation and updating (Handy 1993). Quantitative approaches may be less appropriate when seeking to explore how the changes affect people within the organization. It is vital that leg ulcer projects are seen as the start of a long-term commitment to sustainable service provision. Many projects have discrete time frames and do not continue to evaluate the long-term effects of care beyond the project evaluation period. Some of this will be reflected in the culture of willingness to learn within the organization (Argyris 1990). Moreover, there is a substantial cost of undertaking evaluation, both in financial cost and time required of different staff.

The Riverside Community Leg Ulcer Project was a population-based study that evaluated outcomes in both community and hospital services (Moffatt et al 1992). The evaluation of both services is important as changes that occur in one are likely to impact on the other. As an example of this, increases in patient referrals from one service to the other may benefit the former in terms of reduced patient numbers and resources but may disadvantage the latter, with increased demand. The benefits of the movement of patients may allow for a more efficient overall service, which must be evaluated in both parts of the service. Given the complexity of

hospital contracts, evaluating the effects of these changes may be complex, particularly in care systems that involve multiple agencies. Patients with leg ulceration can be referred to a number of hospital-based specialties, including vascular surgery, dermatology and care of the elderly, and little is known about the most appropriate specialty for each patient group, although most research has been undertaken with vascular surgical support (Moffatt et al 1992, Simon et al 1996, Vowden et al 1997, Adam et al 2003). For evaluation it is important that all these services are involved to observe the real impact on all parts of the leg ulcer service.

Evaluating patient outcomes

Previous studies have relied on outcomes for patients that have been predetermined by health professionals. Patients with leg ulceration are viewed as passive towards the care they receive, with little professional expectation that they would wish to be involved in determining what factors are important to them in the evaluation process (Cullum & Roe 1995). As already discussed, there is a move towards much greater patient involvement in decision-making in health care. Patients are being asked about what services should be provided, where they should be based and increasingly offered choices about how they wish their illness to be managed (McIvor 1991). Quality of life studies have shown the impact that leg ulceration has on patients. Moreover, it has demonstrated the potential improvements that occur with appropriate assessment and treatment, not only in those who experience complete healing but also those patients who improve but fail to heal. This is discussed further in Chapter 30.

While the quality of life literature has used validated tools to determine outcomes of treatment, these have still relied on questions that have been generated by professionals, albeit following studies of patients. Individual patients cannot express choice or indicate the areas of their lives that are most important to them and which aspects they would like to see improved with effective treatment. New phenomenologically based tools allow for expression of the individual's quality of life issues and which aspects they would like to see improved. Care may then be tailored to the individual patient's needs. These tools are often time-consuming to implement and difficult to analyse, making them difficult to incorporate into routine clinical practice. While at present these are seen as research tools, it is hoped that eventually they will be adapted to routine practice. A review of potential outcome measures is given in Table 6.1.

The challenge of effective evaluation

The remit of this chapter does not allow us to give precise details on how the evaluation process should be undertaken, but it is possible to draw upon the literature to provide general principles of effective evaluation. Much discussion has taken place of the potential value of the randomized controlled trial (RCT) compared with pre-versus-postimplementation analysis (Ruckley et al 1995). Both have a place in the evaluation process. The RCT is clearly superior in evaluating individual treatments but may be less valuable for understanding the process of implementation. Pre-versus-post analysis has been criticized because of the difference in the patient groups included in the analysis, particularly in long-term follow-up, which relies on a historical control group. It has been argued that the treatment group will experience better outcomes than can be explained purely by the implementation process, because of differences in case mix or selection of patients who might benefit most from the new system of care (historical controls). In order to counteract this argument, it is essential to record important patient characteristics so that these may be compared before and after the introduction of the new service. Statistical modelling may be used to adjust for such differences, although this is a complex process that would normally require the services of a statistician (Franks & Moffatt 1996). As an example, a number of independent risk factors have been found for complete healing of venous ulceration. These include ulcer duration, ulcer size, mobility and history of deep vein thrombosis (Franks et al 1995a). Implementation projects have shown differences in the risk factor profiles of the pre versus post patient groups and between services. Some of the outcomes from the different services can be explained by the differences in risk factor profiles, although other unknown factors may play

an important role in these outcomes (Franks & Moffatt 1996).

High-quality evaluation requires the collection of consistently high-quality data. It is essential to determine what measures are to be collected and how they will be standardized. As an example of this, we can consider how the classification of aetiology has changed with the introduction of new techniques. Prior to 1990 most assessments of aetiology were based purely on clinical observation of the ulcer and the history of venous disease (Callam et al 1987). With the introduction of Doppler ultrasound it became possible to distinguish with some accuracy the relative contribution of peripheral vascular disease to the ulceration (Cornwall et al 1986, Moffatt et al 1992). With the introduction of photoplethysmography and duplex scanning the presence and distribution of vascular disease has been determined (Adam et al 2003). Alongside improvements in assessment has developed a greater sophistication in the classification of ulceration. From simple categories of venous, mixed and arterial ulceration there are now more complex descriptors of groups, which incorporate other conditions that may be influencing the ulcer aetiology (Nelzen et al 1991b, Moffatt et al 2004).

To allow for comparisons between groups and studies it is essential that information is collected using a common methodology, including ulcer assessment and categorization, and risk factor profile. The development of a minimum data set is an important international challenge that still needs to be addressed. It is also essential that the data are as complete as possible in order that the statistical adjustments mentioned previously can be undertaken.

The time frame for evaluation is often determined by the clinical area and is often very short. Following the Riverside leg ulcer project many services wished to develop similar services based on the same model (Lambourne et al 1996, Thomson et al 1996, Stevens et al 1997, Morrell et al 1998). However, access to funding was frequently time-limited, often to just one year. Thus, time for preimplementation evaluation was very short, frequently too short to evaluate healing rates. The pressure on the health services was to set up a service that would rapidly treat all patients. This meant that comparison of healing rates could not be undertaken,

Table 6.1   Outcome measures used in leg ulcer management

Measure			Comment
Patient	Wound healing	Percentage healed Time to complete healing Reduction in ulcer area	Lack of consensus on most appropriate time to assess healing. Short evaluations may not show effect
	Complications	Infection Wound deterioration	Rarely reported but will have a major influence on patient HRQoL, healing and use of health resources
	Health-related quality of life	Physical ● Pain ● Mobility	Pain is an underreported problem and poorly evaluated. May have a major influence on mobility and social functioning
		Psychological ● Emotional state ● Anxiety ● Depression	Little understanding of how psychological status affects the healing process and how improvements may influence HRQoL and ulcer healing
		Social ● Social isolation ● Role function	Benefits of ulcer healing may not be apparent as changes in social isolation
	Patient satisfaction		Poor development of patient satisfaction tools and their use in leg ulceration
	Patient choice based on informed decisions		Increased political importance but little understanding of how this is used in leg ulcer practice
	Flexible access to care		Related to patient choice. Health services require flexible entry points and clinical pathways between care agencies
Organizational	Integration of leg ulcer services		Services must be able to demonstrate long-term viability
	Care using guidelines of practice		Guidelines require implementation with educational programmes and support in clinical practice
	Rationalization of resources Multidisciplinary deployment		Pragmatic approach to multidisciplinary care
	Integration of services for seamless care		Attention placed on the patient journey between services to provide seamless care
	Appropriate use of educational programmes		Education programmes must reflect current knowledge and skills of professional groups and be relevant and transferable
	Increased knowledge and skills of professionals		
Health Service	Cost-effectiveness	Efficient use of resources Appropriate product usage Lower cost of care	Studies have shown that effective services lead to greater cost-effectiveness, and also a reduction in absolute cost. This is chiefly a consequence of reduced prevalence. The long-term consequence is a healthier population with reduced disability.
	Prevalence reduction	Decreased numbers of patients with ulceration	Little attention is placed on the long-term benefits of systems of care. Deployment of resources must be to those who will benefit from increased intervention

HRQoL, health-related quality of life.

so the key outcome indicator (change in healing rates) could not be determined, limiting the ability of the study to show improved effectiveness (Lambourne et al 1996, Gooch et al 2000).

Evaluation may also require other types of methodology to be used. Qualitative interviews may provide useful information about the patient journey and the multiple methods approach may provide a richer picture of the implementation process. Researchers have struggled to develop appropriate methodologies to evaluate patient satisfaction (Roberts & Tugwell 1987). Few attempts have been made within the leg ulcer literature and there are many complexities that make measures of satisfaction difficult to interpret. Key amongst these is the dependent relationship between patient and professional in a predominantly elderly group unused to expressing opinions on health matters (Bowling 1995).

One of the major challenges that researchers have faced is determining the contribution that leg ulceration makes to the illness burden of patients who may suffer from a number of concurrent conditions influencing their lives (Franks & Moffatt 1998). We are only just beginning to understand the significance of leg ulceration for the psychosocial status of patients because of the predominant focus on clinical parameters alone (Morgan et al 2004). Research has identified a number of social factors that are associated with poor clinical outcomes (Franks et al 1995b). Factors such as low social class, lack of central heating, being male and living alone were all associated with poor healing of venous ulceration. Further work has highlighted the fact that perceived social support is linked to outcome, with those with lowest social support having the poorest outcomes (Moffatt 2001). There is still much work to be undertaken to confirm these results and to try and explain these relationships. The quality of life literature has identified the importance of depression in ulcer healing, yet relatively little is still known about how the patient's psychological status affects healing (Moffatt 2001).

Over the past decade there has been a realization that the development of effective leg ulcers services involves complex change within an organization, and that these initiatives have shown substantial improvement in a wide range of outcomes. At present, we have a limited understanding of the complex interactions that occur within this process. Researchers have attempted to take elements of the organizational approach, believing that these are the key requirements for effective care. The Scottish Leg Ulcer Trial, which randomized health localities to receive either management guidelines alone or guidelines with an educational programme, failed to demonstrate differences in healing rates (Scottish Leg Ulcer Trial Participants 2002). However, no attempt was made to restructure care, nor to evaluate whether the guidelines were used. This illustrates the importance of developing a robust organizational infrastructure for leg ulcer services and a long-term commitment to care provision.

DEVELOPING EDUCATIONAL AND TRAINING PROGRAMMES

Despite the evidence from the Scottish Leg Ulcer Trial, education is seen as an essential component of effective service development. Education programmes must be focused on the key changes required in clinical practice and the knowledge and skill required to complete this transition (Moffatt & Karn 1994). While university-based academic programmes can provide the underpinning knowledge, it is vital that support is available in the clinical setting when these new skills are first applied. Effective education in leg ulcer management requires that practitioners believe that changes in their practice will have tangible benefits for the patients and themselves. It is essential that students are able to learn from their experience in the clinical arena and utilize real life case studies to support their learning process (Ch. 1). The problem-based approach to learning is an example of an educational approach that sets the student in the position of determining what their learning needs are and how they go about achieving these aims. Supported clinical practice is at the heart of the educational approaches in the community clinic programmes through accredited education with clinical nurse specialist support in the clinical environment. In research terms we still do not have evidence as to which types of practitioner can deliver which aspects of care most effectively. In developing education programmes it is important to consider the required competency of the practitioner being trained and how this will be assessed, both academically and in the clinical setting (competency). The educational framework should facilitate the active use of clinical guidelines in guiding clinical decision making (Royal College of Nursing 1998, Scottish Intercollegiate Guidelines Network 1998). Practitioners need to be able to interpret the guidelines in a range of situations from simple to complex and be aware of the limit of their expertise. Educators must be sensitive to the needs of their students and understand where there are difficulties in applying the knowledge to practice.

Ideally education should become a central part of the implementation process and be embedded within the organizational infrastructure (Goble 1994). Education must be seen as a mandatory requirement within leg ulcer services in order that the general level of skill and knowledge is raised and maintained. There are many approaches to delivering education programmes but the key to their success is to consider the ongoing needs of practitioners and their requirement for continual updating and reappraisal of skills. Studies such as the Riverside Community Leg Ulcer Project are examples of initiatives in which formal educational programmes emerged and important partnerships have been developed between universities and clinical services in achieving these aims (Moffatt et al 1992).

With the development of electronic learning many more opportunities exist for students to learn at a distance as well as using interactive web-based facilities that allow for communication with the teacher and also with other students. Given the pressures on time for education, this is a very important development.

In many countries the wound and compression industry plays an important role in educating practitioners in leg ulcer management as well as introducing them to new products. Such initiatives have positive and negative effects. The danger of reliance on industry alone is a potential bias towards specific products produced by the sponsoring company. Reliance on individual wound companies may lead to an unbalanced understanding of the wide range of options available, and companies may be unwilling to properly discuss the negative aspects of their products with clinicians. Not all clinicians are adequately trained in discerning flaws in the arguments presented or in the research that

is being used to support the educational programme. The use of independent clinical experts within the industry training programmes helps to provide a more balanced approach. However, the more inexperienced of these may feel unable to express their reservations about certain products because they are being funded by the sponsoring company. In health-care settings where money is scarce, industry-supported education involving key opinion leaders may be the greatest contribution to wound care education. In health-care settings where contracting with industry is used for the supply of products, an unhealthy alliance may develop that does not develop the critical skills needed for practitioners to understand the evidence basis for practice.

However, there are now healthy partnerships being established between industry and educationalists, including the accreditation through universities of the education provided by these companies. This process allows for a rigorous appraisal of the content, methods of delivery and assessment strategies used. Successful completion of these programmes provides participants with credits towards academic education programmes such as diplomas and degrees, which are valued by the individual practitioners and by the organizations.

In many countries there has been a radical development in the role of wound care and tissue viability specialists. In the UK in the late 1980s few specialists existed. Today, the majority of health-care providers employ a wound care expert. Despite this, there is no mandatory requirement for specialist practitioners to undergo specific educational training to prepare them for this role, unlike the situation in the USA, where for many years the role of the enterostomal therapist (ET) has been well established. In many parts of mainland Europe, no specialist practitioner roles exist. The key attribute of a successful specialist practitioner is their ability to train and empower staff within the organization to provide high-quality care for all patients. There is always the potential danger that specialists will defend their knowledge and skills, thus deskilling the nurses who work under them. The Scottish Leg Ulcer Trial (Scottish Leg Ulcer Trial Participants 2002) suggested that one of the reasons for lack of success was that community nurses treated too few leg ulcer patients in a year to maintain their specialist expertise, and they recommended that patients were treated within clinics run by specialists who had frequent contact with this patient group. Other community-based studies have not experienced this problem, with community nurses treating a much higher proportion of patients within their caseload (Moffatt et al 1992). This underlines the importance of training all staff to an adequate and appropriate level and providing the specialist skills for patients with complex problems.

We consider that education is a vital component of successful change within the establishment of effective leg ulcer services. Organizations must allocate sufficient resources to educate staff if the programme is to produce the improvement in outcomes that have been reported in the literature. No research has been undertaken to identify the best way of educating professionals, and this will be very dependent on the needs of the organization and the practitioners within it.

EXAMPLES OF CARE PROVISION IN DIFFERENT SETTINGS AND HEALTH-CARE STRUCTURES

This section deals with the different approaches to the provision of care for patients suffering from leg ulceration. While this is not an exhaustive list of possible service models, they do illustrate some of the alternative approaches in different health-care systems. We do not advocate any particular model, and research has not been undertaken to demonstrate which is most effective. The success of different models will be dependent on a number of factors, particularly, the health-care structure, funding routes and the role of the interdisciplinary team within the health-care system. As an example of the latter, the roles and responsibilities of different levels of nursing staff and their position and authority within the team varies greatly in different countries. Thus, their contribution as decision-makers will depend on these factors. A list of factors to consider when developing a new service is given in Table 6.2.

Specialist wound care centres

It has been proposed that specialist wound care centres may provide the optimum way forward for wound healing (Gottrup et al 2001). The aim of these centres is to provide standardized wound classification, diagnostics and treatment plans for patients with all types of wound. The centres focus on basic and clinical research, multiprofessional education and quality assurance. As a consequence, they are recognized as national and international centres of excellence. The centres are organized around a hospital service with dedicated inpatient and outpatient services. They are staffed by specialist medical practitioners and specialist nursing teams. In the Danish model, the specialisms include vascular, orthopaedic, gastrointestinal and plastic surgery, together with dermatology, internal medicine and microbiology. The wider multidisciplinary team include podiatrists, physiotherapists, dieticians, occupational therapists and social workers.

The patients attend an initial out-patient visit for assessment and development of a treatment plan (Fig. 6.1). They undergo diagnostic testing, including Doppler scans, angiography and duplex. Patients with minor problems are seen only once, while those with complex problems are seen continuously in the outpatient clinic, with the option of inpatient

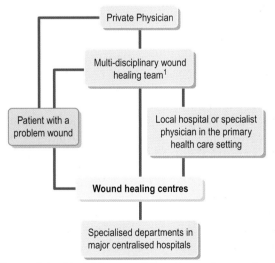

Figure 6.1 Model for organizing of wound care using wound healing centres. * Multidisciplinary team includes one group for each geographical region in the health-care system and consists of specialized educated physicians and nurses from both primary and hospital sectors. (Redrawn from Gottrup et al 2001.)

Table 6.2 Factors to consider when establishing a service.

The size of the problem	Establish the size of the problem in an area. Determine the prevalence, provider of care, place of treatment. The true scale of the problem may not be immediately apparent, with patients being managed in a number of clinical areas
Support and resources	The service will need to be well supported and resourced by management. Managers will need evidence to support proposed improvements in practice. This can come from critical review of the literature or through audit
Multidisciplinary involvement	To ensure that the expertise of all relevant disciplines is available when appropriate to patients
Integration	Integration of acute and community services provides the most effective service for patients
Coordination	A key professional should be responsible for monitoring the service and making sure that new research is implemented into clinical practice
Research-based protocols	The service should deliver care firmly grounded in best practice, as identified from latest research, to all leg ulcer patients
Training	A comprehensive and ongoing training programme will need to be developed that reflects the needs of the practitioner
Accessibility	The service should be flexible in its organization and allow easy access for patients seeking treatment
Transport	A cost-effective reliable transport system will need to be developed if patients are to be brought to clinics
Evaluation	The service will require regular evaluation to ensure that standards are maintained and health outcomes met

care should this be required. Treatments are based on evidence-based algorithms, which include the use of telemedicine for nurses in primary care. The centres act as a focus for education, providing a range from short courses through to multidisciplinary diplomas and masters in wound healing. The Cardiff Wound Healing Institute has a similar structure but also has outreach facilities to the wider hospital and local community, and recently supported the development of community clinics.

The advantages of this model of care include access to specialized teams for the management of patients with complex clinical problems that are proving difficult to manage in routine practice. This model also provides a great opportunity for linking research to practice, and allows for in-depth classification of all wound types and appropriate treatment plans. The ability to admit patients to dedicated inpatient beds is a major advantage in very complex patients. In routine practice these patients are frequently treated in a range of different hospital settings and do not always receive the specialist care they require. The centres benefit from the economy of scale, with large numbers of patients referred. In this environment, specialists can dedicate their time and develop their expertise in problem wounds.

While the centres offer education and training, this can be undertaken in other clinical environments. However, the volume and complexity of the patients in these services provide a rich learning environment that may not be available in routine practice. These centres also have the profile and capacity to attract substantial funding, which allows for a breadth of research ranging from basic science to clinical trials of therapies.

The potential drawbacks of this system include the concentration of resources in one geographical area and the expense of running such a service. It is difficult to know precisely how big an impact these centres make outside their immediate catchment area, although, because of their national profile, this may be considerable. Patients with wounds are frequently immobile, and travelling to a tertiary centre such as this may be problematic, leading to patients with the most difficult wounds remaining in their own homes. For this service to be effective there is a clear need for outreach programmes beyond the local area. There is always the challenge of avoiding the 'ivory tower' syndrome, where ordinary practitioners feel divorced from decisions made in specialist centres. This may be overcome by extensive outreach support and encouragement of practitioners to become engaged in the decision-making process, which draws upon their community expertise. Despite the undoubted success of these centres in caring for complex patients the cost-effectiveness argument still has to be settled.

Community-based leg ulcer services

The epidemiology studies of the 1980s highlighted the fact that over 80% of patients with leg ulceration in the UK were being cared for in the community by the primary health-care team, particularly community (district) nursing staff (Callam et al 1985). The concept of nurse-led community leg ulcer clinics developed from the need to rationalize the care being offered to patients (Moffatt et al 1992). The approach was to provide a locally based leg ulcer service to a geographical population through the development of community clinics based in local health centres throughout the area (Fig. 6.2). Each clinic covered a population of approximately 40 000. The advantage of using health centres was the immediate access to aspects of the wider primary care team such as podiatry and dietetics, and the patients' own general practitioner. The clinics were run by community nurses, who developed a specialty in this field and who were able to treat patients in the clinic and those patients unable to attend clinic in their own home. The clinics were overseen by specialist nurses, who provided a vital link to the acute (hospital) specialties where patients could be referred for investigation and specialist treatment. The link between community and hospital was maintained by the specialist nurses, who worked in both clinical areas and ensured the flow of information between services. Some of the key features were the use of

agreed protocols of care, development of referral criteria and direct nurse referral to hospital specialties. In parallel with these service developments were new innovations in the assessment and management of patients with ulceration, which included use of Doppler ultrasound, pinch skin grafting, sustained compression and a programme to prevent recurrence. This was supported by an educational programme for all relevant staff. The implementation process was multifaceted and followed the procedures and processes outlined earlier in this chapter.

The first service developments using this model were undertaken in the Riverside Community Leg Ulcer Project (Moffatt et al 1992), providing care for 250 000 patients in west London, UK. Over an 18-month period 475 patients with 550 leg ulcers attended the service for treatment. Of these, most (89%) could attend a clinic with transport if required; the remainder were cared for within their own homes using identical assessment and treatment protocols. The overall 12-week healing rate improved from 22% prior to the service implementation to 69% following the development of the new service. Patients who attended at the start of the new service experienced more modest healing (55%), which improved as the clinics developed to 86% at 18 months. This was partly because the patient profile changed, with patients treated in the earlier stages suffering from ulceration of long duration. Those referred later suffered from less chronic ulcers. The changes may have also been the result of improvements in professional practice.

Leg ulceration has a major impact on quality of life. This study was able to show great improvements in the patients' psychiatric morbidity following treatment, the greatest improvement of which was in patients whose ulcers healed completely. At that time, pain was not recognized as a major symptom in venous ulceration. However, this study identified that more than 80% of patients with venous ulceration experienced at least a mild sensation of pain, with 17% experiencing continuous pain from their ulcer (Franks et al 1994). Following treatment 23% experienced pain, with just 1% experiencing continuous pain. These improvements in care were associated with a reduction in the overall cost of the service, with more patients seen (Bosanquet et al 1993). This study became the catalyst for the

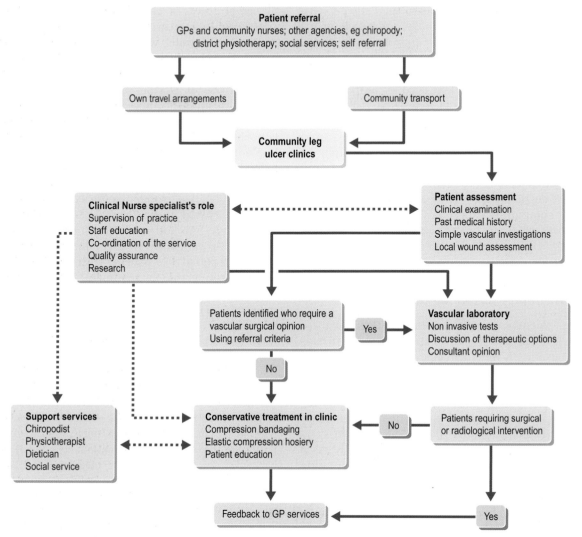

Figure 6.2   The relationship between community leg ulcer clinics and vascular surgical services

development of other similar services, which were developed using a similar framework (Lambourne et al 1996, Thomson et al 1996, Stevens et al 1997, Morrell et al 1998).

The advantages of this model of care include the use of largely existing resources, care of all patients within a geographical area, improvements in professional practice, and access to specialized support through linked services. Particular attention was placed on identifying patients who might experience difficulty in accessing mainstream services. Two groups that were particularly targeted were patients from ethnic minority groups, and the homeless. The disadvantages of this system was the total approach to service change meant that the success of individual components could not be assessed. Also, the model requires a commitment from the acute service in providing support which is not found uniformly. Moreover, changes in the UK health system have made the integration of community and acute services more difficult to achieve due to changes in funding.

Single visit assessment clinic

In the community leg ulcer clinic model, criteria were established for referral for specialist opinion in the acute service (Adam et al 2003). A development of this system is the single visit vascular assessment clinic for all patients provided by the acute service prior to care in the community. Using this model, all patients have access to vascular investigation, with treatment plans based upon the investigations. This model has allowed for greater access to venous surgery and correct diagnosis was achieved in 97% of patients using duplex scanning. Of the 555 patients referred to this acute service, with 689 chronic leg ulcers, venous disease alone was present in 72%, mixed arteriovenous disease in 14.5%, leaving just 15 limbs with pure arterial ulceration. Other non-vascular causes were identified in 50 patients. Overall, superficial venous surgery was performed in 43%. The advantages of this system are access to correct assessment and treatment, the potential for correcting the underlying venous pathology and the potential for influencing the long-term incidence of ulcer recurrence. The disadvantages include the need for a dedicated vascular department alongside the resources required to assess and manage the patients with surgery. We have little evidence about the patients who do not access this service and who remain in the community, or the reasons for this.

OTHER MODELS OF CARE

In this chapter we have outlined some of the current models of care. However, there are alternative approaches to care, which may be useful in certain environments. Most of these other systems revolve around accessing specialist opinion and hospital-based services. The models described so far have shown the greatest benefit in densely populated areas. However, patients in a sparsely populated area may have to travel great distances to access specialist care. A number of approaches have been proposed to overcome this issue, including the use of telemedicine (Dodds 2002).

Telemedicine offers an immediate specialist opinion without the need for patients to travel. In most systems the local practitioner sends a medical history, together with photographs of the wound. While definitive diagnosis may not be possible without specialist investigations and examination, the practitioner does receive guidance on immediate clinical care, and advice on whether specialist intervention is required. Thus, telemedicine acts as a further screening mechanism for referral to specialist centres and as a problem solving facility for practitioners faced with problematic clinical situations. Despite the potential benefits in sparsely populated areas, there has been little evaluation of the potential cost-effectiveness of such systems. Moreover, it is essential that the system offers patient confidentiality through a secure, encrypted system. The equipment costs to establish this service may be high but, once it is in operation, running costs should be relatively low in relation to the volume of patients who benefit from the system.

DISCUSSION

The development of clinical services for patients with leg ulceration has largely developed in an ad hoc manner, with little evaluation of need from a public health perspective. This is not to say that all developments have been inappropriate, just that the evidence supporting them is weak. The reasons for developing these services depend on the emphasis that different professional groups place on aspects of care. As an example, vascular surgeons will focus on surgical interventions while community staff may wish to concentrate on keeping the patient in their own home and providing support to both patients and their families. These foci are not mutually exclusive but should be considered within the context of a multidisciplinary framework that will allow individual practitioners to understand the contribution that other groups make.

To a large extent, services have been developed according to the financial constraints and policy drivers within the health-care system. As an example of this, epidemiological studies in the UK identified that over 80% of patients were cared for by community nursing staff (Callam et al 1985). Any restructuring of care would have to take into consideration the community focus of care delivery in the UK. This was reinforced by changes in the

National Health Service that required greater emphasis on community care of patients and reduction in acute management of all patients. In the USA the health-care structure is more complex because there are multiple agencies working in geographical areas with competition between provider agencies. The care of patients has traditionally been driven by the cost of delivering services to patients rather than the effectiveness of treatment (Ch. 5). This has led in some circumstances to certain products not being made available, as they are perceived to be expensive in terms of unit cost while the potential cost-effectiveness is ignored. There has been little incentive to achieve healing, since payment is dependent on continuing provision of care rather than being outcome-based. Such systems are in danger of suppressing clinical freedom by limiting the availability of products that might be beneficial to patients. Health-care services that rely on medical insurance may lead to two-tier systems, whereby poorer patients with little or no cover are denied best available and newly developed treatments.

The culture of health care is rapidly changing, with an ever-increasing demand for cost efficiency in services that provide for an increasingly elderly population. In many health-care systems there is a much greater requirement for accountability, with more centralized policy control, leading to greater scrutiny of services. It has been suggested that the development and use of clinical guidelines can be seen as an infringement of clinical freedom. However, these guidelines attempt to guide practitioners as to the most clinically effective and cost-effective care. Given the general lack of evidence in leg ulcer management, this remains a major challenge. The current guidelines tend to focus on venous ulceration, for which there is sound clinical evidence on effectiveness (Royal College of Nursing 1998). However, they frequently fail to address the increasing numbers of patients with complex ulceration who fall outside of the recommendations for care.

At present there are no internationally agreed tools for evaluating systems of care for leg ulcer patients. No consensus has been reached on a minimum data set, with different studies using a variety of outcome indicators and different periods of follow up. As an example, early evaluations of treatment focused on the 12-week healing rate (Blair et al 1988a, b), whereas current wisdom is that longer-term follow-up is required in this chronic condition. Also, the benefits of high-cost interventions such as venous surgery are likely to be experienced over a much longer time frame (Adam et al 2003). Similarly, there is a need to evaluate services over a long period. Frequently, implementation projects are undertaken over a short period of time, with little understanding of the benefits that may occur with prolonged evidence-based care. As an example of this, a service providing evidence-based care over an 8-year period experienced a prevalence one-third of that predicted by the epidemiological studies undertaken in the 1980s (Moffatt et al 2004). Continuous monitoring of patient populations also allow us to understand the changing nature of this group, particularly the effect of ageing and changes in the aetiological profile in the population.

Precisely how services should be evaluated is often a matter of debate. The traditional approach to evaluation through randomized clinical trials may appear to be an attractive option. However, there are methodological concerns with this approach, particularly with respect to the complex interactions that occur between trial groups and the difficulty in controlling the many variables that influence the implementation process. An example of this dilemma is found in the Scottish Leg Ulcer Trial. In this trial localities were randomized to receive the Scottish Intercollegiate Guidelines Network (SIGN) leg ulcer guidelines in combination with an educational programme or guidelines alone. Outcomes for this trial were complete healing after 12 weeks of treatment. Baseline healing rates were 30% in both groups, the interventions failing to alter this in either group. The conclusion to this trial was that the educational initiative failed to improve clinical outcomes. This study illustrates how one component of implementation can fail to improve outcome, and reinforces the need for multifaceted implementation, which will lead to real changes in clinical practice through organizational change. This study did not report whether the initiatives influenced professional practice, particularly the adoption of compression therapy.

The alternative to the RCT is the quasi experimental design, where preimplementation services are compared to the postimplementation situation. This design is problematic in its use of historical controls and the difficulty of ensuring comparable populations in both stages of the study. There is evidence in the literature that researchers select patients whom they feel may benefit most from the new interventions.

We believe that there is no correct way of evaluating the development of services. On the one hand the RCT should reduce bias, but on the other it may not provide evidence on how factors influence the successful development of the new service. Both methods may be valuable, and the choice will depend on the precise aims and objectives of the evaluation.

Much of the evaluation so far undertaken has been clinically focused, with little attention to the broader needs of the patients and health services. While there is some evidence of the importance of clinical factors associated with healing, evidence of the impact of social and psychological factors is weak. There is some evidence that poorer healing occurs in those with low perceived social support and those with clinical depression (Franks et al 1994, Moffatt 2001). Other cardiovascular conditions have had much broader evaluations and have highlighted the importance of psychosocial factors in both the development and outcomes of disease (Marmot et al 1984). There may be many factors as yet unknown that influence healing of leg ulceration but lie outside the narrow focus of clinical investigation of risk factors.

There is some evidence that the aetiological profile is changing in leg ulceration, with a higher proportion of patients with complex aetiology and a greater risk of non-healing (Moffatt et al 2004). It is important that mechanisms are developed to evaluate treatment success in these non-healers. There is likely to be a greater emphasis on symptom control and disease management in the future, for which other forms of outcome measurement must be used. Quality of life assessments have already demonstrated that they can be an important outcome measure but have also shown that some groups of patients suffer to a greater extent while others show greater improvements with appropriate care. The challenge will be to understand why these differences occur and how treatment can be focused on these target groups. The area of poorest

evaluation has been in the determination of the relative cost-effectiveness of different models of care. It is essential that models are clinically effective but also fall within the potential financial constraints of the health service. We believe that this will be one of the greatest challenges of the next decade.

This chapter has highlighted the fact that we still have scant research evidence on how new services are best implemented. Health provision is by its nature a dynamic process, adapting to changes in its environment and new demands placed upon it. In this ever-changing climate continuous evaluation may prove difficult. We recognize the importance to a service of a sustainable infrastructure and organizational support. Frequently, services rely on a small group of enthusiastic individuals, with the wider organization failing to take ownership of the service. Embedding the service within the organization is a major goal of successful implementation.

The evidence around the care of patients with chronic leg ulceration has come from highly developed health-care systems in north America, Europe and Australia. The need for services outside these areas has yet to be established. It is unlikely that services designed for the developed world will be appropriate and affordable in the developing world. The health service priorities are likely to be very different, with emphasis still on major causes of mortality, such as infectious disease, and chronic, non-life-threatening conditions low on the health agenda. Wound care products developed for a Western health-care system are frequently not designed for reuse and would be too expensive for use in developing countries. Attempts to tackle leg ulcer care in these countries may require a focus on improving general health and standards of hygiene and involving the patients and families in the care of their wounds.

In conclusion, the development of leg ulcer services is a complex process that relies on many factors, not least the health service culture and the health priorities set within it. There is no one model that will be appropriate for all situations. The evidence to date supports the belief that effective leg ulcer services have a major impact on the health and quality of life of patients and provide benefits for the professionals and organizations delivering care.

References

Adam D J, Naik J, Hartshorne T et al 2003 The diagnosis and management of 689 chronic leg ulcers in a single-visit assessment clinic. European Journal of Vascular and Endovascular Surgery 25:462–468

Andersson E, Hansson C, Swanbeck G 1993 Leg and foot ulcer prevalence and investigation of the peripheral arterial and venous circulation in a randomised elderly population. Acta Dermato-Venereologica (Stockholm) 73: 57–61

Argyris A 1990 Organisational defensive routines: facilitating organizational learning. Addison Wesley, Oxford

Baker S R, Stacey M C, Jopp-McKay A G et al 1991 Epidemiology of chronic venous ulcers. British Journal of Surgery 78: 864–867

Bero L A, Grilli R, Grimshaw J M et al 1998 Closing the gap between research and practice: an overview of systematic reviews of interventions to promote the implementation of research findings. British Medical Journal 317: 465–468

Blair S D, Wright D D I, Backhouse C M et al 1988a Sustained compression and healing of chronic venous ulcers. British Medical Journal 297: 1159–1161

Blair S D, Backhouse C M, Wright D D I et al 1988b Do dressings influence the healing of chronic venous ulcers? Phlebology 3: 129–134

Bosanquet N 1992 Cost of venous ulcers: from maintenance therapy to investment programmes. Phlebology (Suppl 1): 44–46

Bosanquet N, Franks P, Moffatt C et al 1993 Community leg ulcer clinics: cost effectiveness. Health Trends 25: 146–148

Bowling A 1995 Measuring disease. Open University Press, Buckingham

Browse N L, Burnand K G, Lea Thomas M 1988 Diseases of the veins: pathology, diagnosis and treatment. Edward Arnold, London

Callam M J, Ruckley C V, Harper D R, Dale J J 1985 Chronic ulceration of the leg: extent of the problem and provision of care. British Medical Journal 290: 1855–1856

Callam M J, Harper D R, Dale J J, Ruckley C V 1987 Chronic ulcer of the leg: clinical history. British Medical Journal 294; 1389–1391

Callam M J, Harper D R, Dale J J, Ruckley C V 1988 Chronic leg ulceration: socio-economic aspects. Scottish Medical Journal 33: 358–360

Chambers R 2000 Involving patients and the public. How to do it better. Radcliffe primary care. Radcliffe Medical Press, Oxford

Cornwall J V, Dore C J, Lewis J D 1986 Leg ulcers: epidemiology and aetiology. British Journal of Surgery 73: 693–696

Covey S R 1989 The seven habits of highly effective people. Restoring the character ethic. Simon & Schuster, London

Cullum N, Roe B (eds) 1995 Leg ulcers: nursing management. A research based guide. Scutari Press, London

Dobson R 2000 NICE to reconsider evidence on interferon beta. British Medical Journal 321: 1244

Dodds S R 2002 Shared community-hospital care of leg ulcers using an electronic record and telemedicine. International Journal of Lower Extremity Wounds 1: 260–270

European Foundation for Quality Management 2003 The EFQM Excellence Model. European Foundation for Quality Management, Brussels

Evans D, Haines A (eds) 2000 Implementing evidence based changes in healthcare. Radcliffe Medical Press, Oxford

Flanagan M, Rotchell L, Fletcher J, Schofield J 2001 Community nurses', home carers' and patients' perceptions of factors affecting venous leg ulcer recurrence and management of services. Journal of Nursing Management 9:153–159

Franks P J, Moffatt C J 1996 Leg ulcer healing rates: multivariate models to adjust for risk factors for healing (abstract). British Journal of Dermatology 136: 286

Franks P J, Moffatt C J 1998 Who suffers most from leg ulceration? Journal of Wound Care 7: 383–385

Franks P J, Posnett J 2003 Cost effectiveness of compression therapy. In: Understanding compression therapy. EWMA Position Document. Medical Education Partnership, London

Franks P J, Moffatt C J, Oldroyd M et al 1994 Community leg ulcer clinics: effect on quality of life. Phlebology 9: 83–86

Franks P J, Moffatt C J, Connolly M et al 1995a Factors associated with healing leg ulceration with high compression. Age and Ageing 24: 407–410

Franks P J, Bosanquet N, Connolly M et al 1995b Venous ulcer healing: effect of socio-economic factors in London. Journal of Epidemiology and Community Health 49: 385–388

Franks P J, Morton N, Campbell A, Moffatt C J 1997 Leg ulceration and ethnicity. A study in west London. Public Health 111: 327–329

Franks P J, Doherty D C, Moffatt C J 2002 Are socio-demographic factors important in the development of chronic leg ulceration? Ostomy/Wound Management 48: 73–74

Georgiades N, Macdonell R 1998 Leadership for competitive advantage. John Wiley, Chichester

Goble R 1994 Multi-professional education in Europe: overview. In: Leathard A (ed.) Going inter-professional. Routledge, London

Gooch S, Hopkis A, Scott F 2000 Leg ulcer care in east London. In: Evans D, Haines A (eds) Implementing evidence based changes in healthcare. Radcliffe Medical Press, Oxford

Gottrup F, Holstein P, Jorgensen B et al 2001 A new concept of a multi-disciplinary wound healing center and a national expert function of wound healing. Archives of Surgery 136: 765–772

Graham I D, Harrison M B, Moffatt C J, Franks P J 2001 Leg ulcer care: nursing attitudes and knowledge. Canadian Nurse 97(3): 19–24

Handy C 1993 Understanding organizations. Penguin, Harmondsworth

Hinshelwood R D 1987 What happens in groups. Psychoanalysis, the individual and the community. Free Association Books, London

Korn P, Patel S T, Heller J A et al 2002 Why insurers should reimburse for compression stockings in patients with chronic venous statis ulcers. Journal of Vascular Surgery 35: 950–957

Kouzes J M, Posner B Z 1998 Encouraging the heart: a leader's guide to rewarding and recognizing others. Jossey-Bass, San Francisco, CA

Kouzes J M, Posner B Z 2002 The leadership challenge, 3rd edn. Jossey-Bass, San Francisco, CA

Lambourne L A, Moffatt C J, Jones A C et al 1996 Clinical audit and effective change in leg ulcer services. Journal of Wound Care 5: 348–351

Last J M (ed.) 1995 A dictionary of epidemiology, 3rd edn. Oxford University Press, New York

Leathard A 1994 Going inter-professional. Working together for health and welfare. Routledge, London

Lees T A, Lambert D 1992 Prevalence of lower limb ulceration in an urban health district. British Journal of Surgery 79: 1032–1034

Lewin K 1951 Field theory and learning. In : Cartwright D (ed.) Field theory in social science: select theoretical papers. Harper Collins, New York

McIvor S 1991 Obtaining the views of the users of the Health Service. King's Fund Centre for Health Service Development, London

Marmot M G, Shipley M J, Rose G 1984 Inequalities in death. Specific explanations of a general pattern. Lancet 1: 1003–1006

Menzies Lyth I 1989 The dynamics of the social. In: Selected essays, Vol II. Free Association Books, London

Moffatt C J 2001 A study to investigate the relative contribution of clinical and psychosocial factors in the healing of patients with leg ulceration. PhD Thesis, University of London

Moffatt C J 2003 Understanding compression therapy. In: Understanding compression therapy. EWMA Position Document. Medical Education Partnership, London

Moffatt C J, Franks P J 2004 Implementation of leg ulcer services. British Journal of Dermatology (In press)

Moffatt C J, Karn E A 1994 Answering the call for more education: development of an ENB course in leg ulcer management. Professional Nurse 9: 708–712

Moffatt C J, Franks P J, Oldroyd M et al 1992 Community leg ulcer clinics and impact on ulcer healing. British Medical Journal 305: 1389–1392

Moffatt C J, McCullagh L, O'Connor T et al 2003 Randomized trial of four layer and two-layer bandage systems in the management of chronic venous ulceration. Wound Repair and Regeneration 11: 166–171

Moffatt C J, Franks P J, Doherty DC et al 2004 Prevalence of leg ulceration in a London population. Quarterly Journal of Medicine 97: 431–437

Morgan P A, Franks P J, Moffatt C J et al 2004 Illness behavior and social support in patients with chronic venous ulcers. Ostomy/Wound Management 50: 25–32

Morrell C J, Walters S J, Dixon S et al 1998 Cost effectiveness of community leg ulcer clinics: randomised controlled trial. British Medical Journal 316: 1487–1491

Nelzen O, Bergqvist D, Lindhagen A, Hallbook D 1991a Chronic leg ulcers – an underestimated problem in primary health care among elderly patients. Journal of Epidemiology and Community Health 45: 184–187

Nelzen O, Bergqvist D, Lindhagen A 1991b Leg ulcer etiology – a cross sectional population study. Journal of Vascular Surgery 14: 557–564

Roberts J G, Tugwell P 1987 Comparison of questionnaires determining patient satisfaction with medical care. Health Services Research 22: 637–654

Royal College of Nursing 1998 Clinical Practice Guidelines. The management of patients with venous leg ulcers. Royal College of Nursing, London

Ruckley C V, Bale S, Fletcher A 1995 Review of classic research: community clinics for leg ulcers. Journal of Wound Care 4(10):470–472

Scottish Intercollegiate Guidelines Network 1998 The care of patients with chronic leg ulcer (SIGN Publication 26). Scottish Intercollegiate Guidelines Network, Edinburgh

Scottish Leg Ulcer Trial Participants 2002 Effect of a national community intervention programme on healing rates of chronic leg ulcer: a randomised trial. Phlebology 17: 47–53

Senge P M 1990 The fifth discipline. The art and practice of the learning organization. Random House, London

Simon D A, Freak L, Kinsella A et al 1996 Community leg ulcer clinics: a comparative study in two health authorities. British Medical Journal 312: 1648–1651

Stevens J, Harrington M, Franks P J 1997 Audit: a community/hospital leg ulcer service. Journal of Wound Care 6: 62–68

Thomas A 1996 Assessing need. In: Bryar R, Bytheway B (eds) Changing primary health care. Blackwell Science, Oxford

Thomson B, Hooper P, Powell R, Warin A P 1996 Four-layer bandaging and healing rates of venous leg ulcers. Journal of Wound Care 5: 213–216

Vowden K R, Barker A, Vowden P 1997 Leg ulcer management in a nurse-led, hospital-based clinic. Journal of Wound Care 6: 233–236

CHAPTER 7

A framework for patient assessment and care planning

Moya J. Morison, Christine J. Moffatt

INTRODUCTION

Leg ulcers are commonly encountered among patients in both hospital and community settings and can easily develop into chronic lesions of the skin and underlying tissues with inappropriate care. Complications are especially common among patients who are elderly, malnourished, immune-compromised and immobile. It is an accepted principle that the findings from an ongoing process of assessment should form the basis for rational decision-making and care planning. However, there is no universal agreement about the parameters that should be routinely measured and it is all too easy for the assessment process to focus on the wound itself, to the detriment of wider issues such as environmental and social factors that may have a significant impact on the healing process and on the patient's concordance with prescribed treatments.

This chapter aims to provide a clinically useful framework for patient assessment and care planning applicable to patients with leg ulcers and a wide variety of other chronic and acute wounds. It reflects the multidimensional aspects of caring for such patients. The commonalities between the framework presented and a number of other models are discussed.

ASSESSING PATIENTS WITH MULTIPLE HEALTH-CARE NEEDS

It has been estimated that the number of people in the population over the age of 80 years is likely to quadruple in the UK over the next 50 years. Similar trends are being seen in many other developed countries. As people live longer the number of patients presenting with multiple concurrent health-care needs is likely to increase. An example of such a case is that of a frail elderly lady admitted to hospital from a care home for the assessment of her leg ulcers, described below (Case study 1). The case highlights the complex nature of many medical problems where patients (and sometimes other care workers) can present confusing, contradictory and inaccurate information and problems can be compounded by the interaction between a number of concurrent medical conditions. Prioritizing the patients' presenting problems requires sound clinical judgement, and the care of the wound or wounds is clearly only part of a much bigger picture.

Case Study I   An 80-year-old lady with leg ulcers

Mrs Betty Brown is 80 years old and has just been admitted to hospital from the local care home for the assessment of her leg ulcers (Fig. 7.1). On arrival she is found to be doubly incontinent. She has a past medical history of anaemia and chronic obstructive airways disease. She is confused and is unable to give a clear history.

The notes accompanying her are brief and contain some contradictions. According to these

Case Study 1   *An 80-year-old lady with leg ulcers, cont'd*

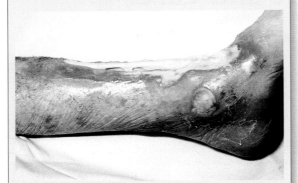

Figure 7.1   An 80-year-old lady with extensive leg ulceration

notes four-layer compression bandage therapy was commenced 3 months earlier in an attempt to heal the leg ulcers. However, the ulcers have become more extensive and sloughy. Betty says that she is very distressed by the intense pain that she experiences on dressing changes. The notes record that she is given paracetamol 500 mg 10 minutes beforehand but that this appears to be having little effect in alleviating her suffering.

On initial assessment Betty is found to have several other ulcers, including a sloughy stage 3 sacral pressure ulcer and superficial stage 2 pressure ulcers on both her elbows. Her skin is extremely dry and fragile. The accompanying notes from the care home state that she has had a poor appetite recently. She is 5 ft 6 in (1.68 m) tall and weighs 8 stone (51 kg).

Her closest relative is a daughter, aged 55, who lives 30 miles away, but she stopped visiting 6 months ago, saying that her mother is abusive and completely uninterested in her wider family. The care home give a different story, saying how distressed the old lady is that she never sees her grandchildren. Betty confides in the nurse who is admitting her that she feels that she has little left to live for. She is apathetic and has ceased to take any interest in her appearance and personal hygiene.

A MODEL TO FACILITATE PATIENT ASSESSMENT AND CARE PLANNING

The basic principles of caring for a patient with a wound have been known for several centuries. The 16th century French surgeon Ambroise Paré stressed the importance of removing the cause of the wound, local wound debridement, the application of a dressing, developing a sound nutritional plan, treating any underlying disease and psychological support. These principles still apply today.

A conceptual framework to aid with patient assessment and care planning is illustrated in Figure 7.2. This model is in two parts. The first section (questions 1–5) stresses the importance of removing the immediate cause of the wound, treating any underlying pathology and more general causes of delayed healing, optimizing the local wound environment and preventing further tissue breakdown. The second section (questions 6–10) encourages the clinician to look at the patient more holistically and to consider: the consequences of the wound for the individual's quality of life; the patient's beliefs about the wound and their perception of the likelihood of a successful outcome to treatment; psychosocial issues that may affect patient concordance with treatment; the patient's need for long-term rehabilitation; and the optimum setting for care. These dimensions are clearly interconnected. Focusing on the wound to the detriment of the whole person is likely to be counterproductive, especially in the longer term, when the responsibility for rehabilitation and health promotion is likely to shift increasingly to the patient and their carers.

Conceptual frameworks and models represent simplifications of reality, rather than being comprehensive representations of it (Hunink 1995). Key concepts are linked schematically, as in Figure 7.2, to indicate tentative or proven relationships. In general, conceptual frameworks cannot be tested as fully as theories, because they are a broader abstraction of reality, but they can be very useful in highlighting what is important, indicating clinical priorities and giving direction and guidance in practical situations. Over the years a number of frameworks and assessment tools have been developed in relation to wound care. They reflect the values, beliefs and perspectives of their authors.

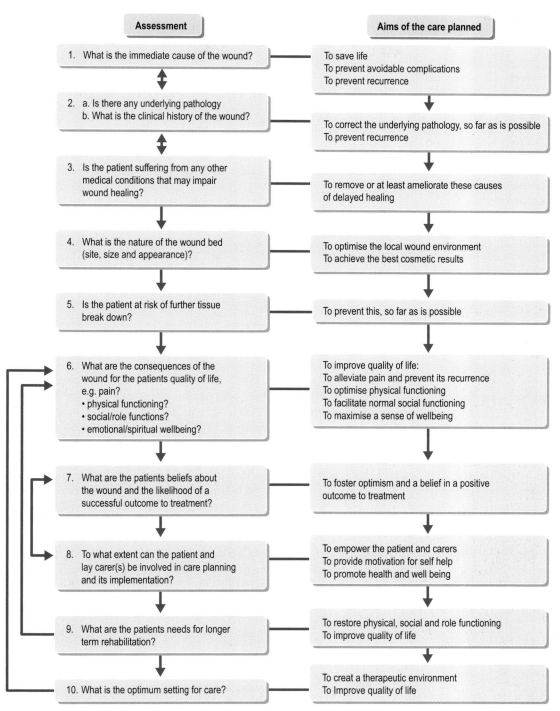

Figure 7.2 A model to facilitate patient assessment and care planning for patients with chronic and acute wounds

Table 7.1 Domains included in some frameworks and models for patient assessment and care planning in the context of wound care

	Figure 7.2	Davis et al 1992	Taylor et al 1999	Sibbald et al 2003	Keast et al 2004
1. Immediate *cause* of wound	✔	✔		✔	[✔]*
2. Underlying *pathology* and *clinical history*	✔	✔	✔	✔	[✔]*
3. *Other medical conditions* that may impair healing	✔	✔	✔	✔	[✔]*
4. The nature of the *wound bed*	✔	✔	✔	✔	✔
5. Risk of *further tissue breakdown*	✔				
6. One or more dimensions of *quality of life*, e.g. pain	✔		✔	✔	✔
7. Patient's *beliefs* about the wound and the likelihood of a successful outcome to treatment	✔				
8. Patient/carer *education* and *involvement* in care planning	✔	✔			
9. *Rehabilitation* needs in longer term	✔	[✔]			
10. Optimum *setting* for care	✔	✔†			

*Adopts model of Sibbald et al (2000, 2003), included for these more 'global' issues.
† The organization and availability of care.

Some are generic, being applicable to a number of wound types, such as: the Wound Organizer (Davis et al 1992) and others are more focused, relating to a specific wound type, such as the Pressure Sore Status Tool (Bates-Jensen et al 1992, 1997), which focuses on the location of the wound and local conditions at the wound site. Dealey (1999) used the Activities of Living model of nursing as a framework for assessing patients with wounds, and stressed the importance of psychological and spiritual as well as physical aspects of care.

At a meeting in June 2002 an expert working group summarized the clinical components of wound bed preparation, along with the underlying cellular environment at each stage (Schultz et al 2003). They designed a model to illustrate the link between clinical observations and underlying cellular abnormalities, linking clinical interventions with their effects at a cellular level (Schultz et al 2003). This model is proving to be highly influential in practice and a number of very useful publications have followed that explore the clinical relevance of the model (Falanga & Harding 2002, Edmonds et al 2004, Falanga 2004, Moffatt et al

2004). Included in the original paper on wound bed preparation that appeared in Schultz et al (2003) is a more wide-ranging model that takes account of the overall health status of the patient and how this may impinge on the wound healing process (Sibbald et al 2000, 2003). It acknowledges the importance of treating the cause of the wound and taking cognisance of patient-centred concerns such as pain and other dimensions of quality of life.

The frameworks summarized in Table 7.1 have a great deal in common but differ in the domains that are made explicit. Frameworks can, perhaps, best be judged by their clinical usefulness in particular situations and can be helpful both as aide memoires and as teaching aids. The sections that follow look at the components of the framework illustrated in Figure 7.2 and draw out some general principles.

What is the immediate cause of the wound?

The immediate cause of a wound may be avoidable or unavoidable, and it may be highly significant and important in itself or it may be relatively trivial.

What is important is that the immediate cause of a wound is sought and, where possible rectified, so that the wound is prevented from recurring. A good example is a diabetic foot ulcer, which may be triggered by ill-fitting footwear. As discussed in Chapter 18, the consequences of wound infection for the diabetic patient can be devastating, perhaps necessitating amputation. Checking a diabetic person's footwear and encouraging the individual and their carers to inspect their feet every day for signs of even the most minor trauma can help to prevent recurrence.

Is there any underlying pathology and what is the clinical history of the wound?

A number of pathological conditions are associated with ulceration in the lower limb (Box 7.1). While infection and blood disorders are uncommon causes of ulceration in the northern hemisphere they are much more common causes of ulceration in tropical countries, as described in Chapter 21.

Identifying the underlying pathology of a leg ulcer is of paramount importance to planning appropriate care. The underlying pathology may be complex and differential diagnosis is imperative, as inappropriate care could precipitate the need for amputation (e.g. if a high level of compression is applied to an ischaemic limb) or could allow an infection to take hold. Assessment of the patient's clinical signs and symptoms and past medical history is an important first step, as described below. Details of further clinical and laboratory investigative techniques are given in the relevant specialist chapters.

Clinical signs and symptoms of venous and arterial ulcers

Clinical signs and symptoms of venous and arterial disorders are summarized in Boxes 7.2 and 7.3. Interpretation of the symptoms of vascular disease requires considerable clinical experience. Problems causing pain with walking, such as arthritis, must be differentiated from arterial insufficiency with associated intermittent claudication. While intermittent claudication most commonly occurs as pain in the calf, high vascular obstruction can cause pain in the buttocks and thighs. Rest pain usually indicates significant arterial stenosis or occlusion.

Box 7.1 *Some causes of leg ulcers*

1. **Principal causes in the developed world**
   - Chronic venous hypertension, usually associated with incompetent valves in the deep and perforating veins
   - Arterial disease, e.g. atherosclerotic occlusion of large vessels leading to tissue ischaemia
   - Combined chronic venous hypertension and arterial disease

2. **More unusual causes in the developed world**
   - Neuropathy, e.g. associated with diabetes mellitus, spina bifida, leprosy
   - Vasculitis, e.g. associated with rheumatoid arthritis, polyarteritis nodosa
   - Malignancy, e.g. squamous cell carcinoma, melanoma, basal cell carcinoma, Kaposi's sarcoma
   - Blood disorders, e.g. sickle-cell disease
   - Infection, e.g. fungal infections, tuberculosis, syphilis, leprosy
   - Metabolic disorders, e.g. pyoderma gangrenosum, pretibial myxoedema
   - Lymphoedema
   - Iatrogenic, e.g. over-tight bandaging, ill-fitting plaster cast.

It decreases with dependency of the lower limb and is made worse by heat, elevation and exercise. The signs and symptoms of acute arterial occlusion are given in Box 7.4. Irreversible damage to skeletal muscle and peripheral nerves occurs rapidly in the absence of adequate collateral circulation. For the diabetic patient peripheral neuropathy is the most common cause of ulceration and is often accompanied by ischaemia. The signs and symptoms of diabetic neuropathy are described in Chapter 18. It is important to note that there are other causes of peripheral neuropathy, including collagen disorders, pernicious anaemia and malignancy affecting the spinal cord. The importance of specialist

Box 7.2   Clinical signs and symptoms of venous problems

- Prominent superficial leg veins or symptoms of varicose veins, such as:
  - Aching or heaviness in the legs, generalized or localized
  - Mild ankle swelling
  - Itching over varices
  - Symptoms caused by thrombophlebitis, such as localized pain, tenderness and redness

- Ankle flare – distension of the tiny veins on the medial aspect of the foot below the malleolus

- Pathological changes to the skin and tissues surrounding the ulcer, including:
  - Pigmentation/staining of the skin around the ulcer
  - Lipodermatosclerosis – hardening of the dermis and underlying subcutaneous fat, which may feel woody
  - Stasis eczema
  - Atrophie blanche – ivory white skin stippled with red dots of dilated capillary loops

Box 7.3   Clinical signs and symptoms of arterial problems

1. **Symptoms**
   - Intermittent claudication
   - Ischaemic rest pain

2. **Signs (many are suggestive of but not specific to ischaemia)**
   - Coldness of the foot
   - Poor tissue perfusion – foot/toes dusky pink when dependent, turning pale when raised above the heart
   - Atrophic, shiny skin
   - Loss of hair on the leg
   - Muscle wasting in calf or thigh
   - Trophic changes in nails
   - Gangrene of toes
   - Loss of pedal pulses

Box 7.4   Clinical signs and symptoms of acute arterial occlusion in the lower limb

- Pain of sudden onset and severe intensity

- Pallor

- Paraesthesia (numbness)

- Pulselessness (absence of pulses below the occlusion)

- Paralysis (sudden weakness in the limb)

- Polar (a cold extremity)

vascular assessment for patients thought to have a significant degree of peripheral arterial disease and for patients with diabetes mellitus cannot be overemphasized. The reader is referred to Chapters 16 and 18 respectively.

For ulcers that prove unresponsive to treatment or have an atypical appearance a more uncommon cause should be considered. The signs and symptoms of ulcers due to malignancy are described in Chapter 19. Ulcers associated with inflammatory disorders are described in Chapter 20. A wide variety of tropical ulcers are described in Chapter 21. Ulcers associated with haematological disorders are discussed in Chapter 22.

The clinical history can also give important clues as to the underlying pathology, as described below.

Clinical history: some indicators of possible venous or arterial involvement

The patient's clinical history can give very important clues in relation to the wound's underlying pathology. Indicators of possible venous and/or arterial problems are summarized in Box 7.5, by way of example.

The patient's clinical history can also indicate the likelihood of delayed healing in some cases.

Box 7.5 *Clinical history – some indicators of possible venous or arterial involvement*

Indicators of possible venous involvement
- Previous thrombogenic events: has the patient ever suffered from one or more of the following:
  - Deep vein thrombosis?
  - Thrombophlebitis?
  - Leg or foot fracture in the affected limb?
- Varicose veins
  - Does the patient have prominent superficial leg veins with signs of valve incompetence?
  - Has the patient ever had any varicose vein surgery or sclerotherapy in the affected leg?

Indicators of possible arterial involvement
- Generalized arterial disease
- Are there any indicators of arterial disease, such as:
  - Previous myocardial infarction?
  - Angina?
  - Transient ischaemic attacks?
  - Intermittent claudication?
  - Cerebrovascular accident?

Margolis et al (1999) found that the failure of venous leg ulcers to heal within 24 weeks was significantly associated with the duration of the wound, a history of venous ligation or stripping and a history of hip or knee replacement surgery, as well as with larger wound area, an ankle brachial pressure index of less than 0.8 and the presence of fibrin on more than 50% of the wound's surface.

The parameters incorporated into the assessment forms of the Scottish Intercollegiate Guidelines Network (SIGN Guidelines 1998) and a computerized database developed and evaluated in Salford (Taylor et al 1999) for the assessment of patients with leg ulcers are summarized in Table 7.2. These include many aspects of the patient's clinical history, described above, and the findings from clinical examination and assessment, described elsewhere. Taylor et al (1999), and Taylor (2002) describe the benefits of their computerized database, which include the generation of reports for research and clinical audit.

Is the patient suffering from any other medical conditions that may impair healing?

Wound healing is likely to be impaired by a number of medical conditions such as diabetes mellitus, circulatory and respiratory disorders. Those factors amenable to correction need to be addressed as part of a comprehensive care plan. An example of a factor that can be highly amenable to improvement is malnutrition. This is a commonly encountered problem, both for hospitalized patients and for debilitated patients living at home. It can lead to delayed wound healing of both acute and chronic wounds (Gray & Cooper 2001, McLaren 2004) yet nutritional assessment and support are often overlooked (Williams 2002, McIlwaine 2003). Optimizing the patient's nutritional status is an important goal of care planning, as described in Chapter 28.

Wound healing in the elderly is qualitatively different from wound healing in a young and fit adult. With increasing age the barrier functions of the skin are altered, there is reduced sensory perception and the individual is increasingly susceptible to trauma. These factors need to be given particular attention, in relation both to skin care and leg ulcer prevention. Elderly patients are also more likely to be suffering from a number of other concurrent medical problems, including cardiovascular and respiratory disease. It is the variety of factors that can lead to delayed healing that makes patient assessment and care planning so challenging (Fig. 7.3).

What is the nature of the wound bed?

Accurate and ongoing assessment of the wound site and of the surrounding skin is essential to planning the most appropriate local wound management and evaluating its effectiveness. Clear and accurate documentation of the findings is essential to ensure that any abnormal changes are picked up quickly and appropriate therapeutic action is taken, as well as ensuring continuity of care. It is also important to be able to recognize when healing is

Table 7.2 Examples of parameters included in the assessment records of patients with leg ulcers

	SIGN Guidelines 1998	Taylor et al 1999
Demographic details	✔	✔
Social circumstances	✔	✔
Current support by health-care professionals	✔	
History of the ulcer	✔	✔
● Length of history	✔	✔
● Duration of current ulcer	✔	✔
Patient history/other diseases/conditions		
● Smoking		✔
● Diabetes	✔	✔
● Rheumatoid arthritis	✔	✔
● Osteoarthritis	✔	
● Claudication	✔	
● Ischaemic heart disease	✔	
● Peripheral vascular disease		✔
● Cerebrovascular accident	✔	
● Previous deep vein thrombosis	✔	✔
● Previous leg fracture	✔	✔
● Previous surgery	✔	
● Treatment of varicose veins		✔
● Obesity		✔
● Pregnancy		✔
Clinical examination/assessments		
● Mobility	✔	✔
● Height/weight/body mass index		✔
● Circumference of ankle and calf	✔	
● Ankle brachial pressure index (ABPI)	✔	✔
● Palpable pulses		✔
● Ankle movement	✔	
● Ulcer position	✔	✔
● Ulcer area	✔	✔
● Oedema	✔	✔
● Cellulitis	✔	
● Dermatitis	✔	
● Condition of surrounding skin		✔
● Slough	✔	✔
● Condition of wound (necrotic, sloughy, infected, granulating, epithelializing)		✔
● Note whether wound swab taken		✔
● Odour	✔	
● Depth	✔	
● Level of pain experienced	✔	✔
● Abnormalities on urinalysis		✔
● Note whether biopsy performed		✔
Investigation of glucose	✔	
Current medication and any allergies	✔	

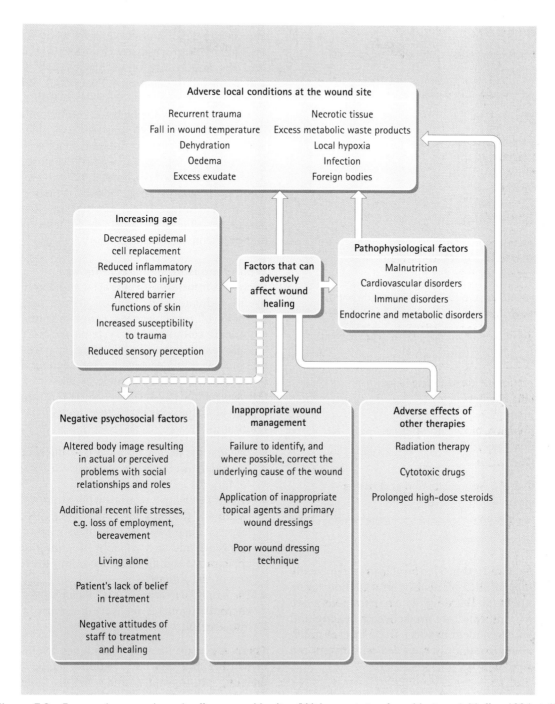

Figure 7.3 Factors that can adversely affect wound healing (With permission from Morison & Moffatt 1994, p. 49)

Box 7.6   Some commonly recorded parameters relating to the wound itself

- Site/position relative to other anatomical structures

- Length, width and surface area

- Depth

- Nature of the wound bed:
  - ◆ Necrotic
  - ◆ Sloughy
  - ◆ Infected
  - ◆ Granulating
  - ◆ Epithelializing

- Exudate type (e.g. serous/serosanguinous/purulent) and estimated volume

- Edges, distinct/indistinct, thickened/rolled under/hyperkeratotic

- Undermining of margins/sinus tract formation

- Odour

- Condition of surrounding skin:
  - ◆ Inflammation
  - ◆ Induration
  - ◆ Oedema, pitting/non-pitting
  - ◆ Dry/flaky
  - ◆ Dermatitis

- Pain at the wound site and at dressing changes

intended to be an aid to the accurate and ongoing recording of the most important parameters. Sterling (1996) found that relevant parameters were documented more frequently when a wound assessment chart was used. Griffith (2004) emphasizes the importance of accurate record keeping and its legal implications. Spencer & Widdows (2000) have shown that where the records are held by the patient this facilitates communication and seamless care for patients with diabetic ulcers, who are being seen by many different health-care professionals. McMath & Harvey (2004) suggest that patient-held records promote patient empowerment by providing a method by which patients and professionals share information. Just what parameters should be routinely recorded is still a matter of considerable debate.

Wound measurement techniques

Decreases in wound surface area and depth can be useful indicators of healing. There are many methods of measurement ranging from highly technical, computerized systems to more basic techniques. However, as you may have discovered for yourself, many problems arise when attempting to measure wounds accurately, by whatever means (Melhuish et al 1994, Oien et al 2002, Samad et al 2002, Flanagan 2003). These include problems relating to:

- *Defining the wound's boundary* – this is observer dependent and so is prone to inaccuracy (Kantor & Margolis 1998)
- *Wound flexibility* – wounds where there is undermining of the skin edge or where the wound is large or deep can be difficult to measure with precision and are capable of changing their appearance significantly according to the position of the patient
- *The natural curvature of the human body* – not all currently available measuring devices take this into account.

There are a number of techniques available for measuring the area of a wound. These include tracing, photography and various computer-assisted means (Lagan et al 2000, Manios et al 2003). One of the simplest, least expensive and clinically most popular methods of assessing the area of a wound is to trace the outline of the wound

progressing well – that is, to be able to recognize the clinical appearance of healthy granulation tissue and epithelium. Deciding which parameters are clinically significant, are predictive of healing and may require treatment has been the subject of much debate. Some commonly recorded parameters are summarized in Box 7.6.

Charting wound healing

There are a number of published wound assessment charts, which vary in the extent to which they have been evaluated and validated. They are

margin on to a clear plastic sheet using an indelible-ink marker. Commercially available plastic measuring tools are available. Tracings can be transferred to the patient's notes and annotated to include the nature of the wound bed, the extent of under-mining of the surrounding skin and the position of the wound relative to other structures. The calculation of wound area can be undertaken using a computer linked to a camera or hand-held scanner. This is a faster and more accurate method than attempting to count centimetre squares on a grid, as these may be incomplete where the grid straddles both the wound and intact tissue. Samad et al (2002) concluded that the measurement of leg ulcer area using computer-aided tracing of digital camera images is more accurate and quicker than contact tracing, provided that appropriate care is exercised when taking the pictures. They suggest that digital images offer considerable advantages over conventional contact tracing where there is shared care between hospital and the community. Digital images can be taken in the patient's home or in a community clinic and transmitted to a remote site for evaluation, reducing the number of patient journeys. Many aspects of the nature can be captured digitally, depending on the image quality.

Deep wounds with undermined areas are a common phenomenon in patients with many wounds left to heal by secondary intention. In these situations it is important to be able to evaluate a wound's progress on a regular basis with some degree of accuracy. However, measurement of the wound area alone may give little indication of the healing that is occurring in the wound bed, which may be accompanied by a significant decrease in the volume of the wound as a whole. The process of granulation is usually accompanied by significant wound contraction as healing progresses.

Plassman & Jones (1998) have described an instrument to measure the area and volume of wounds called MAVIS (Measurement of Area and Volume Instrument System) using colour-coded structured light to produce a three dimensional map of the wound. Plassman & Jones (1998) found that traditional area measurement techniques such as transparency tracings produced results with standard deviations between 4% for large wounds and up to 20% for small wounds of the mean measured value. MAVIS reduced these standard deviations by 3–5%. MAVIS was also found to be superior to using alginate casts for measuring volume. However, the instrument is not suitable for undermined, very deep or very large wounds, the accurate assessment of which remains problematic.

In a study to compare two non-invasive techniques for assessing wound healing: photography and high resolution ultrasound (HRUS), Dyson et al (2003) found that HRUS scanning permitted the quantitative assessment of structural changes deep in the wound, in contrast to photography, which allows recording of changes in the superficial aspects of the wound. These researchers therefore regard photography and the use of high-resolution ultrasound to be complementary. It is also now possible to measure local blood flow, using laser Doppler flowmetry (Timar-Banu et al 2001). These techniques may be of value in helping to evaluate the efficacy of new therapeutic strategies to promote wound healing.

Optimizing the local wound environment

Over the last 20 years there has been a proliferation of new wound dressing products and increasing use of physical therapies such as ultrasound, laser and vacuum-assisted closure.

Wound dressings and cleansing agents   The issues associated with creating the optimum local environment for healing through the use of cleansing agents and the application of dressings are discussed in Chapter 23. Where the wound contains devitalized tissue, debridement is usually indicated, in order to remove a medium for infection, to enable the true extent of tissue damage to be assessed and to facilitate uncomplicated healing. Wounds should be cleansed as necessary, using minimal mechanical force. Irrigation can be useful for cleaning a cavity ulcer. The place of antiseptics in wound management has been the subject of intense debate, while certain historical approaches, such as the use of larval therapy and honey, are experiencing a resurgence of interest and are being re-evaluated for both efficacy and clinical effectiveness. Of the new-generation products, growth factors are currently stimulating intense interest because of their potential to actively stimulate wound healing by modulating endogenous repair processes.

The use of physical modalities Other therapies that are proving of value today include hyperbaric oxygen therapy, pulsed electromagnetic energy (PEME) therapy, vacuum-assisted wound closure and ultrasound. The merits, indications and contraindications of these therapies are discussed in Chapter 26. While many of the published studies involve only a limited number of cases, these physical modalities provide exciting possibilities for the future and deserve closer attention and evaluation now, especially for intractable wounds.

Is the patient at risk of further tissue breakdown?

Every effort should be made to optimize the condition of the patient's skin and to prevent avoidable tissue breakdown. Conditions such as varicose eczema, atrophie blanche and hyperkeratosis may influence the recurrence of ulceration if not adequately addressed.

Sadly for many patients, they will suffer with more than one episode of ulceration, with a proportion having continuous bouts of ulceration over many decades (Callam et al 1987). It is essential that assessment identifies contributing factors that place a patient at increased risk of ulceration. These factors differ between different clinical groups. Patients with venous ulceration are at increased risk if they have had a previous deep vein thrombosis or previous ulcers of long duration (Franks et al 1995a). Concurrent conditions, such as respiratory disease and cardiac failure, which cause lower limb oedema, further increase the risk of recurrence.

Practitioners must assess each episode of ulceration individually. The risk of patients having developed concurrent peripheral vascular disease increases with age. Cornwall found that, in addition to venous disease, 50% of patients with leg ulceration had significant peripheral vascular disease by the time they were over 80 years of age (Cornwall et al 1986). The identification of the patient's arterial status will always remain a key priority in assessing and planning care.

Increasing age is also associated with patients developing complex ulceration due to a number of other contributing aetiologies. Patients may present with a mixed venous arterial ulcer that is further complicated by the presence of diabetes. It is essential that practitioners seek to control all concurrent conditions the patient is suffering from in order to facilitate healing.

Social and psychological issues may also significantly impact on ulcer recurrence (Franks et al 1995b). Wound trauma is a common precipitating factor for recurrent ulceration. Poor mobility and general dexterity compound the risk of traumatic ulceration. Patients living in difficult social situations may find difficulty in reducing risk factors, such as smoking, that they find comfort in. Assessment of the risk of recurrence must include identifying the patient's attitude and understanding of their condition and their willingness to take an active role in managing their own health. Chapter 31 discusses the role that lay beliefs and locus of control play in the health behaviour adopted by patients.

Frail, elderly, immobile patients may also be at high risk of developing a pressure ulcer, as illustrated in Case study 1. A review of approaches to assessing a patient's risk of developing pressure ulcers and the evidence for different methods of prevention and treatment are discussed in Morison 2001. In essence, it is important to assess the risk of one or more pressure ulcers developing and to develop a plan of care that includes: maximizing mobility and activity; planning for patient positioning, transferring and turning; and providing the patient with an appropriate support surface when in bed or a chair.

What are the consequences of the wound for the patient's quality of life?

The model to facilitate a holistic approach to patient assessment and care planning, illustrated in Figure 7.2, emphasizes the importance of gaining a good understanding of the consequences of the wound from the patient's perspective, both currently and in the longer term. Quality of life is a multidimensional construct that includes physical, social, emotional and spiritual dimensions, as described in Chapter 30. Successful treatment can certainly improve patients' quality of life (Franks & Moffatt 1998, Charles 2004).

Pain

Pain is a common and often underestimated problem for patients with wounds (Krasner 1998, Hollinworth & Collier 2000, King 2003, Ryan et al 2003) and at dressing changes (Briggs & Torra i

Bou 2001). Inadequately managed pain can lead to sleep disturbance, irritability, anxiety and depression. Pain is a complex phenomenon that is influenced only in part by the degree of tissue injury or disease, as described in Chapter 29.

Physical functioning

There are a number of well-validated tools to assess physical functioning, such as the ability to mobilize and to carry out normal activities of daily living, including attending to personal hygiene and dressing. In patients with acute or chronic wounds these abilities can be compromised. Many patients with leg ulceration have significantly reduced mobility. This is often directly related to the ulcer and the pain generated by movement. Mobility is further reduced by conditions such as osteoarthritis and rheumatoid arthritis. These compounding factors contribute to delayed healing. Patients with venous ulceration develop progressive loss of ankle movement, many having a completely fixed ankle joint within a short period of time. This has been shown to have a significant effect on wound healing potential (Franks et al 1995c). The length of time that a patient has experienced ulcer episodes is also of importance. Patients who undergo long-term bandaging lose their calf muscle bulk, which directly impacts on the effectiveness of the calf muscle pump in facilitating venous return. The advancing skin changes of lipodermatosclerosis also contribute to reduced ankle movement, with some patients developing equinus deformity due to a shortened Achilles tendon. Foot and gait deformities are common in many patients with varying types of leg ulceration. These complex factors often lead to a loss of general mobility and enforced social isolation and depression. The health-related quality of life literature discussed in Chapter 30 highlights the fact that effective ulcer treatment leads to improvement in symptoms such as pain and reduced mobility as a consequence of ulcer healing.

Social and role functions

Acute and chronic wounds can have both short- and longer-term consequences for the individual in terms of their relationships with others and the performance of their normal social roles of 'husband', 'wife', 'mother', 'friend' or 'work colleague'. Wounds can lead to short- or longer-term loss of independence, and they can lead to financial hardship if they affect the individual's ability to carry on their normal work. A young, otherwise fit man who loses a leg in a motor cycle accident may lose his job, have more restricted recreational opportunities and suffer from loss of self-esteem and altered body image. Even a relatively minor injury can have devastating consequences for anyone whose work involves highly developed psychomotor skills, such as a musician or a surgeon. Assessing the consequences of a wound for the individual is therefore a very important component of both short-term care and longer-term rehabilitation, and may involve many other members of the multidisciplinary team such as physiotherapists and occupational therapists.

Emotional and spiritual wellbeing

The cause of a wound and its physical and social consequences can have a direct bearing on the patient's feelings both about the wound and about themselves.

There is evidence that dedicated leg ulcer clinics can improve the quality of patients' lives, as well as promoting healing (Liew et al 2000).

What are the patient's beliefs about the wound and the likelihood of a successful outcome to treatment?

Beliefs are the lenses through which we view the world. Beliefs are the bedrock of our behaviour.

Wright et al 1996, p.19

There is growing evidence that people's beliefs can be strongly predictive of their behaviour in many health-related domains. A study by Jull et al (2004) investigating factors influencing patient concordance with compression stockings after venous leg ulcer healing found that two factors distinguished those who wore stockings from those who did not 75% of the time:

- The belief that wearing stockings was worthwhile
- The belief that stockings were comfortable to wear.

Commonly cited factors, such as age, sex, difficulty in applying stockings and cosmetic appearance were not significantly related to stocking use in this study. The authors concluded that practitioners should aim to ensure that their communication with patients and patient pamphlets enhanced the perceived value of compression stockings, as this is more likely to result in patient concordance.

Over the last four decades a number of health behaviour models have been developed that encompass belief-related components (Sanderson 2004). For example, the Health Belief Model (Rosenstock 1960, 1990) posits that the likelihood of individuals taking preventative health-related action is a function of four factors, the individual's belief that:

- They are personally susceptible to the condition
- If they were to acquire the condition it would have severe consequences
- Engaging in the health-related behaviour would be beneficial in reducing the threat
- The benefits of taking the action outweigh the costs.

Another well known theory, the Theory of Reasoned Action (Fishbein & Ajzen 1975), holds that attitudes and subjective norms predict behavioural intentions, which are the best predictors of behaviour. This theory has been supported by many subsequent studies (Sutton 1998). In an updated Theory of Planned Behaviour, Ajzen added an additional variable: perceived behavioural control (Ajzen 1991, Madden et al 1992). Together, attitudes, subjective norms and perceived behavioural control predict intention to perform the behaviour, which in turn predicts behaviour (Ajzen 2001).

Five decades of research have established that perceived behavioural control is powerfully predictive of people's motivation and behaviour in many domains, including adaptation to chronic illness and disability (Griffin & Rabkin 1998, Krause et al 1998), pain management (Pellino & Ward 1998), and health-related lifestyle choices (Bennett et al 1998). On the basis of research into perceived control and achievement in schoolchildren, and drawing upon different aspects of perceived control highlighted by studies of the related constructs of locus of control (Lefcourt 1992), learned helplessness (Abramson et al 1978), causal attribution (Weiner 1992) and self-efficacy (Bandura 1989), Skinner (1995) identified two important facets of perceived control: strategy (means–ends) beliefs and capacity (self-agency) beliefs. Strategy beliefs

are the individual's beliefs about 'what it takes' to achieve a particular end, while capacity beliefs are the individual's beliefs about 'having what it takes' to achieve this end. Recent research suggests that perceived behavioural control is a multidimensional construct involving both perceived control and perceived difficulty (Trafimow et al 2002).

A competency framework relating to patients' perceptions of their ability to engage in self-help activities is proposed in Figure 7.4. The model acknowledges the importance of patients' expectations (which in part reflect society's norms), as well as task difficulty, opportunity and the help and support required by patients from health-care professionals. The components of the model are explained in more detail in the explanatory notes to the figure.

In the context of wound care, it is hypothesized that patients who believe that they have control behave in ways that make treatment success more likely. Their sustained engagement in activities that promote healing, such as taking a healthy diet and appropriate exercise, is likely to lead to a better outcome over time. In contrast, it is hypothesized that patients who do not believe that they can influence the outcome may act in ways that forfeit opportunities for exerting control and, through their passivity and avoidance of a task perceived to be difficult, reinforce their own sense of helplessness, which at worst can lead to the strong negative emotion of hopelessness. An example of a patient who has given up attempting to help herself is illustrated in Case study 2.

Case Study 2   *A 40-year-old lady with a diabetic leg ulcer who has 'learned helplessness'*

Maureen Gray has recently been diagnosed with type 2 diabetes. She weighs 22 stone (140 kg) and is finding it increasingly difficult to walk because of breathlessness on exertion. She has three teenage children, who are all known to the police for petty crimes in the community. They regularly play truant from school. Her eldest son Jack is awaiting a court appearance for car theft and driving without a vehicle licence or insurance. Her husband was made redundant 18 months ago when a local factory closed. He spends a good deal of his time in the local bar playing pool with his former work colleagues. Maureen has recently developed a large superficial ulcer on her lower leg. She sees little point in going to see her family physician about it. The health centre is a mile away. The nearest large supermarket is a mile and a half from her house in the opposite direction. For the most part, therefore, Maureen uses the small local store, which has been boarded up because of vandalism. The store carries little fresh fruit or vegetables and Maureen's budget means that she is unable to afford to buy healthy food for her family in any case. The children drift in and out of the house throughout the day and the family rarely sit down together to a meal. The area where Maureen lives is known to be an area of high socioeconomic deprivation. Despite numerous promises by local politicians to improve the physical environment and the facilities for the young people living on the estate, little has happened on the ground and there is a general air of neglect.

A critique of all of the health behaviour models presented above is that they fail to take account of factors such as race, gender and socioeconomic status, as well as broader factors such as a country's public health policy. People who lack health insurance or who are unable to afford a healthy diet may be unable to behave in ways that optimize their health, however much they might want to. More research is needed in this context in relation to wound care. However, what these models do highlight is the multiplicity and complexity of factors that can affect the individual's desire to engage in behaviours that can help their wounds to heal. While such complexity appears daunting, the implications for practice of the model presented in Figure 7.4 are wide-ranging, and worthy of further study. The model encourages clinicians to look beyond the wound to the beliefs and attitudes of the patient with a wound, as these beliefs may be pivotally important in determining patients' optimism and behaviour, including concordance with prescribed treatments and the adoption of a healthier lifestyle.

To what extent can the patient and lay carer be involved in care planning and its implementation?

As noted above, patients' beliefs are likely to be highly predictive of their behaviour. The extent to which patients and carers can be involved in care planning and its implementation also depends upon the values and beliefs of the health professionals responsible for their care (Graham et al 2003, Moffatt 2004). A client-centred approach requires that clinicians believe in the importance of shared responsibility, mutuality and client autonomy, which contrasts with the paternalistic approach underpinned by the belief that the professional always knows best.

The patient's central role

Many patients with wounds may seem to health-care professionals to have little motivation to help themselves (Case study 2). Studies have shown that stress can delay healing in experimentally produced wounds, and Cole-King & Harding (2001) have found a relationship between anxiety and depression and delayed healing in chronic wounds. As Betty Brown's case illustrates (Case study 1), chronic wounds can develop at a time when the patient is least able to help themselves because of illness or disability, and when a chronic wound is slow to heal people can come to believe that they are powerless to influence the situation in a positive way. However, when a client-centred approach is adopted the individual's rights to autonomy and self-determination are fully acknowledged, the health-care professional and the client share responsibility for care planning and the focus shifts from the individual's deficits to facilitating the client's potential for self-help. Naylor (2002) describes the patient's central role in symptom self-assessment for fungating wounds as the cornerstone of effective symptom management and this approach has considerable potential for understanding symptom severity and health-related quality of life issues for patients with other types of chronic wound, such as leg ulcers.

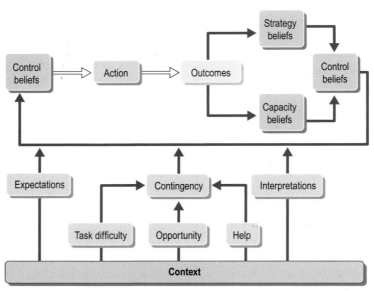

Figure 7.4 Perceived control and perceived helplessness: the sense of competency among patients with wounds and some psychological factors that can determine the extent to which they engage in self-help activities (Adapted from a model by Skinner (1995) in the educational domain)

Explanatory notes

Control beliefs: Patients' (and health-care professionals'!) beliefs about the extent to which they can achieve the desired outcomes, such as wound healing, and prevent undesired events, such as wound breakdown or infection.

Strategy beliefs: Patients' perceptions of what it takes for their wound to heal, e.g. help from health-care professionals, self-help (effort and ability), or luck/unknown.

Capacity beliefs: Patients' perceptions of whether they have what it takes e.g. sufficient help from health-care professionals, the ability to help themselves.

Perceptions of control: A patient's perception of their ability to help the healing process through their own actions.

Outcomes: These can include both wound healing and improvements in the individual's health-related quality of life (HRQoL).

Expectations: The individual's expectations of a successful outcome are influenced by their past experiences, their sense of self-efficacy and their optimism.

Contingency: The contingency between actions and outcomes can be modified by a number of factors, including:

Task difficulty: If a patient perceives a task to be too difficult then they are likely to give up easily and may believe themselves to be helpless to influence the situation in a positive way in the future. This may be exacerbated by a number of factors, such as:

- Unrecognized pathology – if the treatment regimen does not address the underlying pathology of the wound then patients will not experience contingency between their own efforts and the outcome. They may then experience 'learned helplessness', as, no matter how hard they try, the wound fails to heal and their fear of failure becomes self-fulfilling.
- Unrealistic goals – if a health-care professional sets unrealistic goals, for example predicts too short a time for a wound to heal, then the patient will experience non-contingency between action and outcome, as, no matter how hard they try to help themselves, they fail to meet the health-care professional's expectations. They may then lose faith both in the health-care professional and in the treatment!

Figure 7.4, cont'd

Opportunity: Do the patients currently have the opportunity to help themselves, for example:

- Do they have access to a nutritious diet?
- Is their physical environment within the home suitable for them to be functionally independent and to take other self-help measures?

Help: This refers to whether or not patients have access to the resources that they need, for example:

- Appropriate information and explanations from health-care professionals
- Appropriate care and treatment, and non-judgemental monitoring of their progress, by health-care professionals who modify the care planned in the light of the patient's changing circumstances and individual needs and wishes
- The necessary support and help from family, friends and neighbours.

Interpretations: This refers to the patient's interpretation of outcomes (or lack of them) in the short term which can determine the likelihood of action being taken by them again, in the future. The health-care professional's interpretation of events, such as healing or non-healing, can readily be communicated to the patient, either positively or negatively, and can contribute to the patient's own expectations of success or failure in the future.

Involving the patient's family and lay carers

A task that is often neglected is the education and support of family and lay carers. Educational programmes should be structured, organized and comprehensive, and made available to family or care givers as well as to patients (Chapter 32).

Seeing the patient in a wider social context

Although the focus of this chapter is predominantly on the individual, there are many hints in the literature to suggest that society's view of health and health care, and the attitudes of family members, friends and health-care professionals in the local community, have an impact on the nature of the individual's experience of a wound. Individuals are members of families, who are in turn embedded within a local community, set in a wider society. The term 'system' describes 'an integrated whole' in which the parts are interconnected with one another in a complex web of relationships (Fig. 7.5). Systems theory is reflected in a number of models of nursing, such as Neuman's Systems Model, where the client is seen as a unique individual, decision-making is shared and diversity is valued and respected. Family systems theory underpins the move today towards the practice of family nursing in the home.

The aim of care planning should be to take a holistic approach to understanding the unique context within which each individual's wound is to be managed, and to understanding the interaction of a multiplicity of variables on many system levels.

What are the patient's needs for rehabilitation?

Rehabilitation involves restoration of the individual's physical and social functioning, so far as this is possible, and as such build on all of the dimensions of patient assessment and care planning discussed so far.

What is the optimum setting for care?

Patients' social circumstances and the setting for care can have a profound effect on their physical, emotional and social wellbeing. Hospitalization may be essential for patients following trauma or planned surgery because of the specialist facilities and expertise required but care is likely to be costly, both to the provider and to the individual, who may suffer major disruption to their normal life. Care at home is usually associated with more freedom for the individual and often easier access for family and friends, but facilities are more restricted, as is access to health-related services and advice. Deciding on the optimum time to discharge a patient from hospital can be more difficult than it might seem, as there is usually some degree of risk associated with this, especially in the short term. Discharge planning and the organization of home care support services prior to discharge are therefore very important. For some patients a return to their own home will never be possible, and arrangements may need to be made for long-term care, which can have deleterious consequences for the individual's quality of

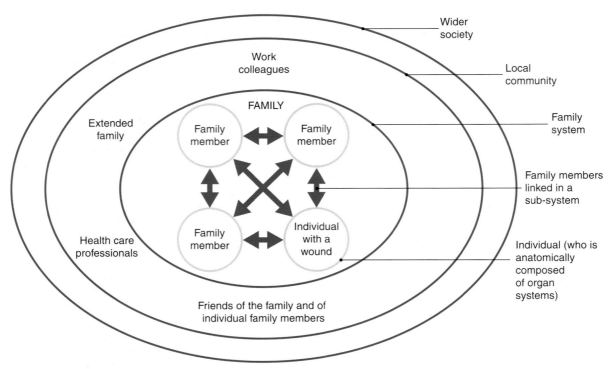

Figure 7.5 The conceptualization of the individual with a leg ulcer, embedded within a family, set in a local community and encompassed by a wider society (With permission from Morison 2001, p. 128)

life and require major adjustments for both them and their carers (Harris and Spence, 2004).

CONCLUSION

Leg ulcers can have a significant impact on an individual's quality of life, including physical and social functioning and the performance of normal social roles. They are often accompanied by pain and discomfort, lowered self-esteem and altered body image, and for some, complications such as sepsis can be life-threatening.

A systematic and holistic approach to patient assessment and care planning is essential for the delivery of care that is effective and meets the needs of the individual and their family. The use of a conceptual framework can facilitate the adoption of a holistic, client-centred approach and can shift the emphasis from the wound towards the patient with a wound.

References

Abramson L Y, Seligman M E P, Teasdale J D 1978 Learned helplessness in humans: critique and reformulation. Journal of Abnormal Psychology 87: 49–74

Ajzen I 1991 The theory of planned behavior. Organizational Behavior and Human Decision Processes 50: 179–211

Ajzen I 2001 Nature and operation of attitudes In: Fiske S T et al (eds) Annual Review of Psychology 52: 27–58

Bandura A 1989 Human agency in social cognitive theory. American Psychologist 44: 1175–1184

Bates-Jensen B M 1997 The Pressure Sore Status Tool a few thousand assessments later. Advances in Wound Care 10: 65–73

Bates-Jensen B M, Vredevoe D L, Brecht M L 1992 The validity and reliability of the Pressure Sore Status Tool. Decubitus 5(6): 80S–86S

Bennett P, Norman P, Murphy S et al 1998 Beliefs about alcohol, health locus of control, value for health and reported consumption in a representative population sample. Health Education Research 13: 25–32

Briggs M, Torra i Bou J E 2001 Pain at wound dressing changes: a guide to management. In: European Wound Management Association (EWMA) position document: pain at dressing changes. Medical Education Partnership, London

Callam M J, Harper D R, Dale J J, Ruckley C V 1987 Chronic ulcer of the leg: clinical history. British Medical Journal 294: 1389–1391

Charles H 2004 Does leg ulcer treatment improve patients' quality of life? Journal of Wound Care 13: 209–213

Cole-King A, Harding K 2001 Psychological factors and delayed healing in chronic wounds. Psychosomatic Medicine 63: 216–220

Cornwall J V, Dore C J, Lewis J D 1986 Leg ulcers: epidemiology and aetiology. British Journal of Surgery 73: 693–695

Davis M H, Dunkley P, Harden R M et al 1992 The wound programme. Centre for Medical Education, University of Dundee, Scotland

Dealey C 1999 The care of wounds: a guide for nurses, 2nd edn. Blackwell Science, Oxford

Dyson M, Moodley S, Verjee L et al 2003 Wound healing assessment using 20 MHz ultrasound and photography. Skin Research and Technology 9: 116–121

Edmonds M, Foster A V M, Vowden P 2004 Wound bed preparation for diabetic foot ulcers. In: European Wound Management Association (EWMA) position document: wound bed preparation in practice. Medical Education Partnership, London, pp 6–11

Falanga V 2004 Wound bed preparation: science applied to practice. In: European Wound Management Association (EWMA) position document: wound bed preparation in practice. Medical Education Partnership, London, pp 2–5

Falanga V, Harding K (eds) 2002 The clinical relevance of wound bed preparation. Springer, Berlin

Fishbein M, Ajzen I 1975 Belief, attitude, intention, and behavior: an introduction to theory and research. Addison-Wesley, Reading, MA

Flanagan M 2003 Wound measurement: can it help us to monitor progression to healing? Journal of Wound Care 12: 189–194

Franks P J, Moffatt C J 1998 Who suffers most from leg ulceration? Journal of Wound Care 7: 383–385

Franks P J, Oldroyd M I, Dickson D et al 1995a Risk factors for leg ulcer recurrence: a randomised controlled trial of two types of compression stocking. Age and Ageing 24: 490–494

Franks P J, Bosanquet N, Connolly M et al 1995b Venous ulcer healing: effect of socio-economic factors in London. Journal of Epidemiology and Community Health 49: 385–388

Franks P J, Moffatt C J, Connolly M et al 1995c Factors associated with healing leg ulceration with high compression. Age and Ageing 24: 407–410

Graham I D, Harrison M B, Shafey M, Keast D 2003 Knowledge and attitudes regarding care of leg ulcers: survey of family physicians. Canadian Family Physician 49: 896–902

Gray D, Cooper P 2001 Nutrition and wound healing: what is the link? Journal of Wound Care 10: 86–89

Griffin K W, Rabkin J G 1998 Perceived control over illness, realistic acceptance, and psychological adjustment in people with AIDS. Journal of Social and Clinical Psychology 17: 407–424

Griffith R 2004 Putting the record straight: the importance of documentation. British Journal of Community Nursing 9: 122–125

Harris J, Spence C 2004, Social and psychological issues. In: Morison M J, Ovington L G, Wilkie K (eds) Chronic wound care: a problem-based learning approach. Mosby, Edinburgh

Hollinworth H, Collier M 2000 Nurses' views about pain and trauma at dressing changes: results of a national survey. Journal of Wound Care 9: 369–373

Hunink G 1995 A study guide to nursing theories. Campion Press, Edinburgh

Jull A B, Mitchell N, Arroll J et al 2004 Factors influencing concordance with compression stockings after venous leg ulcer healing. Journal of Wound Care 13: 90–92

Kantor J, Margolis D J 1998 Efficacy and prognosis value of simple wound measurements. Archives of Dermatology 134: 1571–1574

Keast D H, Bowering C, Evans A et al 2004 MEASURE: a proposed assessment framework for developing best practice recommendations for wound assessment. Wound Repair and Regeneration 12(Suppl): s1–s17

King B 2003 A review of research investigating pain and wound care. Journal of Wound Care 12: 219–223

Krasner D 1998 Painful venous ulcers: themes and stories about their impact on quality of life. Ostomy/Wound Management 44: 38–49

Krause J S, Stanwyck C A, Maides J 1998 Locus of control and life adjustment: relationship among people with spinal cord injury. Rehabilitation Counseling Bulletin 41: 162–172

Lagan K M, Dusoir A E, McDonough S M, Baxter G D 2000 Wound measurement: the comparative reliability of direct versus photographic tracings analysed by planimetry versus digitising techniques. Archives of Physical Medicine and Rehabilitation 81: 1110–1116

Lefcourt H M 1992 Durability and impact of the locus of control construct. Psychology Bulletin 112: 411–414

Liew I H, Law K A, Sinha S N 2000 Do leg ulcer clinics improve patients' quality of life? Journal of Wound Care 9: 423–426

McIlwaine C 2003 Importance of holistic nutritional assessment in wound healing. Journal of Wound Care 12: 285–288

McLaren S 2004 Nutritional screening, assessment and support. In: Morison M, Ovington L, Wilkie K (eds) Chronic wound care: a problem-based learning approach. Mosby, Edinburgh

McMath E, Harvey C 2004 Complex wounds: a partnership approach to patient documentation. British Journal of Nursing: Tissue Viability Supplement 13: s12–s16

Madden T J, Ellen P S, Ajzen I 1992 A comparison of the theory of planned behaviour and the theory of reasoned action. Personality and Social Psychology Bulletin 18: 39

Manios A, Tosca A, Volakakis E et al 2003 Computer-assisted evaluation of wound healing in chronic ulcers. Computers in Biology and Medicine 33: 311–317

Margolis D J, Berlin J A, Strom B L 1999 Risk factors associated with the failure of a venous ulcer to heal. Archives of Dermatology 135: 920–926

Melhuish J M, Plassman P, Harding K 1994 Circumference area and volume of the healing wound. Journal of Wound Care 3: 380–384

Moffatt C J 2004 Perspectives on concordance in leg ulcer management. Journal of Wound Care 13: 243–248

Moffatt C, Morison M, Pina E 2004 Wound bed preparation for venous leg ulcers. In: European Wound Management Association (EWMA) position document: wound bed preparation in practice. Medical Education Partnership, London, pp 12–17

Morison M (ed) 2001 The prevention and treatment of pressure ulcers. Mosby, Edinburgh

Morison M, Moffatt C 1994 A colour guide to the assessment and management of leg ulcers, 2nd edn. Mosby, London

Naylor W 2002 Part 2: Symptom self-assessment in the management of fungating wounds. World Wide Wounds. Available on line at: www.worldwidewounds.com/2002/July

Oien R F, Hakansson A, Hansen B U, Bjellerup M 2002 Measuring the size of ulcers by planimetry: a useful method in the clinical setting. Journal of Wound Care 11: 165–168

Pellino T A, Ward S E 1998 Perceived control mediates the relationship between pain severity and patient satisfaction. Journal of Pain and Symptom Management 15: 110–116

Plassman P, Jones T D 1998 MAVIS: a non-invasive instrument to measure area and volume of wounds. Medical Engineering and Physics 20: 332–338

Rosenstock I M 1960 What research in motivation suggests for public health. American Journal of Public Health 50: 295–301

Rosenstock I M 1990 The health belief model: explaining health behavior through expectancies. In: Glanz F M et al (eds). Health behavior and health education: theory, research and practice. Jossey-Bass, San Francisco, CA, pp 39–62

Ryan S, Eager C, Sibbald G S 2003 Venous leg ulcer pain. Ostomy/Wound Management 49: 16–23

Samad A, Hayes S, French L, Dodds S 2002 Digital imaging versus conventional contact tracing for the objective measurement of venous leg ulcers. Journal of Wound Care 11: 137–140

Sanderson C A 2004 Health psychology. John Wiley, New York

Schultz G S, Sibbald R G, Falanga V et al 2003 Wound bed preparation: a systematic approach to wound management. Wound Repair and Regeneration 11(Suppl): s1–s28

Sibbald R G, Williamson D, Orsted H L et al D 2000 Preparing the wound bed – debridement, bacterial balance, and moisture balance. Ostomy/Wound Management 46: 14–35

Sibbald R G, Orsted H, Schultz G S et al 2003 Preparing the wound bed. Ostomy/Wound Management 49: 24–51

SIGN Guidelines 1998 Leg ulcers: SIGN Guidelines. Scottish Intercollegiate Guidelines Network, Edinburgh

Skinner E A 1995 Perceived control and motivation: stress, coping and competence. Sage, London

Spencer J, Widdows C 2000 Implementation of patient-held records in diabetic foot care. Journal of Wound Care 9: 64–66

Sterling C 1996 Methods of wound assessment documentation. Nursing Standard 11(10): 38–41

Sutton S 1998 predicting and explaining intentions and behaviour. How well are we doing? Journal of Applied Social Psychology 28: 1317–1338

Taylor R J 2002 Mouseyes revisited: upgrading a computer program that aids wound measurement. Journal of Wound Care 11: 213–216

Taylor R J, Taylor A D and Marcuson R W 1999 A computerized leg ulcer database with facilities for reporting and auditing. Journal of Wound Care 8(1): 34–38

Timar-Banu O, Beauregard H, Tousignant J et al 2001 Development of non-invasive and quantitative methodologies for the assessment of chronic ulcers and scars in humans. Wound Repair and Regeneration 9: 123–132

Trafimow D, Finlay K A, Sheeran P, Conner M 2002 Evidence that perceived behavioural control is a multidimensional construct: perceived control and perceived difficulty. British Journal of Social Psychology 41: 101–121

Weiner B 1992 Human motivation: metaphors, theories and research. Sage, London

Williams L 2002 Assessing patients' nutritional needs in the wound-healing process. Journal of Wound Care 11: 225–228

Wright L M, Watson W L, Bell J M 1996 Beliefs: the heart of healing in families and illness. Basic Books, New York

8

Causation of venous leg ulcers

Magnus S. Ågren, Finn Gottrup

INTRODUCTION

Skin ulceration of the lower leg and foot has multiple causes. Venous insufficiency, peripheral arterial disease and diabetes mellitus account for more than 90% of all leg ulcers (Mekkes et al 2003). This chapter will focus on venous leg ulcers, as this is the most common leg ulcer with estimates ranging from 37–81% (Valencia et al 2001, Adam et al 2003b, Briggs & Closs 2003). First the venous anatomy and haemodynamics in the lower leg is briefly described. Following a general summary of the venous system, some vascular pathologies in the superficial and deep systems are presented that lead to ulcer formation. The chapter concludes by reviewing the local circulatory, biochemical and cellular pathophysiological mechanisms that can result in skin breakdown and ulceration.

VENOUS LEG ULCERS

Anatomy and haemodynamics of the vein system in the lower limb

The venous system in the lower limb is anatomically classified by its relationship to the fascia and constitutes the subcutaneous superficial system, the deep system below the muscle fascia and the connecting perforating veins (Caggiati 1999). More than 40 perforators connect the deep and superficial veins.

Important for the venodynamics is the venous pump function of the lower limb. In the upright position a significant amount of blood is translocated to the lower extremity veins. During resting, cyclic muscular action and valves in the veins form a powerful pumping system aiding venous blood return to the heart. The venous pumping system consists of the muscle, the distal calf and the foot pumps (Fig. 8.1). The muscle pumps consist of the anterior, lateral and deep and superficial posterior muscular compartments. Muscular contraction is the main activator of the pump system but passive stretching may also raise intramuscular pressure and promote pumping. Muscle contraction increases the intraluminal blood pressure to more than 100 mmHg, while passive stretching yields one-third of this increase. The pressure in the muscle veins is three times higher than in the superficial veins. Competent venous valves prevent retrograde flow. During the subsequent muscle relaxation the venous pressure falls below the level at rest. This fall in pressure is more pronounced in the deep veins, allowing blood to flow from the superficial to the deep veins. The distal pump is activated by dorsal flexion of the ankle, when the calf muscles are stretched and their distal part descends within the fascial sheath. This movement, together with competent valves, ascertains that venous blood is expelled in a proximal direction. The foot pump is independent of muscular movements (Fig. 8.1). During normal walking the three systems are synchronized to form a complex network of serial and parallel pumps aiding the return of blood to the heart.

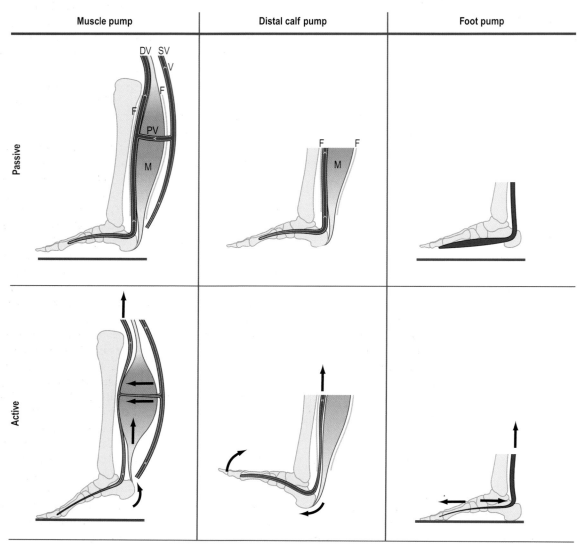

Figure 8.1 Venous pump systems of the foot and calf in relaxed and active state. The muscle pump unit consists of muscles (M) ensheathed by a common fascia (F) and veins within the same compartment. Contraction of the calf muscles (muscle systole), as in plantar flexion of the ankle joint during walking (below), expels blood into the proximal collecting vein. During relaxation (muscle diastole, above) the blood is drained from the superficial veins (SV) into the deep veins (DV) in addition to the arterial inflow, making the pump ready for the subsequent ejection. The distal calf pump is illustrated in the middle. On dorsiflexion of the ankle (passive or active), the bulk of the calf muscle (M) descends within the fascial sheath (F), and expels blood in the distal veins like a piston. The foot vein pump is illustrated to the right. The plantar veins are connected like a bowstring from the base of the fourth metatarsal in front to the medial malleolus. On weight-bearing the tarsometatarsal joints are extended and the tarsal arch is flattened. Thus the veins are stretched, causing them to eject their content of blood. V, venous valve. (From Stranden E 2000 Dynamic leg volume changes when sitting in a locked and free-floating tilt office chair. Ergonomics 43: 421–433, with permission of Taylor & Francis Ltd, http://www.tandf.co.uk/journals.)

Haemodynamic disturbances of the venous system and association with ulcer development

Hippocrates (460–377 BC) was the first person known to describe the association between leg ulcers, enlarged veins and dependency (Adams 1949). He advocated that leg ulcer patients should avoid standing and dangling their leg. Hippocrates introduced 'puncturing' and bandaging for treatment of ulcers and the associated varicose veins. In 1658 William Harvey described the function of the valves of the veins and in 1855 Verneuil described the perforating veins and the associated valves. The role of gravity, prolonged standing and valvular vein insufficiencies were elucidated in the 19th century. Vein ligation, stripping and injection therapy, together with an understanding of the relationship between post-thrombotic damage of the vein and ulcer development, were introduced later in the 19th century.

Different theories have been proposed to explain the development of venous insufficiency (London & Nash 2000). In the normal lower leg in the supine position, blood flows slowly through the veins and the pressure in the ankle is 70–100 mmHg, falling to 10–20 mmHg during walking and about 55 mmHg while sitting. This is achieved through an acceleration of blood flow brought about by the combined action of the venous pumps. If the valves of the superficial and perforator veins are incompetent, blood oscillates up and down in the segments. The resulting retrograde flow in the veins of the lower leg (venous reflux) leads to ambulatory venous hypertension and oedema during exercise. The more extensive and distal the venous reflux, the greater the risk of ulcer formation. The retrograde flow, especially through the saphenofemoral junction, results in a large fraction of blood flowing retrogradely from the deep to the superficial system. Therefore, proximal occlusion of the superficial veins normalizes ambulatory venous pressure (AVP) in the leg and temporarily normalizes the pressure-recovery time after rest. Deep venous incompetence is commonest secondary to previous deep venous thrombosis (DVT). Incompetence of the three venous systems is characterized by ambulatory venous hypertension in the superficial and deep veins. The only effective relief of venous pressure in this condition is elevation of the legs, while exercise only minimally influences AVP. Outflow obstruction may be the result of occluded or partially recanalized veins subsequent to DVT. During muscle contraction the venous pressure may even increase and lead to venous claudication. This venous hypertension leads to distension of the perforators and valve dysfunction. This results in overload of the superficial veins, which is thought to lead to varicose veins.

Whatever the cause of venous insufficiency, the consequence is a decreased ability to reduce venous pressure during exercise, which can eventually develop into an ulcer. Arnoldi & Linderholm (1968) found that skin ulceration occurred if the rise in AVP in the ankle veins exceeded 40–60 mmHg. Only patients with incompetent perforators or an incompetent deep vein system developed raised AVP. In subsequent studies these limits have been refined and if the pressure of a foot vein remains higher than 60 mmHg during walking there is a 50% risk for development of an ulcer, while if the pressure is 45–60 mmHg the risk is 25% and below 45 mmHg the risk is negligible (Shull et al 1979, Nicolaides et al 1993). Likewise, it has been convincingly demonstrated, using duplex ultrasound scanning, that total venous reflux exceeding 10 ml/s predisposes to ulcer development (Vasdekis et al 1989).

About 50–60% of patients with venous leg ulcers show incompetent superficial and perforating vein valves (Ruckley 1993, Kistner 1996, Nelzén et al 1997, Scriven et al 1997, Wong et al 2003). Superficial reflux or primary varices alone cause venous ulcers in a large proportion of these patients (Lees & Lambert 1993, Magnusson et al 2001, Adam et al 2003b). It should be noted that superficial venous reflux may be present in patients without visible varicose veins and influence deep veins, which can aggravate the haemodynamic abnormality further (Scriven et al 1997, Sparks et al 1997, Bergan 1998). Superficial venous surgery also reduces deep venous reflux (Adam et al 2003a). Ablative superficial venous surgery combined with compression therapy reduced the 1-year recurrence rate from 28% to 12% while the 24-week healing rate was not affected by these surgical and conservative procedures (Barwell et al 2004).

The importance, in the pathophysiology of venous ulceration, of isolated incompetent perforating veins has been questioned after recent disappointing results with subfascial endoscopic surgery of lateral perforators (de Rijcke et al 2003). Randomized controlled trials are needed to settle this issue.

About 50% of venous leg ulcer patients have diagnosed deep vein incompetence (Scriven et al 1997, Ruckley et al 2002, Wong et al 2003). A recent case-control study from New Zealand reported that people with a history of DVT were three times more likely to have a leg ulcer than people without a history of venous thrombosis (Walker et al 2003). Surprisingly, former DVT was as common in patients with an ulcer of non-venous origin as in those with a venous ulcer, possibly reflecting mixed aetiologies in leg ulcer patients (Walker et al 2003). However, patients with documented previous DVT can subsequently have normal deep vein function (Scriven et al 1997). It is unclear whether those patients are at the same degree of risk of developing ulceration as patients who have abnormal deep vein function.

Whether venous disease predominantly affects female patients is a matter of debate (Lee et al 2003). Traditionally, it has been assumed that venous leg ulcers are commoner in females than in males. In Western countries an older study showed that the prevalence of varicose veins was less than 19% in men and 44% in women younger than 30 years, while the corresponding figures were 42% and 64% respectively for 50-year-old individuals (Coon et al 1973). More recent studies suggest that there is no gender difference in the risk of developing varicose veins or venous ulceration (Evans et al 1999, Lee et al 2003). The same appears to apply to DVT, as a recent systematic review found a similar incidence of DVT in males and females (Fowkes et al 2003).

Arteriovenous shunting of blood away from nutritive capillaries has been suggested as a reason for ulceration (Malanin et al 1997). Their existence would explain the finding of elevated oxygen tension in varicose veins (Holling et al 1938). However, because no shunting was observed using radioactively labelled microaggregates in patients with varicose veins, arteriovenous shunting is unlikely to be a major factor in the pathogenesis of venous leg ulcers (Lindemayr et al 1972).

Clinical signs and biochemical markers in diagnosis of chronic venous insufficiency

Chronic venous insufficiency (CVI) is manifested by different symptoms and signs. The updating of the CEAP (clinical signs, cause, anatomical distribution and pathophysiological condition) clinical classification for chronic venous disease is a commendable initiative that facilitates interpretation of clinical data (Porter & Moneta 1995). The numerical grading from 0–6 reflects the progressive stages of venous disease severity, eventually leading to cutaneous ulceration (Table 8.1). Corona phlebectatica (ankle flare), corresponding to CEAP class 1, denotes a fan-shaped cluster of small dilated veins radiating down from the Cockett perforator area over the medial side of the ankle and foot that appears to be an early marker for eventual ulceration (Ruckley et al 2002). Class 4 CEAP represents a more advanced stage of CVI in which the pathological and inflammatory changes of the skin are reflected in the clinical signs: pain, oedema, varicose eczema, hyperpigmentation (due to haemosiderin accumulation), atrophie blanche and lipodermatosclerosis. Although lipodermatosclerosis, i.e.

Table 8.1 CEAP* classification of chronic lower extremity venous disease (Porter & Moneta 1995)

Class	Clinical signs
0	No visible or palpable signs of venous disease
1	Telangiectases, reticular veins, malleolar flare
2	Varicose veins
3	Oedema without skin changes
4	Skin changes ascribed to venous disease (e.g. pigmentation, venous eczema, lipodermatosclerosis)
5	Skin changes as defined above with healed ulceration
6	Skin changes as defined above with active ulceration

* Clinical signs (C), cause (E), anatomical distribution (A) and pathophysiological condition (P).

fibrosis in the skin and subcutaneous tissues, is common in venous leg ulcer patients this clinical entity is not exclusively associated with venous insufficiency (Bruce et al 2002). For example, obesity (body mass index >34) was also found to predispose to lipodermatosclerosis in a retrospective study (Bruce et al 2002). Healed and open ulcers due to venous disease fall into CEAP classes 5 and 6 respectively. Clinical examples of the CEAP classes are shown in Figure 8.2.

Systemic biochemical markers of the impact of the venous disease in the lower extremity would also be useful in early detection and diagnosis of CVI. Although plasma levels of vascular endothelial growth factor (VEGF) are increased in all stages of CVD compared with healthy controls, this parameter failed to discriminate the CEAP classes (Howlader & Coleridge Smith 2004). The novel haemosiderin urine test, on the other hand, appears to be more specifically associated with the

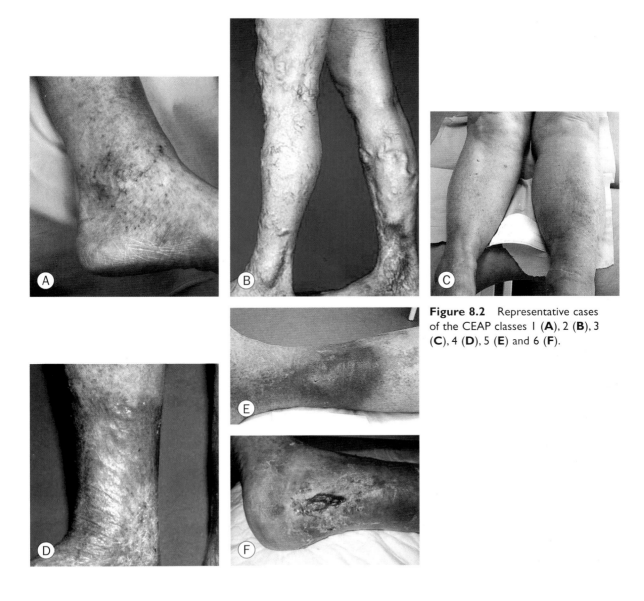

Figure 8.2 Representative cases of the CEAP classes 1 (**A**), 2 (**B**), 3 (**C**), 4 (**D**), 5 (**E**) and 6 (**F**).

CVI categories. Dermal haemosiderin deposition, resulting from extravascular erythrocyte haemolysis, is a characteristic of CVI. Zamboni et al (2003) studied the validity of the test and found a correlation between urine haemosiderin levels and CVI severity according to CEAP. The test showed a 95% diagnostic accuracy (Zamboni et al 2003).

CAUSES OF VENOUS LEG ULCERS

Although the primary cause is venous hypertension resulting from venous disease, only a fraction of patients with CVI develop active skin ulceration (Kistner 1996). Therefore, the pathophysiological mechanism(s) responsible for skin ulceration is still unresolved (Ruckley 1993).

Microcirculatory disturbances

The venous hypertension is transmitted to the nutritional capillaries in the papillary dermis. Capillaries become dilated, convoluted and glomerulus-like (Fagrell 1982, Howlader & Smith 2003). Elegant intravital microscopic investigations of the capillary network in the ankle region have undoubtedly demonstrated the presence of micro-oedema surrounding the small vessels (Fagrell 1982). Gross pathological changes are also observed in the lymphatic capillaries (Eliska & Eliskova 2001). Furthermore, the capillary density is reduced in the gaiter area of advanced lipodermatosclerosis as assessed by videomicroscopy (Luetolf et al 1993, Howlader & Smith 2003). In addition, reduced microvascular perfusion was observed in the skin over the medial malleolus compared with adjacent skin even in healthy volunteers, which may indicate the predisposition of this site for ulcer development (Bull et al 1995).

Fibrin cuff theory

As a result of increased pressure, the capillaries become leaky and macromolecules extravasate, resulting in oedema. In addition, fibrinogen polymerizes on the outside of the vessels, forming pericapillary fibrin cuffs (Browse & Burnand 1982, Falanga et al 1987). This phenomenon appears to occur already in mild CVI without visible skin changes. Pericapillary fibrin cuffs were more abundant in the ankle region than in the thigh of the same patients (Stacey et al 2000). The fibrin matrix that is initially formed is gradually replaced by a more permanent fibrotic structure made up of other extracellular matrix molecules such as fibronectin, laminin, tenascin, type I collagen and type III collagen (Herrick et al 1992). The type IV collagen layer and basal membrane of dermal capillaries are also thickened in legs with venous insufficiency (Peschen et al 1996, Pappas et al 1997). There is controversy as to whether the pericapillary fibrin cuffs are the primary cause of venous ulceration or if their presence is merely a consequence of the ulcer. Balslev et al (1992) observed immunodetectable pericapillary fibrin only in one of 19 patients with venous insufficiency and lipodermatosclerosis and it was equally common in venous and ischaemic leg ulcers.

The 'trap' hypothesis

Falanga & Eaglstein (1993) proposed that macromolecules such as fibrinogen and α_2-macroglobulin leak into the dermis as a result of venous hypertension and then bind or 'trap' growth factors and matrix material that then becomes unavailable for the maintenance of tissue integrity and its repair. The validity of this hypothesis has been questioned (Bollinger 1993) and been tested in an in vitro experiment (Ågren et al 2000). Biopsies from venous leg ulcers and normal skin were first incubated with radiolabelled growth factors and then the release of the growth factors from the tissue explants was measured. Basically, no significant amount of trapping of the growth factors by the chronic ulcer bed was detected because the growth factors were liberated at the rate of normal skin. Although no trapping of growth factors was observed, this in vitro experiment might not correctly mimic the in vivo circumstances in which growth factors are produced within the pericapillary cuffs or taken up from the vasculature.

Does hypoxia exist in the gaiter region?

Disturbances in the microcirculation and the presence of pericapillary cuffs theoretically result in local hypoxia and undernourishment, leading to skin necrosis (Fagrell 1982, Scott & Coleridge Smith 1989, Bollinger 1993). Markedly reduced transcutaneous oxygen tension has also been measured in lipodermatosclerosis and skin contiguous to venous leg ulcers (Falanga et al 1987, Mani et al 1989, Peschen et al 1996). However, lowered transcutaneous oxygen tension does not unequivocally imply impaired exchange of oxygen in the tissue because a decrease in measured transcutaneous oxygen tension may be caused by increased epidermal thickness, oedema or increased metabolism consuming tissue oxygen. Clearance of topical xenon-133 was similar for lipodermatosclerotic and normal skin, suggesting lack of a diffusion barrier (Cheatle et al 1990). Oxygen consumption did not differ between lipodermatosclerotic and normal skin in one study (Stücker et al 2000). Laser Doppler fluxmetry studies recorded higher blood flow in lipodermatosclerotic skin than in normal skin at comparable anatomical sites (Sindrup et al 1987). Increased blood flow was also demonstrated in lipodermatosclerosis by positron emission tomography (Hopkins et al 1983). This paradox, that increased blood flow is present in skin with supposedly decreased oxygenation, suggests that not all venous ulcers can be attributed to poor nutrition of the skin (Vanscheidt et al 1991).

White cell trapping and inflammation

The luminal venous endothelium also undergoes profound changes due to CVI. Ultrastructural studies indicate that the endothelium is actively involved in synthesis of proteins such as endothelial cell adhesion molecules (Pappas et al 1997). Numerous immunohistochemical studies also attest to increased levels of the endothelial cell adhesion molecules ICAM-1, E-selectin and VCAM-1 and their ligands LFA-1 and VLA-4 on leukocytes with progressive stages of CVI in vessel valves and walls (Weyl et al 1996, Takase et al 2000, Rosner et al 2001). Soluble forms of these adhesion molecules are detected at elevated plasma levels in patients with chronic venous disease (Smith 1999). Also, the abnormal haemodynamic conditions in CVI, with sustained venous pressure because of the reduced pressure differential between the arterial and venous systems, effectively trap or slow white blood cells in the microvasculature of the skin (Coleridge Smith et al 1988). In addition, upregulated VEGF expression may increase vascular

permeability (Peschen et al 1998). These cellular, haemodynamic and molecular alterations all aid the infiltration of inflammatory cells into the dermal interstitium. The density of white blood cells is also increased at least seven-fold in CEAP class 4 patients and even more exaggeratedly in class 5 patients compared with normal skin 5 cm proximal to the medial malleolus (Scott et al 1991). An increased number of enlarged lymph nodes around the saphenofemoral junction was observed in patients with class 4–6 CEAP, pointing to an important role of inflammation in CVI (Labropoulos et al 2003).

Coleridge Smith et al (1988) ascribed the increased inflammatory infiltrate to the direct damage to the endothelium caused by sequestered activated neutrophils in the dependent lower leg by their release of reactive oxygen species (Siska et al 1999) and proteinases. This would enable transcapillary diffusion of macromolecules, along with extravasation of erythrocytes, and the formation of fibrin cuffs and haemosiderin deposition in the dermis. Perhaps the accumulation of iron in the diseased skin augments the generation of reactive oxygen species by the Fenton reaction (Ackerman et al 1988, Trenam et al 1992). Also, capillary occlusion by trapped neutrophils would result in focal tissue ischaemia (Fig. 8.3). In support of this hypothesis, the ratio of leg to arm oxygen free radical production of neutrophils from patients with underlying venous disease was highly elevated compared with healthy controls (Whiston et al 1994). The mechanisms that trigger neutrophil activation still remain to be elucidated.

Once initiated, the inflammatory response is perpetuated and is gradually converted into a chronic inflammatory state. Clinically, this is manifested by lipodermatosclerosis with fibrosis in the skin and subcutaneous tissue. Morphologically, the chronic inflammatory infiltrate is predominantly composed of macrophages and lymphocytes (Wilkinson et al 1993, Pappas et al 1997). Mast cells may also contribute to the fibrotic response (Pappas et al 1997). It is likely that different polypeptidic cytokines and growth factors mediate some of these processes. One candidate is the profibrotic and proinflammatory transforming growth factor (TGF)β1, which is also increased at the mRNA and protein levels in the lower leg skin of class 4 patients (Pappas et al 1999).

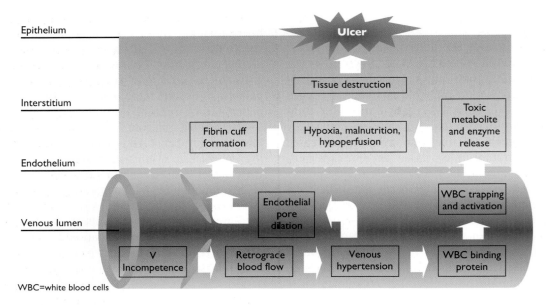

Figure 8.3   White blood cell trapping hypothesis. (From Leach M J 2004 Making sense of the venous leg ulcer debate: a literature review. Journal of Wound Care 13: 52–56, with permission of Emap Healthcare.)

The increased tissue remodelling in lipodermatosclerosis is also coupled with elevated degradative processes, primarily via proteinases. It is thought that excessive local proteolytic activity results in the breakdown of the matrix components of the skin, with the end result of an ulcer.

Role of tissue proteinases

The role of proteinases in the pathogenesis of venous leg ulcers is often discussed because of their tissue-destroying potential. Proteinases have multiple biological functions in skin homeostasis. They not only remodel extracellular matrix proteins but also modulate the bioactivity of cytokines and growth factors by several different mechanisms (Rogalski et al 2002, Stamenkovic 2003).

There are four classes of mammalian proteinase: aspartic proteinases, which require an aspartate residue for activity; cysteine proteinases, which require a cysteine residue for activity; metalloproteinases, including the matrix metalloproteinases (MMPs), which require zinc for activity; and serine proteinases, which require a serine residue for activity. The most pertinent proteinases in skin physiology and remodelling are the serine

proteinases plasmin, urokinase plasminogen activator, tissue-type plasminogen activator and neutrophil elastase, and the MMPs. MMPs are a family of zinc-dependent endopeptidases with 23 human members known to date (Stamenkovic 2003). Collectively, MMPs degrade all extracellular matrix (ECM) proteins.

Overall proteolytic activity, and interstitial collagenase-1 (MMP-1) and the gelatinases MMP-2 and MMP-9 specifically, have been studied in lipodermatosclerotic skin. Degradation of both type I and type IV collagens was increased more than twofold by tissue extracts from lipodermatosclerotic skin compared with normal skin (Herouy et al 1998). The findings indicate increased degradation of the major dermal structural and basement membrane proteins of epidermis and blood vessels in lipodermatosclerosis. The MMPs and possibly also neutrophil elastase appear to be responsible for this increased collagenolysis. MMP-1 makes the initial site-specific cleavage of native collagens and is thought to be the rate-limiting step in interstitial collagen degradation. The gelatinases MMP-2 and MMP-9 (formerly called type IV collagenases) are the major type IV collagen proteinases. In lipodermatosclerosis, MMP-1 protein levels were unaltered while the proteolytic active form of MMP-2 was increased compared with healthy skin (Herouy et al 1998, Saito et al 2001). MMP-2 is constitutively expressed in normal human skin and is capable of cleaving native type I collagen in vitro, albeit slowly and at high levels (Tam et al 2004). Furthermore, TGFβ1 upregulates MMP-2 in cultured human dermal fibroblasts (Kobayashi et al 2003). Surprisingly, the inflammatory-cell-derived MMP-9 did not differ between normal and lipodermatosclerotic skin (Herouy et al 1998, Saito et al 2001). Neutrophil elastase may also be involved in elevation of collagenolysis as it can cleave native type I collagen directly and indirectly by activating latent MMP-2. In addition, neutrophil elastase is capable of converting latent TGFβ1 into active TGFβ1. Increased active TGFβ1 may act as a chemotactic stimulus for invading neutrophils (Ashcroft et al 2000). Also, degradation products of ECM molecules are chemotactic for inflammatory cells, perpetuating the inflammatory process.

Ageing is probably a contributory factor because ulcer formation occurs predominantly in elderly people with atrophic skin. Several endogenous proteinases are increased with ageing because of the combined effect of ultraviolet radiation exposure and intrinsic ageing (Ashcroft et al 1997, Fisher et al 2002). Furthermore, ratios of MMPs and naturally occurring tissue inhibitors of metalloproteinases are also altered in normal skin with intrinsic ageing, favouring the catabolic processes with increased age (Ashcroft et al 1997). Thus, the proteolytic environment in CVI may also be age-dependent, increasing the propensity for ulcer formation of the skin of the lower leg in more elderly patients. Furthermore, increased collagen cross-linking increases the fragility of aged skin (Bailey 1978). Also, epidermal atrophy due to decreased epithelial proliferation and increased apoptosis with ageing increases the risk of skin breakdown (Gilhar et al 2004).

Fibroblasts in chronic venous insufficiency and venous leg ulcers

Fibroblasts serve important physiological functions in the skin. They maintain the homoeostatic balance of the dermal matrix by concurrently producing and degrading collagen and other ECM molecules.

The half-life of collagen is about 15 years in normal human dermis. Fibroblasts also provide paracrine regulation of epidermal homoeostasis. Fibroblasts are quiescent in normal skin but any traumatic or pathological distortion activates their replicative machinery.

CVI appears to influence several biological functions of fibroblasts. The most studied one is in vitro cell replication. For these analyses, resident fibroblasts are isolated from the CVI skin or ulcer and then cultured in vitro. A general feature of cultured fibroblasts is that they are programmed to undergo a certain number of cell divisions. With each cell division fibroblasts gradually lose their ability to proliferate and eventually reach a limit beyond which they are unable to proliferate, termed replicative cellular senescence. However, the existence of cellular senescence in living tissues is still debated in the literature (Hornsby 2002).

Independent research groups have demonstrated that dermal fibroblasts have decreased replicative potential and diminished mitogenic response to several growth factors the more advanced the CVI stage (Mendez et al 1998, Ågren et al 1999, Lal et al 2003, Vasquez et al 2004). Their morphology differs from that of normal dermal fibroblasts and resembles that of senescent cells. One study on venous leg ulcers identified substantial heterogeneity among fibroblasts cultured from chronic venous leg ulcers of varying duration (Ågren et al 1999). The fibroblasts displaying senescent growth behaviour, i.e. irreversible arrest of cell proliferation, were cultured from ulcers older than 3 years, while the fibroblasts from ulcers of less than 3 years' duration grew at almost the same rate as normal dermal fibroblasts (Fig. 8.4). These cell characteristics could be one of the reasons chronic venous ulcers heal slowly, if at all; in other words, the poorer the proliferative capacity of fibroblasts the slower the healing rate of the ulcers. There are clinical findings that support the results with the cultured fibroblasts. In a large cohort of leg ulcer patients in Scotland, it was shown that the more chronic the ulcer the less likely the ulcer is to heal. Particularly interesting was that patients who had had an ulcer for more than 3 years had only a 30% chance of being healed within 12 months of treatment compared with a 80% chance for ulcers of 3 months duration or less (Scottish Leg Ulcer Trial

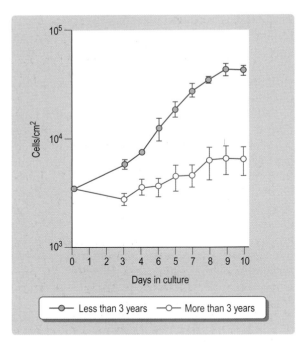

Figure 8.4 Growth kinetics of fibroblasts in vitro isolated from venous leg ulcers of less than 3 years' duration (n = 3) or more than 3 years' duration (n = 5). Wound fibroblasts from venous ulcers older than 3 years grew significantly slower than the fibroblasts derived from the younger venous leg ulcers.

Participants 2002). Furthermore, a positive correlation was found between the percentage of senescent fibroblasts in venous leg ulcers and the time to complete ulcer closure, another clinical correlate (Stanley & Osler 2001). Apart from ulcer duration, ulcer size is an important prognostic determinant of healing (Margolis et al 2004).

Other abnormal fibroblast functions have been observed, for example decreased motility in vitro and accumulation of the cytoskeletal protein α-smooth muscle actin, which are characteristics of myofibroblasts (Raffetto et al 2001). These cells are over-represented in fibrotic tissues, which may suggest that they contribute to some of the features of lipodermatosclerosis. It has been speculated that increased TGFβ1 levels induce these changes. Another, or an additional, inducer of myofibroblasts in skin is tryptase, a unique mast cell serine proteinase that promotes differentiation of normal human dermal fibroblasts into functional myofibroblasts in vitro (Gailit et al 2001).

The underlying mechanisms causing the irreversible phenotypic changes of fibroblasts from skin with chronic venous insufficiency are unknown. Possibly the oxidative stress and the continuous supply of growth-stimulating factors, as a consequence of the chronic inflammation, exhaust the proliferative capacity of fibroblasts. The proinflammatory cytokine tumour necrosis factor (TNF)α increases proliferation and decreases migration of fibroblasts (Leeb et al 2003, Moroguchi et al 2004). Another interesting hypothesis is that increased pressure per se can accelerate fibroblast ageing (Healey et al 2003).

It has been questioned whether the fibroblasts in diseased skin due to venous insufficiency are truly senescent (Stephens et al 2003). Nonetheless, fibroblast alterations are likely to be characteristic rather than causative factors of venous leg ulcers and more research is obviously needed to address this topic. The cellular findings again emphasize the importance of early intervention in CVI patients, otherwise these ulcers are likely to be beyond rescue.

CONCLUSIONS

Venous leg ulcers represent a common health problem with immense socioeconomic impact. Venous hypertension leads to a myriad of microangiopathological changes. In the most severe cases the skin breaks down and an ulcer develops. Several pathophysiological mechanisms have been proposed and are reviewed in this chapter. Does hypoxia, caused by local oedema, pericapillary cuffs and/or neutrophil occlusion, really predispose to ulcer formation? Is the trapping and activation of neutrophils initiating the skin destructive processes? What role do the chronic inflammatory infiltrate and proteinases play in the pathogenesis? Is the altered fibroblast phenotype a feature rather than a cause? None of these isolated hypotheses are without objections and thus the probable answer is that these factors act together. The challenge is to identify patients at risk and intervene early to prevent the occurrence of this in many cases irreversible disease in late stage. To elucidate the precise pathophysiological mechanisms, prospective, longitudinal studies involving a large number of individuals are needed. Until these results are available we have to rely on compression, the only documented prophylactic and effective conservative therapy (Cullum et al 2001).

Acknowledgements

The authors thank Drs Carita Hansson and Monica Kjær for scrutinizing the manuscript and Dr Tonny Karlsmark for providing clinical images.

References

Ackerman Z, Seidenbaum M, Loewenthal E et al 1988 Overload of iron in the skin of patients with varicose ulcers. Possible contributing role of iron accumulation in progression of the disease. Archives of Dermatology 124: 1376–1378

Adam D J, Bello M, Hartshorne T et al 2003a Role of superficial venous surgery in patients with combined superficial and segmental deep venous reflux. European Journal of Vascular and Endovascular Surgery 25: 469–472

Adam D J, Naik J, Hartshorne T et al 2003b The diagnosis and management of 689 chronic leg ulcers in a single-visit assessment clinic. European Journal of Vascular and Endovascular Surgery 25: 462–468

Adams E F 1949 The genuine works of Hippocrates. Sydenham Press, London

Ågren M S, Steenfos H H, Dabelsteen S et al 1999 Proliferation and mitogenic response to PDGF-BB of fibroblasts isolated from chronic venous leg ulcers is ulcer-age dependent. Journal of Investigative Dermatology 112: 463–469

Ågren M S, Eaglstein W H, Ferguson M W et al 2000 Causes and effects of the chronic inflammation in venous leg ulcers. Acta Dermato-Venereologica Supplementum 210: 3–17

Arnoldi C C, Linderholm H 1968 On the pathogenesis of the venous leg ulcer. Acta Chirurgica Scandinavica 134: 427–440

Ashcroft G S, Horan M A, Herrick S E et al 1997 Age-related differences in the temporal and spatial regulation of matrix metalloproteinases (MMPs) in normal skin and acute cutaneous wounds of healthy humans. Cell and Tissue Research 290: 581–591

Ashcroft G S, Lei K, Jin W et al 2000 Secretory leukocyte protease inhibitor mediates non-redundant functions necessary for normal wound healing. Nature Medicine 6: 1147–1153

Bailey A J 1978 Developmental changes of the collagen in normal dermis and in wound healing. Supplementum … ad Thrombosis and Haemostasis 63: 385–388

Balslev E, Thomsen H K, Danielsen L et al 1992 The occurrence of pericapillary fibrin in venous hypertension and ischaemic leg ulcers: a histopathological study. British Journal of Dermatology 126: 582–585

Barwell J R, Davies C E, Deacon J et al 2004 Comparison of surgery and compression with compression alone in chronic venous ulceration (ESCHAR study): randomised controlled trial. Lancet 363: 1854–1859

Bergan J J 1998 Venous insufficiency and perforating veins. British Journal of Surgery 85: 721–722

Bollinger A 1993 A rejected letter to the editors of the Lancet and the need for angiologists to prove their usefulness. Vasa 22: 361–363

Briggs M, Closs S J 2003 The prevalence of leg ulceration: a review of the literature. EWMA Journal 3(2): 14–18, 20

Browse N L, Burnand K G 1982 The cause of venous ulceration. Lancet 2: 243–245

Bruce A J, Bennett D D, Lohse C M et al 2002 Lipodermatosclerosis: review of cases evaluated at Mayo Clinic. Journal of the American Academy of Dermatology 46: 187–192

Bull R, Ansell G, Stanton A W et al 1995 Normal cutaneous microcirculation in gaiter zone (ulcer-susceptible skin) versus nearby regions in healthy young adults. International Journal of Microcirculation Clinical and Experimental 15: 65–74

Caggiati A 1999 The saphenous venous compartments. Surgical and Radiologic Anatomy 21: 29–34

Cheatle T R, McMullin G M, Farrah J et al 1990 Skin damage in chronic venous insufficiency: does an oxygen diffusion barrier really exist? Journal of the Royal Society of Medicine 83: 493–494

Coleridge Smith P D, Thomas P, Scurr J H et al 1988 Causes of venous ulceration: a new hypothesis. British Medical Journal (Clinical Research Edition) 296: 1726–1727

Coon W W, Willis P W III, Keller J B 1973 Venous thromboembolism and other venous disease in the Tecumseh community health study. Circulation 48: 839–846

Cullum N, Nelson E A, Fletcher A W et al 2001 Compression for venous leg ulcers. Cochrane Database Systematic Review, Issue 2, CD000265. Update Software, Oxford

De Rijcke P A, Hop W C, Wittens C H 2003 Subfascial endoscopic perforating vein surgery as treatment for lateral perforating vein incompetence and venous ulceration. Journal of Vascular Surgery 38: 799–803

Eliska O, Eliskova M 2001 Morphology of lymphatics in human venous crural ulcers with lipodermatosclerosis. Lymphology 34: 111–123

Evans C J, Fowkes F G, Ruckley C V et al 1999 Prevalence of varicose veins and chronic venous insufficiency in men and women in the general population: Edinburgh Vein Study. Journal of Epidemiology and Community Health 53(3): 149–153

Fagrell B 1982 Microcirculatory disturbances – the final cause for venous leg ulcers? Vasa 11: 101–103

Falanga V, Eaglstein W H 1993 The 'trap' hypothesis of venous ulceration. Lancet 341: 1006–1008

Falanga V, Moosa H H, Nemeth A J et al 1987 Dermal pericapillary fibrin in venous disease and venous ulceration. Archives of Dermatology 123: 620–623

Fisher G J, Kang S, Varani J et al 2002 Mechanisms of photoaging and chronological skin aging. Archives of Dermatology 138: 1462–1470

Fowkes F J, Price J F, Fowkes F G 2003 Incidence of diagnosed deep vein thrombosis in the general population: systematic review. European Journal of Vascular and Endovascular Surgery 25: 1–5

Gailit J, Marchese M J, Kew R R et al 2001 The differentiation and function of myofibroblasts is regulated by mast cell mediators. Journal of Investigative Dermatology 117: 1113–1119

Gilhar A, Ullmann Y, Karry R et al 2004 Ageing of human epidermis: the role of apoptosis, Fas and telomerase. British Journal of Dermatology 150: 56–63

Healey C, Forgione P, Lounsbury K M et al 2003 A new in vitro model of venous hypertension: the effect of pressure on dermal fibroblasts. Journal of Vascular Surgery 38: 1099–1105

Herouy Y, May A E, Pornschlegel G et al 1998 Lipodermatosclerosis is characterized by elevated expression and activation of matrix metalloproteinases: implications for venous ulcer formation. Journal of Investigative Dermatology 111: 822–827

Herrick S E, Sloan P, McGurk M et al 1992 Sequential changes in histologic pattern and extracellular matrix deposition during the healing of chronic venous ulcers. American Journal of Pathology 141: 1085–1095

Holling H E, Beecher H K, Linton R R 1938 Study of the tendency to edema formation associated with incompetence of valves of communicating veins of the leg. Journal of Clinical Investigation 17: 556–561

Hopkins N F, Spinks T J, Rhodes C G et al 1983 Positron emission tomography in venous ulceration and liposclerosis: study of regional tissue function. British Medical Journal (Clinical Research Edition) 286: 333–336

Hornsby P J 2002 Cellular senescence and tissue aging in vivo. Journals of Gerontology Series A: Biological Sciences and Medical Sciences 57: B251–B256

Howlader M H, Coleridge Smith P D 2004 Relationship of plasma vascular endothelial growth factor to CEAP clinical stage and symptoms in patients with chronic venous disease. European Journal of Vascular and Endovascular Surgery 27: 89–93

Howlader M H, Smith P D 2003 Microangiopathy in chronic venous insufficiency: quantitative assessment by capillary microscopy. European Journal of Vascular and Endovascular Surgery 26: 325–331

Kistner R L 1996 Definitive diagnosis and definitive treatment in chronic venous disease: a concept whose time has come. Journal of Vascular Surgery 24: 703–710

Kobayashi T, Hattori S, Shinkai H 2003 Matrix metalloproteinases-2 and -9 are secreted from human fibroblasts. Acta Dermato-Venereologica 83: 105–107

Labropoulos N, Leder D M, Kang S S et al 2003 Inflammation parallels severity of chronic venous insufficiency. Phlebology/Venous Forum of the Royal Society of Medicine 18: 78–82

Lal B K, Saito S, Pappas P J et al 2003 Altered proliferative responses of dermal fibroblasts to TGF-β1 may contribute to chronic venous stasis ulcer. Journal of Vascular Surgery 37: 1285–1293

Lee A J, Evans C J, Allan P L et al 2003 Lifestyle factors and the risk of varicose veins: Edinburgh Vein Study. Journal of Clinical Epidemiology 56: 171–179

Leeb S N, Vogl D, Gunckel M et al 2003 Reduced migration of fibroblasts in inflammatory bowel disease: role of inflammatory mediators and focal adhesion kinase. Gastroenterology 125: 1341–1354

Lees T A, Lambert D 1993 Patterns of venous reflux in limbs with skin changes associated with chronic venous insufficiency. British Journal of Surgery 80: 725–728

Lindemayr W, Lofferer O, Mostbeck A et al 1972 Arteriovenous shunts in primary varicosis? A critical essay. Vascular Surgery 6: 9–13

London N J, Nash R 2000 ABC of arterial and venous disease. Varicose veins. British Medical Journal 320: 1391–1394

Luetolf O, Bull R H, Bates D O et al 1993 Capillary underperfusion in chronic venous insufficiency: a cause for leg ulceration? British Journal of Dermatology 128: 249–254

Magnusson M B, Nelzén O, Risberg B et al 2001 A colour Doppler ultrasound study of venous reflux in patients with chronic leg ulcers. European Journal of Vascular and Endovascular Surgery 21: 353–360

Malanin K, Haapanen A, Kolari P J et al 1997 The peripheral resistance in arteries of legs is inversely proportional to the severity of chronic venous insufficiency. Acta Dermato-Venereologica 77: 22–25

Mani R, White J E, Barrett D F et al 1989 Tissue oxygenation, venous ulcers and fibrin cuffs. Journal of the Royal Society of Medicine 82: 345–346

Margolis D J, Allen-Taylor L, Hoffstad O et al 2004 The accuracy of venous leg ulcer prognostic models in a wound care system. Wound Repair and Regeneration 12: 163–168

Mekkes J R, Loots M A, Van Der Wal A C et al 2003 Causes, investigation and treatment of leg ulceration. British Journal of Dermatology 148: 388–401

Mendez M V, Stanley A, Phillips T et al 1998 Fibroblasts cultured from distal lower extremities in patients with venous reflux display cellular characteristics of senescence. Journal of Vascular Surgery 28: 1040–1050

Moroguchi A, Ishimura K, Okano K et al 2004 Interleukin-10 suppresses proliferation and remodeling of extracellular matrix of cultured human skin fibroblasts. European Surgical Research 36: 39–44

Nelzén O, Bergqvist D, Lindhagen A 1997 Long-term prognosis for patients with chronic leg ulcers: a prospective cohort study. European Journal of Vascular and Endovascular Surgery 13: 500–508

Nicolaides A N, Hussein M K, Szendro G et al 1993 The relation of venous ulceration with ambulatory venous pressure measurements. Journal of Vascular Surgery 17: 414–419

Pappas P J, DeFouw D O, Venezio L M et al 1997 Morphometric assessment of the dermal microcirculation in patients with chronic venous insufficiency. Journal of Vascular Surgery 26: 784–795

Pappas P J, You R, Rameshwar P et al 1999 Dermal tissue fibrosis in patients with chronic venous insufficiency is associated with increased transforming growth factor-β1 gene expression and protein production. Journal of Vascular Surgery 30: 1129–1145

Peschen M, Zeiske D, Laaff H et al 1996 Clinical histochemical and immunohistochemical investigation of the capillary basal membrane in chronic venous insufficiency. Acta Dermato-Venereologica 76: 433–436

Peschen M, Grenz H, Brand-Saberi B et al 1998 Increased expression of platelet-derived growth factor receptor alpha and beta and vascular endothelial growth factor in the skin of patients with chronic venous insufficiency. Archives of dermatological research 290: 291–297

Porter J M, Moneta G L 1995 Reporting standards in venous disease: an update. International Consensus Committee on Chronic Venous Disease. Journal of Vascular Surgery 21: 635–645

Raffetto J D, Mendez M V, Marien B J et al 2001 Changes in cellular motility and cytoskeletal actin in fibroblasts from patients with chronic venous insufficiency and in neonatal fibroblasts in the presence of chronic wound fluid. Journal of Vascular Surgery 33: 1233–1241

Rogalski C, Meyer-Hoffert U, Proksch E et al 2002 Human leukocyte elastase induces keratinocyte proliferation in vitro and in vivo. Journal of Investigative Dermatology 118: 49–54

Rosner K, Ross C, Karlsmark T et al 2001 Role of LFA-1/ICAM-1, CLA/E-selectin and VLA-4/VCAM-1 pathways in recruiting leukocytes to the various regions of the chronic leg ulcer. Acta Dermato-Venereologica 81: 334–339

Ruckley C V 1993 Does venous reflux matter? Lancet 341: 411–412

Ruckley C V, Evans C J, Allan P L et al 2002 Chronic venous insufficiency: clinical and duplex correlations. The Edinburgh Vein Study of venous disorders in the general population. Journal of Vascular Surgery 36: 520–525

Saito S, Trovato M J, You R et al 2001 Role of matrix metalloproteinases 1, 2, and 9 and tissue inhibitor of matrix metalloproteinase-1 in chronic venous insufficiency. Journal of Vascular Surgery 34: 930–938

Scott H J, Coleridge Smith P D 1989 Tissue oxygenation, venous ulcers and fibrin cuffs. Journal of the Royal Society of Medicine 82: 635–636

Scott H J, Coleridge Smith P D, Scurr J H 1991 Histological study of white blood cells and their association with lipodermatosclerosis and venous ulceration. British Journal of Surgery 78: 210–211

Scottish Leg Ulcer Trial Participants 2002 Effect of a national community intervention programme on healing rates of chronic leg ulcer: randomized controlled trial. Phlebology/Venous Forum of the Royal Society of Medicine 17: 47–53

Scriven J M, Hartshorne T, Bell P R et al 1997 Single-visit venous ulcer assessment clinic: the first year. British Journal of Surgery 84: 334–336

Shull K C, Nicolaides A N, Fernandes e Fernandes J et al 1979 Significance of popliteal reflux in relation to ambulatory venous pressure and ulceration. Archives of Surgery 114: 1304–1306

Sindrup J H, Avnstorp C, Steenfos H H et al 1987 Transcutaneous PO_2 and laser Doppler blood flow measurements in 40 patients with venous leg ulcers. Acta Dermato-Venereologica 67: 160–163

Siska I R, Avram J, Tatu C et al 1999 Some aspects concerning the antioxidant capacity of venous blood in lower limbs varicose veins. Advances in Experimental Medicine and Biology 471: 445–452

Smith P D 1999 Neutrophil activation and mediators of inflammation in chronic venous insufficiency. Journal of Vascular Research 36(Suppl 1): 24–36

Sparks S R, Ballard J L, Bergan J J et al 1997 Early benefits of subfascial endoscopic perforator surgery (SEPS) in healing venous ulcers. Annals of Vascular Surgery 11: 367–373

Stacey M C, Burnand K G, Bhogal B S et al 2000 Pericapillary fibrin deposits and skin hypoxia precede the changes of lipodermatosclerosis in limbs at increased risk of developing a venous ulcer. Cardiovascular Surgery (London) 8: 372–380

Stamenkovic I 2003 Extracellular matrix remodelling: the role of matrix metalloproteinases. Journal of Pathology 200: 448–464

Stanley A, Osler T 2001 Senescence and the healing rates of venous ulcers. Journal of Vascular Surgery 33: 1206–1211

Stephens P, Cook H, Hilton J et al 2003 An analysis of replicative senescence in dermal fibroblasts derived from chronic leg wounds predicts that telomerase therapy would fail to reverse their disease-specific cellular and proteolytic phenotype. Experimental Cell Research 283: 22–35

Stücker M, Falkenberg M, Reuther T et al 2000 Local oxygen content in the skin is increased in chronic venous incompetence. Microvascular Research 59: 99–106

Takase S, Bergan J J, Schmid-Schönbein G 2000 Expression of adhesion molecules and cytokines on saphenous veins in chronic venous insufficiency. Annals of Vascular Surgery 14: 427–435

Tam E M, Moore T R, Butler G S et al 2004 Characterization of the distinct collagen binding, helicase and cleavage mechanisms of matrix metalloproteinase 2 and 14 (gelatinase A and MT1-MMP): the differential roles of the MMP hemopexin c domains and the MMP-2 fibronectin type II modules in collagen triple helicase activities. Journal of Biological Chemistry 279: 43336–43344

Trenam C W, Blake D R, Morris C J 1992 Skin inflammation: reactive oxygen species and the role of iron. Journal of Investigative Dermatology 99: 675–682

Valencia I C, Falabella A, Kirsner R S et al 2001 Chronic venous insufficiency and venous leg ulceration. Journal of the American Academy of Dermatology 44: 401–421

Vanscheidt W, Stengele K, Wokalek H et al 1991 [Peri-capillary fibrin cuffs – an O_2 diffusion block?] Vasa 20: 142–146

Vasdekis S N, Clarke G H, Nicolaides A N 1989 Quantification of venous reflux by means of duplex scanning. Journal of Vascular Surgery 10: 670–677

Vasquez R, Marien B J, Gram C et al 2004 Proliferative capacity of venous ulcer wound fibroblasts in the presence of platelet-derived growth factor. Vascular and endovascular surgery 38: 355–360

Walker N, Rodgers A, Birchall N et al 2003 Leg ulceration as a long-term complication of deep vein thrombosis. Journal of Vascular Surgery 38: 1331–1335

Weyl A, Vanscheidt W, Weiss J M et al 1996 Expression of the adhesion molecules ICAM-1, VCAM-1, and E-selectin and their ligands VLA-4 and LFA-1 in chronic venous leg ulcers. Journal of the American Academy of Dermatology 34: 418–423

Whiston R J, Hallett M B, Davies E V et al 1994 Inappropriate neutrophil activation in venous disease. British Journal of Surgery 81: 695–698

Wilkinson L S, Bunker C, Edwards J C et al 1993 Leukocytes: their role in the etiopathogenesis of skin damage in venous disease. Journal of Vascular Surgery 17: 669–675

Wong J K, Duncan J L, Nichols D M 2003 Whole-leg duplex mapping for varicose veins: observations on patterns of reflux in recurrent and primary legs, with clinical correlation. European Journal of Vascular and Endovascular Surgery 25: 267–275

Zamboni P, Izzo M, Fogato L et al 2003 Urine hemosiderin: a novel marker to assess the severity of chronic venous disease. Journal of Vascular Surgery 37: 132–136

CHAPTER 9

Venous ulcers: patient assessment

Olle P. Nelzén

INTRODUCTION

Patient assessment has become increasingly important in the management of patients with chronic lower limb ulceration. A correct diagnosis at the start of the treatment will allow choice of the most appropriate treatment, thereby minimizing unnecessary delay in achieving leg ulcer healing (Nelzén et al 1991, Norwegian Medicines Control Authority 1995, Nelzén 1999, Ghauri et al 2000). In early studies the examination was more limited and often simply involved inspection of the ulcer, looking for clinical signs of venous disease (Nelzén 1999). However, not all ulcers are pure venous and there are other aetiologies to consider as well. Ulcers of mixed aetiology have proved to be quite common, which underlines the need for a more thorough investigation to disclose all possible factors that might negatively influence healing (Nelzén et al 1991). It is essential that clinicians can make an appropriate assessment and diagnosis of the cause of ulceration in order to select the most appropriate treatment. In addition, a thorough patient assessment may also minimize the risk of future ulcer recurrence (Nelzén 1999). Tailored treatment has without doubt become increasingly important, not least when venous leg ulcers are concerned (Nelzén et al 1991, Barwell et al 2004).

Box 9.1 lists the clinical requirements for first assessment. For primary care these consist of ulcer history, medical history, clinical examination and hand-held Doppler assessments (Norwegian Medicines Control Authority 1995). This basic information will generally give you enough information to be able to make a preliminary diagnosis and to establish a treatment strategy or management plan. The general view for venous ulceration is to offer further diagnostic testing; however, this is not always readily available for all patients (Coleridge Smith 1992, Norwegian Medicines Control Authority 1995, Nicolaides 2000). Colour Doppler ultrasound (CDU), often called duplex scanning, is ideal for providing detailed mapping of the venous dysfunction (Nicolaides 2000). The latter is recommended when venous surgery is considered but can also give valuable information aiding further conservative management. Reassessment is required if the ulcer does not heal according to plan or frequently recurs.

ULCER HISTORY

A number of factors may need to be considered to understand the problem of ulceration in individual patients – first-time or recurrent ulcer, length of ulcer episode, patient reported cause of ulceration, family history of leg ulceration. In addition, it may be helpful to estimate the total number of ulcer episodes.

Information about pain related to the ulcer is important. A description of the type of pain, using a validated pain tool, may help differential diagnosis and identification of patients with arterial insufficiency. Pain has also been identified as a major issue for patients in terms of their health-related quality of life. The issue of pain is described in more detail in Chapter 29.

Box 9.1 *Important components of primary assessment of patients with leg ulcers*

- Medical history
- Ulcer history
- Clinical examination
- Inspection of the ulcer
- Hand held Doppler assessments
  - Arterial
  - Venous

Register what treatments have been given for the ulcer – topical dressings and eventual compression treatment? Try to assess whether effective compression has been used or not. Has the patient had a single or multilayer compression regime or none at all?

MEDICAL HISTORY

For chronic leg ulcers there are some diseases that are more important to know about than others. Cardiovascular diseases are commonly detected among ulcer patients and angina pectoris, myocardial infarction, stroke and hypertension should be asked for. Equally, intermittent claudication is valuable to ask for: does the patient have to stop because of pain upon walking and is the pain relieved after some minutes of resting? Has the patient undergone previous major surgery? You also need to know if the patient is or has been a smoker. Diabetes is commonly detected and it is obviously important to know how it is treated, with insulin, oral drugs, diet or combinations. These are all diseases or conditions raising the likelihood of associated arterial disease in the legs.

For venous ulcers information regarding varicose veins, deep venous thrombosis and previous venous surgery (including varicose vein surgery or sclerotherapy) is of importance. Family history of deep venous thrombosis is an indication of a possible hereditary coagulation disorder, which might require further investigation. Joint disorders can be

of importance by affecting the muscle pumps in the calf and foot negatively. Rheumatoid arthritis may, apart from lowering muscle pump function, also directly be a causative factor through small vessel vasculitis, which sometimes can be the ultimate cause or an additive factor to venous insufficiency.

Knowledge about medication is vital since some drugs may actually case ulceration. Warfarin, for example, can sometimes cause necrotic wounds and some loop-diuretics such as furosemide may cause secondary vasculitis resulting in ulceration.

CLINICAL EXAMINATION

The extent of the clinical examination depends on the professional level of the examiner. A physician ought to perform a regular body assessment, including inspection, palpation and auscultation. A nurse may focus on inspection of the affected limb combined with blood pressure measurements. Apart from this, the investigation should at all times include hand-held Doppler (HHD) assessments of ankle pressures and arm pressures allowing calculation of ankle/brachial pressure index (ABPI). To rely on simply palpation of distal pulses has been shown not to be reliable to rule out arterial insufficiency (Norwegian Medicines Control Authority 1995, Scottish Intercollegiate Guidelines Network 1998, Stacey et al 2002).

Inspection of the limb

Register the location of the ulcer and the number of ulcers, and estimate the size of the ulcer/ulcers. Venous ulcers are most often located in the gaiter area and preferentially medially located. Ulcers of lateral location may also occur but, if ulcers are located on unusual locations, look for differential diagnoses. The size can be measured by tracing of the margins on a transparent plastic sheet, or by measuring the two maximum perpendicular axes, giving the approximate size (length × width) in centimetres (Scottish Intercollegiate Guidelines Network 1998; Ghauri et al 2000). An excellent way to document the size is to use digital photography, but remember to include in the picture some sort of ruler to refer to. By using a length reference the size can be measured later from the picture. There are computer programmes available today where you can use a picture and trace the margins of the ulcer to calculate the ulcer size.

Inspection of the ulcer

Then look at the ulcer by inspecting the edges and the base of the ulcer. Are the edges shallow or punched out and are there signs of epithelialization? What does the base of the ulcer look like? Is it healthy granulating red, covered with yellow slough or are even black necrosis present? If the slough is greenish in colour the ulcer might be colonized or infected with *Pseudomonas*, requiring a swab taken for bacteriological culture. Is the wound wet or is it dry? White softening of the skin margins indicates exudation. Ulcers in legs with heavy oedema are often heavily wet. Ulcers that are deep and exposing tendons are likely not to be of pure venous origin. If you see areas of the ulcer that look strange and differs from the rest of the ulcer, one should be aware of the risk of a carcinoma, which may occasionally develop in venous ulcers. Multiple punch biopsies or even surgical biopsies are advocated under such circumstances.

Inspection of the skin

Well known signs of venous insufficiency are pigmentation, eczema, lipodermatosclerosis and oedema (Fig. 9.1). Visible varicose veins can also indicate a venous component but are not always seen, especially in overweight patients. In such cases, HHD can easily disclose venous insufficiency, as described below. The easiest way to assess whether there is oedema or not is to press your finger against the skin and see if an impression of the skin is the result. If so, we call it a pitting oedema, which is most often caused by venous dysfunction or heart failure. If there is no pitting oedema the swelling can be caused by insufficient drainage of lymph – lymphoedema. Such an oedema only rarely causes ulceration. If the swelling includes the dorsum of the foot this might indicate lymphatic origin. Measuring the circumferences of the calf and gaiter area may be valuable to assess the extent of oedema especially if the swelling is unilateral. Changes of circumferential measurements might be one way of monitoring success of compression treatment.

The nature of the surrounding skin can sometimes indicate inflammatory activity, shifting from

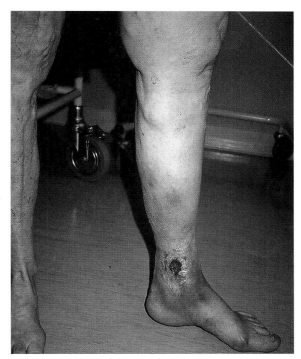

Figure 9.1 A classical venous ulcer with medial location, pigmentation, eczema and visible varicose veins

red to purple depending on the grade of inflammatory activity. A widespread erythema may indicate infection by streptococci, erysipelas, and should result in a bacteriological swab taken and immediate treatment with penicillin. A mixed bluish and red skin border around the ulcer can indicate vasculitis often with areas of skin necrosis surrounding irregularly shaped ulcers. Dry skin with scaling may be caused by a venous eczema. Pigmentation, eczema and fibrosis of the skin and the subcutaneous tissues (lipodermatosclerosis) are all signs indicating possible venous disease. Eczema can sometimes be caused by contact allergy caused by ointments or dressings. If the eczema is defined by the borders of the dressing an allergy might be present.

A simple test of the arterial circulation is to elevate the feet and see if they become pale and then lower the feet into dependency. If the foot or feet turn red with a slight bluish touch, arterial insufficiency may be present; this can be confirmed by performing ABPI measurements.

HAND-HELD DOPPLER INVESTIGATIONS

An HHD is an extremely useful tool that should be used by all health-care professionals who see leg ulcer patients on a regular basis (Norwegian Medicines Control Authority1995, Nelzén 1999). It can give valuable information regarding not only the arterial circulation but also the presence or absence of venous insufficiency in deep and/or superficial veins. Information regarding eventual arterial insufficiency is not only needed to select patients for vascular surgery but is also valuable when deciding what kind of compression regimen to use. Further, if the patient complains of pain as a result of compression treatment it is reassuring for the practitioner to know that it is probably not caused by undetected arterial insufficiency. If normal ABPIs have been recorded it is highly unlikely that impaired arterial circulation is causing the pain. There is a general recommendation that ankle pressures should always be measured in leg ulcer patients, in contrast to venous assessments, which have not yet been widely used. It is acknowledged that training is required to use HHD, but this is readily available at centres seeing large numbers of patients.

The required tools are an HHD, ultrasound gel, a rubber tourniquet and blood pressure cuff (Fig. 9.2). The basic recommendations for primary care applied in Sweden and Norway are to measure ABPIs and to assess if there is reflux (venous insufficiency) in the popliteal vein (Norwegian Medicines Control Authority 1995).

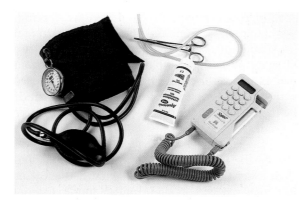

Figure 9.2 Equipment needed to perform assessment with hand-held Doppler

Table 9.1 Interpretation of ankle brachial pressure index levels

ABPI	Interpretation
>0.9	Normal
0.8–0.9	Minor arterial impairment; not likely to influence healing
0.5–0.7	Substantial arterial impairment; may influence healing
<0.5	Critical ischaemia; refer patient to vascular surgeon

How to measure ankle pressure

This is described in detail in Chapter 16. A summary of the interpretation of observed ankle brachial pressure index (ABPI) levels in relation to leg ulceration is shown in Table 9.1.

If the clinical picture indicates possible arterial insufficiency, refer the patient for specialist assessment.

Venous assessment with Doppler

The clinical examination can reveal signs of venous insufficiency, such as varicose veins, pigmentation, eczema, lipodermatosclerosis and oedema, enough to make a venous aetiology highly likely. But the clinical picture can not decide whether the insufficiency engages the deep veins, the superficial veins or both. It is also important to acknowledge that in up to 20% of cases varicose veins may not be visible although there is marked reflux detected by HHD assessment. Recent studies have confirmed the clinical impression that patients with venous ulcers caused by isolated superficial venous insufficiency are best treated with a combination of initial compression treatment and early varicose vein surgery (Nelzén 1999, Barwell et al 2000, 2004). HHD allows for the early selection of appropriate patients (Norwegian Medicines Control Authority 1995, Nelzén 1999). Venous assessment using HHD will not give sufficient information on whether to perform surgery but can act as a screening tool to identify patients who may benefit from surgery. The use of HHD in the community can act as a useful decision-making tool for referral to a specialist vascular unit for CDU. Screening with HHD is rapidly performed and quite easily learned. It is suitable to use this venous screening in conjunction with Doppler assessments of the arterial circulation. This screening can be performed by doctors, nurses or vascular technologists.

Venous screening procedure

Venous screening using HHD is only applicable for patients who have not previously undergone surgery for varicose veins. For patients with recurrent varicose veins a CDU scan is recommended, because of the changed anatomy following surgery (Coleridge Smith 1997, Nicolaides 2000). The patient is preferably examined in a standing position with the leg to be examined not weight-bearing. To detect reflux (venous insufficiency) in the veins, blood flow is simulated by manual compression of the calf muscles. This action forces blood to flow upwards in the major leg veins, which is detected by the Doppler probe as a short flow of blood in the insonated vein segment. Calf muscle compression is used for assessing deep as well as superficial veins (Fig. 9.3).

The veins are insonated at three specific sites: the groin, the medial aspect of the knee and the back of the knee (Fig. 9.4). At the first two sites the competency of the great saphenous vein is tested and in the popliteal fossa competency of the popliteal vein and the small saphenous vein is tested. Finding the saphenous vein in the groin is facilitated by tapping lightly on visible varicosities distally to force blood to flow in the saphenous vein. The saphenofemoral junction is generally found in the groin slightly medial to the palpable pulses in the femoral artery.

With the probe insonating the great saphenous vein, applying calf compression followed by release of compression tests for reflux. If the vein is incompetent a reflux of blood is heard that can last for several seconds. A short reflux lasting less than half a second may be functional, reflecting the time needed for the venous valves to close, and is considered normal. If reflux is confirmed in the saphenous vein on the medial aspect of the knee, great saphenous vein stripping is generally indicated.

The valves of the popliteal vein are crucial for the prognosis of superficial venous surgery. Complete cure can generally only be expected if there is no reflux detected in the popliteal vein. It is therefore extremely important to assess popliteal vein function. The vein is located by using the Doppler probe in the popliteal fossae (Fig. 9.4B). First, locate the pulsating popliteal artery. Second, when you hear the pulses clearly the vein can usually be found since it is running close by the artery. Third, use manual calf compression and listen for

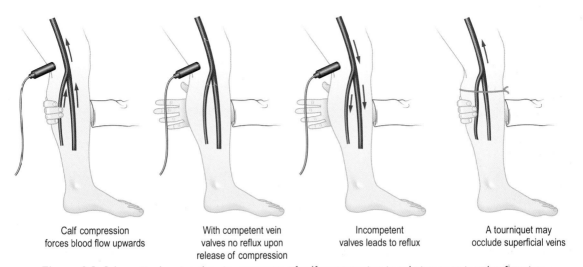

| Calf compression forces blood flow upwards | With competent vein valves no reflux upon release of compression | Incompetent valves leads to reflux | A tourniquet may occlude superficial veins |

Figure 9.3 Schematic drawing showing outcome of calf compression in relation to vein valve function

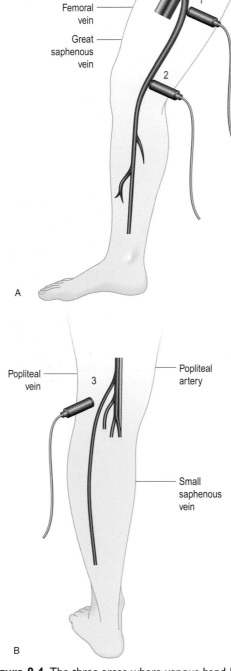

Femoral
artery

Femoral
vein

Great
saphenous
vein

1

2

A

Popliteal
vein

3

Popliteal
artery

Small
saphenous
vein

B

Figure 9.4 The three areas where venous hand-held Doppler screening is performed: (**A**) the groin (1), the medial lower part of the thigh (2) and (**B**) the popliteal fossa (3)

venous blood flow (Fig. 9.5A). When the upward flow of blood has ceased, release the compression and listen for the eventual reflux of blood (Fig. 9.5B). If reflux in the deep veins takes longer than half a second it is considered to indicate significant incompetence.

It can be difficult to determine which vessels are incompetent in the popliteal fossa because of the close proximity of a number of vessels. Reflux can be due to deep venous insufficiency in the popliteal vein, the small saphenous vein or even muscle veins. In order to determine which vessels are involved one can occlude the short saphenous vein with a rubber tourniquet (Figs 9.3, 9.5C). If the reflux in the popliteal fossa disappears with the tourniquet, the reflux probably derives from the short saphenous vein. CDU will give definitive evidence of the site of incompetence and ought to be used regularly in younger patients and in patients where small saphenous vein insufficiency is suspected. A flow chart of the primary venous assessment with hand-held Doppler is shown in Figure 9.6.

ADDITIONAL INVESTIGATIONS

As well as HHD assessment you often need to confirm your findings by using more sophisticated techniques, especially when surgery or another intervention is considered. These techniques can be divided into non-invasive and invasive and there are in addition other techniques, mostly aimed at investigating microcirculatory disturbances. The available additional investigations are listed in Table 9.2.

Non invasive techniques

Colour Doppler ultrasound

Patients with presumed venous ulcers according to the result of the patient assessment described above ought to, if possible, be offered a CDU scan (alternatively called a duplex scan) to map the true nature of their underlying venous dysfunction (Fig. 9.7; Norwegian Medicines Control Authority 1995, Nelzén 1999). This is especially important for patients who may be considered for venous surgery. While venous ulcer healing may occur with compression therapy, venous surgery may prevent

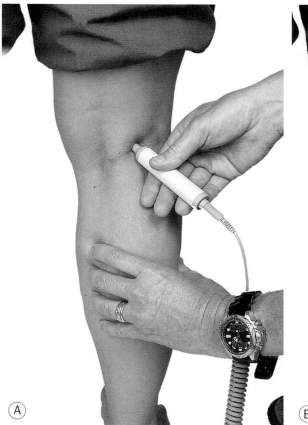

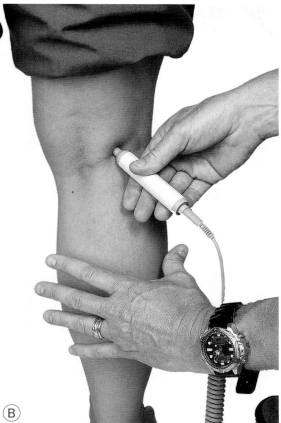

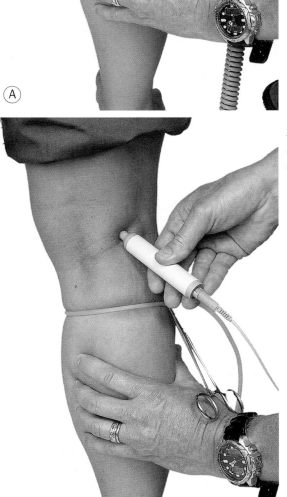

Figure 9.5 (**A**) Calf compression to achieve a proximal flow of venous blood. (**B**) Release of compression to assess for reflux. (**C**) In case of reflux, does occlusion of superficial veins with a tourniquet abolish reflux?

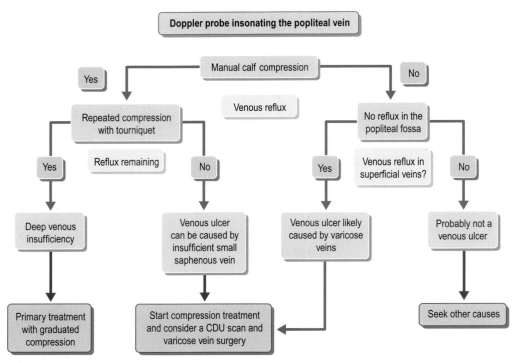

Figure 9.6 Flow chart of the primary venous assessment with hand-held Doppler

Table 9.2 Comparison of different additional techniques to investigate patients with presumed venous ulcers.

Technique of investigation	Anatomical information?	Haemodynamic information?	Invasive?
Colour Doppler ultrasound	Yes	Yes (detailed)	No
Phlebography	Yes	No	Yes
Plethysmography	No	Yes (global)	No
Ambulatory venous pressure	No	Yes (global)	Yes
Magnetic resonance imaging	Yes	No	No
Computed tomography	Yes	No	(Yes)

Detailed, qualitative venous function for all individual venous segments; Global, quantitative data on global venous function of the whole leg only.

recurrence of the venous ulcer and should be considered. A CDU scan is also indicated for patients with recurrent varicose veins after previous venous surgery. In practice it is reasonable to assess almost all patients who are mobile and reasonably healthy with CDU at least once, which is the current recommendation in Scandinavia and the general consensus among experts in the field of venous disease worldwide (Coleridge Smith 1992, Norwegian Medicines Control Authority 1995, Nicolaides 2000). However, access to CDU is highly variable between and within countries. This may lead to the use of alternative methods of venous assessment, which are detailed below.

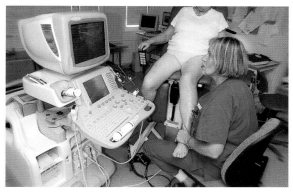

Figure 9.7 Colour Doppler ultrasound examination for venous disease

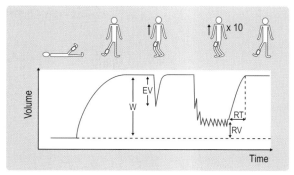

Figure 9.8 An example of a volume curve from a plethysmographic examination, showing the effect of posture and muscle activity. VV, venous volume; EV, expelled volume; RV, residual volume; RT, recovery time

Plethysmography

There are several different techniques for performing this investigation producing a similar result. The most commonly used is probably strain gauge plethysmography; the others are air plethysmography, foot volumetry and light reflection rheography (also called photoplethysmography, PPG; Nicolaides & Miles 1987, Christopoulos et al 1988). These methods are non-invasive and globally measure venous function in the leg. Therefore these methods cannot be used to assess specific veins or segments of veins, because of lack of precision. In clinical practice they offer only limited extra information to a CDU scan but may be useful methods when CDU is unavailable or when venous obstruction is suspected. They can also detect calf muscle pump dysfunction in cases with swelling and no detectable venous reflux, a common problem in venous ulcer patients. The most commonly reported parameter is the venous recovery time (RT) which is a measure of the time to refill distal veins after exercise (usually 10 tiptoes to empty the veins). The shorter the RT the more severe the venous insufficiency. A RT of less than 18 seconds in a standing position is considered pathological. An example of a volume curve produced by these techniques is shown in Figure 9.8.

There are portable devices available that can be used in the community to detect possible venous insufficiency. Using tourniquets to try to distinguish deep from superficial reflux has been shown to be unreliable even in the hands of experienced vascular technologists. Detecting venous reflux by using HHD is easier and a cheaper, since the Doppler is used to measure ankle pressures, which generally can give more valuable information.

Magnetic resonance imaging

This fairly new technique is constantly developing, and today good anatomical images of the venous system can be obtained. It is useful for detecting venous obstruction in pelvic or abdominal veins, especially in patients where phlebography can not be used. However, it cannot at present give functional information. Another drawback is its generally low availability and high cost. An advantage is that it is non-invasive.

Invasive techniques

Ambulatory venous pressure

This is an invasive method of assessing venous pressure in the distal veins of the leg (Kuiper 1964, Nicolaides & Zukowski 1986). Usually, the pressure is measured by cannulating a foot vein. The normal venous pressure in such a vein is in the range 15–30 mmHg. An elevated resting venous pressure indicates venous disease and there is a clear correlation between the severity of venous disease and the degree of elevation of the pressure. Thus leg ulcer patients generally have elevated venous pressures, often in the range 45–85 mmHg. As for the plethysmographic methods, the ambulatory venous pressure (AVP) recovery time can be measured after 10 tiptoe movements. A RT of less than 18 seconds is usually considered pathological. An

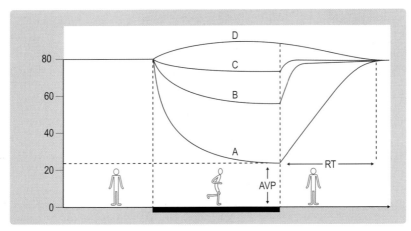

Figure 9.9 Schematic drawing of the ambulatory venous pressure (AVP) in mmHg for (**A**) a normal patient, (**B**) a patient with varicose veins, (**C**) a patient with deep venous insufficiency and (**D**) a patient with deep venous obstruction. RT, recovery time

example of the pressure curves produced is shown in Figure 9.9.

As with the other plethysmographic methods, AVP can only be used to assess global venous function but is probably the most reliable physiological tool for quantifying venous function. It is, however, of limited value in everyday practice since it adds very limited extra information in the clinical situation. Thus it is today normally used only for research purposes in laboratories at hospitals. A further disadvantage is that cannulation of a vein on the dorsum of the foot can be rather painful for the patient.

Phlebography
Ascending and descending phlebography used to be the techniques for investigating patients with venous disorders before CDU became available (Nicolaides 2000). Unlike CDU, phlebography can only give anatomical information and only very limited haemodynamic information can be obtained. Dynamic phlebography can be carried out at certain centres by using a video technique, but is rarely indicated unless deep venous reconstruction is considered. Varicography can be helpful in certain cases of venous malformation or unusual cases of varicose vein recurrence where CDU can not map the situation adequately. Ascending phlebography is still used in the diagnosis of deep vein

thrombosis if CDU is inconclusive. These investigations are invasive and require use of iodine contrast material, which may be harmful to patients with an allergy to iodine or impaired renal function.

Computed tomography
Computed tomography represents the modern way of performing phlebography. It has a similar ability to MRI to provide anatomical information but so far lacks the ability to provide functional information. Furthermore, iodine contrast has to be given and the risk of radiation has to be considered. As for MRI, availability and costs are also important negative factors that restrict the use of this method.

Microcirculatory assessments

Assessment of the microcirculation is seldom of value in venous insufficiency other than for research purposes. Basically, three different techniques have been used to investigate the pathophysiology of venous ulceration.

Laser Doppler
The technique measures movement in the skin and subdermal space and transforms this to an electrical signal. The output is believed to in some way reflect the circulation in the area, arterial and venous, but may also reflect other movements in

the tissue fluids. It has mostly been used to assess the arterial microcirculation and it has currently no place in the diagnosis of venous disease. It is considered simply to be a research tool.

Transcutaneous oxygen pressure measurement

Transcutaneous oxygen pressure measurement assesses the oxygen tension of the tissues surrounding the ulcer. It is a difficult method to use in venous patients for technical reasons and because the oxygen tension varies considerably in the vicinity of the ulcer. It can be low because of lipodermatosclerosis in one area and very high in a neighbouring area with dilated capillaries. The method is of more value in patients with arterial insufficiency and is of little value in patients with venous ulceration. Furthermore, lack of oxygen is not nowadays considered to be of major importance for the development of venous ulcers. This is a technique for research purposes only.

Capillary microscopy

Previous research has shown that patients with venous ulcers have certain characteristic anatomical findings in the capillaries of the foot. These changes are usually monitored by examining the skin at the base of the nails with a special microscope. Typically there are fewer but elongated and very tortuous capillaries in patients with chronic venous insufficiency. The technique is not easily performed and the information gained is of little or no value for clinical purposes. It is strictly a research tool.

Blood samples

There is no need primarily to take blood samples from the routine patient with a typical venous ulcer. If the diagnosis is uncertain or if healing does not proceed as expected upon standard treatment, there might be indications for certain blood samples to be obtained. This screening should look for anaemia, diabetes or elevated inflammatory parameters such as CRP. Rheumatic disease may also sometimes be worth looking for, as well as thrombophilia in patients with presumed postthrombotic limbs.

Biopsies

If malignancy or systemic vasculitis is suspected, multiple biopsies are recommended. There is more detailed discussion of malignant ulceration in Chapter 19.

Venous obstruction

Venous obstruction can sometimes be suspected, especially in patients with a history of previous deep vein thrombosis and severe swelling of the leg. An indication of proximal obstruction is the finding of a continuous flow in the femoral vein in the groin that does not follow respiration. In certain cases, further investigations with invasive technology such as phlebography or functional tests with plethysmography or AVP measurements may be required.

ULCER DIAGNOSIS

The result of the patient assessment ought to provide enough information to be able to set a preliminary ulcer diagnosis. Although venous ulcers are the most common type of chronic leg ulcers there are several differential diagnoses to consider (Nelzén et al 1991, 1999, Ghauri et al 2000). Ulcers of mixed venous and arterial cause are increasingly common, because of ageing populations. Even more complicated cases, with ulcers of multifactorial aetiology, are quite often encountered, where venous insufficiency may be one of several causative factors but not necessarily the dominating factor. The diagnosis forms the basis for the choice of treatment strategy, which should be reassessed if healing does not occur. An example of a classification for clinical use is shown in Table 9.3. This classification is subclassified for venous disease according to the outcome of HHD or CDU scanning, which is helpful in order to select patients in whom early varicose surgery might be a treatment option. The important information is whether the venous insufficiency engages the deep veins, and the popliteal vein in particular, or if it is confined to the superficial venous system only. In the latter case, early varicose vein surgery ought to be considered (Nelzén 1999, Barwell et al 2004).

Table 9.3 Modified leg ulcer classification according to Nelzén et al (1991)

Aetiological group	Definition
1. Venous*	Ulcers caused by venous insufficiency or obstruction without any other causative factor present
2. Mixed venous and arterial*	Ulcers of predominantly venous cause combined with detectable arterial impairment. ABPI generally 0.7–0.9
3. Mixed arterial and venous[†]	Ulcers of predominantly arterial cause combined with a minor venous insufficiency – usually superficial. ABPI generally 0.7 or lower
4. Arterial[†]	Ulcers associated with arterial insufficiency only. ABPI generally 0.7 or lower
5. Arterial and diabetes[†]	Ulcers caused by a combination of arterial insufficiency and diabetic neuropathy – 'neuroischaemic ulcers'. Any sign of arterial insufficiency (non-compressible arteries included) + neuropathy
6. Diabetes	Ulcers caused by neuropathy or diabetes-related skin disorders such as necrobiosis lipoidica diabeticorum
7. Traumatic	Pure trauma-induced ulcers with no other predisposing factor present
8. Pressure	Pure pressure-induced ulcers without any other predisposing factors present
9. Multifactorial A + V + D	Combinations of arterial, venous and diabetic causes, without any of the factors obviously dominating
10. Other multifactorial	Other combinations of aetiological factors with no obviously dominating factor
11. Other single cause	Other single causes of leg ulcers, such as vasculitis, skin tumours, etc.

* Can be subdivided into a) ulcers with deep vein involvement (popliteal vein) and b) ulcers caused by superficial venous insufficiency alone (varicose veins).
† Can be divided into ulcers caused by critical ischaemia (ABPI < 0.5) and ulcers of possible arterial cause.
ABPI, Ankle/brachial pressure index.

DOCUMENTATION

Many units today use some kind of scheme or protocol to document the information gathered during the primary patient assessment (Scottish Intercollegiate Guidelines Network 1998). Digitally stored data and photographs of ulcers greatly enhance patient management, and healing can be more easily followed and documented.

SUMMARY

It should be emphasized that primary patient assessment has become increasingly important in the management of patients with chronic leg ulcers. To secure a preliminary ulcer diagnosis is the primary goal. The diagnosis should be based on medical and ulcer history, inspection and HHD assessments of the arterial and preferably also the venous circulation. A diagnosis of venous ulcer is supported by the typical signs of hypostatic skin changes (pigmentation, eczema and lipodermatosclerosis), and HHD-detected reflux in superficial and/or deep veins. A diagnosis of mixed venous and arterial ulcer is checked by assessing ankle pressures using Doppler and ABPI calculations. It is important to find patients with potentially correctable venous disease early and a prerequisite for this is that the venous function is assessed with at least HHD, preferably supported later by a complete CDU scan to map the venous insufficiency in greater detail. It is important to realize that clinical examination and inspection cannot differentiate a venous ulcer caused by deep vein insufficiency from an ulcer caused by varicose veins. Tailored treatment is today possible for a large group of patients with venous or mixed venous and arterial ulcers, in whom combined use of vascular surgery and conservative compression is likely to result in improved long-term healing and a minimized risk of ulcer recurrence (Nelzén 1999, Barwell et al 2000, 2004). Preliminary selection of such patients can often be made based on the result of a carefully conducted primary patient assessment, as described in this chapter. Patients with clinical and Doppler signs of isolated superficial venous insufficiency can be detected early and ought, if otherwise healthy, to be offered further assessment with CDU scan. Such selection cannot be performed on the basis of clinical symptoms alone.

It is, however, important to bear in mind that all ulcers are not venous and that other diagnoses should be sought if the assessment fails to show evidence of a typical venous nature. By establishing the ulcer diagnosis early, the most appropriate treatment or combinations of treatments are likely to be given to the patient without unnecessary delay. Without a thorough primary assessment, there may be delay in prescribing the most appropriate treatment. It is important to reassess and to question the diagnosis if healing can not be achieved. The assessment ought to serve as a guide as to the best treatment to achieve healing and ideally also the best management strategy to prevent future recurrence of ulceration. The quality of the primary patient assessment is likely to be of great importance for the outcome for the individual patient.

References

Barwell J R, Taylor M, Deacon J et al 2000 Surgical correction of isolated superficial venous reflux reduces long term recurrence rate in chronic venous leg ulcers. European Journal of Vascular and Endovascular Surgery 20: 363–368

Barwell J R, Davies C E, Deacon J et al 2004 Comparison of surgery and compression with compression alone in chronic venous ulceration (ESCHAR study): randomised controlled trial. Lancet 363: 1854–1859

Christopoulos D, Nicolaides A N, Szendro G 1988 Venous reflux: quantification and correlation with the clinical severity of venous disease. British Journal of Surgery 75: 352–356

Coleridge Smith P D 1992 Investigations of Patients with Venous Ulceration. Phlebology Supplement 1: 17–21

Ghauri A S, Taylor M C, Deacon J E et al 2000 Influence of a specialized leg ulcer service on management and outcome. British Journal of Surgery 87: 1048–1056

Kuiper J P 1964 Venous pressure determination (direct method). Dermatologica. 132: 206–217

Nelzén O 1999 How can we improve outcomes for leg ulcer patients? In: Ruckley V, Bradbury A (eds) Venous disease: epidemiology, management and delivery of care. Springer, London, pp 246–253

Nelzén O, Bergqvist D, Lindhagen A 1991 Leg ulcer etiology. A cross sectional population study. Journal of Vascular Surgery 14: 557–564

Nicolaides A N 2000 Investigation of chronic venous insufficiency: a consensus statement. Circulation 102: E126–E163

Nicolaides A N, Miles C 1987 Photoplethysmography in the assessment of venous insufficiency. Journal of Vascular Surgery 5: 405–412

Nicolaides A N, Zukowski A J 1986 The value of dynamic venous pressure measurements. World Journal of Surgery 10: 919–924

Norwegian Medicines Control Authority 1995 Workshop: Treatment of venous leg ulcers: recommendations. Norwegian Medicines Control Authority, Oslo, vol 5, pp 9–32

Scottish Intercollegiate Guidelines Network 1998 The care of patients with chronic leg ulcer. SIGN Publication 26. Scottish Intercollegiate Guidelines Network, Edinburgh

Stacey M et al for the International Leg Ulcer Advisory Board 2002 The use of compression therapy in the treatment of venous leg ulcers: a recommended management pathway. EWMA Journal 2: 3–7

Compression therapy in leg ulcer management

Christine J. Moffatt, Hugo Partsch, Michael Clark

INTRODUCTION

Over the last two decades developments in compression therapy have led to a transformation in the healing rates of venous ulceration (Moffatt et al 1992, Marston et al 1999). There can be few health-care interventions that can make such dramatic claims. Numerous studies across the world have demonstrated at least a doubling of healing rates, with some reporting as much as a threefold improvement in outcome (Effective Health Care 1997). Effective compression also leads to improvements in pain, mobility and general quality of life as a consequence of ulcer healing (Franks et al 1994, 1999). A recently published European position document on compression therapy has highlighted the fact that it is highly cost-effective when delivered in a well coordinated leg ulcer service (EWMA 2003).

Despite these major advances there are great international variations in the use of compression therapy. This is particularly true of those countries where there is little access to the modern compression therapy products required. The major reason for this is the lack of reimbursement for these products, which prevents them being made available to the health-care professionals who treat ulcer patients. Current global initiatives are seeking to challenge these issues in an attempt to introduce internationally agreed standards for compression (EWMA 2003). One of the major challenges ahead is the development of a new classification for compression therapy that takes account of the technological advances in materials that have occurred

and the complexity of the different products and systems in clinical practice. This will involve re-examination of the fundamental scientific principles that underpin compression, in the light of recent research, which challenges many currently held assumptions.

UNDERSTANDING THE PATHOPHYSIOLOGICAL EFFECTS OF COMPRESSION

Compression has been used for many centuries in the treatment of oedema and other venous and lymphatic disorders of the lower limb, but the exact mechanisms of action remain poorly understood. The following section considers the physiological and biochemical effects of compression.

Compression

If an oncotic pressure gradient exists across a semipermeable membrane, such as a capillary wall, water is drawn across the barrier until the concentrations on both sides are equal. (Oncotic pressure is the osmotic pressure created by protein colloids in plasma.) The relationship between these factors is summarized in Starling's equation (Landis & Pappenheimer 1963)

The amount of lymph formed depends upon the permeability of the capillary wall (filtration coefficient) and the gradient of hydrostatic and oncotic pressure between blood and tissue. The hydrostatic pressure difference causes filtration, while the oncotic pressure difference causes reabsorption (Fig. 10.1).

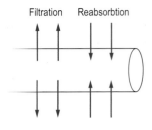

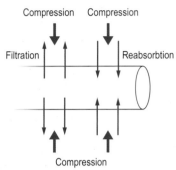

Figure 10.1 Compression works against filtration and promotes absorption

Oedema

Oedema, the accumulation of fluid in extra-vascular tissue, occurs as a result of complex interactions involving the permeability of capillary walls and the hydrostatic and oncotic pressure gradients that exist between the blood vessels and surrounding tissue and the lymphatic drainage.

Starling's equation suggests that the application of external compression will counteract the loss of capillary fluid by increasing local tissue pressure and reinforce reabsorption by squeezing fluid into the veins and lymph vessels. This in turn will help to resolve oedema (Fig. 10.1). Various causes of oedema are identified in Table 10.1.

Depending upon the amount of pressure applied, a compression bandage may influence the internal volume of veins, arteries and lymph vessels. Structures near the surface of the skin are compressed more than the deep vessels. This is because the compressive force is partly dissipated by compression of the surrounding tissues.

In lymphoedema patients nuclear medical investigations have shown that compression removes more water than protein from the tissue, increasing oncotic tissue pressure. This results in a rapid reaccumulation of oedematous fluid if compression is not sustained (Partsch et al 1980).

Effects of compression

Venous system
In a standing individual blood flows slowly through the veins. The venous pressure, which equals the weight of the blood column between the foot and right atrium, is about 80–100 mmHg. During walking, however, blood flow is accelerated by the combined action of the calf muscle pump and the foot pump, which, in patients with competent valves, decreases the volume of venous blood in the foot and reduces venous pressure to about 10–20 mmHg.

If the valves in the large veins become incompetent as a result of primary degeneration or post-thrombotic damage, blood will oscillate up and down in those segments lacking functional valves. The resulting retrograde (backward) flow in the veins of the lower leg (venous reflux) leads to a reduced fall in venous pressure during walking (ambulatory venous hypertension). This causes

Table 10.1 Causes of oedema

Physiology	Possible cause	Effect
↑ Capillary permeability (c)	Cellulitis, arthritis, hormonal cyclic oedema	Inflammatory oedema, 'idiopathic oedema'
↑ Venous (capillary) pressure (P_c)	Heart failure, venous insufficiency dependency syndrome	Cardiac venous oedema
↑ Oncotic tissue pressure (π_t)	Failure of lymph drainage	Lymphoedema
↓ Oncotic capillary pressure (π_c)	Hypoalbuminaemia, nephrotic syndrome, hepatic failure	Hypoproteinaemic syndrome

fluid loss into the tissues and the formation of oedema. Compression of veins with incompetent valves produces an increase in orthograde (towards the heart) flow and a reduction in venous reflux.

The application of adequate levels of compression reduces the diameter of major veins as demonstrated by phlebography and duplex ultrasound (Partsch et al 2000, Partsch & Partsch 2005). This has the effect of reducing local blood volume (Christopoulos et al 1991), by redistributing blood towards central parts of the body. As this can lead to an increase in the preload of the heart and affect cardiac output by about 5% (Mostbeck et al 1977; Fig. 10.2), bilateral bandaging of the thighs and lower legs should be avoided in patients with borderline cardiac function.

Reducing the diameter of major blood vessels will have the secondary effect of increasing flow velocity, provided the arterial flow remains unchanged. The clinical significance of these effects depends upon the relationship between the intra-venous hydrostatic pressure and the degree of external compression applied. In a supine (lying down) individual, pressures in excess of about 10 mmHg over the calf are sufficient to reduce venous diameter. This leads to a marked decrease in blood volume in the lower legs accompanied by a corresponding increase in blood velocity. Pressures in excess of 30 mmHg do not result in a further increase in blood velocity in the large veins or the microcirculation as at this pressure the vessels are maximally emptied and venous volume cannot be reduced any further (Abu-Own et al 1994, Partsch et al 1999).

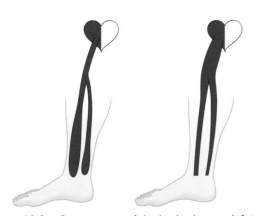

Figure 10.2 Compression of the leg leads to a shift in blood volume with an increase in the preload of the heart

In the upright position, the pressure in the lower leg fluctuates during walking between 20 and 100 mmHg, and therefore much higher levels of compression (e.g. 40–50 mmHg) are required to exert a marked effect upon venous flow.

Arterial circulation

Although it is accepted that compression should never be allowed to impede arterial inflow, there is currently no convincing clinical evidence to indicate what levels of compression may safely be applied to a limb, particularly if there is a risk of arterial impairment.

A systolic ankle pressure below 50–80 mmHg is commonly regarded as a contradiction for high-compression therapy, as is an ankle-brachial pressure index (ABPI) of less than 0.8. Intermittent pneumatic compression systems that exert high pressure peaks in a short time-period followed by long intervals without pressure, aid venous return, reduce oedema and may even help to increase arterial flow by a reactive hyperaemic response (Mayrovitz & Larsen 1997, Dai et al 2002).

Lymphatic system

The function of the lymphatic system is to remove fluid from the interstitial tissues and return it to the venous system. In patients with venous insufficiency, isotopic lymphography shows that prefascial lymphatic drainage is intact or even increased. Subfascial lymph transport is reduced or absent in patients with deep vein thrombosis and deep venous incompetence due to a post-thrombotic syndrome (Partsch 1991).

Short-stretch compression bandages and walking exercises can improve the diminished subfascial lymph transport, but prefascial lymph transport may be decreased because of the reduction of filtration (Lofferer et al 1972). The morphological changes of the lymphatics in lipodermatosclerotic skin, such as fragmentation and extravasation of the contrast medium (dermal backflow), can be normalized with long-term compression (Partsch 1991).

The dramatic reduction of oedema by compression therapy can be explained by the reduction of lymphatic fluid in the tissue, rather than by an improvement of lymphatic transport (Miranda et al 2001).

Microcirculation

Ambulatory venous hypertension in patients with chronic venous insufficiency is the trigger for functional alterations in the endothelium. These alterations are complex and only partially understood. One possibility is that neutrophils become activated, adhere to the endothelial cells and, mediated by the surface exposure of adhesion molecules, produce endothelial injury by releasing cytokines, oxygen free radicals, proteolytic enzymes and platelet activating factors (Smith 1996). Dermal tissue fibrosis (lipodermatosclerosis) is associated with increased transforming growth factor (TGF)β_1 gene expression (Pappas et al 1999); the loss of tissue compliance caused by the fibrosis can lead to reduced skin perfusion and ulceration (Chant 1999). Capillary microthrombosis also contributes to tissue necrosis (Bollinger & Fagrell 1991).

Compression accelerates blood flow in the microcirculation, favours white cell detachment from the endothelium and prevents further adhesion (Abu-Own et al 1994). Capillary filtration is also reduced and reabsorption is increased because of enhanced tissue pressure (Bollinger & Fagrell 1991). In lipodermatosclerotic areas where skin perfusion may be reduced as a result of the strain associated with high tissue pressure (Chant 1999), the use of compression therapy can increase this gradient and improve blood flow. This leads to softened skin (Gniadecka 1995).

Effects on mediators involved in the local inflammatory response may explain both the immediate pain relief that occurs with good compression and subsequent ulcer healing. It has recently been demonstrated, for example, that compression therapy is able to reduce elevated levels of vascular endothelial growth factor and tumour necrosis factor (TNFα) in patients with venous ulcers and that this reduction of serum cytokine levels parallels ulcer healing (Murphy et al 2002). The influence of compression on the tissue injury caused by free radicals, including nitric oxide, requires further investigation (Dai et al 2002).

The application of external compression initiates a variety of complex physiological and biochemical effects involving the venous, arterial and lymphatic systems. Provided that the level of compression does not adversely affect arterial flow and the right application technique and materials are used, the effects of compression can be dramatic, reducing oedema and pain while promoting healing of ulcers caused by venous insufficiency.

Key points

- Compression is the most important component in the conservative treatment of venous leg ulcers and lymphoedema.
- Doppler assessment should always be used before applying compression with frequent reassessment to ensure adequate arterial flow in the limb.
- For ambulant patients with venous insufficiency, high levels of compression (e.g. 40–50 mmHg) are required to produce beneficial haemodynamic effects.
- Impaired lymphatic drainage, secondary to severe chronic venous insufficiency, may be improved by compression.
- Sustained compression is necessary to prevent refilling.

COMPRESSION BANDAGES: PRINCIPLES AND DEFINITIONS

The degree of compression produced by any bandage system over a period of time is determined by complex interactions between four principle factors – the physical structure and elastomeric properties of the bandage, the size and shape of the limb to which it is applied, the skill and technique of the bandager and the nature of any physical activity undertaken by the patient. Difficulties exist in measuring sub-bandage pressure, although international agreement on this issue is being sought.

Determining sub-bandage pressure

Laplace's law

The pressure generated by a bandage immediately following application is determined principally by the tension in the fabric, the number of layers applied and the degree of curvature of the limb. The relationship between these factors is governed by Laplace's law (Box 10.1). The use of this law to calculate or predict sub-bandage pressure has been described by Thomas (2003), although this remains a controversial issue (Melhuish et al 2000).

> **Box 10.1** *Laplace's law*
>
> $P \propto T/R$
>
> - P represents pressure
> - T is tension
> - R is radius
> - $\propto$ is proportional
>
> Applied pressure is directly proportional to the tension in a bandage but inversely proportional to the radius of curvature of the limb to which it is applied (P increases with T but P decreases as R increases).

> **Box 10.2** *Inelastic/elastic bandages*
>
> - Inelastic bandages produce a low resting pressure and high pressure on moving (i.e. create peak pressures)
> - Elastic bandages produce sustained compression with minor variations during walking

Bandage performance

Tension

The tension in a bandage is determined initially by the amount of force applied to the fabric during application. The ability of a bandage to sustain a particular degree of tension (and therefore sub-bandage pressure) is determined by its elastomeric properties, and these in turn are a function of the composition of the yarns and the method of construction.

Extensibility

The ability of a bandage to increase in length in response to an applied force is described as its extensibility (ability to stretch) and it has become common practice across Europe to use terms such as *short-stretch* (minimally extensible, inelastic, passive) and *long-stretch* (highly extensible, elastic, active) to describe this aspect of a bandage's performance.

At some point, once a certain degree of extension is achieved, the physical structure of a bandage will prevent further stretching. This condition is called 'lock-out'. Stemmer and colleagues (1980) suggested that short-stretch bandages should lock out at up to 70% extension (and ideally at 30–40% extension), with long-stretch bandages only locking out at over 140% extension. Unfortunately, they did not suggest what tension should be applied to the bandages in order to achieve these levels of extension, since different bandages may achieve similar extensions when very different

extension forces are applied (Thomas 1990a). Without some form of 'reference' tension, definitions such as long- or short-stretch are relatively meaningless and it is preferable to use the terms elastic or inelastic.

With elastic bandages a small change in extension (as might occur during walking) will result in minor fluctuations in sub-bandage pressure. These bandages are also able to accommodate changes in limb circumference, as occurs when oedema is reduced, with minimal effects on sub-bandage pressure. Conversely, with inelastic bandages large changes in sub-bandage pressure may result from minor changes in calf geometry. These bandages may produce high compression during walking but low resting pressures (Box 10.2).

Power

The amount of force required to cause a specific increase in the length of an elastic bandage is an indicator of the bandage's power (Thomas & Nelson 1998); this characteristic determines the amount of pressure a bandage will produce at a predetermined extension.

Elasticity

The elasticity of a bandage determines its ability to return to its original (unstretched) length as the tension is reduced (Table 10.2). Currently there are no international or European standards relating to the performance of compression bandages. An on-line search of 20 European national standards bodies, conducted in December 2002, identified two national standards related to bandages used to apply limb compression, British Standard (BS) 7505:1995 (British Standards Institute 1995) will

Table 10.2 British bandage pressures

Type BS 7505	Level of compression	Pressure British standard (mmHg)
3A	Light	Up to 20
3B	Light	21–30
3C	Moderate	31–40
3D	High	41–60

be used to illustrate the lack of European agreement on the classification of compression bandage systems. The second standard, from Switzerland, dates back to 1975.

The standards set out test methods for establishing the different aspects of the performance of non-adhesive, fabric-based compression bandages. Of note is that different test methods are used in different countries across Europe.

British standard

Bandages are classified within the standard into one of six categories. Type 1 refers to retention, lightweight, elastic bandages. Type 2 are support bandages (inelastic, short-stretch) and types 3A to 3D are compression bandages (elastic, long-stretch). The four classes of compression bandage are defined according to their ability to apply a specified sub-bandage pressure to a known ankle circumference (23 cm) where the bandage is applied with a 50% overlap between successive layers.

ACHIEVING ADEQUATE PRESSURE

On a normal leg the circumference of the ankle is generally substantially smaller than that of the calf, and it follows from Laplace's law that, if a bandage is applied with constant tension and overlap, the pressures achieved at the gaiter and the calf will be lower than those applied at the ankle. As the circumference of the leg progressively increases, a compression gradient is produced, with the highest pressure on the most distal part of the limb (i.e. the ankle). The consistent formation of this ideal pressure gradient has been difficult to demonstrate practically (Nelson 1996). The failure to demonstrate graduated compression may reflect

Box 10.3 Sub-bandage pressure measurement

Pressure sensors
Large-diameter sensors tend to provide an average value of pressure applied over a large surface area and so do not report peak pressures. Inflexible sensors may record artificially high pressures given their inability to conform to the surface of the leg (point loading of the sensor).

Site of sensor application
A sensor placed over a soft tissue (calf) may return lower pressure readings than a similar sensor placed over a hard site (ankle).

Method of application
The application technique (figure-of-eight or spiral), the number of layers applied and the degree of overlap between layers will affect the pressure applied to the leg.

Position of limb
Pressures are higher when standing and significantly altered during walking (Sockalingham et al 1990).

poor operator technique, the practical problems of maintaining constant tension throughout the bandage during the application process, and poor measurement technique. Factors affecting the measurement of sub-bandage pressure are listed in Box 10.3.

PROBLEM SOLVING

Some of the practical problems associated with bandage application have been addressed by manufacturers, who have included various visual guides to help operators achieve the required tension within the bandage. Advances in textile technology may also help to reduce both inter- and intrabandager variability. One very promising concept is the development of an elastomeric yarn that enables a bandage to achieve relatively constant sub-bandage pressures regardless of minor variations in extension (Moffatt 2002a).

Compression of the lower leg aids the healing of venous leg ulcers. Much is made of sub-bandage pressures in the presentation and evaluation of compression bandages – the values cited (e.g. 40 mmHg at the ankle) are typically given as single values with no apparent variation within and between subjects. In reality, sub-bandage pressures are greatly influenced by several factors, including posture, locomotion and bandage application technique.

The current standards classify individual products but do not define the ways in which these bandages work clinically. In addition, simplistic descriptions of short-stretch (inelastic) and long-stretch (elastic) bandages fail to take account of the huge variations within these two groups and, more importantly, the development of multilayer compression systems that combine materials with different performance characteristics.

Multilayer bandage development is based upon the fact that multiple layers of weak elastic bandages can be used in combination to achieve optimum compression without the inherent risk of using 'high-power' elastic bandages capable of excessive pressure. Multilayer bandages are complex, with some incorporating both elastic and inelastic materials, which provide advantages of both systems: the elastic element provides sustained pressure and the inelastic element provides high pressures during walking and low resting pressures.

At the heart of any new classification must be the ability to translate the technical details about systems into a clinical decision. Optimal levels of compression and best methods of application remain to be determined across Europe, perhaps within the framework of developing a European-wide standard for the testing and classification of bandage systems (Box 10.4).

APPLICATION ISSUES IN COMPRESSION THERAPY

Much attention has been placed on the development and evaluation of compression systems but relatively little on how different applications may influence their effectiveness. Some bandages systems, such as four-layer, have been developed with a defined application technique and as new bandages are being developed more attention is being placed on the most effective technique for individual products (Moffatt 2002b). Simple spiral techniques are frequently used in the UK, USA and Canada but more complex techniques are reported from mainland Europe. Irrespective of the application technique adopted there are important principles that apply to the correct application of all systems. While standardization of techniques may be beneficial, nevertheless the individual requirements of patients must always be considered if compression is to be effective and well tolerated by the patient.

Assessment issues

The assessment of patients with leg ulceration is described in Chapter 7.

Preparing the patient for compression

It is essential that the patient understands that compression therapy is the most important part of their treatment. Research has shown that patients frequently fail to understand the underlying cause of their ulcer and how this is causing their delayed healing (Edwards et al 2002). Their beliefs about their illness are of great importance in their ability to adhere with compression. This is discussed further in Chapter 31. Acceptance of compression will also be influenced by their previous experiences of ulcer treatments, as well as their current needs and hopes for the future. Too often when they decide on the compression bandage regime, practitioners fail to take account of the complex issues that the

---

Box 10.4   *Classification requirements for bandages*

- Characteristics of extensibility, power and elasticity affect the amount of pressure a bandage will apply and how long it will be sustained

- The current classification system refers to individual bandages and does not adequately reflect the physiological effects of multilayer bandaging systems

- A Europe-wide standard for the testing and classification of bandage systems is required

patient may be facing. Patients may find attending for regular treatment a significant burden if they are working, and self-care regimes should be considered in these cases (Philips et al 1994). Symptom control during compression is also of great importance. While pain has been shown to improve with compression therapy, during the first few weeks pain levels may increase (Franks & Moffatt 1998). Advice on taking regular analgesia and the use of elevation and exercise may influence whether patients will persevere (Buchmann 1997).

There are variations in opinion as to the correct patient positioning for bandaging. However, the clinical condition of the patient will often determine this. Many patients will be unable to lie flat and will require bandaging in a chair. The patient should be in the best position possible to prevent the practitioner from stooping and to allow full access to the limb. Patients who are very immobile or who have heavy limbs should be bandaged by two people to ensure evenness of application.

Care of the skin

Before each compression bandage is applied it is important to examine the skin for any signs of varicose eczema or loss of skin integrity. Patients who wear bandages for prolonged periods of time may develop extensive build-up of dead epithelial cells, particularly if paraffin-based products are used regularly and are not washed from the skin at each dressing change. Regular washing of the limb in warm water with an emollient helps to remove excess exudate and reduce the odour from the ulcer, thus rendering a 'socially' clean limb for the patient. The skin should be regularly examined for signs of pressure damage. Vulnerable sites include the tibial crest, the dorsum of the foot and the Achilles tendon. Early signs of pressure damage may include erythema progressing to purple discoloration and ulceration (Fig. 10.3). Bandage slippage creates bands of oedema above the level of the bandage and indentation beneath the area of slippage due to the tourniquet effect created by the bandage (Fig. 10.4). Uneven application of compression can be seen in the collection of bands of oedema at areas where the compression is inadequate (Fig. 10.5). Common problem areas include the dorsum of the foot, because of over-tight

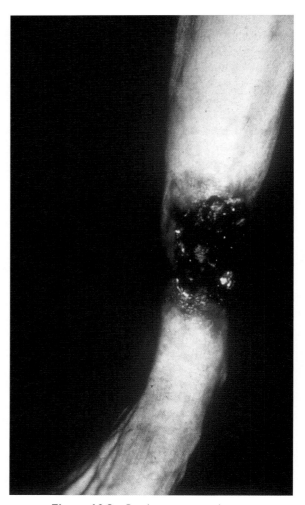

Figure 10.3 Bandage pressure damage

bandaging around the ankle, and the mid calf, because of over-tightening (extending) of elastic bandages. Foot deformities should be noted in order that modifications can be made to the application technique.

Applying compression to the foot

There is considerable debate about whether compression should be applied to the foot or whether it should commence around the ankle. This debate arises from concern that the foot is particularly vulnerable to pressure damage because it does not have the layers of subcutaneous and fatty tissue afforded as protection to the leg. However, provided

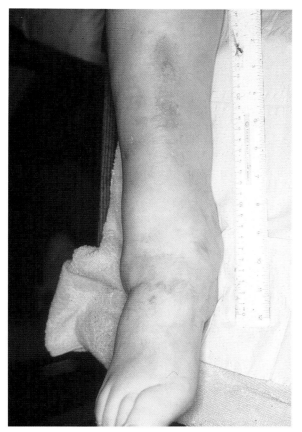

Figure 10.4 Bandage slippage creating a tourniquet effect

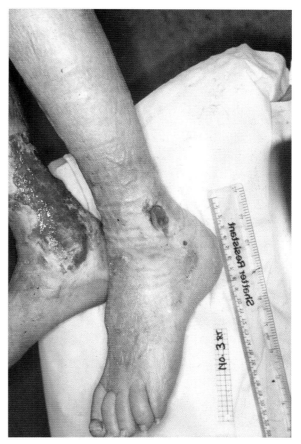

Figure 10.5 Bands of oedema formation due to poor bandaging technique

that the practitioner identifies any vulnerable areas, there is no reason why compression cannot be safely applied over a suitable padding, which will cushion and protect the limb from pressure damage. It is now an internationally agreed criteria that all compression bandages should be applied from the base of the toes over a suitable underlayer (EWMA 2003).

The forefoot is particularly vulnerable to the collection of oedema, and this situation can be exacerbated when there is over-tight bandaging around the ankle creating a tourniquet effect (Fig. 10.6). Toe bandaging may be required if the toes appear oedematous or sausage like in appearance, with enhanced skin folds (Fig. 10.7). Toe lymphoedema may develop without other obvious signs in the limb. It is frequently seen in patients with a long history of bandaging for ulceration and

may be a consequence of trapped oedema in the foot leading to localized secondary skin and lymphatic changes. Mycosis is a common accompaniment and may lead to repeated episodes of bacterial infection. The technique for toe bandaging is presented in Box 10.5.

Protection of foot deformities

Foot deformities such as hallux valgus are frequently found in patients with leg ulceration and require extra protection. Equinus deformity causes a significant reduction in venous return and is associated with delayed ulcer healing (Moffatt et al 2001). Particular care should be taken when bandaging these limbs as exceedingly high pressure can be applied over the dorsum of the foot, leading to

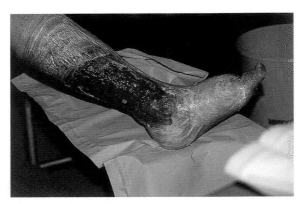

Figure 10.6 Forefoot oedema due to overtight bandaging around the ankle

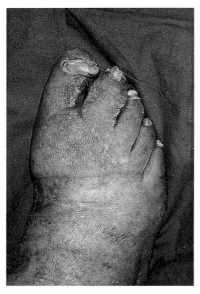

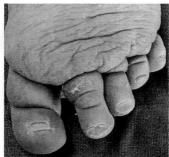

Figure 10.7 Toe swelling (lymphoedema) requiring toe bandaging

ulceration (Fig. 10.8). The foot can be protected by the addition of extra layers of wool padding. Synthetic padding maintains its cushioning effect better than cotton padding because the fibres retain their loft even when wet. However, synthetic fibres may lead to allergies and should be used with caution over a cotton tubular bandage that extends well above and below the padding. Superior underpadding is now being developed for use beneath compression bandages (Moffatt 2002b).

Thin foam bandages can be used as an alternative to wool underpadding and are used extensively in lymphoedema multilayer bandaging. These are applied in a spiral using the same application technique as for wool padding and are particularly useful in preventing slippage. Care must be taken in their application. If they are applied too tightly they can cause constricting bands of trapped oedema and tissue necrosis. They have the advantage that they can be washed and sterilized.

Areas at risk of pressure damage can be protected by individually cut pieces of foam that spread the pressure away from the area at risk. Pressure damage may result from inappropriate footwear when bandages are forced into an unsuitable, tight shoe. Patients should be encouraged to avoid vanity and wear a shoe that provides adequate support for the foot and ankle and is large enough to encompass the bandage without disruption. Trainers are often a suitable choice but may be unpopular in older patients. If the patient has a significant gait deformity they should be referred for an orthotic assessment and a custom-made pair of shoes should be provided.

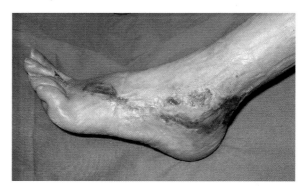

Figure 10.8 Danger of compression damage in equinus foot deformity

> ### Box 10.5 *Bandaging oedematous toes*
>
> 1. Wrap the big toe, making sure that the bandage starts at the middle of the nail
>
> 2. If the patient finds that the bandage irritates the crease of the toes on the plantar side, cover with a small piece of foam with the edges cut to avoid trauma
>
> 3. Bandage the remaining toes (2–4), anchoring each turn around the foot
>
> 4. Make sure the base of each toe is well covered
>
> 5. The fourth toe can be bandaged to the fifth toe or the fifth toe can be left free
>
> 6. If there are extensive skin folds these can be cushioned with a small piece of a foam dressing cut to size

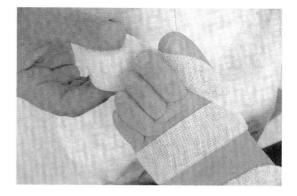

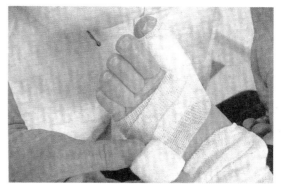

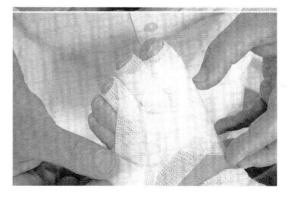

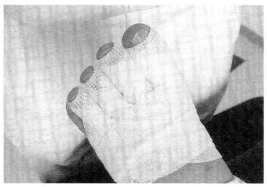

Removal of forefoot oedema can be problematic (Fig. 10.9). Methods to reduce this include changing the bandage application technique and the use of tailor-made foam pads. Minimal oedema may be removed by the simple addition of an extra layer of bandage to increase the sub bandage pressure over the affected area. Over-extension of the bandage should be avoided as it is passed around the ankle, as this may prevent drainage. Foam padding cut to the shape of the dorsum of the foot applies localized pressure and can be very effective. Care should be taken to ensure that the foam is cut to fit into the toe creases and that the edges are bevelled to avoid friction or pressure damage (Fig. 10.9). The pad should then be firmly bandaged in place. While most compression therapy involves the use of 10 cm width bandages, narrower bandages may also be useful around the foot and can be applied in a figure of eight or spica technique to increase pressure.

Ulceration occurring in the retromalleolar area can be very hard to heal (Asmussen & Strossenreuther 2003; Fig. 10.10). This is because of the lack of pressure that can be applied directly to the ulcer. Many patients with ulceration in this area have

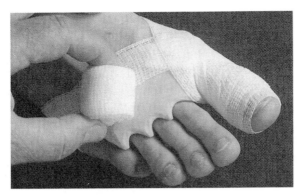

Figure 10.9 Using bevelled shaped foam to reduce forefoot oedema. Reproduced with permission of BSN and Lohmann Rauscher

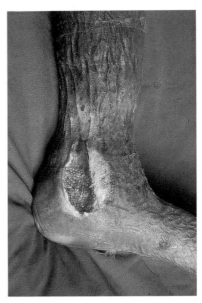

Figure 10.10 Retromalleolar ulceration is difficult to heal due to the lack of direct pressure to the ulcer

restricted ankle mobility (Helliwell & Cheesbrough 1994). This is in part due to the prolonged lack of ankle movement, as ulcers in this area can be particularly painful and changes in the subcutaneous tissues further reduce movement. The addition of wool padding helps to redistribute the pressure more evenly around the ankle. Kidney-shaped foam pads can be applied over the protective padding to increase pressure in this area (Fig. 10.11). If these are not available a secondary dressing pad can be folded in half and cut to the correct size. Care should be taken to ensure the pads are correctly positioned as slippage may cause pressure damage over the malleoli. Adaptions to the bandage technique may also be helpful. The stirrup technique, using a narrow bandage, allows for extra pressure to be directly applied to this area. When the bandage has been applied to the foot and ankle it is important to check that the patient has good ankle movement.

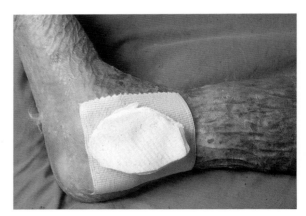

Figure 10.11 Applying pressure to retromalleolar ulceration to enhance local pressure

Bandaging the ankle

The application technique for applying bandages to the foot and leg is shown in Figures 10.12 and 10.13. The ankle should be bandaged using a figure of eight technique to allow for freedom of ankle movement. The heel and Achilles tendon area must be carefully bandaged. Failure to do this can lead to localized oedema formation and bandage slippage, which may cause extensive pressure damage involving loss of the tendon. Care should

be taken when bandaging the ankle to avoid over-extension of the bandage as it is passed around the ankle. This can be particularly problematic if the practitioner has to hold the limb while applying the bandage. The dorsal tendon area is also an area that is vulnerable to high pressure and necrosis. Extra protection may be given with wool padding or a piece of foam that has a central slit cut to allow

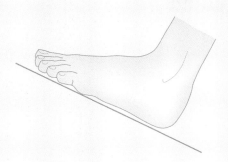

(a) Position the foot in a comfortable position, at a right angle to the leg.

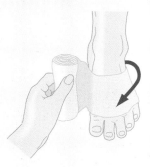

(b) Begin by making two anchoring turns around the foot. Be sure to include the base of the toes.

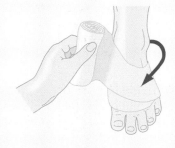

(c) Next take a high turn above the heel.

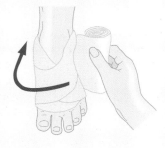

(d) Then fill the base of the foot with a low turn. From here, the bandage can be applied in a spiral as in this figure or in a figure of eight (Figure 15.13).

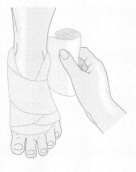

(e) Apply the bandage in a spiral, ensuring there is a 50% overlap.

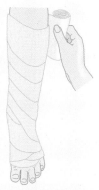

(f) Ensure the bandage is applied right up to the tibial tuberosity.

Figure 10.12 Application of compression bandage using a spiral technique

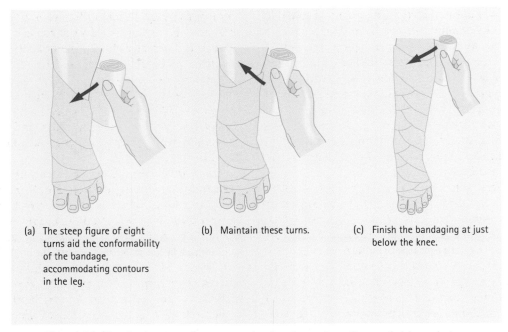

(a) The steep figure of eight turns aid the conformability of the bandage, accommodating contours in the leg.

(b) Maintain these turns.

(c) Finish the bandaging at just below the knee.

Figure 10.13 Application of a compression bandage using a figure of eight technique

movement. A thin hydrocolloid dressing may also be useful if the skin in this area is particularly vulnerable. Bandages should not be cut to reduce pressure over the front of the foot as this may change the overall compression level and lead to rapid deterioration of the bandage.

Bandaging the limb

Most patients with venous ulceration only require bandaging to the knee. However, in patients with accompanying lymphoedema that extends to the thigh, full-length bandaging is required. This is discussed more fully in Chapter 14. A long-established principle in graduated compression is the need to achieve a pressure gradient of 50–60% between the ankle and knee. Laplace's law implies that when a bandage is applied with even tension the greatest pressure is applied at the ankle, with the narrowest radius, and the least pressure at the calf, with the largest radius. Therefore in patients with a normal limb shape a natural gradient of pressure should be applied. Research has shown, however, that even experienced bandagers rarely achieve the pressure gradient (Nelson 1996). A common

problem is tightening of the bandage mid-calf, causing a tourniquet effect. Patients with inverted-champagne-bottle-shaped legs and those with thin limbs and a loss of gradient are particularly at risk of inadequate compression. Measurement of the ankle circumference is an important aspect of assessment, which should identify small and large limbs that require a change in application of the bandage or the selection of a bandage system designed for the size of limb.

Despite these issues, high healing rates have been reported over the last 15 years with compression therapy (Moffatt et al 1992). This raises an important question about whether direct pressure to the limb is more important than achieving the correct gradient, which is one example of the principles of compression that require re-evaluation.

European recommendations on compression state that bandaging should be applied with maximal dorsiflexion of the foot. In other areas, such as the UK and USA, the limb is bandaged at rest. Research has not been undertaken to prove which method is best. The bandage should always extend over the gastrocnemius muscle to avoid slippage. The practitioner should be able to place a finger above the bandage in the popliteal space to ensure full movement of the knee. Some authors report that, when layers of bandaging are applied, the direction of bandaging should be changed: the first layer is applied in a clockwise direction, the second in an anti clockwise direction (Asmussen & Strossenreuther 2003). They also suggest that, when bandaging the calf muscle, the muscles are pushed in a medial direction to ensure that the ankle joint (the talocrural joint) will have its full range of movement.

The tibial crest is an area at risk of pressure damage, particularly in those with thin limbs. Men with a normal limb shape may also be at risk because the tibial crest is exposed, with little overlying subcutaneous or fatty tissue to provide protection. This area can be protected by the addition of extra wool padding pleated over the area, or foam padding placed on either side of the tibial crest to distribute the pressure away from the bony prominence. Thin limbs may benefit from additional padding in the calf region to create a more natural limb gradient.

The two main techniques for bandaging the limb are the simple spiral and the figure of eight or spica technique (Fig. 10.13). The spiral bandage is generally applied with a 50% extension when using elastic bandages and a 50% overlap to ensure evenness if two layers of bandage are applied all the way up the limb. The figure of eight bandage is also applied with the same overlap and extension and, because of the increased number of layers, gives a higher pressure than the same bandage applied using a spiral technique (Thomas 1990a). A figure of eight application can be very useful when bandaging a disproportionate limb. Because of the extra pressure applied using this method, great care should be taken when applying strong, elastic, single-layer bandages, as very high pressures may be applied. It is essential that the bandage manufacturer's instructions are carefully read before application.

Many bandage companies have recognized the danger of over-extension of elastic bandages and have sought to address this. Bandage symbols provide a useful guide to the practitioner as to how much the bandage has been stretched. Examples include rectangles becoming squares and ovals becoming circles. Research has shown that while these may be useful they do not replace the effectiveness of correct training (Nelson 1996). Other advances include the development of bandages containing sophisticated elastomers that prevent pressure peaks occurring with over extension (Proguide™). The pressure applied by this product plateaus at around 50% extension and does not increase in pressure with further extension (Moffatt 2002b).

Inelastic bandages are applied using a variety of techniques, although simple spiral and figure of eight technique are frequently chosen. Because of the requirement to produce a rigid structure around the calf, these bandages are applied at full extension (although they have a limited extension range). Multilayer systems such as four-layer bandaging incorporate spiral and figure of eight techniques to produce an accumulative level of compression. The complexities of the different products and techniques of application highlight the urgent need to reclassify bandages in a useful manner for practitioners.

USING COMPRESSION FOR PROBLEM AREAS

Coping with bandage slippage

Compression is also effective at dealing with problem areas of the limb. Lymphoedema experts report the value of using ridged foam to stimulate softening of fibrotic tissue beneath compression (Asmussen & Strossenreuther 2003). Dealing with bandage slippage can be a significant problem for the patient and professional and may lead to the need for frequent bandage re-applications. Bandage slippage may lead to tissue damage and extending of the ulcerated area. A number of techniques can be employed to reduce this. The use of extra padding to recontour the limb to a normal shape has already been discussed, but can also be useful in reducing slippage. A figure of eight technique helps to anchor the bandage around the calf and the use of cohesive bandages, both elastic and inelastic (e.g. Actico™, Coban™, Coplus™), is also very effective. Small horizontal strips of foam 6–8 cm wide and 0.5 cm thick can be wrapped around the limb in between the outer layers of bandage, which are applied in a figure of eight (Asmussen & Strossenreuther 2003). Practical steps such as the application of a cotton liner over the finished bandage can also help to prevent movement. The greatest slippage is likely to occur when using cotton or inelastic bandages, which cannot 'follow through' when the oedema is removed and the limb is reduced in size. Because of the recoil in elastic bandages they are more able to cope with changes, although some slippage may still occur in very obese patients or during the early stages of treatment.

In patients with a large calf in proportion to the ankle, greater pressure may be required in the calf area. Increased pressure can be achieved in a number of ways

- Increasing the bandage extension
- Increasing the degree of overlap
- Increasing the number of layers.

Bandages should be replaced if severe slippage occurs to ensure that they are having a therapeutic effect.

When to use thigh-length bandaging

Full-length bandaging may be required for patients with lymphoedema, deep vein thrombosis or superficial thrombophlebitis extending into the thigh. Compression therapy is only one component of effective lymphoedema management, which is discussed in Chapter 14. The calf can be bandaged in a sitting or lying position and the patient's thigh is then bandaged while standing with their knee flexed. It is often easier to bandage the lower and upper leg as individual sections. A protective cotton liner, wool padding or foam should be applied to the upper limb and a foam pad should be placed behind the knee to avoid friction. The knee should be bandaged with a figure of eight to allow freedom of movement. Because of the increased circumference of the thigh it is useful to use a figure of eight bandage technique here also to give adequate compression. Complex techniques using tailored foam are reported in the literature but should not be attempted without training. Glues are available to help prevent slippage but should be used with extreme caution in venous ulcer patients because of the high risk of contact allergy.

EVALUATING THE EFFECTIVENESS OF COMPRESSION

It is important to continuously evaluate the progress the patient is making and to adapt the compression if changes are required. Care must be taken to ensure that the correct bandage or system is used throughout treatment. Removal of oedema from the limb will often give an indented effect but there should be no signs of pressure damage. The bandage or system should also be capable of managing large amounts of exudate. The skin and ulcer should be evaluated for signs of maceration, which would suggest that exudate management is inadequate. Of great importance is to determine how comfortable the patient has found the bandage and to modify any areas that have caused discomfort. The same applies to adhesive bandages which are excellent for compression therapy of the thigh.

INTERNATIONAL ALGORITHM

An international algorithm has been developed as one of several initiatives aimed at developing international agreement on the use of compression and as a stimulus to begin the process of developing a new classification for compression therapy (EWMA 2003; Fig. 10.14). An international expert panel of clinicians and academics (the International Leg Ulcer Advisory Board) was established to undertake this work. The aim was to produce a treatment pathway that reflected the current state of knowledge and was of practical use to clinicians. The group drew on over 150 published papers, Cochrane systematic reviews and published guidelines. Many of the areas did not have robust evidence and in theses cases consensus of expert opinion was used to clarify issues.

Assessment

The correct assessment of ulceration has already been discussed in Chapter 7. The algorithm highlights the importance of being certain about the underlying aetiology before compression is commenced. The use of non invasive procedures, such as recording of an ABPI, are considered mandatory (Vowden et al 1996). The confirmation and correction of venous disease by surgery should be performed wherever possible. The true value of venous

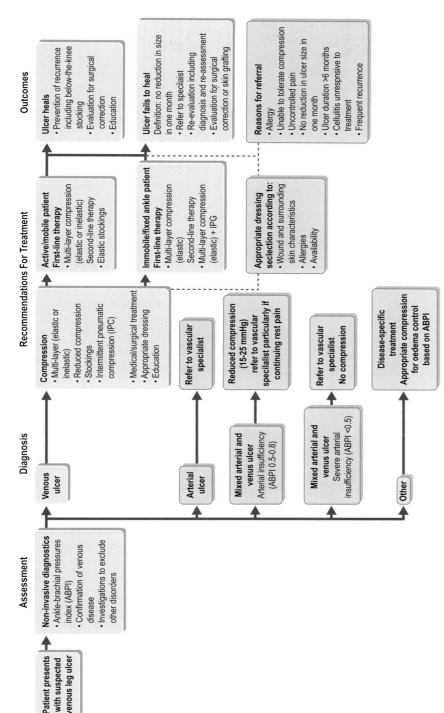

Figure 10.14 A recommended treatment pathway developed by the Leg Ulcer Advisory Board for the use of compression therapy in venous leg ulcers

surgery in ulcer healing and recurrence has yet to be fully determined (Ghauri et al 1998, Barwell et al 2000). While venous ulceration forms the largest group, ulcers of other aetiology should also be excluded. This is particularly important with an ageing population, where the chance of concurrent conditions affecting the ulcer increases significantly (Nelzén et al 1994).

Diagnosis

The algorithm divides ulceration into several categories that relate to the choice of compression.

Venous ulcer

This refers to a patient with an uncomplicated venous ulcer with little evidence of arterial disease (ABPI >0.8). It also excludes patients with complex medical conditions. The level of mobility is not included at this stage in the algorithm.

Arterial ulcer

Compression should never be used in patients with severe peripheral vascular disease and an ABPI below 0.5 unless under strict medical management and close observation. Referral to a vascular surgeon is required.

Mixed arterial and venous ulcer

There are two categories used to describe patients with venous ulceration accompanied by arterial disease. The difference between these groups is extremely important. Patients with an ABPI 0.5–0.8 have medium levels of arterial involvement but may safely tolerate the use of low levels of compression (15–25 mmHg; Moffatt et al 1992). The second group have more advanced arterial disease with an ABPI <0.5. In this group referral to a vascular surgeon is required and compression is not recommended. It is important to remember that the arterial status of these patients may change rapidly. A sudden increase in pain or inability to wear compression may indicate that the peripheral vascular disease has advanced and reassessment with Doppler should be undertaken. There are great variations in the tolerance of compression in this patient group. If pain, particularly at night, is a major factor, the practitioner should consider

using an inelastic bandage with a low resting pressure.

Other

This category includes patients with diabetic foot ulceration and other rarer aetiologies such as vasculitis and skin cancers. These require full investigation and the appropriate treatment for the condition. In some situations concurrent oedema may delay healing. Compression may be useful in these cases but should be prescribed after checking the ABPI and after ensuring that there are no other contraindications to compression, such as extensive microcirculatory failure, which may be seen in a range of disorders including diabetes mellitus and rheumatoid arthritis.

Recommendation for compression

The algorithm recommends the use of either elastic or inelastic multilayer systems as first-line treatment in venous ulceration. The difficulties of classifying the different bandages and systems have already been discussed. The research review came to a number of conclusions: the use of compression was more effective than no compression; high compression (35–45 mmHg) was more effective than low compression (15–25 mmHg); elastic or inelastic multilayer systems were more effective than single-layer systems (Cullum et al 2001).

Multilayer elastic

Multilayer elastic systems consist of a wool padding layer with a combination of three or four elastic bandages to provide sustained compression. Many of these systems have a cohesive outer layer that provides rigidity and prevents slippage. A number of two-layer bandaging systems have been developed that consist of a wool padding layer and a high-compression elastic bandage. Excessively high pressure can be applied with some single-layer elastic bandages if they are inappropriately applied or used on a very small limb.

Multilayer inelastic

Multi layer inelastic systems may comprise a wool padding underlayer and a number of layers of a cotton bandage applied at full stretch to the limb.

Advances of this system (Actico™) include the use of a two-layer system of wool padding and a cohesive inelastic bandage that provides compression and prevents the slippage associated with this type of bandage. A recent study found that the healing rates with this system were comparable to the traditional four layer bandage (Franks et al 2003).

Other multilayer inelastic bandages include the Pütterbandage consisting of two layers of cotton bandages and the Rosidal which additionally uses a padding layer of polyurethane foam. These bandages can be washed and reused.

Reduced compression

Reduced levels of compression (15–25 mmHg) are indicated as a secondary approach to the treatment of venous ulceration (Arthur & Lewis 2000). While it is acknowledged that lower levels of pressure may not be efficacious as higher levels, there are some patients who cannot tolerate high pressure and experience severe pain. Reduced compression may also be used in the initial stages of treatment, progressing to high compression as the patient's tolerance increases.

Stockings

The true potential of using stockings in the healing phase of ulceration has not been adequately explored (Cullum et al 2001). There are a number of advantages in their use, particularly in younger patients who wish to have greater control over their ulcer and who do not wish for the inconvenience of weekly attendance for treatment. Stockings, if correctly measured and fitted, provide an adequate level of compression and are aesthetically more pleasing than wearing bandaging. Patients may shower and remove them at night and they may be a very cost-effective way of providing compression in this small group.

However they are not suitable for all patients with leg ulceration. They require a high degree of manual dexterity to apply and remove and, because of the large number of elderly, frail patients with poor manual dexterity, they cannot be uniformly used. Older patients in particular may not want the responsibility of looking after their own ulcer but prefer the health-care professional to do so. Stockings are not suitable for large ulcers with high

levels of exudate, as it is difficult to apply an adequate underlayer. The main indication for compression stockings is to prevention ulcer recurrence or the development of oedema that may predispose the patient to developing a recurrent ulcer. Hosiery is also used to reduce the swelling after a deep vein thrombosis and to maintain limb volume, prevent oedema formation and reduce skin changes and complications in the patient with lymphoedema.

Intermittent pneumatic compression

The role of intermittent pneumatic compression in the treatment of venous disease has been the subject of a systematic review (Mani et al 2001). The main conclusions are that there is insufficient evidence to date to suggest that it should be used in routine practice. However in the small number of studies undertaken there were promising indications that it may be beneficial in the healing of resistant ulceration when used in combination with compression therapy. Clinicians are frequently faced with immobile patients who cannot elevate their limb or go to bed at night. In these cases, anecdotal reports would suggest that intermittent pneumatic compression may be very helpful and avoid the need for hospitalization that occurs frequently in this patient group.

Active and immobile patients

A major factor influencing the healing of venous ulceration is the patient's level of general mobility and the degree of ankle function. The algorithm considers the specific recommendations for active and immobile patients. These recommendations draw on research that has examined the physiological changes occurring with different compression materials and the risk factor analyses that have been undertaken on venous ulcer studies (Partsch 1991, Franks et al 1995a, Margolis et al 2000).

Active/Mobile

Active, mobile patients can be treated with either elastic or inelastic multilayer systems. The role of stockings has already been discussed.

Immobile/fixed ankle joint

Immobile patients often provide the greatest challenge to the health-care professional. The algorithm recommends the use of elastic multilayer bandaging for this group. Elastic compression will provide a sustained level of compression even if the patient cannot move. Inelastic bandages rely on calf movement to provide a high working pressure but have a relatively low resting pressure, which may lead to the formation of oedema. Little research has been undertaken to define which compression systems should be used in mobile and immobile patients. The recommendations rely heavily on theoretical assumptions rather than outcome studies. In a recent randomized controlled trial of an elastic multilayer system versus an inelastic multilayer system, a subgroup analysis revealed a surprising result, with immobile patients healing better in the inelastic regime than the elastic (Franks et al 2003).

The importance of the correct medical and surgical treatment are highlighted in this algorithm and are discussed further in Chapters 11, 12 and 13. While there is little evidence to suggest that simple dressings enhance ulcer healing, inappropriate selection of dressings may be a major factor in delaying healing and is examined in Chapter 23. There is increasing recognition of the role patients may play in their care. They should understand their condition and treatment and how they can influence their progress through the adoption of health education strategies (Chapter 32).

Outcomes

Compression therapy has been shown to greatly improve the healing rates of venous ulcers. The literature reports a wide range of healing rates from as low as 30% to over 75% at 12 weeks (Moffatt et al 1992, Scottish Leg Ulcer Trial Participants 2002). It is often difficult to identify why these differences occur; however, a number of clinical risk factors have been identified that affect outcome. These include: the size and duration of the ulcer, general and ankle mobility and, in some studies, popliteal reflux (Franks et al 1995a, Brittenden et al 1998, Chetter et al 2001). There may be many other clinical and psychosocial issues that affect healing but have not yet been identified.

Ulcer heals

Within the algorithm there are a number of priorities for managing the patient when the ulcer heals. Patients should be fitted with the highest class of below-knee hosiery they can manage to help prevent recurrence. Patients should be seen regularly to check their skin and hosiery and surgical correction of superficial varicose veins should be considered (Barwell et al 2000). While traditional surgery has involved the superficial venous system, recent work has shown benefit in patients with concurrent segmental deep vein involvement (Adam et al 2003). The patient should be cognisant with the fact that he has a life long condition which may recur if he fails to look after his legs and seek immediate treatment if an ulcer recurs.

Ulcer fails to heal

The algorithm recommends re- assessment and referral if there is no reduction in the ulcer size within one month. Many studies have found that patients have suffered with an ulcer for may years without appropriate referral having taken place (Callam et al 1987, Nelzén 1997). Specialist intervention may be required to determine whether surgical correction or skin grafting is needed. Contact dermatitis and chronic episodes of infection may require further investigation. Failure to heal may also be linked to a deterioration in the patient's general health status or level of mobility. Some of the problems causing delayed healing cannot be effectively changed. A small proportion of patients may have to adjust to the reality of living with an ulcer. The difficulties of coping with ulceration and adjustment to illness are discussed further in Chapter 31.

Managing recurrence

Factors influencing venous ulcer recurrence

While research relating to recurrence of ulceration remains sparse, studies suggest that the rate of recurrence is high (Erickson et al 1995, Moffatt & Dorman 1995, McDaniel et al 2002). Compliance with wearing compression hosiery has been shown to affect the rate of recurrence (Erickson et al 1995). A randomized controlled trial of compression hosiery (class II, 18–24 mmHg) identified a number of factors associated with ulcer recurrence. These independent risk factors were: the previous size of the ulcer (>10 cm), a history of deep vein thrombosis and unsuitability for stockings (Franks et al 1995b). Other authors have also found increased recurrence rates in patients who have had a previous deep vein thrombosis (Stacey et al 1991). These factors indicate that the severity of the underlying disease may be an important factor to consider. Johnson identified that patients reported difficulties in the use of compression hosiery (Johnson 1988), and Travers found that, of 32 women, 17 did not wear their stockings at all, while 60% found the cosmetic appearance unacceptable (Travers et al 1990). Other factors they identified included friable skin, difficulty in applying and removing stockings and skin irritation. A large randomized controlled trial of class II (18–24 mmHg) and class III (25–35 mmHg) hosiery found that the recurrence rate was lowest in the class III group but compliance was found to be problematic (Harper et al 1995).

A systematic review of randomized controlled trials in ulcer recurrence found weak evidence that compression hosiery reduced recurrence and recommended further research in this area (Nelson 2001). Current recommendations, based on the limited research available and expert opinion, suggest that patients should be fitted with the highest level of compression they can tolerate, provided that compliance is good.

Professionals may be fatalistic in their attitudes to ulcer recurrence and delegate this task to less qualified staff (Flanagan et al 2001). Effective recurrence programmes should be an integral part of all leg ulcer services. Creative approaches to this include the development of leg clubs, which encourage patient participation and long-term follow-up in a relaxed environment (Fassiadis et al 2002). Programmes involving carers and health-care assistants can be useful, particularly in the frail immobile group. The patients should also be regularly assessed by a trained health-care professional to ensure that any changes in their medical condition or arterial status are identified. Any change in symptoms such as pain or numbness should immediately be reported and a regular ABPI should be performed. Effective education of patients should emphasize the importance of seeking medical advice immediately there is an ulcer, as the longer the

ulcer is present the greater the chance of delayed healing (Franks et al 1995a). Complete ulcer healing is a vital component of cost-effective care (Korn et al 2002). This is discussed further in Chapter 5.

Patient assessment

A detailed patient history can identify whether the patient is at increased risk of ulcer recurrence. Table 10.3 outlines some of the factors that should be considered before fitting with hosiery. In addition to a clinical history, the practitioner should assess factors that may influence their adherence to hosiery. These will include the patient's attitude to their health, the ownership they have of their condition and their level of motivation. An account of the patient's knowledge and understanding of their treatment will assist in the development of an individualized patient education programme. Many of the problems with hosiery can be overcome by knowledgeable and imaginative clinical management (Moffatt & Dorman 1995).

Classification of hosiery

In order for recurrence to be reduced to a minimum it is essential that the practitioner understands the current classifications for compression hosiery. The reasons for the difference in the way hosiery is classified in different countries have already been discussed. Patients with a healed venous ulcer should be fitted with the highest class of hosiery they can tolerate and safely apply (Table 10.4). In the UK a pressure of at least 18–24 mmHg is recommended while a higher pressure of 25–35 mHg is preferred. Using the German classification the degree of compression recommended for this patient group is higher, with a class III stocking giving a pressure of 34–46 mmHg. Research has not yet been undertaken to determine the exact range of pressure that is most beneficial in preventing recurrence. However in the clinical setting it is important to remember that applying a low level of compression is better than none at all. If patients have problems with application and removal, two lower-class stockings can be used to apply accumulative pressure.

Circular and flat knit hosiery

With the development of new technologies there are considerable advances in the production of

Table 10.3 Assessment issues in recurrence

Assessment	Notes	Action
Check for skin integrity	Allow a few weeks following healing to ensure the epithelium is robust	Note potential skin problems such as varicose eczema or contact dermatitis
Ensure adequate arterial supply	Record an ankle to brachial pressure index (ABPI) – this should be >0.8	Inability to record an ABPI – check for easily palpated pulses and vascular symptoms
Check for known allergies	Rubber or elastane found in hosiery are common allergens	Application of a cotton liner usually solves these problems; consider hosiery with a high cotton content
Examine foot and leg for deformities	Use protection over vulnerable sites	Ensure that deformities do not require a custom-made stocking
Measure for hosiery	Following agreed protocol, decide whether circular-knit or flat-knit hosiery is required	Consider range of hosiery available for individual patient needs – consider garments with zippers if dexterity is a problem
Disproportionate limbs may require custom-made hosiery	Follow custom-made protocol to ensure correct fit	Consider whether garment should have an open or closed toe
Assess patient understanding	This process should begin at the time of first ulcer assessment	Patients need to understand that they are potentially ulcer patients for life
Check manual dexterity	Ensure that you observe the patient applying and removing the hosiery	Use the adaptive aids available and consider the role of family and carers
Check footwear	Check that shoes fit well	Check the patient after 1 week to ensure that no problems have emerged

Table 10.4 British and German classification for compression hosiery

	Pressure applied	Recommended use
United Kingdom		
Class I	14–17 mmHg	Varicose veins, mild oedema
Class II	18–24 mmHg	Moderate/severe varicose veins, prevention of ulcer recurrence
Class III	25–35 mmHg	Gross varices, post-phlebitic limb, leg ulcer recurrence, lymphoedema
Germany RAL		
Class I	18–21 mmHg	Minor varicose veins, early varices during pregnancy; not suitable for oedema
Class II	23–32 mmHg	Varicose veins with oedema, post-traumatic swelling, significant varicose veins during pregnancy
Class III	34–46 mmHg	Chronic venous insufficiency, secondary varicose veins, extensive oedema, recurrence
Class IV	>40 mmHg	Lymphoedema

compression hosiery. There are two methods for making compression garments and it is important to understand how these manufacturing processes affect the choice of garments. Circular-knit garments are knitted on a cylinder and have no seam. This type of stocking can be made thinner and finer and may be particularly useful in low-risk patients who do not develop significant oedema. They are less suitable if high levels of compression are required or oedema develops, as the circular nature of the knitting process may cause the development of tight bands within the oedematous region. The use of thin microfibres within hosiery allow for the production of sheer, silky garments that are very attractive to patients who are concerned with their appearance.

Stockings produced by a flat-knit machine are knit row by row using a knitting pattern and, when the garment is complete, are sewn together. These garments can be made in unlimited shapes and sizes. They are particularly used in the management of lymphoedema patients, who often have gross limb deformities. Many garments of this type have an inelastic component and are particularly useful for controlling oedema reduction because of the increased stiffness within the garment. When measured correctly, these garments can give an almost perfect fit to each individual limb, even in extreme body shapes. They are also available in a wide range of ready-made garments.

The choice of product available to practitioners will vary between countries. In many parts of the world hosiery is not reimbursed and patients will be forced to buy their own. In the UK the range of products available in the community through the drug tariff reimbursement is different from the products that can be prescribed in a hospital setting, many of which comply to the higher levels of compression seen in Europe.

Measuring the limb

The accurate measurement of the limb should always be carefully recorded (Moffatt & O'Hare 1995). When two limbs are involved, both limbs should be measured separately. The optimum time for measurement is at the beginning of the day or immediately after the compression bandage has been removed. It is essential not to measure for hosiery while oedema is present. Many of the reported problems with hosiery relate to inaccurate measurement or the wrong prescription. While many patients' limbs will be adequately accommodated by the standard sizes available, some patients with disproportionate limbs may require a custom-made stocking. Care should be taken to ensure that the hosiery is of sufficient length for tall patients. When using open-toed stockings it is important to check that they are long enough, otherwise bands of oedema may develop over the forefoot. It is generally accepted by clinicians that, in venous ulcer management, below knee stockings are as effective as those that are thigh-length (Lawrence & Kakkar 1980). Thigh-length stockings are required in a number of clinical situations: when oedema extends to the thigh, when varicosities are present in the thigh region, when oedema accumulates around the knee joint or arthritic changes make below-knee stockings uncomfortable for the patient to wear.

The limb is ready for the application of hosiery once the ulcer has completely epithelialized and has regained some of its tensile strength. Often, the trauma of application and removal damages friable skin and it is advisable to wait a few weeks after the ulcer has healed before commencing hosiery. Measurement can be undertaken using a measuring board, which the patient places their foot flat against. If this is not available the patient can be measured in the standing position with the calf muscle contracted. In immobile patients who are unable to stand, two people should undertake the procedure to ensure accuracy of the measurement. Figure 10.15 shows the different points on the limb that should be measured with the tape measure. In very immobile patients, garments containing zippers should be considered, and in those who complain of slippage a product with siliconized bands at the top of the garment can be helpful. Patients who develop oedema and repeated ulcer recurrence in the retromalleolar region may benefit from hosiery containing silicone padding in this area. This applies pressure to the perforating veins and, by increasing local pressure to the area, reduces oedema. The decision to prescribe open or closed toecaps is often a matter of patient preference. Care should be taken in patients with hallux

Measurement for custom made stockings

a Metatarsal small toe joint,
   foot in dorsiflexion

h Around heel following ankle
   crease, foot in dorsiflexion

b Smallest ankle point above
   medial malleolus

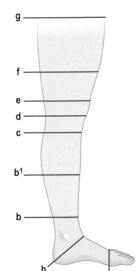

Measurement for ready made stockings

- Use a tape measure
a measure the ankle
   circumference at narrowest
   point
b measure the calf at
   widest point
c for thigh length measure
   at widest point

- Check these mesurements
  fall within the given range for
  stocking type (measurement
  outside range requires made-
  to measure stocking)

- Measurement d and e are
  important for excessively tall or
  short patients

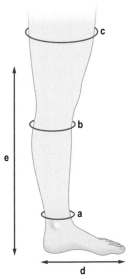

Figure 10.15 Measurement chart for compression
hosiery

valgus as bands of pressure over this area may cause tissue necrosis. When using the very high levels of compression, authors have recommended using open- rather than closed-toe garments (Asmussen & Strossenreuther 2003). While removal of compression hosiery at night is the preferred option, in those who are unable to do so it may be left in place for a week. The leg can then be washed and creamed and a clean stocking can be reapplied.

Fitting the stocking

Patients must be carefully instructed on how to take care of their leg and thus reduce the chance of recurrence. This must include the daily application of emollients and avoidance of products that may cause an allergic reaction, or those with paraffin, which may cause deterioration of the garment. A cotton tubular liner may be useful if the skin is friable or the stocking causes local erythema or irritation. If this situation persists, a stocking with a high cotton content may be used. Managing the transition from high-compression bandaging to hosiery may be difficult. Oedema may occur if the pressure applied by the stocking is considerably less than that applied by the bandage. Regular follow-up is required in this important phase. Application and removal techniques should be observed to ensure that the patient will be able to manage on their return home, and information leaflets can be provided to give instructions (Fig. 10.16). A number of useful aids are available to assist with this. Rubber washing-up gloves and slip mats are also helpful. Common problems observed in these patients include overstretching of the stocking over the calf, turning down the top of the stocking, causing a ridge, and pressure damage over the dorsum of the foot due to ridges in the stocking. The patient should be informed about the care of the stocking and that it will need to be replaced at least 6-monthly. Tears, ladders or holes will affect the overall performance.

Particular care should be taken with patients who are mentally frail and may push the stocking down. In some cases these vulnerable patients may best be managed with a multi-layer bandage systems with a cohesive outer layer that prevents the patient tampering with it while providing sustained compression.

Compression stockings

In order to provide firm support and stop your legs becoming swollen, your stockings should feel firm and be worn every day. You can take them off at night but you should put them on again first thing every morning before your legs become swollen.

Because they need to be firm-fitting, your stockings will take a little longer to put on than ordinary stockings or socks. Regular use of a moisturising cream will help you get them on and keep your skin in good condition. The drawings below show how to apply a stocking with an open toe.

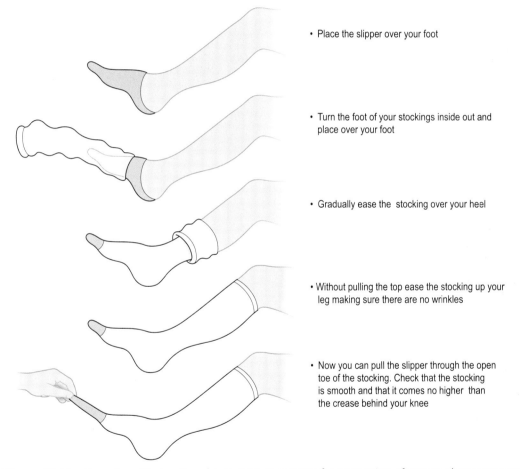

- Place the slipper over your foot

- Turn the foot of your stockings inside out and place over your foot

- Gradually ease the stocking over your heel

- Without pulling the top ease the stocking up your leg making sure there are no wrinkles

- Now you can pull the slipper through the open toe of the stocking. Check that the stocking is smooth and that it comes no higher than the crease behind your knee

Figure 10.16   Examples of instruction sheets given to patients for prevention of venous ulcer recurrence

illustration continued on following page

Whenever you can, raise your legs.

Get your legs as high as you can. Don't sit upright with your legs hanging down.

The best position would be with your legs level with your chest. Perhaps you could lie on a sofa with your legs on a pillow on the arm.

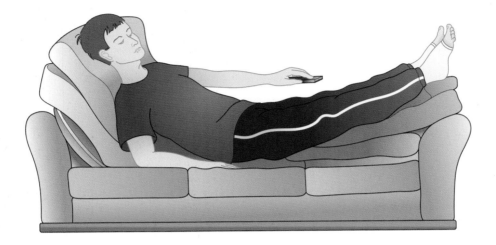

If your legs feel tight or they ache, this is probably because you have not been moving much. Go for a walk or at the very least do the following foot exercises.

- Point your toe towards the floor and then bring your foot back as far as far as you can. Repeat this exercise at least ten times.

- Move your toes in the circular motion, making as big a circle as you can. You can try this exercise in both a clockwise and anticlockwise direction. Repeat this exercise at least ten times.

Whatever you do. don't take your stockings off.

Figure 10.16, cont'd

CONCLUSION

The potential value that compression may play in improving the outcome for patients with leg ulceration on an international basis has yet to be realized. In countries that have invested in the development of improved services a glimpse of this potential can be viewed (Moffatt et al 1992). This chapter highlights the complexity of understanding compression therapy, both the scientific principles underpinning its use and the art of careful, patient-centred application. As new technologies develop in this field, the need for a new international classification of compression therapy becomes more urgent. Individual practitioners already have the potential to make dramatic improvements in the lives of their patients and families and reduce the huge burden of suffering associated with leg ulceration.

References

Abu-Own A, Shami S K, Chittenden S J et al 1994 Microangiopathy of the skin and the effect of leg compression in patients with chronic venous insufficiency. Journal of Vascular Surgery 19: 1074–1083

Adam D J, Bello M, Hartshorne T, London N J 2003 Role of superficial venous surgery with combined superficial and segmental deep venous reflux. European Journal of Vascular and Endovascular Surgery 25: 469–472

Arthur J, Lewis P 2000 When is reduced compression bandaging safe and effective? Journal of Wound Care 9: 467–471

Asmussen P D, Strossenreuther R H K 2003 Compression therapy. In: Foldi M, Fold E, Kubik S (eds) Textbook of lymphology for physicians and lymphoedema therapists. Urban & Fischer, San Francisco, CA

Barwell J R, Taylor M, Deacon J, Ghauri A S 2000 Surgical correction of isolated venous reflux reduces long term recurrence rate in chronic venous leg ulcers. European Journal Vascular and Endovascular Surgery 20: 263–268

Bollinger A, Fagrell B 1991 Clinical capillaroscopy. Hofgrefe & Huber, New York

British Standards Institute 1995 Specification for the elastic properties of flat, nonadhesive, extensible fabric bandages. BS 7505:1995. British Standards Institute, London

Brittenden J, Bradbury A W, Allan P L, Prescott R J 1998 Popliteal vein reflux reduces the healing of chronic venous ulcers. British Journal of Surgery 85: 60–62

Buchmann W F 1997 Adherence: a matter of self-efficacy and power. Journal of Advanced Nursing 26: 132–137

Callam M J, Harper D R, Dale J J, Ruckley C V 1987 Chronic ulcer of the leg :clinical history. British Medical Journal 294: 1389–1391

Chant A 1999 The biomechanics of leg ulceration. Annals of the Royal College of Surgeons of England 81: 80–85

Chetter I, Spark J, Goulding V et al 2001 Is there a relationship between the aetiology and healing rates of lower limb venous ulcers? Phlebology 16: 47–48

Christopoulos D C, Nicolaides A N, Belcaro G, Kalodiki E 1991 Venous hypertensive microangiopathy in relation to clinical severity and effect of elastic compression. Journal of Dermatologic and Surgical Oncology 17: 809–813

Clark M 2003 Compression bandages: principles and definitions. In: European Wound Management Association (eds) Position document: understanding compression therapy. Medical Education Partnership, London, pp 5–7

Cullum N A, Nelson E A, Fletcher A W, Sheldon T A 2001 Compression for venous leg ulcers (Cochrane review). In: The Cochrane Library. Update Software, Oxford

Dai G, Tsukurov O, Chen M et al 2002 Endothelial nitric oxide production during in-vitro simulation of external limb compression. American Journal of Physiology, Heart Circulation Physiology 282: H2066–H2075

Deutsches Institut für Gütesicherung und Kennzeichnung Medizinische Kompressionsstrümpfe 1987 RAL-GZ 387. Beuth-Verlag, Berlin

Edwards L M, Moffatt C J, Franks P J 2002 An exploration of patients' understanding of leg ulceration. Journal of Wound Care 11: 35–39

Effective Health Care 1997 Compression therapy for venous leg ulcers. Effective Health Care 3(4)

Erickson C A, Lanza D J, Karp D L, Edwards J W 1995 Healing of venous ulcers in an ambulatory care programme : the roles of chronic insufficiency and patient compliance. Journal of Vascular Surgery 22: 629–636

Fassiadis N, Godby C, Agland L, Law N 2002 Preventing venous ulcer recurrence: the impact of the well leg clinic. Phlebology 17: 134–136

Flanagan M, Rotchell L, Fletcher J, Scofield J 2001 Community nurses', home carers', and patients' perceptions of factors affecting venous leg ulcer recurrence and management of services. Journal of Nursing Management 9: 153–159 May

Franks P J, Moffatt C J 1998 Who suffers most from leg ulceration? Journal of Wound Care 7: 383–385

Franks P J, Moffatt C J, Connolly M et al 1994 Community leg ulcer clinics: effect on quality of life. Phlebology 9: 83–86

Franks P J, Moffatt C J, Connolly M et al 1995a Factors associated with healing leg ulceration and high compression. Age and Ageing 24: 407–410

Franks P J, Oldroyd M I, Dickson D et al 1995b Risk factors for leg ulcer recurrence :a randomised trial of two types of compression stocking. Age and Ageing 24: 407–410

Franks P J, Bosanquet N, Brown D et al 1999 Perceived health in a randomised controlled trial of single and multi-layer bandaging. European Journal of Vascular and Endovascular Surgery 17: 155–159

Franks P J, Moody M, Moffatt C J 2003 Randomised trial comparing four layer with cohesive short stretch compression bandaging in the management of chronic venous ulceration. Tissue Viability Society, Blackpool

Ghauri A S, Nyamekye I, Grabs A J, Farndon J R 1998 Influence of a specialised leg ulcer service and venous surgery on the outcomes of venous leg ulcers. European Journal Vascular and Endovascular Surgery 16: 238–244

Gniadecka M 1995 Dermal oedema in lipodermatosclerosis: distribution, effects of posture and compressive therapy evaluated by high frequency ultrasonography. Acta Dermato-Venereologica 75: 120–124

Harper D R, Nelson E A, Gibson B et al 1995 A prospective randomised controlled trial of Class 2 and Class 3 elastic compression in the prevention of venous ulceration. Phlebology Supplement 1: 872–873

Helliwell P S, Cheesbrough M J 1994 Arthropathica ulcerosa: a study of reduced ankle movement in association with chronic leg ulceration. Journal of Rheumatology 21: 1512–1514

Johnson G V 1988 Elastic stockings. British Medical Journal 296: 720

Korn P, Patel S T, Heller J A et al 2002 Why insurers should reimburse for compression stockings in patients with chronic venous stasis. Journal of Vascular Surgery 35: 950–957

Landis E M, Pappenheimer J R 1963 Exchange of substances through the capillary wall. In: Handbook of physiology circulation. American Physiology Society, Washington, sect 2, p II

Lawrence D, Kakkar V V 1980 Graduated static external compression of the lower limb :a physiological assessment. British Journal of Surgery 67: 119–121

Lofferer O, Mostbeck A, Partsch H 1972 [Nuclear medicine diagnosis of lymphatic transport disorders of the lower extremities.] Vasa 1: 94–102

McDaniel H B, Marston W A, Farber M A, Mendes R R 2002 Recurrence of chronic venous ulcers on the basis of clinical, etiologic, anatomic, and pathophysiologic criteria and air plethysmography. Journal of Vascular Surgery 35: 723–728

Mani R, Vowden K, Nelson E A 2001 Intermittent compression for the treatment of venous leg ulcers (protocol for a Cochrane review). In : The Cochrane Library. Update Software, Oxford

Margolis D J, Berlin J A, Strom B L 2000 Which venous ulcers will heal with limb compression bandaging? American Journal of Medicine 109: 15–19

Marston W A, Carlin R E, Passman M A et al 1999 Healing rates and cost efficacy of outpatient compression treatment for leg ulcers associated with chronic venous insufficiency. Journal of Vascular Surgery 30: 491–498

Mayrovitz H N, Larsen P B 1997 Effects of compression bandaging on leg pulsatile blood flow. Clinical Physiology 17: 105–117

Melhuish J M, Clark M, Williams R J, Harding K G 2000 The physics of sub-bandage pressure measurement. Journal of Wound Care 9: 308–310

Miranda F Jr, Perez M C, Castiglioni M L, Juliano Y 2001 Effect of sequential intermittent pneumatic compression on both leg lymphedema volume and on lymph transport as semi-quantitatively evaluated by lymphoscintigraphy. Lymphology 34: 135–141

Moffatt C J 2002a Oral presentation: Lo stato dell'arte della terpia compressiva (Varistretch® compression). III Congresso Nazione AIUC, Italy, November

Moffatt C J 2002b La terapia elastocompressiva nella gestione delle ulcere dell'arto inferiore: domande e risposte. III Congresso Nazionale AIUC, Italy, November

Moffatt C J, Dorman M C 1995 Recurrence of leg ulcers within a community ulcer service. Journal of Wound Care 4: 57–61

Moffatt C J, O'Hare L 1995 Graduated compression hosiery for venous ulceration. Journal of Wound Care 4: 32–37

Moffatt C J, Franks P J, Oldroyd M et al 1992 Community clinics for leg ulcers and impact on healing. British Medical Journal 305:1389–1392

Moffatt C J, Doherty D C, Franks P J 2001 Clinical risk factors for leg ulceration : a case control study. International Angiology 20: 2(Suppl 1): 115

Mostbeck A, Partsch H, Peschl L 1977 [Alteration of blood volume distribution throughout the body resulting from physical and pharmacological interventions.] Vasa 6: 137–141

Murphy M A, Joyce W P, Condron C, Bouchier-Hayes D 2002 A reduction in serum cytokine levels parallels healing of venous ulcers in patients undergoing compression therapy. European Journal of Endovascular Surgery 23: 349–352

Nelson E A 1996 Compression bandaging in the treatment of venous ulcers. Journal of Wound Care 5: 415–418

Nelson E A 2001 Systematic reviews of prevention of venous ulcer recurrence. Phlebology 16: 20–23

Nelzén O 1997 Patients with chronic leg ulcers: aspects of epidemiology, aetiology, clinical history, prognosis and choice of treatment. Skaraborg County Leg and Foot ulcer study, Slafus, Uppsala University, Paper VII. Uppsala University, Uppsala

Nelzén O, Berqvist D, Lindhagen A 1994 Venous and non venous leg ulcers: clinical history and appearance in a population study. British Journal of Surgery 81: 182–187

Pappas P J, You R, Rameshwar P, Gorti R 1999 Dermal tissue fibrosis in patients with chronic venous insufficiency is associated with increased transforming growth factor-beta1 gene expression and protein production. Journal of Vascular Surgery 30: 1129–1145

Partsch B, Partsch H 2005 Calf compression pressure required to achieve venous closure from supine to standing positions. Journal of Vascular Surgery 42: 734–738

Partsch H 1991 Compression therapy of the legs. A review. Journal of Dermatologic Surgery and Oncology 17: 799–805

Partsch H 2003 Understanding the pathophysiological effects of compression. In: European Wound Management Association (eds) Position document: understanding compression therapy. Medical Education Partnership, London, pp 2–4

Partsch H, Mostbeck A, Leitner G 1980 Experimental investigations on the effect of intermittent pneumatic compression (Lymphapress) in lymphoedema. Phlebologie und Proktologie 9: 6566

Partsch H, Menzinger G, Mostbeck A 1999 Inelastic leg compression is more effective to reduce deep venous refluxes than elastic bandages. Dermatologic Surgery 25: 695–700

Partsch H, Rabe E, Stemmer R 2000 Compression therapy of the extremities. Editions Phlébologiques Françaises, Paris, pp 789–795

Philips T, Stanton B, Provan A, Lew R 1994 A study of impact of leg ulcers on quality of life: financial, social and psychologic implications. Journal of the American Academy of Dermatology 31: 49–53

Scottish Leg Ulcer Trial Participants 2002 Effect of a national community intervention programme on healing rates of chronic leg ulcer: a randomised trial. Phlebology 17: 47–53

Smith P D 1996 The microcirculation in venous hypertension. Cardiovascular Research 32: 789–795

Sockalingham S, Barbenel J C, Queen D 1990 Ambulatory monitoring of the pressures beneath compression bandages. Care Science and Practice 8(2): 75–78

Stacey M C, Burnand K G, Lea Thomas M, Pattison M 1991 The influence of phlebographic abnormalities on the natural history of venous ulceration. British Journal of Surgery 78: 868–871

Stemmer R, Marescaux J, Furderer C 1980 [Compression therapy of the lower extremities particularly with compression stockings.] Hautarzt 31: 355–365

Thomas S 1990a Bandages and bandaging. The science behind the art. Care Science and Practice 8: 57–60

Thomas S M 1990b Wound management and dressings. Pharmaceutical Press, London

Thomas S 2003 The use of the Laplace equation in the calculation of sub-bandage pressure. Available on line at: www.worldwidewounds.com

Thomas S, Nelson A E 1998 Graduated external compression in the treatment of venous disease. Journal of Wound Care 78(Suppl): 1–4

Travers J P, Harrison J D, Makin D S 1990 Post operative use of compression stockings in preventing recurrence of varicose veins. Paper presented to the Venous Forum of the Royal Society of Medicine, London 7(8): 383–385

Vowden K R, Goulding V, Vowden P 1996 Hand-held Doppler assessment for peripheral vascula r disease. Journal of Wound Care 5: 125–128

CHAPTER

11

Surgery and sclerotherapy in the management of venous ulcers

Peter Vowden, Kathryn Vowden

INTRODUCTION

Varicose veins, dilated, lengthened and tortuous superficial veins, are the most common representation of venous disease and are present in 25–33% of the female population and between 10% and 20% of men, the prevalence rising with increasing age (da Silva et al 1974, Evans et al 1999). A true estimate of the prevalence of varicose veins is difficult to determine (Evans et al 1999). Varicose veins are probably the most common condition presenting to general and vascular surgeons. Over 50 000 patients are admitted to hospitals in the UK each year for the treatment of varicose veins or their complications (Hobbs 1991).

Venous hypertension, a direct result of chronic venous insufficiency, may be caused by either superficial or deep venous disease, or a combination of both, and is responsible for a variety of symptoms and signs. Symptoms may include cramps, particularly nocturnal cramps, itching, swelling, leg tiredness and pain, while the signs may range from increased venous skin markings (telangiectasia, reticular veins, varicose veins and varix) and oedema to skin changes such as pigmentation, eczema, lipodermatosclerosis, atrophie blanche and ulceration. In addition to these signs, varicose veins may be complicated by thrombosis and inflammation, superficial thrombophlebitis or bleeding. Unfortunately data from the Edinburgh Vein Study concluded that in patients with varicose veins no particular pattern of symptoms was useful in predicting future skin changes or ulceration (Evans et al 1997, 1999).

VENOUS ANATOMY

The veins of the lower limb are grouped into the superficial veins, those lying within the skin and subcutaneous tissues, and the deep veins, those lying deep to fascia within the muscles. Junctional, perforating or communicating veins bridge the fascia, linking the two systems. The superficial venous system is further divided into the long or greater saphenous vein and its tributaries and the short or lesser saphenous vein and its tributaries. The origin of the long saphenous vein is at the medial end of the dorsal venous arch of the foot, from where it passes just in front of the medial malleolus and then runs a course along the medial aspect of the calf, knee and thigh to reach its termination in the groin at the saphenofemoral junction. The short saphenous system, which starts at the lateral end of the dorsal venous arch, passes behind the lateral malleolus, from where it extends along the posterior aspect of the calf, draining into the deep venous system in the popliteal fossa at the saphenopopliteal junction. The two superficial systems do not function in isolation and are joined by interconnecting subcutaneous veins such as Giacomini's vein, which can run as an upward extension of the short saphenous vein joining either the proximal long saphenous vein or the deep profunda femoris vein. Incompetence in these veins linking the long and short saphenous systems can effect the distribution of varicosities. In addition to the two major junctions, the saphenofemoral and saphenopopliteal junctions, the superficial venous network drains into the deep venous system through a series of perforating or communicating veins. The majority of superficial veins, junctional and perforating veins, and deep veins have valves that direct flow initially towards the deep venous system and then back to the heart. Some veins within muscles are, however, valveless sinuses.

The vein wall is made up of three layers: the tunica intima, the inner most layer; the media; and the adventitia. The proportion of smooth muscle, elastin and collagen in the wall varies according to the location and size of the vein. Venous valves consist of two leaflets made from folds in the intima reinforced by a layer of connective tissue. Valve numbers increase towards the periphery: the inferior vena cava and common iliac veins rarely have valves and up to one-quarter of common femoral veins are valveless. It has been suggested that proximal valve paucity may contribute to the development of progressive descending valvular incompetence and lead to the development of varicose veins in some people (Browse et al 1988). The long saphenous vein contains between three and seven valves while the perforating veins usually contain only a single valve. Valvular competence is the key to calf muscle pump function, the prevention of venous reflux and the control of ambulatory venous hydrostatic pressure.

VENOUS PATHOPHYSIOLOGY

Venous return

Veins do not, in themselves, have an innate capacity to propel blood back to the heart. Venous return is dependent upon the compressive force on the deep veins derived from the action of the surrounding lower limb musculature and the compression of the venous plexus in the foot, and is aided by changes in intra-abdominal and thoracic pressure and by limb elevation, which allows gravity to assist venous return. The one-way valves within the deep veins prevent reflux of blood down into the limb, while valves within the perforating veins prevent the reflux of blood back into the superficial venous system during standing or muscle contraction. As well as actively propelling blood back towards the heart, exercise reduces the ambulatory venous pressure in the distal venous system and provides a method to drain blood from the dermal venous plexus and the larger skin veins.

The calf muscle pump

The popliteal vein, which acts as the outflow channel for the calf muscle veins and the short saphenous system, is frequently referred to as the gatekeeper for the calf muscle pump (Brittenden et al 1998). The function of the calf muscle pump is dependent on two elements: mobility (both of the individual and of the ankle joint) and a functional set of venous valves within both the deep and the perforating veins. If the function of either is impaired, venous return will be compromised and the ambulatory venous pressure will be increased. Limb elevation, even in the presence of failure of both mechanisms, will enhance venous return and reduce venous hydrostatic pressure.

The association between reduced patient and ankle mobility and delayed venous leg ulcer healing and increase in ulcer recurrence is well recognized, and this indicates the importance of a functional calf muscle pump in leg ulcer management. Brittenden and co-workers (1998) noted a link between popliteal vein reflux as measured by duplex ultrasound and an increasing incidence of venous ulceration, while Barwell et al (2000a) have indicated that a link may exist between popliteal reflux and ulcer healing.

The microcirculation

The microcirculation acts as the interphase between the arterial and venous systems and provides a zone for both gaseous and nutritional exchange. Flow within the microcirculation is dependent upon the arteriovenous pressure gradient, the resistance of the capillary bed, the viscosity of the blood, red cell deformability and an intact local response that controls capillary flow by increasing the activity of the precapillary sphincter.

Both venous reflux and venous outflow obstruction increase venous hydrostatic pressure and result in venous hypertension. This alters the balance between osmotic and oncotic pressures within the capillary–venular bed and predisposes to oedema formation. This is described in more detail in Chapter 8). Chant (1999) also suggests that a number of purely mechanical factors related to the relationship between capillary and tissue pressures come into play in the gaiter area that create an environment in which ulceration and delayed healing are almost inevitable. Figure 11.1 indicates

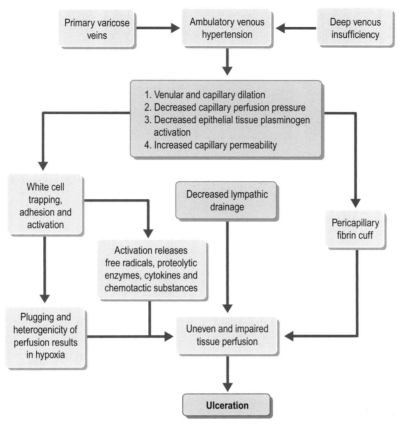

Figure 11.1 Proposed explanation for the development of venous ulceration in the presence of chronic venous disease

a possible mechanism for the development of venous ulceration in the presence of chronic venous disease.

ASSESSMENT OF VENOUS DISEASE

Assessment of the impact of venous disease is usually based on the patient's description of symptoms and a physical inspection of the limb and superficial venous system. While this may give an indication of the underlying pathology, it generally provides insufficient information for the accurate classification, diagnosis and treatment of the patient's venous disease. The presence of lower limb ulceration alone does not define a patient as having venous disease.

Information may be supplemented by conducting a more detailed examination, such as Trendelenburg testing, to establish the site(s) of junctional incompetence and reflux. More reliable evidence can, however, be obtained using the hand-held Doppler. When managing patients with potential complex venous disease, such as those with a history of limb trauma or a previous deep vein thrombosis, a secondary complication of venous disease such as venous ulceration, or recurrent varicose veins, more detailed anatomical and functional information should be obtained using colour flow duplex ultrasonography (Campbell et al 1997, Darke et al 1997). This investigation has the advantage of providing information on the status of both the deep and superficial venous systems (Fig. 11.2) and is particularly useful in assessing the reflux and patency status of the veins in the popliteal fossa and when planning surgery for recurrent varicose veins (Ch. 11). The level of information provided by

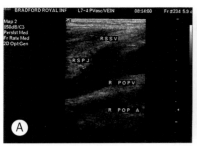 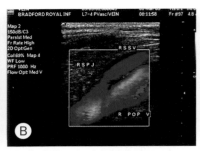 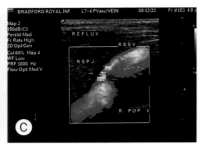

Figure 11.2 (**A**) Greyscale ultrasound image showing popliteal artery and vein and the saphenopopliteal junction. (**B**) Colour flow image of the same area at rest. (**C**) Reflux into the short saphenous system on calf compression and relaxation demonstrating valvular incompetence and the absence of reflux into the popliteal vein below the saphenopopliteal junction.

clinical examination supported by hand-held Doppler assessment, supplemented when necessary by colour flow duplex ultrasonography, is usually more than adequate to safely conduct superficial venous surgery and only rarely is additional information required from venography, plethysmography or venous pressure measurements. The role and methods for these tests has been reviewed in more detail by Vowden (1998). Figure 11.3 outlines the investigation pathway for a patient with superficial venous disease (Ch. 9). Photoplethysmography can, however, provide useful information in some patients on the deep and superficial venous systems when access to ultrasound is limited, and may assist in selecting which patients with venous leg ulceration to refer for consideration of surgery (Moffatt et al 2001). Further information is also necessary before undertaking venous reconstructive surgery such as venous bypass (e.g. the Palma crossover operation (Tibbs 1993)) to overcome a venous outflow obstruction or venous valve reconstruction or transplantation (Neglen & Raju 2003, Tripathi et al 2004), which, although still experimental, may offer a way to correct venous reflux.

CLASSIFICATION OF VENOUS DISEASE

Varicose veins may be classified into dilated venules (thread or spider veins), primary varicose veins, which may be localized or related to junctional valvular incompetence, and secondary varicose veins, which may follow deep vein thrombosis or be associated with arteriovenous fistulae or congenital abnormalities such as Klippel–Trenaunay syndrome (Tibbs et al 1997). Alternative, more detailed classification systems exist such as the CEAP (*c*linical, *e*tiological, *a*natomical and *p*athophysiological factors) classification (Bergan 1999; Box 11.1). This system is a descriptive classification, whereas venous severity scoring and quality of life scores are instruments for longitudinal research to assess outcomes (Eklof et al 2004). A simplified system has been proposed but still needs validation (Bergan 1999, Cornu-Thenard et al 2004).

CONSERVATIVE MANAGEMENT OF VENOUS DISEASE

The non-invasive management of chronic venous insufficiency is based on three strategies:

- Elevation of the limb
- The use of compression hosiery
  - ◆ Simple varicose veins: European Class I–II hosiery
  - ◆ Complicated venous disease: European Class II hosiery
- Pharmacology
  - ◆ Agents to reduce aching and cramps, such as quinine
  - ◆ Agents to increase venous tone, such as micronized purified flavonoid fraction (Daflon 500; Pinjala et al 2004)) or horse chestnut extract (Pittler & Ernst 2004). It has been suggested that such agents may be used cost

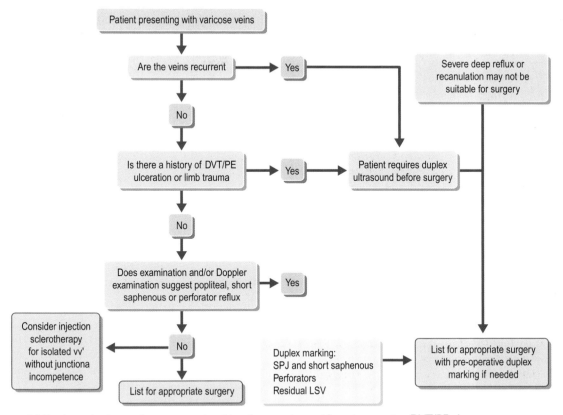

Figure 11.3 Investigation and treatment algorithm for a patient with varicose veins. DVT/PE, deep venous thrombosis/pulmonary embolism; LSV, long saphenous vein; SPJ, saphenofemoral junction; vv, varicose veins

effectively as an adjunct in the management of venous ulcer disease (Simka & Majewski 2003)

- Oxpentifylline (Trental) has also been suggested as an adjuvant therapy (Colgan et al 1990) but later work by Dale et al (1999) found no significant benefit (Chapter 13).

Compression, whether in the form of hosiery, bandaging, a compression device such as Circaid or intermittent pneumatic compression, is and will remain the mainstay of treatment of chronic venous hypertension. Compression is an effective method of both treating a venous ulcer and preventing recurrence. It is, however, a lifelong treatment option, as it does not correct the underlying disease process: it simply reduces the long-term complications of chronic venous hypertension.

VENOUS SURGERY

Venous surgery for superficial varicosities and/or junctional or communicating vein reflux

Superficial venous surgery consists of three components. The first and most important is the ligation and division of incompetent perforating or junctional veins, the second is the removal of the major stem veins that feed refluxed blood from the site of junctional incompetence to the cutaneous varicosities. The third aspect, frequently the most important to the patient, is the cosmetic element to the surgery, the removal of the cutaneous varicosities. For an effective long-term outcome all three elements must be completed; failure to do so results in a higher rate of recurrence.

Box 11.1 *The CEAP classification*

'C': clinical findings

Usually easily seen on physical examination

- C0 = No visible venous disease
- C1 = Telangiectatic or reticular veins (superficial spider veins)
- C2 = Varicose veins
- C3 = Oedema
- C4 = Skin changes without ulceration (e.g. pigmentation or lipodermatosclerosis)
- C5 = Skin changes with healed ulceration
- C6 = Skin changes with active ulceration

After this number, the letter 'a' is assigned if the patient is asymptomatic, and the letter 's' is assigned if the patient experiences symptoms. An additional number may follow the 's' to denote the severity of the symptom. More than one number may be assigned if the patient has several findings on clinical examination.

'E': aetiology of the venous disease

- 'c' for congenital disease
- 'p' for primary disease (not due to another cause)
- 's' for secondary venous disease, usually due to prior deep vein thrombosis

'A': anatomical findings

Usually based on duplex ultrasound examination, the code referring to the site of disease.

Superficial veins (As)

1. Telangiectasias or reticular veins
2. Long (greater) saphenous vein – above the knee
3. Long (greater) saphenous vein – below the knee
4. Short (lesser) saphenous vein
5. Non-saphenous

Deep veins (Ad)

1. Inferior vena cava
2. Common iliac vein
3. Internal iliac vein
4. External iliac vein
5. Pelvic veins: gonadal, broad ligament, etc.
6. Common femoral vein
7. Deep femoral vein
8. Superficial femoral vein
9. Popliteal vein
10. Crural veins: anterior tibial, posterior tibial, peroneal
11. Muscular veins: gastrocnemius, soleus, etc.

Perforating veins

1. Thigh
2. Calf

'P': pathophysiological component

- 'r' for reflux
- 'o' for obstruction
- 'r,o' for both reflux and obstruction

In addition, a disability score for chronic venous insufficiency may be used, with

- 0 denoting a patient who is asymptomatic and thus has no disability
- 1 denoting a patient who is symptomatic but can function without a support device
- 2 denoting a patient who can work an 8-hour day *only* with a support device
- 3 denoting a patient who is unable to work even with a support device

Example: A patient with an active, painful venous leg ulcer who is unable to work, who has a history of deep vein thrombosis and has, on duplex ultrasound examination, reflux in the deep system with patient recannulation of the superficial femoral vein and long saphenous reflux would be coded as:

$$C_{6s}E_sA_{52,3}Ad_8P_{ro3}$$

Surgery to communicating veins

Junctional ligation Incompetence at the saphenofemoral junction is the most common cause of superficial varicosities. The junction, which lies deep to the saphenous opening, has a fairly constant position and lies below the fascia lata and is covered by the cribriform fascia. The junction may exist in a number of anatomical configurations (Donnelly et al 2005); it is therefore important that the anatomy is carefully defined to ensure that all branches from the junction are ligated and divided and that the common femoral vein is not damaged or narrowed. Once divided, it has been suggested that the saphenous opening should be closed to reduce the incidence of neovascularization and subsequent recurrent varicose veins (Earnshaw et al 1998).

Saphenopopliteal junctional incompetence is a less common cause of superficial varicosities but is more difficult to manage. The location of the junction within the popliteal fossa is variable both in its surface location, depth and anatomical configuration; it is therefore valuable to have the junction marked preoperatively with duplex ultrasound. Even so, the close proximity of several major nerves within the popliteal fossa and, at times, difficult access increase the risk of both nerve and vein damage.

Re-exploration of either junction for recurrent varicose veins may be a challenging operation and carries with it a higher risk of complications. It is again aided by accurate preoperative duplex assessment.

An alternative approach to junctional incompetence is to attempt to restore a functional valve and thus to prevent reflux. Lane et al (2002) have reported on the success of this method in the treatment of mild to moderate junctional incompetence.

Perforator surgery   Perforating veins, which act as direct communications between the deep and superficial venous systems, exist throughout the leg but tend to be concentrated in the medial gaiter area and lower third of the thigh. They often communicate with the long or short saphenous veins through tributaries rather than joining the main trunk and may therefore not be removed when the saphenous vein itself is stripped or ablated. They can conveniently be identified and marked by preoperative duplex examination. A number of options exist for their management. When only a few are present they can be ligated directly through a small incision placed over the perforator. When multiple perforators are present it may be more convenient to ligate the perforators endoscopically (subfascial endoscopic perforator surgery – SEPS). The subfascial space in the calf is developed through a small incision placed in the upper medial calf. Perforating

veins can be seen crossing this space and can be ligated endoscopically. The advantage of this procedure is that it allows perforators over a wide area to be ligated and avoids incisions in the potentially compromised or ulcerated gaiter area skin (Baron et al 2004, Sybrandy et al 2001). Surgical alternatives to this technique include the Linton and Cocket procedures (Tibbs 1993). Perforator surgery has been successfully combined with skin grafting in the management of recalcitrant venous ulcers (Baron et al 2004).

Removal of the long and short saphenous veins

If the proximal main vein of the long and short saphenous systems is left intact there is a higher incidence of recurrent varicosities (Winterborn et al 2004). For the short saphenous system it may be sufficient to excise the proximal 10–12 cm of the short saphenous vein; for the long saphenous system it is usual to strip the long saphenous vein to the level of the knee. Several stripping techniques exist; the most common use either an olive or an inversion technique (Wilson et al 1997) to remove the vein. To reduce the risk of cutaneous nerve damage, stripping is usually from groin to knee; even so, the saphenous nerve may be damaged leaving the patient with some discomfort or numbness in the distribution of the nerve (Holme et al 1990). When the long saphenous itself is bifid or other major branches exist from the junction, these branches can also be managed by stripping.

Any residual saphenous vein can act as a source for recurrent varicosities. When this is the case the vein can be accurately located by duplex ultrasonography and any residual vein stripped or removed by stab avulsions.

Surgery to cutaneous varicosities

Cutaneous varicosities can conveniently be removed using a phlebectomy hook through small 3–5 mm incisions placed directly over the varicosities. Larger varicosities may be ligated but the majority can simply be avulsed. These small incisions are usually closed with suture strips and leave little residual mark or scar. Alternative techniques have been suggested (Scavee et al 2003, Aremu et al 2004), and surgery can be performed under tourniquet to reduce bruising.

Postoperative management

Superficial venous surgery can usually be performed as a day case. Patients are usually discharged in a light compression bandage and are encouraged to mobilize. Common practice is usually to leave bandages in place for a week, after which patients are encouraged to use light compression hosiery. Those with a history of venous ulceration are generally prescribed European class II stockings and are instructed to wear them long-term to further reduce the risk of recurrent ulceration.

The role of superficial venous surgery in the management of venous ulceration

Numerous studies have demonstrated that superficial reflux alone may be present in 50% or more of patients with venous ulceration (Cornwall et al 1986, Grabs et al 1996, Vowden et al 2001). These, and those patients with evidence of only minimal deep reflux, may benefit from venous surgery in the management of their ulcer disease.

Surgery and ulcer healing Barwell et al (2004) were unable to show any advantage of superficial venous surgery over and above conventional compression bandaging in the healing of venous ulceration, a result supported by our own observations. Iafrati et al (2002) have, however, found an improvement in both healing and recurrence rates with aggressive superficial and perforator (SEPS) surgery, a result supported by Bianchi et al (2003). Adam et al (2003) support this view and also found that surgery could successfully be applied even in the presence of deep reflux, with the correction of limited deep reflux in some patients. In our hands early surgery does seem to be associated with a higher incidence of complications, in particular wound infection and cellulitis. Improved healing has, however, been reported when SEPS has been combined with grafting in the management of recalcitrant ulcers associated with perforator incompetence (Sybrandy et al 2001).

Surgery and ulcer recurrence The mainstay of ulcer recurrence prevention is the use of compression hosiery after ulcer healing. However, ulcer recurrence rates can be depressingly high even in regular hosiery users (Mayberry et al 1991, Dinn & Henry 1992, Moffatt & Franks 1995), recurrence rates of between 28% and 69% being reported over a 12–18-month period (Monk & Sarkany 1982, Moffatt & Dorman 1995). Recurrence rates are higher in patients with poor mobility or with larger initial ulcers (Vowden & Vowden 2004) or in those with a poor record of hosiery usage (Samson & Showalter 1996). Recurrence rates tend to be highest in the initial 3 months after healing (Moffatt & Dorman 1995) and this is supported by our own experience, where 25% of recurrence occurred in the first 90 days and 59% in the first year (Vowden & Vowden 2004). To be of maximum benefit in reducing ulcer recurrence, surgery, should be undertaken as soon after ulcer healing as is practical.

The potential value of superficial venous surgery as a method of reducing ulcer recurrence has been suggested for a number of years. Darke & Penfold (1992) indicated the advantage of surgery and since then several studies have supported this view (DePalma & Kowallek 1996, Ghauri et al 1998, Barwell et al 2000b, McDaniel et al 2002). However, until recently, data from controlled trials were lacking. The ESCHAR study (Barwell et al 2004) demonstrated a marked reduction in ulcer recurrence in the surgically treated group and our own experience is that targeted venous surgery can markedly reduce the level of ulcer recurrence (Vowden & Vowden 2004). Surgery can be performed under local, regional or general anaesthesia and is therefore applicable to most patients with venous ulceration and superficial venous disease. There is as yet little evidence relating to the use of endovenous surgery in the prevention of ulcer recurrence but, providing all sites of junctional incompetence can be eliminated, it should be as effective as conventional venous surgery. Perforator surgery has been linked to a marked reduction in ulcer recurrence whether performed by an open or endoscopic method (Sybrandy et al 2001). Further trials are necessary, however, before the role of SEPS in the management of venous ulcer disease can be confirmed (Tenbrook et al 2004).

Deep vein surgery

Scott et al (2004) have recently reviewed the role of surgery in the management of deep venous insufficiency. A variety of procedures have been attempted ranging from superficial venous surgery, through perforator surgery (SEPS) to deep venous reconstruction. The latter has included valvuloplasty, transplantation and transposition (Jamieson & Chinnick 1997, Perrin 2000). Few randomized studies have been undertaken and, for the majority of reports, patient numbers are low. Scott et al (2004) conclude that the optimal surgery for patients with deep venous insufficiency remains unclear. This opinion is supported by Hardy et al (2004) in their Cochrane review.

ENDOVASCULAR THERAPY

Sclerotherapy

Conventional sclerotherapy has been practised for decades and is the injection of aqueous solutions into abnormally dilated or cosmetically unacceptable veins. These solutions irritate and damage the endothelial lining of the treated vein, causing it to thrombose, fibrose, stenose and then hopefully be absorbed by surrounding tissue. A number of different agents are used, including ethanolamine oleate and sodium tetradecyl sulphate (Soumian & Davies 2004). Those recommended by the consensus conference (Anon 1997) on sclerotherapy of varicose veins of the lower limb are:

- Chromated glycerine, 25–100%
- Polidocanol, 0.2–1%
- Sodium salicylate, 6–12%
- Hypertonic glucose.

The technique is best suited to the management of isolated varicosities not associated with junctional reflux and postsurgical recurrent or residual varicosities once residual junctional incompetence has been excluded. Sclerotherapy is also effective in the management of telangiectasias, spider veins and reticular veins. The chosen sclerosant is injected, using a small (25–33G) needle, into the selected vein(s) or telangiectasia. An initial test dose is recommended to check for adverse reactions. Compression can be used but may not affect outcome (Fraser et al 1985).

A number of different methods have been described for injecting veins. These include; Fegan's method (Fegan 1963), Tournay's method (1997) and Sigg's method (Sigg & Zelikovski 1975). Good comparative data between sclerotherapy and sur-

gery are limited but most show a high recurrence rate of varicosities (20–70%) after sclerotherapy (Soumian & Davies 2004).

Sclerotherapy must be performed with caution as allergy can occur. The majority of side effects are, however, minor and include hyperpigmentation, pruritus and neovascularization, all of which affect the cosmetic outcome. Rare major complications include blistering, ulceration, thrombophlebitis and deep vein thrombosis and intra-arterial injection. The outcome and complication risk may be improved by using duplex-ultrasound-guided injections (Kanter et al 1995, Min & Navarro 2000).

Sclerotherapy has been suggested as an adjunct to compression in the management of venous ulceration, with improvement reported in both healing and recurrence rates (Queral et al 1990, Labas et al 2002).

Foam sclerotherapy is a recent development in the treatment of venous disease that has great promise and offers a number of advantages over conventional sclerotherapy (Yamaki et al 2004), although only a few non-randomized studies have been published to date and long-term outcome data are still lacking (Soumian & Davies 2004). A number of foam-generating techniques have been described (Cabrera & Garcia-Olmedo 2000, Frullini 2000, Tessari et al 2001, Frullini and Cavezzi 2002). Sclerosing foam is a non-equilibrated dispersion of gas bubbles in a sclerosing solution, the foam being made of tiny bubbles covered with a tension-active liquid, the smaller the bubbles the more active the foam. The foam preparations appear to have a number of advantages over conventional sclerosants in that they enhance the effectiveness of the sclerosant, allowing the use of a lower dose, which in turn increases safety. Extravasation of the foam is better tolerated than the liquid sclerosant, while the presence of air in the sclerosant increases the accuracy of duplex-guided sclerotherapy. Complications similar to those encountered with conventional sclerotherapy are described. The potential respiratory complications are still unclear (Soumian & Davies 2004).

Endovenous radiofrequency ablation

Radiofrequency energy generates heat and has been used for some time in a controlled fashion to ablate abnormal conducting tissue in the heart to treat arrhythmias (Olgin et al 1997). The technique has been modified to allow ablation of abnormal veins. A catheter is passed along the vein under ultrasound control to the site of the most proximal incompetent valve, usually the saphenofemoral junction. The radiofrequency energy heats the vein wall to a controlled 85°C using a catheter electrode in a controlled feedback loop and this ablates the vein as the catheter is withdrawn at approximately 3 cm/min. The VNUS (VNUS Medical Technologies, Sunnyvale, CA) is the most common system used. The procedure can be performed under local or general anaesthesia. To reduce the risk of local thermal injury in the tissue surrounding the vein and the overlying skin, the procedure is usually performed under tumescent anaesthesia, the perivenous tissues and the subfascial space being infiltrated with saline or a dilute local anaesthetic solution.

The results reported with this technique are encouraging, with initial closure rates of the long saphenous vein of between 93% and 100% being reported (Fassiadis et al 2002, Goldman & Amiry 2002, Weiss & Weiss 2002). Later results are also good, with a 2-year follow-up closure rate of 90% and a symptom improvement score of 95% (Weiss & Weiss 2002, Pichot et al 2004). Early comparative data are encouraging and may indicate a long-term place for this technique in the management of varicose veins (Lurie et al 2003), and therefore potentially venous ulceration. Complications include bruising, tenderness, paraesthesia, phlebitis, skin burns and deep vein thrombosis. Minor residual veins left after main trunk ablation can be managed by local phlebectomies or by injection sclerotherapy.

Endovenous laser therapy

A procedure similar to that described for radiofrequency ablation is followed but in the case of laser therapy the vein wall is heated with 810 nm or 940 nm wavelength laser energy delivered via a laser fibre. The results are also similar to other endovenous techniques (Min et al 2003) but a higher complication rate has been described by some authors (Soumian & Davies 2004). Proebstle et al (2003) have reported the success of endovenous laser therapy in the management of short saphenous reflux, including patients with healed and open ulcers.

Endovenous therapy requires the presence of a skilled ultrasonographer, a duplex machine and expensive radiofrequency or laser equipment. Further randomized clinical trials comparing conventional surgery with endovenous techniques are needed before the widespread adoption of these methods. It has, however, been suggested that these techniques might play a role in the management of venous ulceration and the prevention of recurrence (Welch 2004).

CONCLUSION

Superficial venous reflux, whether in isolation or in combination with deep reflux, is a correctable cause of venous ulceration. Surgical intervention may contribute to ulcer healing, particularly in recalcitrant ulceration. There is increasingly sound evidence that superficial venous surgery has an important role to play in the prevention of ulcer recurrence. However, if maximal benefit is to accrue intervention should be undertaken soon after ulcer healing.

The role of less invasive endovenous therapy in the management of venous ulceration is as yet unclear. Early results in the management of uncomplicated primary varicose veins are encouraging and these treatments may have a future role to play in improving both the healing and recurrence rate for venous ulceration.

References

Adam D J, Bello M, Hartshorne T, London N J 2003 Role of superficial venous surgery in patients with combined superficial and segmental deep venous reflux. European Journal of Vascular and Endovascular Surgery 25: 469–472

Anon 1997 Consensus conference on sclerotherapy of varicose veins of the lower limb. Phlebology 12: 2–160

Aremu M A, Mahendran B, Butcher W et al 2004 Prospective randomized controlled trial:

conventional versus powered phlebectomy. Journal of Vascular Surgery 39: 88–94

Baron H C, Wayne M G, Santiago C A, Grossi R 2004 Endoscopic subfascial perforator vein surgery for patients with severe, chronic venous insufficiency. Vascular and Endovascular Surgery 38: 439–442

Barwell J R, Ghauri A S K, Taylor M et al 2000a Risk factors for healing and recurrence of chronic venous leg ulcers. Phlebology 15: 49–52

Barwell J R, Taylor M, Deacon J et al 2000b Surgical correction of isolated superficial venous reflux reduces long- term recurrence rate in chronic venous leg ulcers. European Journal of Vascular and Endovascular Surgery 20: 363–368

Barwell J R, Davies C E, Deacon J et al 2004 Comparison of surgery and compression with compression alone in chronic venous ulceration (ESCHAR study): randomised controlled trial. Lancet 363: 1854–1859

Bergan J J 1999 How should venous disease be classified? In: Ruckley C V, Fowkes F G R, Bradbury A W (eds) Venous disease. Springer-Verlag, London, pp 73–79

Bianchi C, Ballard J L, Abou-Zamzam A M, Teruya T H 2003 Subfascial endoscopic perforator vein surgery combined with saphenous vein ablation: results and critical analysis. Journal of Vascular Surgery 38: 67–71

Brittenden J, Bradbury A W, Allan P L et al 1998 Popliteal vein reflux reduces the healing of chronic venous ulcer. British Journal of Surgery 85: 60–62

Browse N L, Burnand K G, Thomas M L 1988 Disease of the veins: pathology, diagnosis and treatment. Edward Arnold, London

Cabrera J J, Garcia-Olmedo M A 2000 Treatment of varicose long saphenous veins with sclerosant in microfoam: longterm outcomes. Phlebology 15: 19–23

Campbell W B, Niblett P G, Ridler B M et al 1997 Hand-held Doppler as a screening test in primary varicose veins. British Journal of Surgery 84: 1541–1543

Chant A 1999 The biomechanics of leg ulceration. Annals of the Royal College of Surgeons of England 81: 80–85

Colgan M P, Dormandy J A, Jones P W, Schraibman I G, Shanik D G, Young R A 1990 Oxpentifylline treatment of venous ulcers of the leg. British Medical Journal 300: 972–975

Cornu-Thenard A, Uhl J F, Carpentier P H 2004 Do we need a better classification than CEAP? Acta Chirurgica Belgica 104: 276–282

Cornwall J V, Dore C J, Lewis J D 1986 Leg ulcers: epidemiology and aetiology. British Journal of Surgery 73: 693–696

Dale J J, Ruckley C V, Harper D R, Gibson B, Nelson E A, Prescott R J 1999 Randomised double blind placebo controlled trial of pentoxifylline in the treatment of venous leg ulcers. British Medical Journal 319: 875–878

Darke S G, Penfold C 1992 Venous ulceration and saphenous ligation. European Journal of Vascular Surgery 6: 4–9

Darke S G, Vetrivel S, Foy D M et al 1997 A comparison of duplex scanning and continuous wave Doppler in the assessment of primary and uncomplicated varicose veins. European Journal of Vascular and Endovascular Surgery 14: 457–461

Da Silva A, Widmer L K, Martin H et al 1974 Varicose veins and chronic venous insufficiency. Vasa 3: 118–125

DePalma R G, Kowallek D L 1996 Venous ulceration: a cross-over study from nonoperative to operative treatment. Journal of Vascular Surgery 24: 788–792

Dinn E, Henry M 1992 Treatment of venous ulceration by injection sclerotherapy and compression hosiery: a 5-year study. Phlebology 7: 23–26

Donnelly M, Tierney S, Feeley T M 2005 Anatomical variation at the saphenofemoral junction. British Journal of Surgery 92: 322–325

Earnshaw J J, Davies B, Harradine K, Heather B P 1998 Preliminary results of PTFE patch saphenoplasty to prevent neovascularization leading to recurrent varicose veins. Phlebology 13: 10–13

Eklof B, Rutherford R B, Bergan J J et al 2004 Revision of the CEAP classification for chronic venous disorders: consensus statement. Journal of Vascular Surgery 40: 1248–1252

Evans C J, Fowkes F G R, Ruckley C V et al 1997 Edinburgh Vein Study: methods and response in a survey of venous disease in the general population. Phlebology 12: 127–135

Evans C J, Lee A J, Ruckley C V, Fowkes F R G 1999 How common is venous disease in the general population? In: Ruckley C V, Fowkes F G R, Bradbury A W (eds) Venous disease. Springer-Verlag, London, pp 3–14

Fassiadis N, Kianifard B, Holdstock J M, Whiteley M S 2002 Ultrasound changes at the saphenofemoral junction and in the long saphenous vein during the first year after VNUS closure. International Angiology 21: 272–274

Fegan W G 1963 Continuous compression technique of injecting varicose veins. Lancet 2: 109–112

Fraser I A, Perry E P, Hatton M, Watkin D F 1985 Prolonged bandaging is not required following sclerotherapy of varicose veins. British Journal of Surgery 72: 488–490

Frullini A 2000 New technique in producing sclerosing foam in a disposable syringe. Dermatologic Surgery 26: 705–706

Frullini A, Cavezzi A 2002 Sclerosing foam in the treatment of varicose veins and telangiectases: history and analysis of safety and complications. Dermatologic Surgery 28: 11–15

Ghauri A S, Nyamekye I, Grabs A J et al 1998 Influence of a specialised leg ulcer service and venous surgery on the outcome of venous leg ulcers. European Journal of Vascular and Endovascular Surgery 16: 238–244

Goldman M P, Amiry S 2002 Closure of the greater saphenous vein with endoluminal radiofrequency thermal heating of the vein wall in combination with ambulatory phlebectomy: 50 patients with more than 6-month follow-up. Dermatologic Surgery 28: 29–31

Grabs A J, Wakely M C, Nyamekye I et al 1996 Colour duplex ultrasonography in the rational management of chronic venous leg ulcers. British Journal of Surgery 83: 1380–1382

Hardy S C, Riding G, Abidia A 2004 Surgery for deep venous incompetence. Cochrane Database Systematic Revues, CD001097. Update Software, Oxford

Hobbs J T 1991 ABC of vascular diseases. Varicose veins. British Medical Journal 303: 707–710

Holme J B, Skajaa K, Holme K 1990 Incidence of lesions of the saphenous nerve after partial or complete stripping of the long saphenous vein. Acta Chirurgica Scandinavica 156: 145–148

Iafrati M D, Pare G J, O'Donnell T F, Estes J 2002 Is the nihilistic approach to surgical reduction of superficial and perforator vein incompetence for venous ulcer justified? Journal of Vascular Surgery 36: 1167–1174

Jamieson W G, Chinnick B 1997 Clinical results of deep venous valvular repair for chronic venous insufficiency. Canadian Journal of Surgery 40: 294–299

Kanter A, Gardner M, Isaacs M 1995 Identification of arteriovenous anastomoses by duplex ultrasound. Implications for the treatment of varicose veins. Dermatologic Surgery 21: 885–9

Labas P, Ohradka B, Cambal M, Martinicky D 2002 The treatment of venous leg ulcers by compression sclerotherapy. Bratislavske lekarske listy 103: 442–446

Lane R J, Cuzzilla M L, Coroneos J C 2002 The treatment of varicose veins with external stenting to the saphenofemoral junction. Vascular and Endovascular Surgery 36: 179–192

Lurie F, Creton D, Eklof B et al 2003 Prospective randomized study of endovenous radiofrequency obliteration (closure procedure) versus ligation and stripping in a selected patient population (EVOLVeS Study). Journal of Vascular Surgery 38: 207–214

McDaniel H B, Marston W A, Farber M A et al 2002 Recurrence of chronic venous ulcers on the basis of clinical, etiologic, anatomic, and pathophysiologic criteria and air plethysmography. Journal of Vascular Surgery 35: 723–728

Mayberry J C, Moneta G L, Taylor L M Jr, Porter J M 1991 Fifteen-year results of ambulatory compression therapy for chronic venous ulcers. Surgery 109: 575–581

Min R J, Navarro L 2000 Transcatheter duplex ultrasound-guided sclerotherapy for treatment of greater saphenous vein reflux: preliminary report. Dermatologic Surgery 26: 410–414

Min R J, Khilnani N, Zimmet S E 2003 Endovenous laser treatment of saphenous vein reflux: long-term results. Journal of Vascular and Interventional Radiology 14: 991–996

Moffatt C J, Dorman M C 1995 Recurrence of leg ulcers within a community ulcer service. Journal of Wound Care 4: 57–61

Moffatt C, Franks P 1995 The problem of recurrence in patients with leg ulceration. Journal of Tissue Viability 5: 64–66

Moffatt C J, Doherty D C, Franks PJ 2001 Non-invasive investigations of venous pathology in leg ulceration: a population study. In: 11th Conference of the European Wound Management Association, Dublin, Ireland. European Wound Management Association, London

Monk B E, Sarkany I 1982 Outcome of treatment of venous stasis ulcers. Clinical and Experimental Dermatology 7: 397–400

Neglen P, Raju S 2003 Venous reflux repair with cryopreserved vein valves. Journal of Vascular Surgery 37: 552–557

Olgin J E, Kalman J M, Chin M et al 1997 Electrophysiological effects of long, linear atrial lesions placed under intracardiac ultrasound guidance. Circulation 96: 2715–2721

Perrin M 2000 Reconstructive surgery for deep venous reflux: a report on 144 cases. Cardiovascular Surgery 8: 246–255

Pichot O, Kabnick L S, Creton D et al 2004 Duplex ultrasound scan findings two years after great saphenous vein radiofrequency endovenous obliteration. Journal of Vascular Surgery 39: 189–195

Pinjala R K, Abraham T K, Chadha S K et al 2004 Long-term treatment of chronic venous insufficiency of the leg with micronized purified flavanoid fraction in the primary care setting. Phlebology 19: 179–184

Pittler M H, Ernst E 2004 Horse chestnut seed extract for chronic venous insufficiency. Cochrane Database of Systematic Revues, CD003230. Update Software, Oxford

Proebstle T M, Gul D, Kargl A, Knop J 2003 Endovenous laser treatment of the lesser saphenous vein with a 940-nm diode laser: early results. Dermatologic Surgery 29: 357–361

Queral L A, Criado F J, Lilly M P, Rudolphi D 1990 The role of sclerotherapy as an adjunct to Unna's boot for treating venous ulcers: a prospective study. Journal of Vascular Surgery 11: 572–575

Samson R H, Showalter D P 1996 Stockings and the prevention of recurrent venous ulcers. Dermatologic Surgery 22: 373–376

Scavee V, Lesceu O, Theys S et al 2003 Hook phlebectomy versus transilluminated powered phlebectomy for varicose vein surgery: early results. European Journal of Vascular and Endovascular Surgery 25: 473–475

Scott N A, Corabian P, Forbes T L, Hardy S C 2004 Surgical treatment for chronic deep venous insufficiency. Phlebology 19: 109–119

Sigg K, Zelikovski A 1975 'Quick treatment' – a modified method of sclerotherapy of varicose veins. Vasa 4: 73–78

Simka M, Majewski E 2003 The social and economic burden of venous leg ulcers: focus on the role of micronized purified flavonoid fraction adjuvant therapy. American Journal of Clinical Dermatology 4: 573–581

Soumian S, Davies A H 2004 Endovenous management of varicose veins. Phlebology 19: 163–169

Sybrandy J E, van Gent W B, Pierik E G, Wittens C H 2001 Endoscopic versus open subfascial division of incompetent perforating veins in the treatment of venous leg ulceration: long-term follow-up. Journal of Vascular Surgery 33: 1028–1032

Tenbrook J A Jr, Iafrati M D, O'Donnell T F Jr et al 2004 Systematic review of outcomes after surgical management of venous disease incorporating subfascial endoscopic perforator surgery. Journal of Vascular Surgery 39: 583–589

Tessari L, Cavezzi A, Frullini A 2001 Preliminary experience with a new sclerosing foam in the treatment of varicose veins. Dermatologic Surgery 27: 58–60

Tibbs D J 1993 Varicose veins and related disorders. Butterworth-Heinemann, London

Tibbs D J, Fletcher E W 1983 Direction of flow in superficial veins as a guide to venous disorders in lower limbs. Surgery 93: 758–767

Tripathi R, Sieunarine K, Abbas M, Durrani N 2004 Deep venous valve reconstruction for non-healing leg ulcers: techniques and results. Australian and New Zealand Journal of Surgery 74: 34–39

Vowden P 1998 The investigation of venous disease. Journal of Wound Care 7: 143–147

Vowden K, Vowden P 2004 Abstract. Ulcer recurrence profiles: Implication for service provision. In: Wounds UK Harrogate 2004. Wounds UK, Aberdeen.

Vowden K R, Goulden V, Wilkinson D, Vowden P 2001 Venous disease in leg ulceration as revealed by Duplex ultrasound: influence on healing and recurrence. In: 11th European Conference on Advances in Wound Management, Dublin, Ireland. European Wound Management Association, London

Weiss R A, Weiss M A 2002 Controlled radiofrequency endovenous occlusion using a unique radiofrequency catheter under duplex guidance to eliminate saphenous varicose vein reflux: a 2-year follow-up. Dermatologic Surgery 28: 38–42

Welch H J 2004 Surgical options for the treatment of venous ulcers. Vascular and Endovascular Surgery 38: 195–202

Wilson S, Pryke S, Scott R et al 1997 'Inversion' stripping of the long saphenous vein. Phlebology 12: 91–95

Winterborn R J, Foy C, Earnshaw J J 2004 Causes of varicose vein recurrence: late results of a randomized controlled trial of stripping the long saphenous vein. Journal of Vascular Surgery 40: 634–639

Yamaki T, Nozaki M, Iwasaka S 2004 Comparative study of duplex-guided foam sclerotherapy and duplex-guided liquid sclerotherapy for the treatment of superficial venous insufficiency. Dermatologic Surgery 30: 718–722; discussion 722

12

Surgical treatment to cover skin defects, including skin grafting and tissue extension

Luc Téot

INTRODUCTION

The surgical management of leg ulcer is poorly developed, with most medical input coming from dermatologists. Surgery is usually only contemplated for patients presenting with large, hard to heal or recurrent ulcers, where skin grafting following sharp debridement is usually proposed.

Pinch skin grafting was proposed more than 135 years ago and, for a large proportion of European dermatologists, is the standard technique for closure of a venous leg ulcer. Extensive surgical excision of the lipodermatosclerotic area followed by skin grafting was initially undertaken by Schmeller & Gaber (2000) and redefined more recently by Gottrup (2004). More recently the use of skin substitutes (cellularized or non-cellularized) has been popularized by Falanga & Sabolinski (1999), although no surgical wound treatment in venous leg ulcer can completely obviate the necessity of wearing compression.

Surgical preparation of the wound bed includes mechanical and sharp debridement; the use of negative pressure therapy and biosurgery; the appropriate indications for dermal and epidermal substitutes; correct planning and skin grafting technique; indications and the proper surgical techniques for flaps (including recent developments in prefabricated flaps); and the appropriate use of tissue extension. This chapter will also include the future possible applications of gene therapy.

WOUND BED PREPARATION
Surgical debridement

Surgical debridement is usually undertaken in the operating theatre and is different from sharp debridement undertaken at the bedside or in a clinic because of the size of the ulcer. Electro-cauterization may be used to stop bleeding, and analgesia is tailored to the patient's pain. Excision depth is variable, depending on the amount of fibrin tissue to be resected before obtaining a uniformly bleeding wound bed.

Techniques

Superficial excision using water jets   Recently a new tool was designed and proposed as a high-pressure debriding agent. The Versajet system is based on the application of a high-pressure water jet tangential to the surface of the wound. The water and debris are collected back into the handpiece by a curved metal piece acting in a similar way to a curette. The machine can be used at different water pressure levels. No published clinical series are available on this product at present. Other water jet systems using high pressure (e.g. Debritom) are currently under evaluation. Recent results have been reported in trials using ultra-sound-assisted wound treatment (Palmier & Trial 2004).

Superficial excision using ultrasound Local application of ultrasound has recently been proposed to excise fibrotic tissue. This technique is now under evaluation in terms of reduction of pain and the precise destruction of the fibrinous tissues.

Excision of the necrotic/fibrotic tissues: the shaving technique In this technique, the aim is to excise a minimum amount of tissue and to perform a tangential excision to expose a uniformly vascularized bed. The shaving technique should limit the loss of blood. Expert evaluation of the quality of the bed prepared by such techniques is required. This technique has been extensively used in Germany for 20 years. The necrotic and fibrous tissues are widely removed, the lipodermatosclerotic area being partially or totally removed. Perfectly vascularized granulation tissue should be obtained before applying a split-thickness skin graft. This technique requires general anaesthesia. Schmeller & Gaber evaluated the long-term effects of shave therapy in non-healing venous leg ulcers. 41 patients with 75 recalcitrant leg ulcers caused by primary deep vein incompetence or post-thrombotic syndrome were operated on using shave therapy. The average follow-up period was 2 years and 5 months. The healing rate was 76% for ulcers associated with primary deep vein incompetence and 58% for ulcers associated with post-thrombotic syndrome. One-third of the cases presented were recurrent ulcers but these ulcers were reduced by 80–90% of their original size. In 'non-healing' venous leg ulcers due to deep venous insufficiency, shave therapy yields favourable long-term results. Because it is only a symptomatic treatment that does not reduce pathological refluxes, continuous compression of the lower leg has to be maintained after surgery.

Excision to the fascia This technique is more ambitious and is comparable to the strategy of excision–grafting used in burns surgery. The aim is to remove all the necrotic and fibrous tissues, and also the lipodermatosclerotic area under and around the leg ulceration. In some cases, a large circumferential excision of the skin is undertaken, treating both the consequence and the cause of chronic venous disease, as perforator veins can be excised and removed in the same operation. This technique represents one way of radically excising large ulcers. It is usually indicated when calcifications are present, requiring the excision to be undertaken at different depths. No lymphatic obstruction has been reported and the deep venous system seems efficient enough to prevent excessive congestion and oedema of the limb after excision to the fascia.

Indications

A small venous leg ulcer will not be a candidate for extensive surgical debridement. A progressive, staged debridement using non-surgical techniques will be preferred to a sharp, extensive, painful excision because of the intense pain provoked by tissue incision or resection. Sharp debridement can be limited to a simple curettage of the ulcer after pain prevention using EMLA cream 30 minutes beforehand. Premedication can be given 1 hour before surgery in large venous leg ulcers. Alternatively, surgical debridement can be carried out under general anaesthesia immediately before undertaking the covering technique.

Sharp debridement is not appropriate for arterial ulcers because of the risk of creating necrotic areas on the edges of the sharp debridement. Arterial ulcer debridement should only be performed when an operative protocol of revascularization can be programmed. In some cases, the vascular surgeon will not schedule the patient for bypass or angioplasty, because of obstacles in the distal vascular bed. Surgical debridement should not be performed in this situation. In necrotic angiodermatitis, rapid superficial debridement followed by skin grafting is proposed by some in order to manage the extreme pain usually associated with this condition.

Negative pressure therapy

Technique

Negative pressure (VAC) therapy is performed by application of a piece of polyurethane foam cut to the volume of the wound, covered with adhesive film and linked to an aspirating machine (Téot et al 2004; Fig. 12.1). This technique is employed mainly in traumatic situations but may also be used for chronic wounds presenting with cavities, such as pressure ulcers. The VAC technique is frequently used in diabetic ulcers and in chronic leg ulcers because of its antibacterial properties.

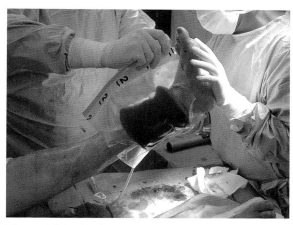

Figure 12.1 Negative pressure therapy: application of the foam after skin grafting

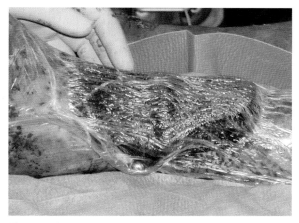

Figure 12.2 Negative pressure therapy: retraction of the foam when a low pressure is applied (55 mmHg)

VAC therapy can be applied as a wound bed preparation technique, prior to skin grafting. The pressure to be applied can be varied between 50 and 200 mmHg, with the standard level being 125 mmHg (Fig. 12.2). The negative pressure can be applied over fibrous tissues and exposed structures such as tendons and bones (lateral or medial malleoli) after limited surgical debridement. The length of use depends on the vascular status of the patient, pure venous leg ulcers responding better to the treatment than arterial ulcers. Explanations for the spectacular promotion of granulation tissue achieved are numerous. In their pioneering experi-

mental article, Morykwas et al (1997) explained the fibroblast stimulation by an antibacterial action but recent work has shown that bacteria remain present in the wound after VAC application. Some authors have shown that VAC therapy promotes vascular endothelial growth factor expression (Téot et al 2004).

Indications

Venous leg ulcers   VAC has mainly been applied as a technique promoting the granulation tissue and control of oedema. These effects have been clinically proven, although no randomized controlled trials have been undertaken. In a recent prospective, controlled, open, non-comparative study, Loree at al (2004) assessed the effectiveness of topical negative pressure in the fibrinous debridement of chronic leg ulcers. The median percentage reduction in fibrinous tissue was 28% on day 3 and 40% on day 6. VAC therapy was considered to be rapid and effective in promoting angiogenesis and the formation of healthy tissue.

Different modes of treatment and types of foam have been developed for use in VAC therapy. An ambulatory unit has been proposed and has demonstrated its usefulness in the management of leg ulcers. This technique allows the patient some mobility, the negative pressure being applied permanently over the leg ulcer, with the pump and battery being suspended from a belt.

Arterial ulcers   VAC therapy can be considered as an interim measure, limiting the risks of infection but, because of the absence of vascularization in the underlying structures, not allowing the promotion of granulation tissue.

Skin grafting   VAC is more commonly used as a mean of fixing a skin graft (Chang et al 2001, Webb & Schmidt 2001). In this indication, the pressure level must be low (about 55 mmHg). The machine is easy to use, allowing for different levels of pressure and varying modes of action, i.e. intermittent or continuous. Perforated polyvinyl pads are cut to the exact size of the area to be covered, and fixed using adhesive films. Negative pressure therapy can also be applied in the postoperative period over a dermal substitute in the same way as over a skin graft.

Biosurgery

Techniques

Since the 19th century, the use of maggots has been promoted for the debridement of chronic wounds. Leg ulcers were included in these series (Sherman 2003) and the efficacy of maggots in removing fibrinous tissues was confirmed. The development of a bag to contain the maggots was considered as a refinement compared to free maggots directly delivered into the wound. Complications are limited to allergic reactions. Although most authors acknowledge the antiseptic properties of the maggots' secretions, they are not active against some bacteria, including *Pseudomonas*. Maggots are better used after mechanical debridement (curettage). They are changed every 2–3 days.

Indications

The usual indications for larval therapy is diabetic foot debridement, but the indications are rapidly extending, biosurgery having demonstrated some efficiency in acute and chronic situations.

These results are convincing Health Authorities that maggots may be a useful tool in wound management. In Denmark, maggots are considered to be first-line debriding therapy in diabetic foot ulceration.

Larval debridement therapy has been shown anecdotally to clear ulcers of necrotic slough (Wayman et al 2001). It has been compared directly with 'modern' therapies in a randomized control study comparing the application of larvae and hydrogel. Effective debridement occurred with a maximum of one larval application in six of six patients. Four of the six patients in the hydrogel group still required dressings at 1 month. The median cost of treatment of the larval group was half that of the control group ($p < 0.05$). This study confirms both the clinical efficacy and cost-effectiveness of larval therapy in the debridement of sloughy venous ulcers.

Biosurgery was also used in a recent clinical study for debridement in 30 patients with chronic leg ulcers of mixed origin (Wollina et al 2002). The effect of a single application of maggots for 1–4 days was evaluated by a clinical wound score and contact-free spectroscopy. Side-effects were recorded. Debridement was rapid and selective, and well tolerated in most patients. The wound secretion was temporarily increased. 12 out of 30 patients reported temporary pain but only two needed analgesic treatment. Other side-effects included venous bleeding in one patient. Oxygenation is the possible mechanism invoked to explain these rapid results.

When is surgical debridement required?

In most cases, debridement is proposed by nurses or doctors when dealing with an unusual situation where the usual techniques of debridement are not appropriate, for example when the amount of necrotic tissue is too large to be removed in a single stage. This is dependent on the availability of surgical facilities, the knowledge of the professionals and the capacity for the patient to be treated close to their home. When the fibrotic tissue is large, adherent and recurrent, the need for surgical resection is high but poorly understood and not always undertaken by professionals. Steed et al (1996) demonstrated in a randomized control trial the value of having a wound cleaned of debris, foreign tissues and necrotic areas.

Surgical debridement can be applied to prevent or treat infection, especially in ulcers where there are difficulties in the diagnosis of a local infection. Dolynchuk developed an algorithm for debridement, defining situations where surgical debridement was necessary. Usually, surgical debridement undertaken by a surgeon is followed immediately by a covering technique, the so-called excision–grafting technique.

SURGICAL COVERING TECHNIQUES

Skin substitutes

Skin substitutes represent the future of burns coverage. Some solutions are already available on the market, but all of them have limitations. These products are discussed in detail in Chapter 24.

Skin grafting

Techniques

Skin grafting can be undertaken using different types of graft: allografts originating from tissue banks or autologous skin grafts (partial thickness, expanded or not, full-thickness) from the patient.

Allogenic skin Allogenic skin is a living tissue originating from cadavers and pre-mortem situations. Legislation is not universally identical and in some countries this solution is not permitted. Allogenic skin can be used either fresh or cryopreserved, tissue banks freezing and storing these products. Usually, this skin is subject to rejection, starting during the second week after application, although only the epidermal layer, which contains immunologically active cells, is liable to rejection. The dermis will adhere to the underlying wound to create a good support for any type of epidermal coverage. Usually, autologous keratinocyte cultures are used to cover the alloderm. Potentially, a cadaver allograft could transmit viral diseases.

Pinch skin grafts Pinch skin grafts (small pieces of full-thickness skin) are the most common method used in some European countries to treat venous leg ulcer. This technique is easy to perform and does not need an operating room. Results show a graft take of 70–90% with a recurrence rate of less than 30% 3 months postoperatively, representing a good outcome for the closure of small venous leg ulcers.

The Baux technique uses scalpel incisions in the granulation tissue and inserts the pinch skin grafts in these holes. This 'burying' technique is proposed in cases of difficult to heal leg ulcers.

The preoperative period requires precise care. There is a significant risk of infection after grafting and the granulation tissue has to be well prepared. Some authors recommend the use of antiseptics such as povidone iodine during this period; others support the use of silver dressing. No consensus exists on this issue but the immediate preoperative period is critical in ensuring the future of the skin graft. Systemic antibiotics administered during the surgical period as a one-shot bolus are sometimes proposed to combat the risk of infection after the surgical procedure.

Management in the postoperative period includes the following:

- *The dressing* should be non-adherent and conformable. The position of the pinch skin grafts should be clearly indicated on the outside of the dressing (using a marker). There is a high risk of removing pinch skin grafts during the first dressing change if an adherent dressing is used. Several non-adherent dressings are available on the market. The first dressing change is usually performed after 3 days, the second dressing after 5 days
- *Compression* should be minimal during this period, and ideally the patient should remain lying in bed with the legs elevated
- *Haematoma prevention* can be achieved by strict control of haemostasis during the surgical procedure. Anticoagulant agents and salicylic acids should be stopped before surgery (given again the day after skin grafting)
- *Discharge* is completed after 1 week and allowed only when compression can be reapplied correctly.

Complications during this period can include:

- *Immediate infection of the pinch skin grafts*: This is a consequence of technical failure or poor postoperative management
- *Movement of the dressing with displacement of the pinch skin grafts* is due to the same causes. It is important to reiterate that these small pieces of skin are just maintained over the recipient site by the dressing itself. No stitches are possible and the only way to prevent any movement is to fix the dressing properly.

Long term complications are associated with:

- Poor compliance of the patient with compression bandages
- Local infection
- Recurrence of the disease because of a poor scar; hyperkeratinization of the area can be observed after skin grafting
- 30–40% of skin grafts fail during the first 3 months after surgery.

Large full-thickness skin grafts Large, full-thickness grafts are only occasionally used in venous leg ulcers (Fig. 12.3), even though their use may be indicated in badly vascularized areas such as over the ankle joint.

In large venous leg ulcer, mesh grafting is usually performed after a long period of non-healing (more than a year), treatment having conformed to the usual standard of care. This technique requires

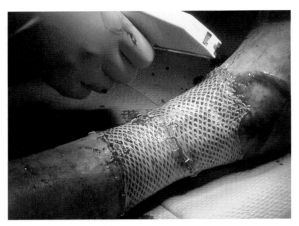

Figure 12.3 Split-thickness skin graft

hospitalization for 6 days, a surgical procedure performed under general anaesthesia and a postoperative period.

When to perform a skin graft?

Skin grafting involves a surgical procedure in which a piece of skin will be harvested from the patient's body and put over a wound. Several consequences can be expected, for example a permanent scar at the donor site area and a tendency for the graft to be rejected linked to difficulties with local revascularization or diffusion nutrition of this small piece of tissue. Local infection has also been evoked as a possible cause of rejection.

Skin grafting is indicated when the granulation tissue covers the whole wound, without any remaining necrotic tissue or undermined zones. In most cases, this visual criterion is enough to prevent any important local complications. Some authors have proposed undertaking a bacteriological count before grafting, with a limit of 10^5 bacteria per cubic millimetre, proposed as a consequence of observations of bacteriological counts prior to skin grafting. It is also important to determine the visual characteristics of the wound bed. The criteria for grafting are that the wound is red; that it bleeds uniformly on contact; and that there is no important exudate; no undermined lateral area and no hypergranulation.

Skin grafting is not indicated when islands of keratinization occur. In this situation, cortisone locally applied on tulle can be used to promote keratinization. Povidone iodine has also been pro-

posed. The underlying tissue can also be formed by an artificial dermis. In this case the skin graft should be thin enough to accelerate the take of the graft over poorly vascularized tissue.

Flap surgery

Techniques

Angiosomes   Angiosomes (anatomical correspondence between skin areas and vascular sources) were defined anatomically during the 1930s by the extensive anatomical works of Salmon. Angiosomes represent the vascular territories corresponding to each part of the human body, especially the muscles and the skin. This means that it is possible to pediculize a flap including one or several components, to rotate it or transplant it in another location on the body using microsurgical techniques.

Local random flaps   Local random flaps were proposed as coverage for limited defects. They comprise advancement flaps, rotation flaps and Z-plasties and their basic principle is to maintain random vascularization. Most of these flaps are usually proposed for coverage of small defects or to treat skin retraction, and exceptionally for leg ulcer coverage.

Regional pedicled flaps   Regional pedicled flaps are based on anatomical work undertaken since the 1970s by plastic surgeons. Each muscle and piece of skin on the body surface is characterized in terms of the source and type of its vascularization. An atlas including this classification is now freely available throughout the world. Several flaps can cover a skin defect from a leg ulcer, such as the distally based supramalleolar flap; the reverse sural flap (venous or arterial) and, more proximally, the sural muscle flap; the gemellus muscle flap and the extensor brevis muscle flap. These flaps can combine muscle, skin and aponeurosis in the same transfer.

Microsurgically revascularized flaps are a solution few propose in leg ulcer coverage. Some authors use a proximally revascularized thin flap, such as the antebrachial aponeurotic flap. Prefabricated flaps are a variant of the last one, where angiogenic stimulation coming from a skin expander is promoted and captured by a vascular carrier surgically installed under the skin expander. These are extreme solutions when no skin is available, for instance in post-traumatic situations.

Indications

Flap surgery is indicated in large tissue defects, when deep tissues are exposed, such as bone, tendons or major blood vessels. In exceptional cases of complicated venous leg ulcer where infection or large areas of necrotic occur, these techniques may be used. Normally, however, these techniques should be reserved for traumatic loss of tissue. Some clinical series have described their use in diabetic foot ulceration, when the loss of tissue is substantial, exposing joints or bony surfaces.

Skin and tissue expansion

Technique

Skin expansion was proposed two decades ago in order to promote skin enlargement, either before the use of expanded skin as a skin graft (bank expansion) or so that the extra skin obtained could be used as the source of a regional flap. The angiogenic capacities of skin expansion are linked to progressive stimulation of vessel formation using a silicone expander implanted under the surface of the skin at the junction between the fatty tissue and the muscle aponeurosis. The expander is progressively inflated with sterile saline through the channel of a valve, which is also implanted under the skin separately from the silicone balloon and joined to it by a tube. At regular intervals injections are performed through the skin above the valve and the enlargement of the skin surface progresses in a similar way to the abdominal skin of a pregnant woman.

Indications

This technique has been used extensively in skin defects of the skull, and in scar situations where the surrounding skin can be expanded easily. Technical requirements are linked to the resistance of the underlying structure on which the expander is located. Expansion is more effective when the underlying structures are hard tissues capable of resisting pressure. This resistance allows the skin to be projected outwards rather than the expander penetrating into the tissues. In open wounds, very few reports of use of skin expansion are found,

because of the high risk of infection presented by the foreign bodies full of inert liquid and by the chronic wound itself. The risk of infection is always important in skin expansion. Other possible complications relate to risk of skin perforation from inside to outside during expansion. The rate of inflation must be determined precisely before injection. Usually, two injections per week are undertaken, the quantity of injected liquid being determined by the final volume of expansion required and the capacity of the skin for expansion. The shape of the expansion and the quality of its surface can be modulated by the surgeon.

In venous leg ulcers, and more generally in reconstructive surgery of the lower limb, there are few indications for skin expansion, as it is not always successful because of the lack of counter-pressure underneath the expander, the high risk of infection and the poor vascularization associated with leg ulcers.

GENE THERAPY

Gene therapy, even though it largely remains a technique for the future, offers alternative treatment solutions (Eriksson et al 1998, Eriksson 2004). It is now possible to label cells in the tissues, transfect them in vitro and transplant them back into wounds (Kolodka et al 1998). Other authors prefer to transfect cells in the wound itself using the in vivo gene transfer method (Eriksson et al 1998). Growth factors encoding genes present an important interest when compared with topical application. Gene transfer offers the advantage of a continuous delivery of growth factors for a period of time that depends on the technique.

Morgan et al (1987) cultivated keratinocytes that had previously been transfected and transplanted them on to nude mice. Later, Andreatta-van Leyen et al (1993) proposed a genetically bioengineered bandage. Eming et al (1998) proposed seeding genetically modified human keratinocytes over-expressing platelet-derived growth factor PDGF-α into skin grafts. These techniques are now being developed in the laboratory to enhance wound healing by upregulation of deficient situations. Control of fibrosis and of delivery during necrotic process of negative factors in the wound are also under investigation.

CLINICAL SITUATIONS SEEN BY SURGEONS

Cellulitis

Patients with cellulitis are sent to surgeons because of the dramatic consequences of a generalized infection and the possibility of rapid and extensive debridement. In fact, cellulitis is a contraindication for surgery, as the risk of bacterial spread is high. These cases are better treated by general antibiotics, except when an abscess is observed clinically or using ultrasound.

Lipodermatosclerosis

Patients suffering from leg ulcers for a long period of time or having several recurrences are often referred to surgeons. These patients, if still young, can have their ulcer excised and covered using skin grafts and/or dermal substitutes.

Malignant transformation

Squamous cell cancer can develop after a period of years (usually more than 10) in a chronic venous leg ulcer. Treatment should consist of wide resection of the skin tumour (>2 cm from the margins) followed by either immediate or delayed reconstruction, depending on the safety of the margins during the resection. A specialized check-up, looking for metastatic lesions, should be planned. Complementary treatment (radiotherapy) is sometimes necessary, although this may lead to delayed healing (Ch. 19).

DISCUSSION

Venous ulcers affect up to 2.5 million patients per year in the USA and 2 million in Europe. Although not usually fatal, these chronic wounds severely affect patients' quality of life because of impaired mobility and substantial loss of productivity. These venous ulcers are small initially but, as they are often undertreated, they tend to progress to larger ulcers, often associated with serious complications including exudate, erythema, cellulitis, dermatitis, pain and possible malignancy. In many cases ulcers recur. Cellulitis is often seen by surgeons, as the situation is critical in ambulatory medicine. Extensive surgical excision and grafting is a rarely chosen option. Published series are small, and indicate around 30% recurrence. Most professionals involved in the management of elderly patients who are unable to withstand long haemorrhagic surgery will opt for a simple skin graft. The choice between pinch skin graft and expanded partial-thickness skin grafts is linked to their availability and the surgeon's expertise with a dermatome. These technical difficulties limit the surgical options. The use of dermal substitutes in dermal stabilization has yet to be realized. This technique looks promising, because of the complete replacement of the dermal component. The option of skin constructs will also certainly bring new interesting results in coverage of venous leg ulcers and could decrease the high rate of recurrence. The cost of these techniques may limit their use and reduce the therapeutic options.

References

Andreatta-van Leyen S, Smith D J, Bulgrin J P et al 1993 Delivery of growth factor to wounds using a genetically engineered biological bandage. Journal of Biomedical Materials Research 27: 1201–1208

Chang K P, Tsaii C C, Lin T M et al 2001 An alternative dressing for skin graft immobilization: Negative pressure dressing. Burns 27: 839–842

Eming S A, Medalie D A, Tompkins R G et al 1998 Genetically modified human keratinocytes overexpressing PDGF-A enhance the performance of a composite skin graft. Human Gene Therapy 9: 529–539

Eriksson E, Yao F, Svensjo T 1998 In vivo gene transfer to skin and wound by microseeding Journal of Surgical Research 78: 85–91

Eriksson E 2004 Gene therapy in wounds. In: Téot L, Banwell P, Ziegler U (eds) Surgery in wounds. Springer-Verlag, Berlin

Falanga V, Sabolinski M L 1999 A bilayered living skin construct (Apligraf) accelerates complete closure of hard to heal venous ulcers. Wound Repair and Regeneration 7: 201–207

Gottrup F 2004 Venous ulcer surgery. In: Téot L, Banwell P, Ziegler U (eds) Surgery in wounds. Springer-Verlag, Berlin

Kolodka T M, Garlick J A, Taichman L B 1998 Evidence for keratinocyte stem cells in vitro: long term engraftment and persistence of transgene expression from retrovirus-transduced keratinocytes. Proceedings of the National Academy of Sciences of the USA 95: 4356–4361

Loree S, Dompmartin A, Penven K et al 2004 Is vacuum assisted closure a valid technique for debriding chronic leg ulcers? Journal of Wound Care 13: 249–252

Morgan J R, Barrandon Y, Green H, Mulligan R C 1987 Expression of an exogenous growth hormone gene by transplantable human epidermal cells. Science 237: 1476–1479

Morykwas M J, Argenta L C, Shelton-Brown E I, McGuirt W 1997 Vacuum-assisted closure: a new method for wound control and treatment: animal studies and basic foundation. Annals of Plastic Surgery 38: 553–562

Palmier S, Trial C 2004 Mechanical debridement using waterjets. In: Téot L, Banwell P, Ziegler U (eds) Surgery in wounds. Springer-Verlag, Berlin

Schmeller W, Gaber Y 2000 Surgical removal of ulcer and lipodermatosclerosis followed by split-skin grafting (shave therapy) yields good long-term results in 'non-healing' venous leg ulcers. Acta Dermato-Venereologica 80: 267–271

Sherman R A 2003 Maggot therapy for treating diabetic foot ulcers unresponsive to conventional therapy. Diabetes Care 26: 446–451

Steed D L, Donohoe D, Webster M W, Lindsley L 1996 Effect of extensive debridement and treatment on the healing of diabetic foot ulcers. Diabetic Ulcer Study Group. Journal of the American College of Surgeons 183: 61–64

Téot L, Otman S, Giovannini U 2004 The use of negative pressure therapy in managing wounds. European Tissue Repair Society Focus Meeting on Topical Negative Pressure Therapy, London, December 2003

Wayman J, Nirojogi V, Walker A et al 2001 The cost effectiveness of larval therapy in venous ulcers. Journal of Tissue Viability 11: 51

Webb L X, Schmidt U 2001 Wound management with vacuum therapy. Unfallchirurgie 104: 918–926

Wollina U, Liebold K, Schmidt W D et al 2002 Biosurgery supports granulation and debridement in chronic wounds–clinical data and remittance spectroscopy measurement. International Journal of Dermatology 41: 635–639

An overview of pharmacological treatment options for venous leg ulcers

Andrew Jull

INTRODUCTION

Sustained venous hypertension is widely accepted as the essential biomechanical disturbance in chronic venous insufficiency. How this disturbance then leads to ulceration in some patients has yet to be completely characterized. The principal microcirculatory hypotheses in the last 25 years (described in Ch. 8) have been those of the pericapillary fibrin cuff formation that prevents tissue oxygenation (Browse & Burnand 1982) and the more enduring theory of leukocyte sequestration ('white cell trapping'; Coleridge Smith et al 1988, Coleridge Smith 2002), which causes the activation of leukocytes, fibrin cuff formation and the release of proinflammatory mediators and free radicals, with subsequent tissue damage. The investigation of pharmacological means for treating venous ulceration has in many respects been driven by the hypotheses of the condition's pathogenesis. In this chapter only investigations of systemic pharmacological regimens have been included, although there have a number of trials of topical drug treatments that are also congruent with the microcirculatory hypotheses (Roelens 1989, Salim 1991, La Marca et al 1999, Senet et al 2003). The drugs are listed here alphabetically by their generic names.

ASPIRIN

Pharmacology and suggested mechanism of action

Aspirin is a non-steroidal anti-inflammatory salicylate that blocks thromboxane A_2 formation and thus inhibits platelet activation (Bjornson & Raasen

2003). The action of aspirin in ulcer healing is unknown, although it has been suggested that its effect is derived from the suppression of inflammation, perhaps enhanced by the inhibition of platelet activity (Ibbotson et al 1995).

Evidence

One randomized controlled trial (Layton et al 1994, Layton 1994) investigated the effect of aspirin on healing in venous leg ulceration. 20 patients from a hospital dermatology clinic with ulcers larger than 2 cm^2 were enrolled, 10 in each arm. The treatment consisted of 300 mg daily of enteric-coated aspirin, or a placebo, both as an adjuvant to long-stretch compression bandages. The main outcome was ulcer size; where the participant had more than one ulcer ($n = 12$), the combined surface area of all ulcers was calculated. The mean surface area of ulcers in the aspirin group decreased from 16.5 cm^2 at baseline to 10 cm^2 following 4 months of treatment. The placebo-treated group was unchanged from a mean surface area of 14.3 cm^2 after 4 months. Complete healing was reported in 50% (5/10) of patients treated with aspirin, giving a number needed to treat (NNT) of 2. (NNT estimates the number of patients that must be treated in order to achieve one more healed patient with a venous ulcer.) However, the confidence interval (CI) around the treatment effect was wide (absolute difference 50%, 95% CI 19–81%, NNT 2, 95% CI 1–5). *Strengths and limitations:* Blinding and randomization were employed, and the intervention was an adjuvant to compression bandaging, the mainstay of venous ulcer therapy. Unfortunately, the trial enrolled few patients, and any difference between the groups could well have been random variation. In addition, the duration of follow-up was probably insufficient. *Funding source*: Not reported.

Adverse effects

No side effects were experienced by participants in Layton et al 1994, nor were any adverse effects reported in an investigation of the activity of aspirin in venous leg ulceration (Ibbotson et al 1995). However, aspirin has been associated with an increased risk of gastric ulceration during prolonged therapy, although the risk appears reduced with the use of enteric-coated products (Hawthorne et al 1991). Aspirin also increases the risk of haemorrhagic stroke (He et al 1998), although the increase in risk is small (from a baseline of 12 strokes per 10 000 people to 26 strokes per 10 000 people when treated with aspirin). Aspirin may be also associated with iron deficiency anaemia in the elderly, although this association is derived from preliminary research (Black & Fraser 1999).

Summary

Current evidence suggests that the use of aspirin might provide additional benefit to compression therapy. However, this evidence should be interpreted very cautiously. Further trials are necessary before the effect of aspirin on venous leg ulcer healing can be considered to have been determined. *US Food and Drug Administration (FDA) approved for venous disease*: Not indicated. *British National Formulary*: Not indicated for venous disease.

CINNARIZINE

Pharmacology and suggested mechanism of action

Cinnarizine is a histamine antagonist, with a calcium-channel-blocking activity (Roncaglioni & Vanderleest 2002, Sweetman 2002). It is primarily used in the palliation of motion sickness, and the nausea and vertigo associated with Ménière's disease (Sweetman 2002). The action of cinnar-izine in ulcer healing is unknown, although it has been suggested that its effect is derived from the suppression of histamine and other inflammatory substances (Aussems & Mulls 1970).

Evidence

One randomized controlled trial (Aussens & Muls 1970) has evaluated the effect of cinnarizine in leg ulcers, following an earlier report that the antihistamine improved healing times (Jacobs 1968). A total of 53 outpatients with ulcers were enrolled in the trial, the majority (44, 83%) having a venous aetiology; other causes were listed as capillaritis (2, 4%), arteritis (3, 5%), radiodermatitis (1, 2%) diabetes (2, 4%) and trauma (1, 2%). Participants were assigned to receive 50 mg cinnarizine three times daily, or a matching placebo, for 8 weeks, in addition to the most appropriate treatment regimen for their ulcer. 25 participants with venous ulcers were assigned to the treatment group, 19 to the control group. 97% (43) of participants with venous ulcers were treated with compression, receiving either elastic bandaging (27) or Unna's boot (16), as well as the randomized treatment. The main outcome measure was healing time. The median healing time was 6 weeks in the cinnarizine group compared to 8 weeks in the placebo group ($p < 0.01$). 19 participants (68%) assigned to the treatment group and seven (28%) assigned to the placebo group were estimated to have healed by 8 weeks (absolute difference 40%, 95% CI 15–65, NNT 3, 95% CI 2–7). *Strengths and limitations*: Although the trial employed random allocation and blinding, the heterogenous nature of the sample, the relatively small numbers enrolled and the short duration of follow-up are limitations to establishing the effect of cinnarizine. *Funding source*: Not reported.

Adverse effects

Those participants receiving cinnarizine experienced the only side effects reported in Aussems & Muls 1970. One participant suffered diarrhoea, a second a skin rash. Headache (Pianese et al 2002) and increased sleepiness (Nicholson et al 2002) have been reported in other blinded trials. More seriously, cinnarizine has been reported to induce parkinsonism (Gimenez-Roldan & Mateo 1991).

Summary

Current evidence suggests that the use of cinnarizine might provide additional benefit to compression therapy in terms of the proportion of healed ulcers at 8 weeks. However, this evidence should be interpreted very cautiously and further trials are necessary before cinnarizine can be considered as an adjuvant treatment for venous ulcers. *FDA approved for venous disease*: Not indicated. *British National Formulary*: Not indicated for venous disease.

MICRONIZED PURIFIED FLAVONOID FRACTION

Pharmacology and suggested mechanism of action

Micronized purified flavonoid fraction (MPFF) is a semisynthetic flavonoid consisting of 90% diosmin and 10% hesperidin synthesized from a citrus species, *Rutaceae aurantieae* (Lyseng-Williamson & Perry 2003). Flavonoids are oxygen free-radical scavengers, or antioxidants. The action of MPFF in ulcer healing is unknown, although it has been suggested that its effect is derived from anti-inflammatory effects, possibly through reduction in leukocyte and endothelial activation (Coleridge Smith 2000).

Evidence

Three randomized controlled trials have reported investigations into the effect of MPFF in venous leg ulceration (Guilhou et al 1997, Glinski et al 1999, Roztocil et al 2003). The largest trial (Roztocil et al 2003) enrolled 150 patients from 17 centres in the Czech and Slovak Republics, 82 patients in the treatment group and 68 patients in the control group. The treatment consisted of 1 g daily of MPFF for up to 24 weeks, in addition to compression. The trial was open-label and the control group simply received compression bandaging. A standard topical treatment regimen (chloraminum, normal saline and silver nitrate solution for cleansing the ulcer and Vaseline, zinc paste, normal saline and potassium solution for the area surrounding the ulcer) was employed in both groups,

with the addition of local antibiotics or steroids for up to 5 days, if indicated. The primary outcomes were the proportion of healed ulcers at 6 months and time to complete healing. 53 (64.6%) participants in the treatment and 28 participants (41.2%) in the control group healed after 24 weeks treatment (absolute difference 23.5%, 95% CI 7.8–36.1%, NNT 4, 95% CI 3–13). Time to healing significantly favoured the treatment group (137 days v 166 days, $p = 0.04$). *Strengths and limitations:* Random allocation was employed and the intervention was an adjuvant to the mainstay of venous ulcer therapy. Although the topical treatments employed in this trial do not follow the recommendations of recent clinical practice guidelines, this would not have had a differential effect on the trial results as both groups of participants were exposed to the same regimen. Allocation concealment was not described and the control group did not receive placebo medication. This design could lead to selection and attribution biases. *Funding source:* Not reported.

The second similarly sized trial (Glinski et al 1999) enrolled 140 patients from ten dermatology clinics in nine Polish cities, 71 patients in the treatment group and 69 patients in the control group. The treatment consisted of 1 g daily of MPFF for 24 weeks, as an adjuvant to long-stretch compression bandaging. The control group simply received compression bandaging, which in both groups was applied by the participants themselves. A standard topical treatment regimen was employed (Twice daily saline compresses with either silver nitrate or chlorhexidine solution, and silver sulfadiazine ointment applied overnight). The main outcome was complete healing and secondary outcomes were percentage reduction in ulcer area, percentages experiencing symptoms associated with chronic venous insufficiency (CVI) and a cost-effectiveness analysis using a health service perspective. 33 participants (46.5%) in the treatment group healed at 24 weeks compared with 19 participants (27.5%) in the control group (absolute difference 20%, 95% CI 3–35%, NNT 5, 95% CI 3–31). Reduction in ulcer area was also significantly different between the groups, as was discomfort, although there was no difference between the groups for other symptoms of CVI (pain, heavy legs or nocturnal cramps). The cost-effectiveness ratio also favoured the treatment group at €1026.2 per healed ulcer (1998 terms) compared with €1871.8 per healed ulcer for the control group. *Strengths and limitations:* Random allocation was employed and the intervention was an adjuvant to the mainstay of venous ulcer therapy. Although the topical treatments employed in this trial do not follow the recommendations of recent clinical practice guidelines, this is unlikely to have had a differential effect on the trial results as both groups of participants were exposed to the same regimen. Allocation concealment was not described and the control group did not receive placebo medication. This design could lead to selection and attribution biases. However, the main outcome measure was determined using an objective measure (photography and planimetry) that was unlikely to be influenced by a lack of blinding, and all patients were included in the analysis. *Funding source:* Not reported.

The third randomized trial (Guilhou et al 1997) employed a stronger design using blinding. The trial was conducted in nine sites in France, which enrolled 107 patients, 55 in the treatment group and 52 in the placebo group. Randomization was stratified for ulcer size (<10 cm², >10 cm²) and participants received either 1 g of MPFF or matching placebo daily for 2 months as an adjuvant to elastic compression. The main outcome was complete healing of the reference ulcer. Secondary endpoints included percentage of ulcer area healed, total number of healed ulcers where the participant had multiple ulcers, and symptoms of chronic venous insufficiency. There was a non-significant difference in complete healing, with 14 participants (25.5%) in the treatment group completely healed at 2 months compared with six participants (11.5%) in the placebo group (absolute difference 14%, 95% CI −0.5–28.3%). *Strengths and limitations:* The trial was blinded, with randomization stratified for a well known prognostic factor (ulcer size) and the intervention was an adjuvant to the mainstay of venous ulcer therapy. The two groups were broadly similar, although fewer participants in the treatment group had deep venous insufficiency. However, follow-up was for the relatively short period of time of 8 weeks and reporting survival analysis over a longer period of follow-up would

more clearly reveal differences in healing rates over time. *Funding source:* Not reported.

Adverse effects

No side effects were reported in Glinski et al 1999 or Roztocil et al 2003, and those receiving MPFF in Guilhou et al 1997 experienced only mild side effects, such as fatigue, headaches and gastrointestinal disturbance. An analysis of studies involving 2850 participants treated with MPFF (Meyer 1994) found the incidence of side effects to be 10%, the majority being gastrointestinal effects such as abdominal and epigastric pain, gastric discomfort, nausea, dyspepsia, vomiting and diarrhoea. The other main group of adverse effects is autonomic effects such as insomnia, drowsiness, vertigo, headache, tiredness, anxiety, cramps, palpitations and hypotension.

Summary

When the trials are combined in a meta-analysis (Fig. 13.1), the relative risk (RR) of complete healing was about two-thirds more when patients were treated with MPFF in addition to compression (100/206 v 53/189, RR 1.69, 95% CI 1.30–2.19). Although the treatment effect of MPFF is significant, the three trials were quite different in duration and further trials are necessary before the effect of MPFF on ulcer healing can be completely assured. However, current evidence is strongly suggests that MPFF provides additional benefit when used as an adjuvant to compression for healing venous leg ulcers and that the addition of MPFF to a patient's regimen would be a cost-effective adjunct from a health service perspective. *FDA approved for venous disease:* No. *British National Formulary:* Drug not included.

GRANULOCYTE–MACROPHAGE COLONY STIMULATING FACTOR

Pharmacology and suggested mechanism of action

Granulocyte–macrophage colony-stimulating factor (GM-CSF) is a recombinant haemopoietic growth factor derived from *Escherichia coli* (Henke 2001). GM-CSF stimulates the activation of white cells, especially granulocytes, macrophages and mono-

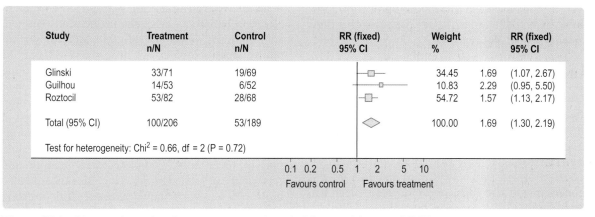

Study	Treatment n/N	Control n/N	RR (fixed) 95% CI	Weight %	RR (fixed) 95% CI
Glinski	33/71	19/69		34.45	1.69 (1.07, 2.67)
Guilhou	14/53	6/52		10.83	2.29 (0.95, 5.50)
Roztocil	53/82	28/68		54.72	1.57 (1.13, 2.17)
Total (95% CI)	100/206	53/189		100.00	1.69 (1.30, 2.19)

Test for heterogeneity: $Chi^2 = 0.66$, df = 2 (P = 0.72)

0.1 0.2   0.5   1   2   5   10

Favours control   Favours treatment

Figure 13.1 Meta-analysis of trials using micronized purified flavonoid fraction (MPFF) as an adjuvant to compression for treatment of venous leg for venous leg ulcers

cytes (Sweetman 2002) and promotes the migration and proliferation of endothelial cells (Bussolino et al 1989). GM-CSF may participate in the regulation of normal wound healing and it has been suggested that its use in chronic wounds may enhance normal inflammatory and granulation responses (Da Costa et al 1997).

Evidence

Two randomized controlled trials have investigated the effect of GM-CSF on leg ulcers. However, one trial (Da Costa et al 1997) enrolled 25 participants with venous or ischaemic leg ulcers and it is not possible to discern from this report what the rates of healing were for the venous ulcer group. The same authors conducted a second trial (Da Costa et al 1999) that enrolled 60 participants from a single hospital in Portugal. The trial aimed to determine the effect of two different doses (200 or 400 µg) of GM-CSF on venous ulcer healing in comparison to placebo. Participants were randomly assigned to either GM-CSF injected subcutaneously into four sites around the reference ulcer, 0.5 cm from the edge of the lesion, or placebo treatment was given weekly for 4 weeks, or until the ulcer closed, whichever occurred first. Participants assigned to placebo received matching injections. Participants were followed up for 12 weeks for the primary endpoint, with a final contact at 6 months to evaluate

for ulcer recurrence. 21 participants were randomly assigned to placebo, 21 to the 200 µg dose and 19 to the 400 µg dose; all participants received four-layer compression bandaging. The primary outcomes were complete healing of the reference ulcer and a greater than 50% reduction in ulcer area. Other outcomes were time to healing, 6-month recurrence rates and adverse effects. 58% (23/40) of participants in the GM-CSF arms had completely healed reference ulcers at 12 weeks, 57% (12/21) who received the 200 µg dose and 61% (11/19) who received the 400 µg dose. 19% (4/21) of participants in the placebo arm healed (absolute difference 36.5%, 95% CI 12.6–60.3%, NNT 3, 95% CI 2–8). There was no significant difference in healing rates between the two doses of GM-CSF, but the 400 µg was associated with faster healing times. *Strengths and limitations:* This pragmatic trial used GM-CSF as an adjuvant to a widely used system of compression bandaging. The trial employed random allocation and was blinded. Local treatment was standardized and those receiving the treatment were broadly equivalent at baseline to participants on placebo, although the average ulcer size was smaller in the placebo group and duration of the ulcer prior to treatment was also shorter. However, this difference at baseline would have benefited the placebo group if it did have an impact on the results. Although the participants were followed up for 12 weeks, reporting survival analysis over a longer period of follow-up would more clearly reveal differences in healing rates over time. *Funding source:* Not reported.

Adverse effects

Itching was the only side effect reported in the early trial (Da Costa et al 1997), but more side effects were reported in the GM-CSF treated groups (26% in the 200 µg arm, 38% in 400 µg arm) in the later trial (Da Costa et al 1999) than in the placebo group (9%). All side effects were rated as mild to moderate and the most common side effect was lumbar pain (15%), followed by malaise (13%).

Summary

Current evidence suggests that GM-CSF is a safe and promising treatment that appears to provide additional benefit to compression therapy in terms of the proportion of healed ulcers at 12 weeks after 4 weeks of treatment. However, further trials are necessary before this effect can be assured and the cost-effectiveness of GM-CSF as an adjuvant to compression therapy needs to be established before its use could be broadly applied. *FDA approved for venous disease:* No. *British National Formulary:* Not indicated for venous disease.

IFETROBAN

Pharmacology and suggested mechanism of action

Thromboxane (TxA_2) is one of the prostanoids (Sweetman 2002), along with the prostaglandins, both being products of arachidonic acid. TxA_2 is known to induce platelet aggregation, whereas the prostaglandins prevent platelet aggregation. Blockade of platelet activation could theoretically be achieved by TxA_2 inhibition (Rosenfeld et al 2001). Ifetroban sodium is such a TxA_2 inhibitor.

Evidence

One randomized controlled trial (Lyon et al 1998) investigated the effect of the TxA_2 inhibitor ifetroban on venous ulcer healing. The trial enrolled 203 eligible patients from 36 centres into a two-phase trial. During the lead-in phase, all par-

ticipants were given an oral placebo for 4 weeks to establish adherence with the medication regimen. 165 patients remained eligible for the second phase, were stratified by ulcer size (<10 cm^2 or >10 cm^2) and randomized to receive either 250 mg ifetroban or a matching placebo daily, in addition to compression (Unna's boot and elastic compression wrap), for 12 weeks. Outcomes to be evaluated at the 12-week endpoint included percentage change in ulcer area, time required to achieve a 50% reduction in ulcer area, complete ulcer healing and recurrence of healed ulcers. The index ulcer healed in 46 (55.4%) participants in the treatment group and 44 (53.6%) participants in the control group (absolute difference 1.8%, 95% CI −13.4–17%) *Strengths and limitations:* This explanatory trial employed random allocation as well as blinding; the two groups were similar at baseline and the treatment was an adjuvant to compression. However, the duration of treatment and follow-up may have been insufficient to establish a difference between ifetroban and placebo. *Funding sources:* Bristol-Myers Squibb and ConvaTec Corporation.

Adverse effects

No significant side effects occurred during the study by Lyon et al (1998). Minor side effects were not reported.

Summary

Current evidence suggests that the use of ifetroban does not appear to provide additional benefit to compression therapy in terms of the proportion of healed ulcers at 12 weeks. Although further trials would be necessary before a lack of effect can be truly assumed, the marginal increment in healing rates is likely to be too small to attract further investigation. *FDA approved for venous disease:* Drug not included. *British National Formulary:* Drug not included.

MESOGLYCAN

Pharmacology and suggested mechanism of action

Mesoglycan is a heparinoid derived from calf aorta and is composed primarily of heparan sulphate and dermatan sulphate. Heparinoids include highly sulphated polysaccharides and are also known as glucosaminoglycans, glycosaminoglycan polysulphated compounds, sulphated mucopolysaccharides and sulphated glucosaminoglycans. Although mesoglycan is thought to have antithrombotic and antiplatelet activities (Sweetman 2002), its action in venous ulcer healing remains unknown. It has been suggested that that mesoglycan's ability to inhibit white cell activation, prevent fibrin formation and promote fibrinolysis, or the proliferative action of heparan and dermatan sulphate in epithelialization, may promote ulcer healing (Arosio et al 2001)

Evidence

One randomized controlled trial (Arosio et al 2001) investigated the effect of mesoglycan in the treatment of venous leg ulcers. The trial enrolled 183 eligible outpatients from 18 hospital departments of vascular or general surgery in Italy. The trial aimed to determine the effect of mesoglycan, as an adjuvant to compression, on time to ulcer healing. Active treatment consisted of mesoglycan 30 mg injected intramuscularly every day for 3 weeks, followed by oral mesoglycan 50 mg daily until 24 weeks of treatment was completed. Matching placebos for both the intramuscular injections and tablets were employed. Randomization was stratified by centre; 92 participants were randomized to receive mesoglycan and 91 participants to receive the placebo treatment, in addition to compression (short-stretch elastic bandages and zinc oxide elastic or inelastic bandages). Other components of wound care were at the discretion of the local investigator. The main outcome was time to healing of the reference ulcer, as indicated by complete ulcer epithelialization. Other outcomes included ulcer pain, health-related quality of life as measured by the Medical Outcomes Short Form 36 (SF36) questionnaire, and adverse events. 89% (82) of participants treated with mesoglycan and 76% (69) of participants treated with placebo healed within 24 weeks (absolute difference 13.3%, 95% CI 2.5–24.2%, NNT 8, 95% CI 4–41). Median time to healing was 64 days for participants on mesoglycan and 70 days for those receiving the placebo. *Strengths and limitations:* This pragmatic trial used mesoglycan as an adjuvant to a treatment regimen that was adapted to changes in the participant's condition. The trial employed random allocation, was blinded and followed up participants for a sufficiently long period to establish healing times. Those receiving the treatment were broadly equivalent at baseline to participants on placebo. *Funding source:* Mediolanum Farmaceutici.

Adverse effects

Arosio et al (2001) found that the tolerability profile was similar in both the mesoglycan and placebo arms (8% v 7% of participants). While serious adverse events were reported in both arms, none of these were likely to be related to the treatment. Elsewhere (Nobili 1999) local cutaneous reactions associated with injections and gastrointestinal disturbances, such as nausea and vomiting, have been reported.

Summary

Current evidence suggests that mesoglycan provides additional benefit to compression therapy in terms of the proportion of healed ulcers after 24 weeks of treatment. However, the cost-effectiveness of mesoglycan as an adjuvant to compression therapy needs to be determined before the benefits of its use can be considered assured. *FDA approved for venous disease:* No. *British Formulary:* Drug not included.

PENTOXIFYLLINE

Pharmacology and suggested mechanism of action

Pentoxifylline is a methylxanthine derivative and a haemorrheological agent (Samlaska & Winfield 1994). Its microcirculatory effect in venous ulcer healing is unknown, although, among its many effects, pentoxifylline has been shown to inhibit leukocyte adhesion (Neuner et al 1997, Krakauer 2000), reduce free radical expression (Ciuffetti et al 1994) and reduce platelet aggregation (Ward & Clissold 1987).

Evidence

One systematic review (Jull et al 2000, 2002) of randomized controlled trials has investigated the effect of pentoxifylline on healing in chronic leg ulcers. The review employed an extensive search strategy that included 19 electronic databases, hand searching of conference proceedings and 38 journals. Attempts were also made to locate unpublished studies by contacting the manufacturer of pentoxifylline. To be included, studies had to be randomized controlled trials that included patients with venous leg ulcers and compared pentoxifylline against a placebo or a comparison treatment. In addition, an objective outcome measure had to be reported. Nine trials were identified, five of which (Schurmann & Eberhardt 1986, Colgan et al 1990, Barbarino 1992, Dale et al 1999, Falanga et al 1999) compared pentoxifylline to placebo, with compression as a standard treatment in both groups. Three trials (Weitgasser 1983, Arenas & Atoche 1988, Herdy et al 1997) compared pentoxifylline alone to placebo, and one trial (Apollonio & Angeletti 1992) compared pentoxifylline to defibrotide. In the trials that used compression as a background treatment, 243 participants received pentoxifylline as an adjuvant to compression bandaging, mostly in three doses of 400 mg per day for between 8 and 24 weeks. 204 participants received a matching placebo in addition to compression. Those who received pentoxifylline in addition to compression were a third more likely to heal within the treatment period than those who received placebo (155/243 v 96/204, RR 1.30, 95%CI 1.10–1.54). In the trials where pentoxifylline was compared to placebo without compression as a background treatment, 54 participants received pentoxifylline in three doses of 400 mg daily for between 8 weeks and 6 months, compared to 48 participants who received a matching placebo. Participants who received pentoxifylline were more than twice as likely to heal or substantially improve than those who received the placebo (RR 2.42, 95% CI 1.34–4.35). *Strengths and limitations:* The review employed a rigorous methodology, with extensive searching, assessment of trials against appropriate inclusion criteria, and data extraction from the source trials being independently reviewed. However, different systems of compression were employed in each trial, introducing methodological heterogeneity, although such heterogeneity may well have led to an underestimation of treatment effect rather than over-estimation. *Funding source:* Centre for Evidence Based Nursing, Aotearoa.

Adverse effects

Eight trials (Weitgasser 1983, Arenas & Atoche 1988, Colgan et al 1990, Barbarino 1992, Herdy et al 1997, Dale et al 1999, Falanga et al 1999, Herdy et al 2002) involving participants with venous ulceration reported adverse events. 17% of participants receiving pentoxifylline (and 12% receiving a placebo) reported side effects, mostly headaches and gastrointestinal disturbances.

Summary

Two further trials (Belcaro et al 2002, de Sanctis et al 2002), which employed compression as a standard background treatment, have been published and a third (Pizarro et al 1996), published in 1996, has been located since the systematic review was last updated. It is not clear from one report (de Sanctis et al 2002) whether it is a 12-month follow-up from the 6-month study (Belcaro et al 2002), or whether different participants were recruited into a 6-month and 12-month trial. Therefore only the 6-month report will be considered here. When the two trials that used compression as a background treatment are included in a meta-analysis (Fig. 13.2), participants receiving pentoxifylline in addition to compression were 50% more likely to heal than those receiving placebo (221/351 v 126/317, RR 1.59, 95% CI 1.15–2.18). Pentoxifylline in addition to compression does appear to increase healing rates. An abstract (Bosanquet et al 1995) suggests that pentoxifylline is a cost-effective adjuvant to compression with a healed ulcer costing US$2190 (1995 terms) compared with US$2570 when treated with compression alone. However, the lack of detail in this abstract prevents a full appraisal of the economic analysis. *FDA approved for venous disease:* No. *British National Formulary:* Unlicensed indication where compression alone is insufficient.

PROSTAGLANDIN E₁

Pharmacology and suggested mechanism of action

Prostaglandin (PGE_1) is a member of the prostanoid family (Sweetman 2002), along with thromboxane A_2 inhibitors, and is one of 20 naturally occurring

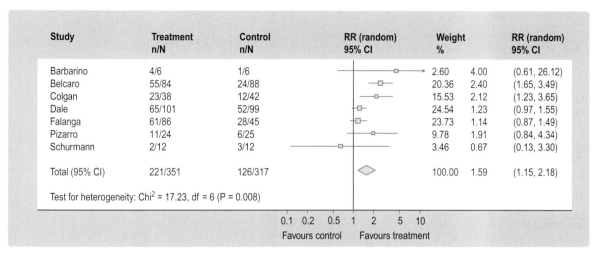

Study	Treatment n/N	Control n/N	RR (random) 95% CI	Weight %	RR (random) 95% CI
Barbarino	4/6	1/6		2.60 4.00	(0.61, 26.12)
Belcaro	55/84	24/88		20.36 2.40	(1.65, 3.49)
Colgan	23/38	12/42		15.53 2.12	(1.23, 3.65)
Dale	65/101	52/99		24.54 1.23	(0.97, 1.55)
Falanga	61/86	28/45		23.73 1.14	(0.87, 1.49)
Pizarro	11/24	6/25		9.78 1.91	(0.84, 4.34)
Schurmann	2/12	3/12		3.46 0.67	(0.13, 3.30)
Total (95% CI)	221/351	126/317		100.00 1.59	(1.15, 2.18)

Test for heterogeneity: Chi^2 = 17.23, df = 6 (P = 0.008)

0.1 0.2 0.5 1 2 5 10

Favours control   Favours treatment

Figure 13.2 Meta-analysis of trials using pentoxifylline as an adjuvant to compression for treatment of venous leg ulcers

prostaglandins (Massoud 2002). The action of PGE_1 in venous ulcer healing remains unknown, although PGE_1 is known to have microcirculatory effects on white cell activation, platelet aggregation and vasodilatation (Coleridge Smith 2002).

Evidence

One randomized controlled trial (Rudofsky 1989) has investigated the effect of PGE_1 on venous leg ulcers that were resistant to healing after 4 months of treatment by other means. 44 patients at a university clinic underwent a 14-day washout period during which drugs for venous disorders were discontinued. At the end of the washout period, the participants were randomized to receive either 180 µg PGE_1 daily by intravenous infusion over 3 hours, or a matching placebo. This treatment was administered until the ulcers healed, or dermoplasty became feasible, or for 6 weeks, whichever was the sooner. The treatment was delivered as an adjuvant to compression bandaging. Participants also received secondary therapeutics, such as antibiotics, as required. The trial collected data on several outcomes, including complete healing, venous volume, venous capacity, transcutaneous Po_2 (tcPo_2), symptoms of venous insufficiency and adverse effects of the treatment. 40% (8/20) of participants treated with PGE_1 had healed by the trial's end compared with 9% (2/22) of those

treated with placebo (absolute difference 31%, 95%CI 6.3–55.5%, NNT 3, 95% CI 2–16). No participant reported any side effects to the treatment. *Strengths and limitations:* This trial was a pragmatic trial as PGE_1 was an adjuvant to compression and a regimen that could be adapted to changes in the participant's condition. Allocation to treatment was described as random and the trial employed blinding. However, data on the baseline characteristics were not presented, making it difficult to determine if the groups were similar at the start of the trial. Furthermore, two participants were excluded from the analysis because insufficient data was collected, although it was not identified which group the participants were excluded from. A sensitivity analysis using the worst-case scenario (including the participants as treatment failures in the denominator of the treatment arm) suggests that the trial results were robust to the exclusion of these participants, although the treatment effect was reduced slightly, with the lower bound of the confidence interval moving closer to no difference between the groups (absolute difference 27.7%, 95% CI 3.9–50.7%, NNT 4, 95% CI 2–26). The short duration of the trial was an additional limitation and establishing ulcer survival over a longer period of follow-up would more clearly reveal differences in healing rates over time. *Funding source:* Not reported.

Adverse effects

No side effects occurred in the study by Rudofsky (1989). In a trial (Toyota et al 1993) of PGE_1 versus placebo for patients with diabetic neuropathy, where two-thirds of the patients in each arm also had diabetic leg ulcers, the tolerability profile was similar. Seven percent of patients in the treatment group and 5% of patients in the placebo group reported side effects, most of which were mild. Side effects in the treatment group included light-headedness, heartburn, stiffness, retinal haemorrhage, anorexia, constipation and itching.

Summary

Current evidence suggests that prostaglandin E_1 is a safe treatment that may provide additional benefit to compression therapy in terms of the proportion of healed ulcers after 6 weeks of treatment. However, further trials over longer terms are necessary to confirm the effect of PGE_1. In addition, the cost-effectiveness of PGE_1 as an adjuvant to compression therapy needs to be determined before the benefits of its use can be considered assured. *FDA approved for venous disease:* Not indicated. *British National Formulary:* Not indicated for venous disease.

RUTOSIDES

Pharmacology and suggested mechanism of action

Hydroxyethylrutosides are a mixture of semisynthetic flavonoids often obtained from buckwheat, the Chinese pagoda plant and the leaves of some eucalyptus trees. Hydroxyethylrutosides have been shown to reduce capillary permeability and oedema (Wadworth & Faulds 1992).

Evidence

Two randomized controlled trials (Mann 1981, Stegmann et al 1986) have investigated the effect of rutosides in venous ulceration. The larger trial (Stegmann et al 1986) enrolled 107 patients with leg ulcers that were due to chronic venous insufficiency or post-thrombotic syndrome. The trial aimed to determine the effect of Venuron as an adjuvant to compression on ulcer healing. Active treatment consisted of 1 g of oral Venuron taken twice daily for 6 weeks. It is not reported whether a matching placebo or blinding was employed. 55 patients were randomized to receive the treatment in addition to compression (two-layer bandage). Participants were also managed with secondary treatments, such as antibiotics or topical corticosteroids, as required. The primary outcome was healing at 6 weeks. 47% (26/55) of those treated with Venuron and compression and 33% (17/52) of those treated with compression alone healed (absolute difference 14.6%, 95% CI −3.8–32.9%, NNT 7, 95% CI −27–3). *Strengths and limitations:* This was a pragmatic trial with a rutoside as an adjuvant to a standard compression regimen, and local treatment that could be adapted to changes in the participant's condition. The groups appeared to be broadly equivalent at baseline. However, a placebo does not appear to have been used, nor blinding employed, and participants were only followed up for a short period. Reporting survival analysis over a longer treatment period might more clearly reveal differences in healing rates over time. *Funding source:* Not reported.

A second smaller trial (Mann 1981) enrolled 28 patients with venous leg ulcers. The trial aimed to determine the effect of rutosides as an adjuvant to compression on ulcer healing. 14 patients were randomly allocated to receive 1 g of oral Paroven daily for 3 months and the remaining group received a matching placebo. Compression consisted of tubinette and an Elastoweb bandage. Participants were also managed with secondary treatments as required. The primary outcome was healing at 12 weeks. One patient in each arm healed during the follow-up period. *Strengths and limitations:* This was a pragmatic trial with a rutoside as an adjuvant to a standard compression regimen, and local treatment that could be adapted to changes in the participant's condition. Healing over time was reported, and the groups appeared to be broadly equivalent at baseline. The trial was blinded, and the treatment and placebo groups were similar at baseline. Although the participants were followed up for 3 months, reporting survival analysis over a longer period of follow-up would more clearly reveal differences in healing rates over time, as simply reporting the proportion of ulcers healed after a short period of follow-up can be misleading. *Funding source*: Drug and placebo provided by Zyma (UK) Ltd.

Adverse effects

Hydroxyethylrutosides have been evaluated in numerous clinical trials for the symptoms of chronic venous insufficiency and are generally well tolerated. The incidence of adverse events has been similar in both placebo and treatment arms in randomized controlled trials, and gastrointestinal disturbances, headache, dizziness and pruritus are the commonly reported side effects (Wadworth & Faulds 1992).

Summary

When the two trials were combined in a meta-analysis (Fig. 13.3), ulcer healing was about 37% more likely to occur when patients were treated with a rutoside compared to placebo (26/69 v 18/66, RR 1.37, 95% CI 0.85–2.21), although this result is not significant. Currently, it remains possible that taking rutosides might improve ulcer healing, but further trials are necessary before the drug's effect on venous leg ulcer healing can be considered to have been determined. *FDA approved for venous disease*: Drug not included. *British National Formulary*: Indicated for relief of symptoms of oedema associated with chronic venous insufficiency.

STANOZOLOL

Pharmacology and suggested mechanism of action

Stanozolol is a synthetic derivative of testosterone and an anabolic steroid that has a fibrinolytic action (Murr & Rogers 2003). Although the action of stanozolol in venous ulcer healing is unknown, the microcirculatory action against fibrin combined with increased rates of ulcer healing in a small crossover trial investigating the treatment of lipodermatosclerosis (Burnand et al 1980) suggested sufficient justification for assuming that stanozolol might have a role in venous ulcer healing.

Evidence

One randomized controlled trial (Layer et al 1986, Northeast et al 1989) has investigated the effect of stanozolol in venous ulceration. The trial aimed to determine the effect of stanozolol as an adjuvant to compression on venous ulcer healing time. 126 patients who presented to a hospital-based clinic in England and met the inclusion criteria were enrolled in the trial. The participants were stratified by ulcer size (<2 cm^2, 2–5 cm^2, >5 cm^2) and randomized to receive either 5 mg stanozolol twice daily or a matching placebo, in addition to compression (Calaband bandages covered with a crepe bandage and held in place by Tubigrip). Participants were also managed with secondary treatments,

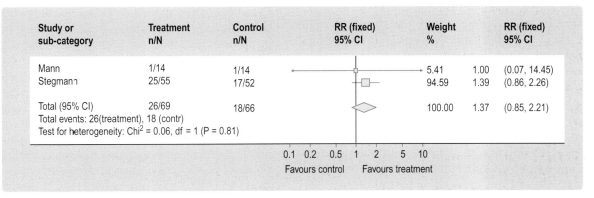

Study or sub-category	Treatment n/N	Control n/N	RR (fixed) 95% CI	Weight %	RR (fixed) 95% CI
Mann	1/14	1/14		5.41	1.00 (0.07, 14.45)
Stegmann	25/55	17/52		94.59	1.39 (0.86, 2.26)
Total (95% CI)	26/69	18/66		100.00	1.37 (0.85, 2.21)
Total events: 26(treatment), 18 (contr)					
Test for heterogeneity: Chi^2 = 0.06, df = 1 (P = 0.81)					

0.1 0.2 0.5 1 2 5 10
Favours control   Favours treatment

Figure 13.3 Meta-analysis of trials using hydroxyethylrutosides as an adjuvant to compression for treatment of venous leg ulcers

such as antibiotics or topical corticosteroids as required. The duration of treatment was until ulcer healing or 12 months. The primary outcome was healing time. 86% (44/51) of those treated with stanozolol and 80% (44/55) of those treated with placebo healed (absolute difference 6.3%, 95% CI −7.9−20%, NNT 16, 95% CI −13−5). *Strengths and limitations:* This was a pragmatic trial with stanozolol as an adjuvant to a standard compression regimen and local treatment that could be adapted to changes in the participant's condition. The trial employed random allocation (with stratification to ensure that the groups were balanced for a key prognostic variable), was blinded, used intention to treat analysis and followed up participants for a sufficiently long period in order to establish healing times. *Funding sources:* Sterling Research Laboratories and Research Endowment Fund of St Thomas' Hospital.

Adverse effects

Three patients in each group reported side effects in Northeast et al 1989, although the actual effects are not reported. However, no participant withdrew from the study because of side effects. In a previous study of stanozolol for treatment of venous lipodermatosclerosis, headaches and irregular light menstruation were the only side effects (Burnand et al 1980). Elsewhere, however, there have been reports of stanozolol interacting with anticoagulants (Murr & Rogers 2003).

Summary

Current evidence suggests that stanozolol does not provide additional benefit to compression therapy in terms of healing time or proportion of patients with healed ulcers after 60 weeks of treatment. Although further trials would be necessary before a lack of effect can be truly assumed, the marginal increment in healing rates is likely to be too small to attract further investigation. The apparent lack of effect on healing time should not be confused with the effect stanozolol has in the treatment of lipodermatosclerosis (Burnand et al 1980, McMullin et al 1991). *FDA approved for venous disease:* Not indicated. *British National Formulary:* Drug not included.

SULODEXIDE

Pharmacology and suggested mechanism of action

Sulodexide is a heparinoid, consisting of dermatan sulphate and low-molecular-weight heparin, that is derived from porcine intestinal mucosa (Sweetman 2002). Heparinoids include highly sulphated polysaccharides and are also known as glucosaminoglycans, glycosaminoglycan polysulphated compounds, sulphated mucopolysaccharides and sulphated glucosaminoglycans. The action of sulodexide in venous ulcer healing is unknown, although the drug is considered to have antithrombotic and antiplatelet actions (Mutschler & Roncaglioni 2002).

Evidence

Two randomized controlled trials (Scondotto et al 1999, Coccheri et al 2002) have investigated the effect of sulodexide in venous ulceration. A third controlled trial (Kucharzewski et al 2003) employed a quasi-random method of allocating participants to treatment, but has been included here. The largest trial (Coccheri et al 2002) enrolled 235 patients aged 18–75 years, with leg ulcers that were due to chronic venous insufficiency and measured more than 2 cm in diameter. The trial involved 31 centres in Italy and aimed to evaluate the effect of sulodexide as an adjuvant to compression on ulcer healing. 121 patients were randomized to receive sulodexide, administered as 60 mg intramuscularly for 20 days followed by 100 mg orally once per day for 70 days. 114 participants were allocated to a matching placebo treatment. Compression according to local standards was commenced on all participants following randomization, but adherence fell to approximately 85% in both groups over the duration of the trial. A variety of compression systems were employed: short-stretch bandages, self-adherent bandages, zinc oxide bandages (either alone or in conjunction with another bandage), and four-layer bandages. The primary outcome was ulcer healing at 2 months, as indicated by complete epithelialization. Other outcomes were ulcer healing at 3 months, reduction in ulcer area and adverse events. Analysis was by intention to treat, although five participants were excluded from the analysis as they withdrew after randomization but before treatment commenced. 52% (63) of the participants on sulodexide and 32% (36) of those allocated to placebo completely healed at 3 months (absolute difference 20.5%, 95% CI 8.2–32.8%, NNT 5, 95% CI 5–12). The frequency of adverse events in the sulodexide group did not significantly differ from that of the placebo group (19.1% v 15.4%). *Strengths and limitations:* This pragmatic trial used sulodexide as an adjuvant to the treatment regimens employed in local centres. The trial employed random allocation, was blinded, used intention to treat analysis and the treatment and placebo groups were similar at baseline. Although the participants were followed up for 3 months, reporting survival analysis over a longer period of follow-up would more clearly reveal differences in healing rates over time as simply reporting the proportion of ulcers healed after a short period of follow-up can be misleading. *Funding source:* Not reported.

A second smaller trial (Scondotto et al 1999) also aimed to determine the effect of sulodexide as an adjuvant to compression on ulcer healing. 94 patients were enrolled. 52 participants were randomized to receive sulodexide, administered as 60 mg intramuscularly for 30 days followed by 50 mg orally twice per day for 30 days. 42 participants were allocated to standard treatment, which consisted of short-stretch bandaging. The primary outcome was the percentage of ulcers healed at 2 months as indicated by complete epithelialization. The secondary endpoint was mean time to healing. 30 participants (69%) in the sulodexide group had healed compared with 15 participants (36%) on standard care (absolute difference 33.5%, 95%CI 14.3–52.7%, NNT 3, 95%CI 2–7). Mean healing time was 72 days for the sulodexide group and 110 days for the standard care group, although this difference was not statistically significant. *Strengths and limitations:* The trial employed random allocation, and the treatment was an adjuvant to compression. However, the trial was open-label, with no independent verification of healing reported. Further, the treatment and control groups did differ at baseline in terms of the depth of ulcers, with more of the deeper ulcers allocated to sulodexide. However, such a difference would have favoured the control group. Participants were only followed up for the 2 months of treatment. Reporting survival analysis over a longer treatment period might

more clearly reveal differences in healing rates over time. *Funding source:* Not reported.

A third trial (Kucharzewski et al 2003) also aimed to determine the effect of sulodexide as an adjuvant to compression on venous ulcer healing time. 44 patients were enrolled. The trial employed pseudo-randomization to allocate 23 participants to treatment with sulodexide in addition to compression by Unna's boot. 21 participants were allocated to compression by Unna's boot alone. At 10 weeks all participants (100%) receiving sulodexide had healed compared with nine participants (42.8%) in the control group (absolute difference 57.4%, 95% CI 36–78.6%, NNT 2, 95% CI 1–3). *Strengths and limitations:* The treatment was an adjuvant to compression, healing over time was reported and the groups appeared to be broadly equivalent at baseline. However, allocation to treatment was not random and may have introduced selection bias. In addition, blinding was not employed and participants were only followed up for a short period. Reporting survival analysis over a longer treatment period might more clearly reveal differences in healing rates over time. *Funding source:* Not reported.

Adverse effects

Sulodexide is generally well tolerated. In a double-blind, double-dummy trial (Saviano et al 1993), participants were randomized to receive either 25 mg or 50 mg twice per day, or 100 mg once daily. On average 10% of participants reported an adverse event, the majority of which were considered to be mild and lasted less than 24 hours. Nausea, heartburn, epigastric pain and dyspepsia were the only side effects reported and there was no evidence of a dose-related effect.

Summary

Combining the three trials in a meta-analysis (Fig. 13.4), complete healing was about three-quarters more likely to occur when patients were treated with a sulodexide in addition to compression compared to placebo (RR 1.74, 95%CI 1.38–2.20). The two smaller trials produced larger results, probably as a consequence of the number of participants and the use of less rigorous methods than the larger trial. However, the relative risk of healing at 3 months was 1.65 (95%CI 1.20–2.27) in the

Study	Treatment n/N	Control n/N	RR (fixed) 95% CI	Weight %	RR (fixed) 95% CI
Coccheri	63/121	36/114		58.77	1.65 (1.20, 2.27)
Kucharzewski	23/23	9/21		14.92	2.33 (1.42, 3.82)
Scondotto	30/52	15/42		26.31	1.62 (1.01, 2.58)
Total (95% CI)	116/196	60/177		100.00	1.74 (1.38, 2.20)
Test for heterogeneity: Chi^2 = 1.56, df = 2 (P = 0.46)					

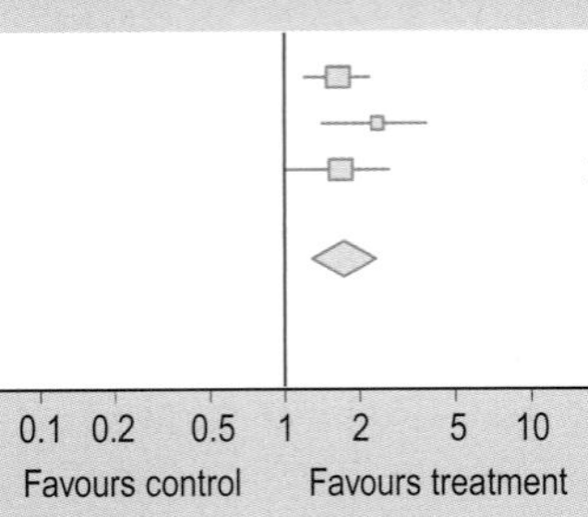

```
          0.1 0.2   0.5  1   2    5   10
            Favours control   Favours treatment
```

Figure 13.4 Meta-analysis of trials using sulodexide as an adjuvant to compression for treatment of venous leg ulcers

larger trial, a figure that is not greatly different from that of the smaller trials. Sulodexide in addition to compression appears to increase the likelihood of healing by about 40%, as indicated by the lower parameter of the confidence interval. However, the cost-effectiveness of sulodexide as an adjuvant to compression therapy needs to be determined before the benefits of its use can be considered assured. *FDA approved for venous disease:* No. *British National Formulary:* Drug not included.

ZINC SULPHATE

Pharmacology and suggested mechanism of action

Zinc is an essential trace element that, although present in minute quantities (30 mmol) in an adult, is a component of more than 50 enzymes (Davidson & Eastwood 1986). The action of zinc in venous ulcer healing is unknown.

Evidence

One systematic review (Wilkinson & Hawke 1998) of randomized controlled trials has investigated the effect of oral zinc sulphate on healing in chronic leg ulcers. The review employed an extensive search strategy that included 19 electronic databases, hand searching of five journals and conference proceedings. Attempts were made to locate unpublished studies by contacting a manufacturer of zinc tablets and searching databases of grey literature. To be included, studies had to be randomized controlled trials that included patients with venous or arterial leg ulcers and compared oral zinc sulphate against a placebo or no intervention. In addition, an objective outcome measure, such as complete healing, had to be reported. Six trials were identified, four of which (Greaves & Ive 1972, Haeger et al 1972, Hallbook & Lanner 1972, Phillips et al 1977) enrolled only participants with venous leg ulcers. Sixty-five participants received zinc sulphate in doses that ranged from 200 mg three times per day to 220 mg twice per day for between 12 weeks and 40 weeks. This is the equivalent of 50 mg elemental zinc per tablet. Seventy-six participants received a matching placebo. The trial durations varied, with participants receiving treatment for between 12 and 40 weeks depending on the follow-up period. The trials were not pooled in a meta-analysis, but the individual relative risks ranged from 1.01 to 1.50 although no result reached significance. *Strengths and limitations:* The systematic review employed a rigorous methodology, with extensive searching, assessment of trials against appropriate inclusion criteria, and two reviewers independently extracting the data from source trials. However, the review was limited by the poor quality of the included trials and the small numbers of participants included in the trial reports, at least two of which recruited more participants than they reported on. Additionally, the trial reports in most cases lacked useful information on co-interventions, such as effective compression bandaging. *Funding source:* Institute of Health Sciences, Oxford.

Adverse effects

The most common side effects of zinc salts are gastrointestinal disturbances (Sweetman 2002), such as abdominal pain, dyspepsia and diarrhoea, which are most apparent when zinc is taken on an empty stomach. Zinc tablets and multivitamins containing zinc may impair the absorption of common antibiotics (Anonymous 2003). There have been reports of zinc being associated with copper deficiency (Fosmire 1990) and dyslipidaemia (Hooper et al 1980), although other reports do not support these studies (Chandra 1984, Samman & Roberts 1987).

Summary

When the four trials were combined in a meta-analysis (Fig. 13.5), ulcer healing was about 20% more likely to occur when patients were treated with a zinc sulphate compared to placebo (33/65 v 33/76, RR 1.22, 95% CI 0.88–1.68), although this result is not significant. Currently, it remains possible that taking zinc sulphate could improve healing, but any additional benefit as an adjuvant to compression has not been determined. Although one trial (Hallbook & Lanner 1972) did suggest that zinc-deficient patients might attract the most benefit from oral zinc supplementation, the lack of a definitive test (Wood 2000) makes identifying this group of patients difficult except where the deficiency is severe. Further trials are necessary before the effect of zinc sulphate on venous leg ulcer healing can be assured. *FDA approved for venous disease:* No. *British National Formulary:* Zinc salts broadly indicated only where the patient is zinc-deficient.

Case Study 1   *Possible drug treatment for a venous leg ulcer*

You have been treating Daphne, a 69-year-old woman with a venous leg ulcer, for 8 weeks. Daphne's first leg ulcer appeared approximately 7 years ago, and she has had two episodes of recurrence since then. She expresses frustration that her ulcers seem to take forever to heal, and wishes there was something she could do to speed things up. Her notes reveal that the last ulcer took 7 months to heal despite being smaller than her current ulcer. Daphne's ulcer has a clean base and no signs of infection, and the maximum length and width, corrected for the area of an ellipse, indicates that the ulcer is about $7cm^2$ in size. This is only slightly smaller than when you first began treatment. You acknowledge Daphne's frustration and suggest that you return on your next visit with information about other treatments that might help her. She is enthusiastic about this idea.

When you return to the clinic, you set aside some time to review the clinic's wound resource manual, which contains reviews of pharmacological treatments for leg ulcers. You also scrutinize *Clinical Evidence*, which you know contains a summary of the evidence for venous ulcer treatments, effective or otherwise, and is updated every 6 months. You find that a number of pharmacological agents have been investigated for their effect on venous ulcers.

Although several drugs, such as sulodexide, mesoglycan, GM-CSF and PGE_1 are promising adjuvants to compression for venous leg ulcers, only MPFF (Daflon) and pentoxifylline (Trental) have been subject to investigations of their cost-effectiveness. Both these drugs seem to be cost-effective in comparison to treatment with compression alone. These drugs may not be appropriate adjuvants for every patient with a venous ulcer, but might usefully be employed where patients are less likely to heal after prolonged treatment with effective bandaging. A validated prediction rule found that patients with ulcer area of more than $5cm^2$, which had been present for 6 or more months prior to treatment, had a reduced likelihood of healing even after 24-weeks of compression (Margolis et al 2000). Daphne's ulcer is $7cm^2$ but has been present for less than 6 months. However, she does have a history of prolonged healing. You resolve to investigate the availability of both Daflon and Trental with a view to recommending their use to Daphne.

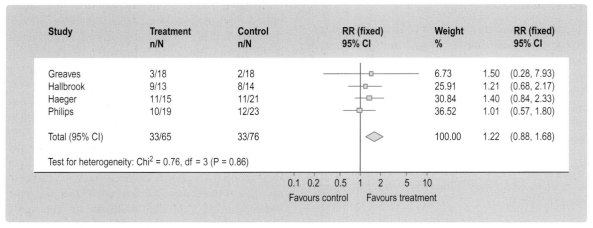

Study	Treatment n/N	Control n/N	RR (fixed) 95% CI	Weight %	RR (fixed) 95% CI
Greaves	3/18	2/18		6.73	1.50 (0.28, 7.93)
Hallbrook	9/13	8/14		25.91	1.21 (0.68, 2.17)
Haeger	11/15	11/21		30.84	1.40 (0.84, 2.33)
Philips	10/19	12/23		36.52	1.01 (0.57, 1.80)
Total (95% CI)	33/65	33/76		100.00	1.22 (0.88, 1.68)

Test for heterogeneity: Chi^2 = 0.76, df = 3 (P = 0.86)

0.1 0.2   0.5   1   2   5   10

Favours control   Favours treatment

Figure 13.5   Meta-analysis of trials using zinc sulphate for treatment of venous leg ulcers

References

Anonymous 2003. Zinc salts. In: Hutchison T A, Shahan D R (eds) DRUGDEX® System. MICROMEDEX, Greenwood Village, CO

Apollonio A, Angeletti R 1992 Terapia conservativa delle ulcere flebostatiche (confronto tra pentossifillina defibrotide impiegati per via generale) [Conservative treatment of venous leg ulcers (pentoxifylline versus defibrotide)]. Giornale Italiano di Angiologia 12: 153–156

Arenas R, Atoche C 1988 Postthrombotic leg ulcers: safety and efficacy of treatment with pentoxifylline (double-blind study in 30 patients). Dermatología Revista Mexicana Segunda Época 32: 34–38

Arosio E, Ferrari G, Santoro L et al 2001 A placebo-controlled, double-blind study of mesoglycan in the treatment of chronic venous ulcers. European Journal of Vascular and Endovascular Surgery 22: 365–372

Aussems J, Muls M 1970 Evaluation of the therapeutic efficacy of cinnarizine (Stugeron) in the treatment of crural ulcers. Clinical Trials Journal 7: 273–276

Barbarino C 1992 Pentoxifylline in the treatment of venous leg ulcers. Current Medical Research and Opinion 12: 547–551

Belcaro G, Cesarone M R, Nicolaides A N et al 2002 Treatment of venous ulcers with pentoxifylline: a 6-month randomized, double-blind, placebo controlled trial. Angiology 53(Suppl 1): S45–S47

Bjornson D C, Raasen R C 2003 Aspirin. In: Hutchison T A, Shahan D R (eds) DRUGDEX® System. MICROMEDEX, Greenwood Village, CO

Black D A, Fraser C M 1999 Iron deficiency anaemia and aspirin use in old age. British Journal of General Practice 49: 729–730

Bosanquet N, Franks P J, Brown D et al 1995 Cost effectiveness of oxpentifylline in venous ulcer healing. Phlebology 10(Suppl 1) 1: 36

Browse N L, Burnand KG 1982 The cause of venous ulceration. Lancet 2: 243–245

Burnand K, Clemenson G, Morland M et al 1980 Venous lipodermatosclerosis: treatment by fibrinolytic enhancement and elastic compression. British Medical Journal 280: 7–11

Bussolino F, Wang J M, Defilippi P et al 1989 Granulocyte- and granulocyte–macrophage-colony stimulating factors induce human endothelial cells to migrate and proliferate. Nature 337: 471–473

Chandra R K 1984 Excessive intake of zinc impairs immune responses. Journal of the American Medical Association 252: 1443–1446

Ciuffetti G, Paltriccia R, Lombardini R et al 1994 Treating peripheral arterial occlusive disease: pentoxifylline vs exercise. International Angiology 13: 33–39

Coccheri S, Scondotto G, Agnelli G et al 2002 Randomised, double blind, multicentre, placebo controlled study of Sulodexide in the treatment of venous leg ulcers. Thrombosis and Haemostasis 87: 947–952

Coleridge Smith P D 2000 Micronized purified flavonoid fraction and the treatment of chronic venous insufficiency. Microcirculation 7: S35–S40

Coleridge Smith P D 2002 Deleterious effects of white cells in the course of skin damage in CVI. International Angiology. 21(Suppl 1): 26–32

Coleridge Smith P D, Thomas P, Scurr J H, Dormandy J A 1988 Causes of venous ulceration: a new hypothesis. British Medical Journal 296: 1726–1727

Colgan M P, Dormandy J A, Jones P W et al 1990 Oxpentifylline treatment of venous ulcers of the leg. British Medical Journal 300: 972–975

Da Costa R M, Jesus F M, Aniceto C, Mendes M 1997 Double-blind randomized placebo-controlled trial of use of granulocyte-macrophage colony-stimulating factor in chronic leg ulcers. American Journal of Surgery 173: 165–168

Da Costa R M, Jesus F M R, Aniceto C, Mendes M 1999 Randomized, double-blind, placebo-controlled, dose-ranging study of granulocyte–macrophage colony stimulating factor in patients with chronic venous leg ulcers. Wound Repair and Regeneration 7: 17–25

Dale J, Ruckley C, Harper D et al 1999 Randomised, double blind placebo controlled trial of pentoxifylline in the treatment of venous leg ulcers. British Medical Journal 319: 875–878

Davidson R, Eastwood M A (eds) 1986 Human nutrition and dietetics, 8th edn. Churchill Livingstone, Edinburgh

De Sanctis M T, Belcaro G, Cesarone M R et al 2002 Treatment of venous ulcers with pentoxifylline: a 12-month, double-blind, placebo controlled trial. Microcirculation and healing. Angiology 53(Suppl 1): S49–S51

Falanga V, Fujitani R M, Diaz C et al 1999 Systemic treatment of venous leg ulcers with high doses of pentoxifylline; efficacy in a randomized, placebo-controlled trial. Wound Repair and Regeneration 7: 208–213

Fosmire G J 1990 Zinc toxicity. American Journal of Clinical Nutrition 51: 225–227

Gimenez-Roldan S, Mateo D 1991 Cinnarizine-induced parkinsonism. Susceptibility related to aging and essential tremor. Clinical Neuropharmacology 14: 156–164

Glinski W, Chodynicka B, Roszkiewicz J et al 1999 The beneficial augmentative effect of micronised purified flavonoid fraction (MPFF) on healing of leg ulcers: an open, multicentre, controlled, randomised study. Phlebology 14: 151–157

Greaves M, Ive F 1972 Double-blind trial of zinc sulphate in the treatment of chronic venous leg ulceration. British Journal of Dermatology 87: 632–634

Guilhou J J, Dereure O, Marzin L et al 1997 Efficacy of Daflon 500 mg in venous leg ulcer healing: a double-blind, randomized, controlled versus placebo trial in 107 patients. Angiology 48: 77–85

Haeger K, Lanner E, Mannsson P O 1972 Oral zinc sulphate in the treatment of venous ulcers. Vasa 1: 62–69

Hallbrook T, Lanner E 1972 Serum-zinc and healing of venous leg ulcers. Lancet 2: 780–782

Hawthorne A B, Mahida Y R, Cole A T, Hawkey C J 1991 Aspirin-induced gastric mucosal damage: prevention by enteric-coating and relation to prostaglandin synthesis. British Journal of Clinical Pharmacology 32: 77–83

He J, Whelton P K, Vu B, Klag M J 1998 Aspirin and risk of hemorrhagic stroke: a meta-analysis of randomized controlled trials. Journal of the American Medical Association 280: 1930–1935

Henke P N D 2001 Molgramostim. In: Hutchison T A, Shahan D R (eds) DRUGDEX® System. MICROMEDEX, Greenwood Village, CO

Herdy C D C, Thomaz J B, Souza S R et al 1997 Acao da pentoxifilina na cicatrizacao das ulceras de estase: Um estudo clinico-comparativo [Efficacy of pentoxifylline in the healing of venous ulcers: A comparative clinical study]. Arquivos Brasileiros de Medicina 71: 157–161

Hooper P L, Visconti L, Garry P J, Johnson G E 1980 Zinc lowers high-density-lipoprotein-cholesterol levels. Journal of the American Medical Association 244: 1960–1961

Ibbotson S H, Layton A M, Davies J A, Goodfield M J D 1995 The effect of aspirin on haemostatic activity in the treatment of chronic venous leg ulceration. British Journal of Dermatology 132: 422–426

Jacobs A 1968 The treatment of crural ulcers with cinnarizine. Ars Medici 23: 799–802

Jull A B, Waters J, Arroll B 2000 Oral pentoxifylline for treatment of venous leg ulcers (Cochrane Review). In: The Cochrane Library, Issue 2. Update Software, Oxford

Jull A B, Waters J, Arroll B 2002 Pentoxifylline for treatment of venous leg ulcers: a systematic review. Lancet 359: 1550–1554

Krakauer T 2000 Pentoxifylline inhibits ICAM-1 expression and chemokine production induced proinflammatory cytokines in human pulmonary epithelial cells. Immunopharmacology 46: 253–261

Kucharzewski M, Franek A, Koziolek H 2003 Treatment of venous ulcers with sulodexide. Phlebologie 5: 115–120

La Marca G, Pumilia G, Martino A 1999 Effectiveness of mesoglycan topical treatment of leg ulcers in subjects with chronic venous insufficiency. Minerva Cardioangiologica 47: 315–319

Layer G T, Stacey M C, Burnand K G 1986 Stanozolol and the treatment of venous ulceration – an interim report. Phlebology 1: 197–203

Layton A M 1994 Treatment of chronic leg ulcers [author's reply]. Lancet 344: 1513

Layton A M, Ibbotson S H, Davies A J, Goodfield M J 1994 Randomised trial of oral aspirin for chronic venous leg ulcers. Lancet 344: 164–165

Lyon R T, Veith F J, Bolton L, Machado F 1998 Clinical benchmark for healing of chronic venous ulcers. American Journal of Surgery 176: 172–175

Lyseng-Williamson K A, Perry C M 2003 Micronised purified flavonoid fraction: a review of its use in chronic venous insufficiency, venous ulcers and haemorrhoids. Drugs 63: 71–100

McMullin G M, Watkin G T, Coleridge Smith P D, Scurr J H 1991 Efficacy of fibrinolytic enhancement with stanozolol in the treatment of venous insufficiency. Australian and New Zealand Journal of Surgery 61: 306–309

Mann R J 1981 A double blind trial of oral O. B-hydroxyethyl rutosides for stasis leg ulcers. British Journal of Clinical Practice 35: 79–81

Margolis D J, Berlin J A, Strom B L 2000 Which venous leg ulcers will heal with limb compression bandages? American Journal of Medicine 109: 15–19

Massoud N 2002 Alprostadil. In: Hutchison T A, Shahan D R (eds) DRUGDEX® System. MICROMEDEX, Greenwood Village, CO

Meyer O C 1994 Safety and security of Daflon 500 mg in venous insufficiency and hemorrhoidal disease. Angiology 45: 579–584

Murri N, Rogers D 2003 Stanozolol. In: Hutchison T A, Shahan D R (eds) DRUGDEX® System. MICROMEDEX, Greenwood Village, CO

Mutschler E, Roncaglioni C 2002 Sulodexide. In: Hutchison T A, Shahan D R (eds) DRUGDEX® System. MICROMEDEX, Greenwood Village, CO

Neuner P, Klosner G, Pourmojib M et al 1997 Pentoxifylline in vivo and in vitro down-regulates the expression of the intercellular adhesion molecule-1 in monocytes. Immunology 90: 435–439

Nicholson A, Stone B, Turner C, Mills S L 2002 Central effects of cinnarizine: restricted use in aircrew. Aviation, Space and Environmental Medicine 73: 570–574

Nobili A 1999 Mesoglycan: In: Hutchison T A, Shahan D R (eds) DRUGDEX® System. MICROMEDEX, Greenwood Village, CO

Northeast A D R, Layer G T, Stacey M et al 1989 The effect of fibrinolytic enhancement on venous ulcer healing. In: Davy A, Stemmer R (eds) Phlebologie '89. John Libbey Eurotext, Montrouge

Phillips A, Davidson M, Greaves M 1977 Venous leg ulceration: evaluation of zinc treatment, serum zinc and rate of healing. Clinical and Experimental Dermatology 2: 395–399

Pianese C P, Hidalgo L O, Gonzalez R H et al 2002 New approaches to the management of peripheral vertigo: efficacy and safety of two calcium antagonists in a 12-week, multinational, double-blind study. Otology & Neurotology 23: 357–363

Pizarro I, Aburto I, Parra J et al 1996 Ulceras venosas de las piernas: en busca del mejor tratamentio. Revista Chilena de Cirugia 48: 453–460

Roelens P 1989 Double-blind placebo-controlled study with topical 2% ketanserin ointment in the treatment of venous ulcers. Dermatologica 178: 98–102

Roncaglioni C, Vander Leest J 2002 Cinnarizine. In: Hutchison T A, Shahan D R (eds) DRUGDEX® System. MICROMEDEX, Greenwood Village, CO

Rosenfeld L, Grover G J, Stier C T 2001 Ifetroban sodium: an effective TxA_2/PGH_2 receptor antagonist. Cardiovascular Drug Reviews 19: 97–115

Roztocil K, Stvrtinova V, Strejcek J 2003 Efficacy of a 6-month treatment with Daflon 500 mg in patients with venous leg ulcers associated with chronic venous insufficiency. International Angiology 22: 24–31

Rudofsky G 1989 Intravenous prostaglandin E_1 in the treatment of venous ulcers – a double-blind, placebo controlled trial. Vasa Supplementum 28: 39–43

Salim A S 1991 The role of oxygen-derived free radicals in the management of venous (varicose) ulceration: a new approach. World Journal of Surgery 15: 264–269

Samlaska P, Winfield E A 1994 Pentoxifylline. Journal of the American Academy of Dermatology 30: 603–621

Samman S, Roberst D C K 1987 The effect of zinc supplements on plasma zinc and copper levels and reported symptoms in healthy volunteers. Medical Journal of Australia 146: 246–249

Saviano M, Maleti O, Liguri L 1993 Double-blind, double-dummy, randomized, multicentre clinical assessment of the efficacy, tolerability and dose-effect relationship of sulodexide in chronic venous insufficiency. Current Medical Research and Opinion 13: 96–108

Schurmann W, Eberhardt R 1986 Wirksamkeit von Pentoxifyllin als Zusatz zu Kompressions- und Lokaltherapie bei Patienten mit Ulcus cruris varicosum/postthromboticum [The efficacy of pentoxifylline added to topical therapy in patients with varicose and postthrombotic ulcers]. Therapiewoche 36: 2343–2345

Scondotto G, Aloisi D, Ferrari P, Martini L 1999 Treatment of venous leg ulcers with sulodexide. Angiology 50: 883–889

Senet P, Bon F X, Benbunan M et al 2003. Randomized trial and local biological effect of autologous platelets used as adjuvant therapy for chronic venous leg ulcers. Journal of Vascular Surgery 38: 1342–1348

Stegmann W, Hubner K, Deichmann B, Muller B 1986 Efficacy of O-(β-hydroxyethyl)-rutosides in the treatment of venous varicose ulcer. Therapiewoche 36: 1828–1833

Sweetman S (ed.) 2002 Martindale: the complete drug reference, 33rd edn. Pharmaceutical Press, London

Toyota T, Hirata Y, Ikeda Y et al 1993 Lipo-PGE1, a new lipid-encapsulated preparation of prostaglandin E1: placebo-and prostaglandin E1-controlled multicenter trials in patients with diabetic neuropathy and leg ulcers. Prostaglandins 46: 453–468

Wadworth A N, Faulds D 1992 Hydroxyethylrutosides: a review of its pharmacology, and therapeutic efficacy in venous insufficiency and related disorders. Drugs 44: 1013–1032

Ward A, Clissold S P 1987 Pentoxifylline: a review of its pharmacodynamic and pharmacokinetic properties and its therapeutic efficacy. Drugs 34: 50–97

Weitgasser H 1983 The use of pentoxifylline (Trental 400) in the treatment of leg ulcers: results of a double-blind trial. Pharmatherapeutica 3(Suppl 1): 143–151

Wilkinson E, Hawke C 1998 Does oral zinc aid the healing of chronic leg ulcers? Archives of Dermatology 134: 1556–1560

Wood R J 2000 Assessment of marginal zinc status in humans. Journal of Nutrition 130(5S Suppl): 1350S–1354S

Lymphoedema of the lower limb: causation, assessment and management

Anne F. Williams, Peter Mortimer

INTRODUCTION

Lymphoedema of the lower limb presents as persistent swelling, confined to the leg/s or also affecting the lower abdomen and genital area. Evidence suggests that venous and lymphatic insufficiency coexist in some patients (Bull et al 1993, Brautigam et al 1998) and the significance of lymphatic failure in chronic venous disease may not be fully recognized. Not only does the presence of oedema influence ulcer healing, but chronic venous ulceration will also damage local lymphatics increasing the potential for lymphoedema to develop. Additionally, a grossly oedematous leg, with stretched and fragile skin, is at risk of skin damage and ulceration.

This chapter will explore the problem of lower limb lymphoedema, overviewing epidemiological and aetiological factors, underlying pathophysiology and mechanisms associated with oedema formation. The psychosocial impact of lymphoedema on the individual will be discussed and the assessment and management of people with lymphoedema described, with particular reference to conservative management approaches.

Lymphoedema is defined as an oedema of more than 3 months duration that does not reduce on elevation (Moffatt et al 2003) and results from a failure in the lymphatic system. However, in reality the picture is often more complex, as some patients with chronic swelling exhibit a mixed aetiology compounded by other factors such as obesity, immobility, cardiac failure or advanced malignancy. As a result the term 'chronic oedema' is often used to reflect the multifaceted nature of this condition (British Lymphology Society 2001a).

EPIDEMIOLOGY

The prevalence literature relating to lower limb lymphoedema is limited and the extent of the problem is not clear and may be greatly underestimated (Moffatt et al 2003). This is probably due to several factors including the difficulties in classifying the various types of primary lymphoedema (Browse & Stewart 1985) and the problems with establishing aetiology in patients with lower limb swelling (Blankfield et al 1998). In the UK many lymphoedema services have developed for people with cancer-related lymphoedema while the problem of non-cancer lymphoedema appears to remain under-recognized (Lymphoedema Framework Project 2002).

A prevalence study in the UK used a case ascertainment method and reported a crude lymphoedema prevalence rate of 1.33/1000, rising to 5.4/1000 in the over-65-year-old group (Moffatt et al 2003). Within the total patient group, 90% of the men and 51.2% of the women had leg swelling.

Studies of cancer-related lymphoedema have identified lower limb lymphoedema in 40% of patients following groin dissection (Shaw & Rumball 1990), 47% of women following treatment for vulval cancer (Ryan et al 2003) and 41% of women following cervical cancer treatment (Werngren-Elgström & Lidman 1994). A review of the literature identified 6–20% developing leg lymphoedema following groin dissection for malignant melanoma (Hughes & Thomas 1999) and more recently a figure of 29% has been reported in this same patient group (Serpell et al 2003). Henningsohn et al (2002) have identified heaviness in the legs or lower abdomen in 23% of men following radical radiotherapy for urinary bladder carcinoma and an earlier study reported lymphoedema in 18% of men following pelvic lymphadenectomy for prostate cancer (Lieskovsky et al 1980).

In one study, Moffatt et al (2004) identified chronic oedema in 35% of patients with leg ulceration. A further study of 689 chronic leg ulcers showed 17 patients to have ulceration due to lymphoedema and 11 patients due to 'mixed lymphoedema and venous reflux' (Adam et al 2003). In this study lower limb venous duplex scan was performed to assess venous disease, although it is not clear how the diagnosis of lymphoedema was established. Prasad et al (1990) have also reported oedema in 55% of patients with leg ulceration.

There are some difficulties in comparing the various epidemiological studies, as methods used for identifying and quantifying lymphoedema vary and there is no standard definition of lymphoedema (Williams et al (2005). Equally there are no data on the incidence of genital and/or trunk oedema in these patients. It is clear, however, that lymphoedema may be a significant problem in some patient groups and that additional studies are required to identify aetiological and risk factors.

THE LYMPHATIC SYSTEM

The lymphatic system has an important role in fluid balance, removing water, large molecules and particles from the interstitial tissues and returning them to the vascular circulation. It also has an immune function, filtering bacteria and other particulate matter through the lymph nodes, where lymphocytes are produced and phagocytosis takes place. Nutritionally, the intestinal lymphatics absorb digested fats and the lymph system transports them to the blood stream.

Lymphatic vessels are present in most organs of the body, although not in nervous tissue. They are slightly bigger and more permeable than blood vessels and there are valves present within many of the larger lymphatics. At the microcirculatory level, a network of blind-ended initial lymphatics is present in the upper dermis. These are thin-walled and are highly permeable to proteins and to particulate matter. They contain flap valves that allow fluid to enter but close when the pressure rises within the lymphatic. Elastic fibres and anchoring filaments support the initial lymphatics in the surrounding tissues and facilitate the dilation of the flap valves in response to changing tissue pressures (Ryan & de Berker 1995).

Lymph drains from the initial lymphatics into a plexus of pre-collectors in the deeper papillary dermis and then into collector vessels. The collectors gradually increase in size and the larger vessels have two or three layers of smooth muscle cells. They contain unidirectional valves and each segment between two valves is called a lymphangion. These vessels are contractile and lymph propulsion is enhanced by tissue movement, skeletal muscle activity, pulsation of adjacent arteries and changing intrathoracic and intra-abdominal pressures, influenced by breathing (Vaqas & Ryan 2003). The lymph vessels empty proximally and this creates a pressure gradient that exerts a suction effect, enhancing drainage from distal lymphatics.

There are over 600 lymph nodes in the body. Lymph is drained via the main collectors through regional lymph node groups and on to larger vessels such as the thoracic and right lymphatic ducts, from where it is returned to the venous circulation (Fig. 14.1). Regions or territories of the skin are drained via specific lymphatic pathways through regional collectors and lymph nodes. The skin lymph drainage territories (lymphatic basins) are divided by 'watersheds', which represent areas of potential anastomoses between the various groups of regional lymph nodes.

Lymph nodes are situated at superficial and deep levels and range from 0.2–3 cm in diameter (Földi et al 2003). The superficial inguinal lymph nodes lie parallel to the saphenous vein and drain the entire superficial lymphatic network of the lower extremity and the anterior and lateral abdominal wall to the level of the umbilicus, gluteal region, external genitals and perineal region. The deep lymph nodes lie medially to the femoral vein and drain the deep lymphatics of the lower extremity and the genitalia. These shared drainage routes explain why leg, trunk and genital oedema may coexist following inguinal lymphadenectomy.

PATHOPHYSIOLOGY UNDERLYING OEDEMA FORMATION

The blood capillary wall is a semipermeable membrane and fluid continually moves between blood capillary and interstitial tissues. Four main

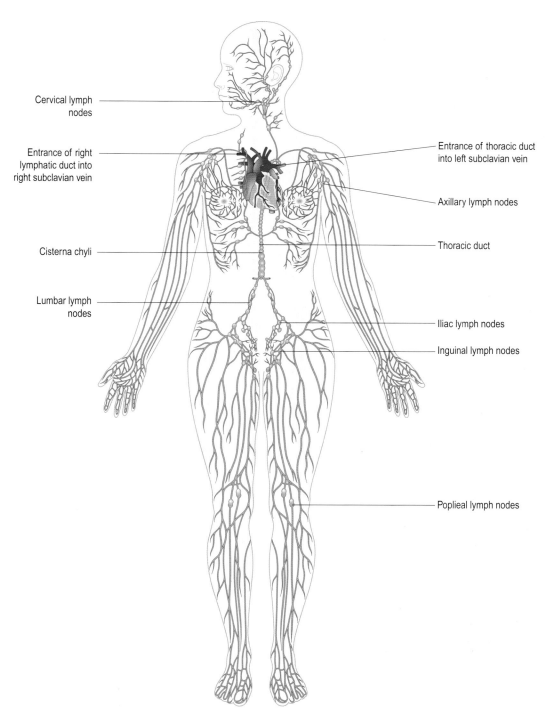

Figure 14.1 The lymphatic system, showing large lymphatics and lymph node groups

pressures influence the rate of filtration across the capillary membrane: the capillary hydrostatic pressure, the interstitial hydrostatic pressure, the plasma colloid osmotic pressure and the interstitial colloid osmotic pressure (Stanton 2000). These pressures or forces form the basis of the Starling principle of fluid exchange.

The ability to return the excess fluid and other substances from the interstitial tissues to the vascular circulation is defined as the transport capacity of the lymphatic system (Földi 1989). Fluid accumulates in the tissues when lymph drainage capacity is compromised. Proteins remain in the interstitial fluid and there is a proliferation of macrophages. An inflammatory response ensues, producing an excess of fibroblasts and collagen fibres, with destruction of the elastic fibres. This results in a non-pitting lymphoedema characterized by tissue fibrosis, skin problems and risk of infection (Figure 14.2).

If the capillary filtration rate exceeds the lymphatic drainage capacity for a sufficient period of time, oedema will also develop as the lymphatic system becomes overwhelmed by the excess capillary filtrate. This can result from venous hypertension, cardiac failure, prolonged immobility and

Table 14.1 Stages of lymphoedema (International Society of Lymphology 2003)

Stage	Description
Stage 0	Latent or subclinical condition where swelling is not evident despite impaired lymph transport; can exist for many years
Stage I	Early accumulation of fluid that reduces with elevation; excess volume of <20%
Stage II	Accumulation of fluid with pitting and does not reduce on elevation; at later stages may be non-pitting; excess volume of 20–40%
Stage III	Non-pitting swelling with trophic skin changes; excess volume of >40%

local inflammatory conditions and ulceration. The release of substances such as histamine increases capillary permeability, as they cause endothelial junctions in the blood capillary to open, moving more fluid into the tissues. Inflammatory processes also cause obliteration of lymphatics due to lymphangitis and lymphangiothrombosis.

Oedema also develops in hypoproteinaemia where the reduction in plasma colloid osmotic pressure raises the net capillary filtration rate. This type of oedema may be more generalized, with ascites, and is associated with nutritional malabsorption, excessive loss of urinary protein due to nephrotic syndrome, protein-losing enteropathy, hepatic cirrhosis and metastases. Proteins such as albumin are synthesized in the liver and oedema usually occurs when the plasma protein concentration is below 27 g/litre.

Okeke et al (2004) discuss the controversies surrounding lymphoedema development and suggest that re-evaluation of the microcirculatory processes leading to oedema is required. Arm lymphoedema secondary to breast cancer has been associated with increased arterial inflow (Svensson et al 1994) and low interstitial protein concentration (Bates et al 1993) but the mechanisms underlying these findings are unclear. Angiogenic factors have been hypothesized as leading to an increase in capillary filtration rate in arm swelling (Mellor et al 2002), although how this relates to leg oedema has not been established.

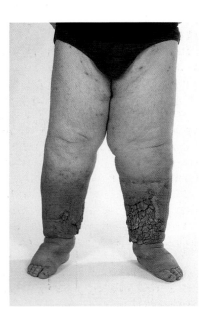

Figure 14.2 Lymphoedema with associated skin changes: papillomatosis and hyperkeratosis

CHRONIC VENOUS DISEASE AND THE LYMPHATIC SYSTEM

The literature provides some insight into the relationship between chronic venous insufficiency and oedema. Gniadecka (1996) used skin ultrasound in patients with different types of oedema and showed those with severe venous hypertension and lipodermatosclerosis to have oedema confined to the papillary dermis, suggesting this is due to increased capillary permeability. Evidence also suggests that venous hypertension and lymphoedema may coexist (Wheatley et al 1996, Kim et al 1999, Adam et al 2003, Vaqas & Ryan 2003). Wheatley et al (1996) assessed 32 patients with leg oedema using duplex Doppler sonography and lymphoscintigraphy. The study identified 50% with lymphatic abnormalities, 50% with abnormal Doppler studies and six patients with combined lymphatic and venous abnormalities.

Impaired lymph drainage appears to be a contributory factor in chronic venous disease. Bull et al (1993) used quantitative lymphoscintigraphy and identified significantly reduced lymph drainage in ulcerated limbs and also in patients with chronic venous disease with no history of ulceration. Impaired lymph drainage has also been identified in early post-thrombotic syndrome (Brautigam et al 1998). An earlier study highlighted lymphatic damage around the site of infected venous ulcers and dermal lymphatic abnormalities in areas of atrophie blanche (Bollinger et al 1982). Clearly lymphatic insufficiency is not a causal factor but does contribute to oedema formation in chronic venous disease.

CLASSIFICATION OF OEDEMAS

In 1957 Kinmonth et al described a clinical classification for primary and secondary lymphoedema describing the associated lymphographic abnormalities (Kinmonth et al 1957). Since then, Browse & Stewart (1985) published another classification system and this has recently been further refined (Browse 2003). Problems remain, however, with a lymphoedema classification system based on aetiology, as the functional and physiological processes resulting in lymphoedema are not always easily established. Growing knowledge of genetic factors in lymphoedema is providing greater insight into these conditions, although the terms 'primary' and 'secondary' lymphoedema continue to provide a useful framework.

Primary lymphoedema is a result of an intrinsic abnormality or insufficiency in the lymphatic system. It affects all ages and is referred to as *lymphoedema congenita* when present at birth or developing within the first year. Milroy's disease is a term used to describe congenital, hereditary lymphoedema and appears to be associated with a failure in lymphangiogenesis due to an inactivation of the *VEGFR3* gene (Burnand & Mortimer 2003). Other genetic forms of lymphoedema include the lymphoedema–distichiasis syndrome caused by mutations in *FOXC2*, in which a double row of eyelashes is also present (Brice et al 2002). Genetic syndromes such as Klippel–Trenaunay and Turner's are also associated with primary lymphoedema.

Abnormalities may be present at birth but not manifest until later life. Meige's disease is a term used to describe primary familial lymphoedema that develops after puberty. This is a form of *lymphoedema praecox* (Browse & Stewart 1985) and commonly presents in females around puberty or pregnancy. Onset can be related to a minor injury and in the initial stages may be mistaken for swelling due to a muscle sprain. *Lymphoedema tarda* identifies a lymphoedema occurring later in life, usually after 35 years.

Lymphatic abnormalities in primary lymphoedema include an absence of lymphatics (aplasia), reduced numbers of lymphatics (hypoplasia), lymph node fibrosis or valvular incompetence associated with dilated, tortuous vessels (Box 14.1). Lymphoedema presenting in adulthood is more likely to reflect an acquired condition in which lymphatics become obliterated, leading to an obstruction, although the exact processes underlying this are unclear (Browse 2003). Distal obliteration is the most common type, occurring in 80% of cases, mainly females, and initially presenting as bilateral mild ankle swelling with slow progression. Proximal obliteration occurs in 10% of cases and is often unilateral, affecting males and females and involving the whole leg, often starting proximally (Kinmonth and Wolfe 1980).

Secondary lymphoedema is due to damage or changes in the lymphatics resulting from an external cause (Box 14.2). Filarial lymphoedema is endemic in countries such as India (Campisi 1999) and is due to infestation with filaria. Other infective diseases such as tuberculosis can cause lymph node fibrosis. Cancer-related swelling generally results from surgery and radiotherapy. Risk may be increased by postsurgical complications such as seroma and infection (Gaarenstroom et al 2003). Tumour recurrence should also be considered in lymphoedema of a progressive nature. Non-cancer-related aetiologies include trauma, infection and inflammatory conditions, all of which damage lymphatics.

Other conditions, such as lipoedema, are mistaken for lymphoedema (Fig. 14.3). Lipoedema is characterized by a distinctive distribution of excess subcutaneous tissue in the legs, buttocks and arms. The swelling is bilateral, the tissues are soft, tender and bruise easily (Harwood et al 1996) and a band of fat is present above the ankle, although the feet are rarely swollen in the early stages. Weight loss does little to improve the condition. In the longer term, lymphoedema can develop (lipoedema–lymphoedema syndrome).

Cyclical or idiopathic oedemas also occur in women and may present as generalized fluid retention and weight gain compounded by oliguria and constipation (Földi et al 2003). Some are affected by the menstrual cycle and may be triggered by stress. The potential for oedema in conditions associated with hypoproteinaemia has previously been described. Although these are not lymphatic in origin, they can occur in patients who already have lymphoedema, and further complicate the swelling.

Box 14.1   Abnormalities in primary lymphoedema (Adapted from Browse 2003)

Genetically determined abnormalities
1. Aplasia, malformation and valvular incompetence of the central lymph trunks, e.g. thoracic duct
2. Aplasia, hypoplasia or dilatation and valvular incompetence in lymphatic vessels of the limb

Acquired
3. Obliteration of lymphatics – this may be distal or proximal lymphatics, or a combination
4. Obstruction at level of lymph nodes due to fibrosis

Box 14.2   Causes of secondary lymphoedema

- Cancer – surgery, radiotherapy fibrosis, tumour obstruction

- Infection, inflammation
  - Lymphangitis, lymphangiothrombosis, erysipelas
  - Lymphatic filariasis, leprosy, tuberculosis
  - Inflammatory conditions, e.g. rheumatoid arthritis, dermatitis

- Trauma, e.g. burns, orthopaedic surgery, arterial bypass

- Chronic venous disease, post-thrombotic syndrome, ulceration

- Reduced mobility, paralysis

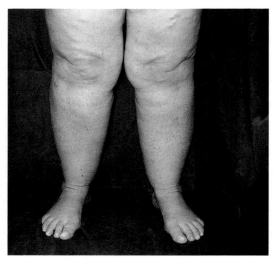

Figure 14.3   Lipoedema

QUALITY OF LIFE

Studies of quality of life in breast-cancer-related lymphoedema identify problems with body image, clothing and social relationships (Woods 1993), symptoms of pain, stiffness and restricted mobility (Poole & Fallowfield 2002). Literature on leg swelling is limited, although it is reasonable to assume that there may be some similarities in the experience of both groups. Sitzia & Sobrido (1997) showed that pain scores in leg lymphoedema were higher than in arm swelling and Moffatt et al (2003) reported pain and discomfort as a problem. The latter study also showed that oedema had affected employment status in 9% of individuals with chronic oedema.

A study of six women with primary lymphoedema of the lower limb highlighted the distress experienced by these women, particularly in the early stages of their condition when a diagnosis was not forthcoming (Williams et al 2004). Frustration with the lack of information available from health professionals and difficulties with social relationships, feelings of isolation and depression, anxiety about keeping the swelling hidden and being unable to wear skirts were also described.

ASSESSMENT ISSUES

Successful management of lymphoedema depends on establishing the diagnosis and identifying coexisting and contributory factors in order to develop an individualized plan of treatment and care. A comprehensive and structured assessment (Box 14.3), complemented by appropriate investigations (Table 14.2), is important to determine suitability for lymphoedema treatment. Problems such as deep venous thrombosis, cardiac failure, diabetes, thyroid dysfunction and hypoproteinaemia should be identified prior to referral to a lymphoedema centre and a referral pathway may be a useful tool in this process (Forth Valley 2002). An assessment

Table 14.2 Investigations

Investigation	Description
Isotope lymphography or lymphoscintigraphy	Injection of a radio-labelled protein, usually technetium-99m, to the interstitium Provides images of lymphatics and lymph nodes Quantifies lymph flow by monitoring radiocolloid uptake and transit times using a gamma camera Less invasive than oil contrast lymphography and can be used on the limb, trunk and head areas Will differentiate between oedema of lymphatic, venous origin and lipoedema in some patients
Contrast lymphography or lymphangiography	Identifies large lymph vessel abnormalities Useful for assessing chylous reflux and thoracic duct injury Invasive and has largely been replaced by lymphoscintigraphy
Computed tomography (CT)	Identifies soft tissue changes such as skin thickening and increased fat density Honeycomb effect seen between the muscle and subcutis, due to thickening and fibrosis between the fat lobules Can determine differential diagnosis of lymphoedema in an oedema of unknown aetiology
Ultrasound	Not widely used in lymphoedema Identifies thickening of the subcutis and dermis Skin ultrasound shows oedema in dermis
Magnetic resonance imaging (MRI)	Honeycomb pattern in subcutis and dermal thickening seen in lymphoedematous limb Differentiates between lymphoedema, lipoedema and venous oedema

Box 14.3 *Examples of the assessment criteria used in lymphoedema*

Medical history
- Medical conditions, including cardiac, renal, hepatic, vascular and endocrine
- Cancer diagnosis and treatment
- Past surgery; complications such as wound infection or seroma
- Medications, such as steroids and hormonal therapies, that may cause fluid retention
- Symptoms associated with swelling

Details of the oedema
- Precipitating factors
- Progression and duration of swelling
- History of infection
- Past treatments for lymphoedema
- Past treatments for infection
- Pattern of swelling over the day: does it go down overnight?

Clinical examination
- Site of swelling: regional, whole limb (body chart can be used)
- Trunk or genital oedema
- Condition of the skin, tissues, nails
- Stemmer's sign – inability to pinch skin at base of second toe because of fibrosis

Measurement
- Limb volume of each limb
- Excess and percentage excess limb volume
- Volume of proximal and distal segments
- Degree of shape distortion
- Weight, height, body mass index

Psychosocial assessment
- Family and social network
- Feelings about having lymphoedema
- Employment status
- Changes and adjustments made to lifestyle and job
- Sources of information
- Goals for the short- and long-term future

Factors affecting outcome
- Vascular complications
- Pain
- High body weight
- Recurrent infection or chronic skin condition
- Immobility, sedentary lifestyle
- Lack of support
- Active malignancy

of psychological status, with identification of patient goals and factors that may affect outcome, is also important in establishing a patient centred plan of treatment and care.

Investigations

Ascertaining a clinical diagnosis can be difficult, particularly in primary lymphoedema, and investigations may be required (Tiwari et al 2003; Table 14.2). However, results can be inconclusive and may not influence the treatment plan. A differential diagnosis is important to exclude vascular abnormalities and Doppler ultrasound is particularly useful to exclude venous reflux (Stanton et al 2000).

Hand-held Doppler, used to assess ankle brachial pressure index prior to compression therapy, may provide unreliable results in a grossly oedematous limb. A 5 MHz Doppler probe should be used and referral for specialist vascular assessment should be considered. Pulse oximetry appears to offer an alternative method for assessing arterial status in these patients (Bianchi & Douglas 2002). Further work is required to explore the validity and reliability of Doppler and pulse oximetry investigations in the grossly swollen and fibrotic limb and these are used as part of a comprehensive assessment in ascertaining suitability for compression bandaging in these patients.

Outcome measures

Quantifiable measures used to assess and monitor lymphoedema include calculation of limb volume and identification of shape distortion (Badger 1997, Stanton et al 2000). Commonly, skin circumferential measurements are taken at 4 cm intervals along the limb and are used to calculate the volume of the limb as a cylinder ($V_{\text{limb}} = \Sigma\, Z^2/\pi$). Affected and non-affected limb volumes are compared in a unilateral oedema and the results are expressed as an excess and percentage excess volume. Additional calculations of proximal and distal limb segments allows for calculation of the proximal:distal (P:D) ratios of each limb. A difference of more than 0.1 when comparing the Proximal: Distal (P:D) ratio of each leg in a patient with unilateral oedema has been found to reflect shape distortion (Badger 1997).

Skin and tissue changes are more difficult to quantify. Tissue tonometry, skinfold calipers and bioimpedance measures are used mainly in lymphoedema research (Stanton et al 2000) and their clinical validity and reliability need further investigation. Further work is also required to explore measures for trunk and genital oedema. Work is ongoing into a condition-specific quality of life tool for lower limb lymphoedema (Williams 2002).

MANAGEMENT OF LYMPHOEDEMA

Conservative management of lymphoedema combines four main treatment strategies: skin and preventative care, exercise, massage and compression therapy (Földi et al 2003). A number of patients will require a two-phase approach commencing with the intensive treatment phase often referred to as decongestive lymphatic therapy (DLT) or complex decongestive therapy (CDT), followed by a maintenance phase. Others move directly into the maintenance phase.

- Decongestive (intensive) phase:
  - ◆ Skin and preventative care
  - ◆ Manual lymphatic drainage
  - ◆ Multilayer lymphoedema bandaging
  - ◆ Isotonic exercises
- Maintenance phase:
  - ◆ Skin and preventative care
  - ◆ Simple lymphatic drainage
  - ◆ Lymphoedema hosiery
  - ◆ Isotonic exercises

The intensive phase consists of daily treatment over 2–4 weeks to reduce swelling of the limb and/or trunk, normalize limb shape and improve skin and tissue condition. The focus of the maintenance phase is rehabilitation and self-management in order to achieve stability and prevent complications. In patients with advanced disease, treatment aims are palliative and the programme is modified (EWMA 2005). Treatment decisions are made according to the criteria listed in Table 14.3 and the individual needs of the patient.

There is a growing evidence base for lymphoedema treatment although much of this is limited to breast cancer-related swelling. Studies of DLT in patients with lower limb lymphoedema provide some insight (Boris et al 1994, Ko et al 1998) but results are not easily comparable. A quality of life study showed significant changes in pain, physical mobility scores and energy following treatment (Sitzia & Sobrido 1997) but highlighted the limitations of a non-condition-specific tool.

Table 14.3 Example of criteria used in treatment decisions (British Lymphology Society 2001b)

	Intensive phase	Maintenance phase
Site of swelling (body chart may be used)	Limb and/or trunk, genitalia	Confined to limb
Limb size	Limb volume excess >20% compared to unaffected limb	Limb volume excess < 20% compared to unaffected limb
Limb shape	Shape distortion identified by P:D ratio difference of >0.1	No shape distortion
Condition of skin and tissues	Subcutaneous tissue is predominantly fibrotic and non-pitting; skin damage/problems	Predominantly soft and pitting, skin is healthy and intact
Other pathology	History of recurrent infection; vascular problems	No complicating factors

MANAGEMENT STRATEGIES

Skin care

Skin and tissue changes in lymphoedema lead to recurrent infection and poor treatment response if not addressed. The epidermis becomes overstretched and dry and underlying tissues become fibrosed. Problems such as dermatitis, folliculitis, lymphangiectasia (overfilled bulging lymph vessels on skin surface), papillomatosis and hyperkeratosis occur (Table 14.4, Fig. 14.4). Lipodermatosclerosis is a result of oedema in chronic venous disease, where subcutaneous tissues become fibrosed, predisposing to ulceration (Vowden 1998).

Macerated areas can develop within skin folds and lymphoedematous skin is vulnerable to injury and ulceration. Ulcerated areas require careful assessment to establish the underlying cause and exclude malignancy. Lymphorrhoea, the leaking of lymph from the skin, is distressing for patients and can be controlled with measures such as bandaging (Ling et al 1997). Tissue viability and dermatology specialists provide additional expertise in the management of these patients.

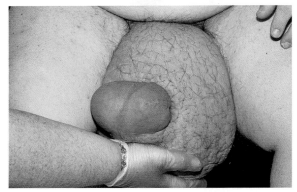

Figure 14.4 Genital oedema showing swelling of the scrotum and penis with papillomatosis present on the scrotum.

Table 14.4 Skin and tissue problems in lymphoedema

Problem	Description	Management
Dry skin	Skin stretching causes splitting of epidermis	Daily washing and moisturizing using emollients; ointment such as 50/50 white soft paraffin/liquid paraffin under bandages
Dermatitis	Contact dermatitis caused by irritant such as leaking lymph or allergic reaction	Avoid substances causing problem. Use bland emollients and topical corticosteroids in short term
Hyperkeratosis	Increased thickening of the stratum corneum resulting in thickened, scaly skin	Use of emollients and possible use of a keratolytic agent. Avoid sharp debridement as this can damage the skin and lead to infection. A hydrocolloid dressing applied for several days can help to lift hyperkeratotic layers
Lymphangiectasia	Dilated skin lymphatics bulging from the skin, look like blisters and may leak	Respond to pressure of bandages but may be persistent
Papillomatosis	A cobblestone appearance on the skin due to lymphangiectasia followed by fibrosis	Responds to pressure of bandages
Lymphorrhoea	Leaking of lymph from the skin	Palliative bandaging used with appropriate dressings; usually resolves in 2–3 days but may reoccur
Folliculitis	Inflammation of hair follicles due to poor skin hygiene or oils trapped in follicle, may be exacerbated by compression therapy	Meticulous skin hygiene, use of emollients; care when applying moisturizer; final stroking should be downwards in direction of hair growth

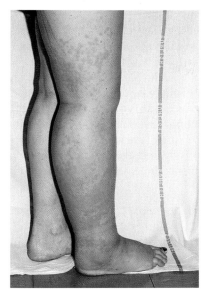

Figure 14.5 Acute inflammatory episode in a patient with lymphoedema

Management of infection

Fungal and bacterial infections are common in lower limb swelling. Acute inflammatory episodes, often called cellulitis or erysipelas, affect 30% of patients (Mortimer 2000) and are characterized by redness, heat and systemic flu-like symptoms (Fig. 14.5). Lymphangitis also presents as red streaking along the lymphatics of the limb. The term *acute inflammatory episode* reflects the current debate on whether attacks are truly infective (Badger et al 2003), although antibiotics are usually the first-line treatment. Either amoxicillin 500 mg 8 hourly, co-amoxiclav 625 mg 8 hourly or clindamycin 600 mg 6 hourly is currently recommended over a 2-week period. If infection occurs, lymphoedema treatments are stopped until acute symptoms subside. Rest and supported elevation and hydration are advised.

A low-grade, non-specific inflammation can lead to poorly controlled lymphoedema. Inflammation may subside following decongestion of the limb, although long-term antibiotic therapy may be required, particularly if there is a history of recurrent acute infection. In this instance, phenoxymethylpenicillin 500 mg daily or 1 g if body weight is more than 75 kg can be used or erythromycin 250–500 mg daily if allergy to penicillin exists.

General advice on skin care and prevention of skin injury will minimize the risk of complications:

- Daily meticulous washing using an emollient, dry carefully, especially between toes
- Moisturizing daily with unperfumed, non-lanolin-based cream
- Avoiding risk of injury such as blister, scratch, insect bite, sunburn, wet shave
- Treating skin breaks with antiseptic
- Checking for fungal infection, especially in skin folds and between toes.

Compression therapy

Hosiery garments

Compression garments are used to control and, where possible, reduce the swelling. Physiologically they improve venous and lymphatic drainage by reducing hydrostatic pressures in lymphatic and venous capillaries and maximizing the muscle pump.

Circular-knit garments, widely used in vascular disease, are used in mild lymphoedema, when the limb is a regular shape. However, they are designed to fit a standard leg shape and in a poorly shaped limb they can lead to skin damage and further distortion as they create a tourniquet effect in the deep skin folds. Although this can be addressed to some degree by a custom-made garment, circular-knit garments should be used with care in lymphoedema as the fine, soft fabric is not always suitable. Additionally, it is unclear whether the compression profile of stockings designed for venous disease is relevant to lymphoedema management.

Custom-made flat-knit garments are increasingly being used in lymphoedema and provide rigidity that accommodates poor shape. They have been shown to be effective in reducing deep venous reflux (Partsch et al 1999) and may enhance the function of lymphatics by ensuring a greater variation between resting and working pressures (Figure 14.6). The open, wide-mesh stitch pattern and higher cotton content also provide air permeability and reduce perspiration (Hampton 2003).

Garments are now available on drug tariff in the UK. These are now based on a European standard of compression, as the drug tariff has adopted a new classification for lymphoedema garment which is based on European recommendations (Ref.

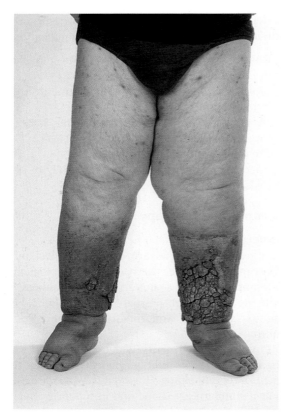

Figure 14.6   Flat-knit compression hosiery garment for lymphoedema (Courtesy of BSN Medical Ltd)

Reichs Ausschuss etc). Custom-made garments are available for genital and truncal swelling and are cobined with or provided separately from the stockings. Other accessories such as toecaps are also available.

Patients are taught how to apply the garments to avoid damaging the materials. Rubber gloves can be used and the garment is never pulled from the top as this overstretches the material. Once applied, the material should be evenly distributed over the limb and should not be folded over at the top. A variety of garment applicators are available.

Multilayer lymphoedema bandaging

Bandaging is used to reduce limb size, normalize limb shape and improve skin and tissue condition (Williams and Keller 2005). A study by Badger et al

(2000) has shown that bandaging for 3 weeks, prior to fitting hosiery garments, is more effective in reducing lymphoedema than hosiery alone (Fig. 14.7).

Physiologically, bandages have the same effects as hosiery but can forcibly move fluid through tissue spaces towards the root of the limb. Inelastic, short- or non-stretch bandages provide high working and low resting pressures and enhance lymph drainage. They can also be used to address underlying problems such as fibrosis. The following layers are used:

- *Stockinette*: Loose cotton lining material to protect the skin and absorb sweat
- *Digit bandaging*: 4 cm conforming bandage such as Mollelast (Vernon Carus) or similar bandage to reduce toe swelling and prevent fluid being pushed distally (Fig. 14.8)
- *Padding*: Foam or wadding to protect bony areas and pad out the limb to achieve a cylindrical shape prior to applying the main bandages
- *Inelastic, low-stretch bandages*: Rosidal K, Comprilan or Actico cohesive bandages, used in layers and applied as spiral and/or figure of eight to provide rigidity. Bandages can also be used over the hip if there is oedema on the trunk or root of the limb.

The four-layer bandaging system used in the management of leg ulceration is unsuitable for most patients with lymphoedema and can lead to problems with toe and knee swelling (Todd et al 2003). Bandaging should usually extend to above the knee and is commonly full leg length. To accommodate the change in limb shape and size as an oedema reduces, the bandages should be changed regularly and often daily in the initial stages of treatment. Application of cohesive bandages may prevent bandage slippage.

Modified and reduced pressure bandaging systems are used in patients with advanced cancer, in those with chronic venous disease and oedema, in patients with dependency oedema and in the elderly and infirm (EWMA 2005). In advanced cancer, for example, palliative bandaging is used to alleviate symptoms such as lymphorrhoea, pain and reduced mobility and function. It is important that patients and practitioners have realistic expectations of what

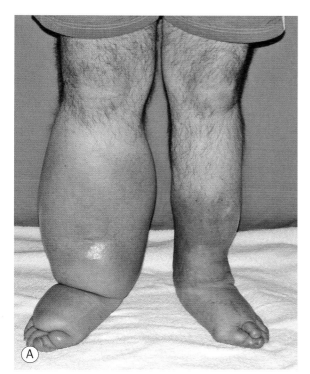 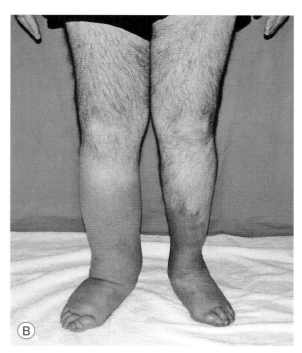

Figure 14.7 Lymphoedema (**A**) before and (**B**) after decongestive lymphatic therapy. (Courtesy of An Arm & a Leg, Intensive In-patient Lymphoedema Clinics)

can be achieved with palliative bandaging, particularly in patients with advanced malignancy and systemic problems such as venous obstruction, hypoproteinaemia and renal failure. Key principles of palliative care, with a focus on quality of life and symptom relief, are important. If there is generalized oedema it may be inappropriate to direct fluid to other areas such as the genitalia. Bandaging may be contraindicated in the presence of superior and inferior vena cava obstruction, cardiac failure, acute infection, active untreated malignancy and acute deep venous thrombosis.

Palliative bandaging is provided using stockinette, padding and one layer of a non-elastic, short-stretch bandage. It may be appropriate to bandage to below or just above the knee in these patients. Bandages such as K-lite may also be used. Toes should usually be bandaged and care is taken as the root of the swollen toe is vulnerable to pressure and should be protected with a small piece of wadding placed under the bandage.

Manual lymphatic drainage

Manual lymphatic drainage (MLD) is a gentle, specialized type of massage developed in France by Emil Vodder in the 1930s. Since then, several other methods of MLD have developed, although they all follow the same principles (Casley-Smith & Casley-Smith 1997, Leduc & Leduc 2000, Földi et al 2003). The aim of MLD is to redirect excess fluid from oedematous areas towards healthy regional lymph nodes (Fig. 14.1). Fluid is moved across the anastomoses in the watersheds between the territories of lymph drainage. Studies have shown that massage strongly influences lymph flow (Mortimer et al 1990) and MLD has been found to be effective in reducing limb volume in women with breast cancer (Johansson et al 1999, Williams et al 2002).

MLD allows collateral lymph drainage routes to become established and is important in midline oedema, for example in the genital area. Limb swelling may be better controlled if the trunk has

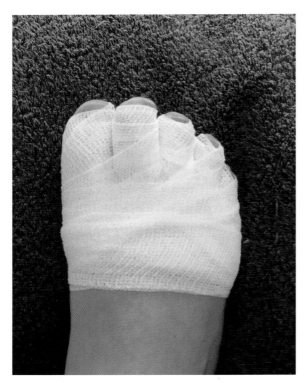

Figure 14.8   Toe bandaging

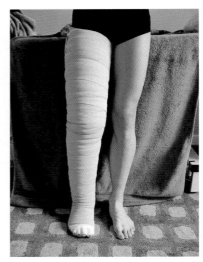

Figure 14.9   Multilayer lymphoedema bandaging

Exercise

The term 'exercise' is used in lymphoedema to refer to various different activities, including passive, assisted movements, daily recreational activities and active exercise programmes. Walking and swimming are particularly useful in leg swelling. The needs, abilities and motivation of each individual with lymphoedema vary considerably according to age and general health of the patient and some will require referral to physiotherapy.

The aim of exercise in lymphoedema is to improve mobility, joint flexibility and skeletal muscle function to enhance venous and lymphatic return (Hughes 2000). Patients should always exercise while wearing hosiery garments, except in water. Those with a dependent limb or poor mobility are a particular challenge. They are often overweight and may have reduced ankle mobility, a problem already associated with poor ulcer healing (Barwell et al 2001).

Other treatments for lymphoedema

Intermittent pneumatic compression pumps are not widely used for lymphoedema. They should only be applied after manual lymphatic drainage massage has decongested the trunk area, as they encourage fluid congestion at the root of the limb and increase the risk of genital oedema (Boris et al 1998). Pumps may have a role in the management

been decongested. Other indications for MLD include scarring, fibrosis and chronic ulceration, particularly where oedema is present. Hutzschenreuter et al (1989) studied patients with arterial disease and showed MLD to increase blood flow in arterioles, capillaries and veins.

A modified form of MLD has developed in the UK, called simple lymphatic drainage (SLD) (British Lymphology Society 1999). It is designed to be taught to patients and their carers. MLD and SLD treatment of leg lymphoedema commences proximally and centrally to clear the way ahead prior to draining the distal areas. Neck and axillary lymph nodes are treated, followed by the unaffected and affected side of the trunk and then the limb. Breathing techniques are also taught, as the changes in intrathoracic and intra-abdominal pressures brought about by inspiration and expiration increase flow from the central lymph trunks into the venous system (Vaqas & Ryan 2003).

of below-knee oedema associated with chronic venous disease but patients should always be closely monitored and instructed to avoid high pressures.

Diuretics are not routinely indicated for lymphoedema and the prolonged use of diuretics may lead to secondary hyperaldosteronism (Földi et al 2003). However, in patients with advanced disease, complicated by cardiac failure and hypoproteinaemia, short-term use of potassium-sparing diuretics may be indicated.

CONCLUSION

Lymphoedema is a complex condition that may coexist with chronic venous disease and ulceration.

Patients require careful assessment and a comprehensive management programme. Ideally this should be provided through a specialist lymphoedema treatment centre in conjunction with generalist colleagues in other settings such as primary care. In the UK, lymphoedema services are fragmented and inequitable and currently there is no national strategy for service provision. Lymphoedema services are predominately nurse- and/or physiotherapy-led and different models for service provision need to be evaluated. As this is a chronic condition, people with lymphoedema become experts in their treatment and health professionals need to work closely with patients to achieve appropriate goals.

References

Adam D J, Maik J, Hartshorne T et al 2003 The diagnosis and management of 689 chronic leg ulcers in a single-visit assessment clinic. European Journal of Vascular and Endovascular Surgery 25: 462–8

Badger C 1997 A study of the efficacy of multi-layer bandaging and elastic hosiery in the treatment of lymphoedema and their effects on the swollen limb. PhD Thesis, Institute of Cancer Research, London

Badger C M A, Peacock J L, Mortimer P S 2000 A randomised, controlled, parallel-group clinical trial comparing multilayer bandaging followed by hosiery versus hosiery alone in the treatment of patients with lymphoedema of the limb. Cancer 88: 2832–2837

Badger C, Seers K, Preston N, Mortimer P 2003 Antibiotics/anti-inflammatories for reducing acute inflammatory episodes in lymphoedema of the limbs (Protocol for a Cochrane Review). In: The Cochrane Library, Issue 3. Update Software, Oxford

Barwell J R, Taylor M, Deacon J et al 2001 Ankle motility is a risk factor for healing of chronic leg ulcers. Phlebology 16: 38–40

Bates D O, Levick J R, Mortimer P S 1993 Change in macromolecular composition of interstitial fluid from swollen arms after breast cancer treatment, and its implications. Clinical Science 85: 737–746

Bianchi J, Douglas S 2002 Pulse oximetry: vascular assessment in patients with leg ulcers. Wound Care September: 23–28

Blankfield R P, Finkelhor R S, Alexander J J et al 1998 Etiology and diagnosis of bilateral leg edema in primary care. American Journal of Medicine 105: 192–197

Bollinger A, Paster G, Hoffmann U, Franzeck U K 1982 Fluorescence microlymphology in chronic venous incompetence. International Angiology 8: 234–236

Boris M, Weindorf S, Lasinski B, Boris G 1994 Lymphedema reduction by non-invasive complex lymphedema therapy. Oncology 8: 95–106

Boris M, Weindorf S, Lasinski B B 1998 The risk of genital edema after external pump compression for lower limb lymphedema. Lymphology 31: 15–20

Brautigam P, Földi E, Schaiper I et al 1998 Analysis of lymphatic drainage in various forms of leg edema using two compartment lymphoscintigraphy. Lymphology 31: 43–55

Brice G, Mansour S, Bell R et al 2002 Analysis of the phenotypic abnormalities in lymphoedema-distichiasis syndrome in 74 patients with FOXC2 mutations or linkage to 16q24. Journal of Medical Genetics 39: 472–483

British Lymphology Society 1999 Manual lymphatic drainage (MLD) and simple lymphatic drainage (SLD) – guidelines for health professionals. British Lymphology Society, Caterham, Surrey

British Lymphology Society 2001a Clinical definitions. British Lymphology Society, Caterham, Surrey

British Lymphology Society 2001b Chronic oedema population and needs. British Lymphology Society, Caterham, Surrey

Browse N 2003 Aetiology and classification of lymphoedema. In: Browse N, Burnand K G, Mortimer P S (eds) Diseases of the lymphatics. Edward Arnold, London, pp151–156

Browse N L, Stewart G 1985 Lymphoedema: pathophysiology and classification. Journal of Cardiovascular Surgery 26: 91–106

Bull R H, Gane J N, Evans J E et al 1993 Abnormal lymph drainage in patients with chronic venous leg ulcers. Journal of the American Academy of Dermatology 28: 585–590

Burnand K G, Mortimer P S 2003 Lymphangiogenesis and the genetics of lymphoedema. In: Browse N, Burnand K G, Mortimer P S (eds) Diseases of the lymphatics. Edward Arnold, London, pp 102–109

Campisi C 1999 Global incidence of tropical and non-tropical lymphoedema (editorial). International Angiology 18: 3–5

Casley-Smith J R, Casley Smith J R 1997 Modern treatment for lymphoedema, 5th edn. Lymphoedema Association of Australia, Malvern, South Australia

EWMA (2005) European Wound Management Association (EWMA) Focus Document: Lymphoedema bandaging in practice. London MEP Ltd.

Földi M 1989 The lymphoedema chaos: a lancet. Annals of Plastic Surgery 22: 505–515

Földi M, Földi E, Kubik S (eds) 2003 Textbook of lymphology for physicians and lymphedema therapists. Urban & Fischer, Munich

Forth Valley 2002 Referral pathway for lymphoedema. Forth Valley Health Board, Stirling

Gaarenstroom K N, Kenter G G, Trimbos J B et al 2003 Postoperative complications after vulvectomy and inguinofemoral lymphadenectomy using separate groin incisions. International Journal of Gynaecological Cancer 13: 522–527

Gniadecka M 1996 Localization of dermal edema in lipodermatosclerosis, lymphedema, and cardiac insufficiency. Journal of the American Academy of Dermatology 35: 37–41

Hampton S 2003 Elvarex compression garments in the management of lymphoedema. British Journal of Nursing 12: 925–926, 928–929

Harwood C A, Bull R H, Evans J, Mortimer P S 1996 Lymphatic and venous function in lipoedema. British Journal of Dermatology 134: 1–6

Henningsohn L, Wijkström H, Dickman P W et al 2002 Distressful symptoms after radical radiotherapy for urinary bladder cancer. Radiotherapy and Oncology 62: 215–225

Hughes K 2000 Exercise and lymphoedema. In: Twycross R, Jenns K, Todd J (eds) Lymphoedema. Radcliffe Medical Press, Oxford, ch 10

Hughes T M, Thomas J M 1999 Combined inguinal and pelvic lymph node dissection for stage 111 melanoma. British Journal of Surgery 86: 1493–1498

Hutzschenreuter P, Brümmer H, Ebberfeld K 1989 Experimental and clinical studies of the mechanisms of effect of manual lymph drainage therapy. Journal of Lymphology 13: 62–64

International Society of Lymphology 2003 The diagnosis and treatment of peripheral lymphedema. Consensus Document of the International Society of Lymphology. Lymphology 36: 84–91

Johansson K, Albertsson M, Ingvar C, Ekdahl C 1999 Effects of compression bandaging with or without manual lymph drainage treatment in patients with postoperative arm lymphedema. Lymphology 32: 103–110

Kim P I, Huh S, Huang J H et al 1999 Venous dynamics in leg lymphoedema. Lymphology 32: 11–14

Kinmonth J B, Wolfe J H 1980 Fibrosis in the lymph nodes in primary lymphoedema. Histological and clinical studies in 74 patients with lower-limb oedema. Annals of the Royal College of Surgeons of England 62: 344–354

Kinmonth J B, Taylor G W, Tracey G D, Marsh J D 1957 Primary lymphoedema: clinical and lymphangiographic studies of a series of 107 patients in which the lower limbs were affected. British Journal of Surgery 45: 1–10

Ko D S C, Lerner R, Klose G, Cosimi A B 1998 Effective treatment of lymphedema of the extremities. Archives of Surgery 133: 452–458

Leduc A, Leduc O 2000 Manual lymphatic drainage. In: Twycross R, Jenns K, Todd J (eds) Lymphoedema. Radcliffe Medical Press, Oxford, ch 12

Lieskovsky G, Skinner D G, Weisenburger T 1980 Pelvic lymphadenectomy in the management of carcinoma of the prostate. Journal of Urology 124: 635–638

Ling J, Duncan A, Laverty D, Hardy J 1997 Lymphorrhoea in palliative care. European Journal of Palliative Care 4: 50–52

Lymphoedema Framework Project 2003 Lymphoedema Framework Conference: Towards a national framework for lymphoedema management – a participative event on 18 April 2002. Lymphoedema Framework Journal, Autumn 6–8

Mellor R H, Stanton A W B, Menadue L et al 2002 Evidence for dermal angiogenesis in breast cancer related lymphoedema demonstrated using dual site fluorescence angiography. Microcirculation 9: 207–219

Moffatt C J, Franks P J, Doherty D C et al 2003 Lymphoedema: an underestimated health problem. Quarterly Journal of Medicine 96: 731–738

Moffatt C J, Franks P J, Doherty DC et al (2004) Prevalence of leg ulceration in a London population QJM 97 431-7.

Mortimer P 2000 Acute inflammatory episodes. In: Tywcross R, Jenns K, Todd J (eds) Lymphoedema. Radcliffe Medical Press, Oxford, ch 9

Mortimer P S, Simmonds R, Rezvani M et al 1990 The measurement of skin lymph flow by isotope clearance- reliability, reproducibility, injection dynamics, and the effect of massage. Journal of Investigative Dermatology 95: 677–682

Okeke A A, Bates D O, Gillant D A 2004 Lymphoedema in urological cancer. European Urology 45: 18–25

Partsch H, Menzinger G, Mostbeck A (1999) Inelastic leg compression is more effective to reduce deep venous refluxes than elastic bandages. Dermatologic Surgery 25: 695–700

Poole K, Fallowfield L J 2002 The psychological impact of post-operative arm morbidity following axillary surgery for breast cancer: a critical review. Breast 11: 81–87

Prasad A, Ali-Khan A, Mortimer P S 1990 Leg ulcers and oedema: a study exploring the prevalence, aetiology and possible significance of oedema in leg ulcers. Phlebology 5: 181–187

Reichs-Ausschuss für Lieferbedingungen 1987 RAL-GZ 387 Medical compression hosiery. Deutsches Institut für Gütesicherung und Kennzeichnung, St Augustin, Germany

Ryan T J, de Berker D 1995 The interstitium, the connective tissue environment of the lymphatic, and angiogenesis in human skin. Clinics in Dermatology 13: 451–458

Ryan M, Stainton M C, Slaytor E K et al 2003 Aetiology and prevalence of lower limb lymphoedema following treatment for gynaecological cancer. Australian and New Zealand Journal of Obstetrics and Gynaecology 43: 148–151

Serpell J W, Carne P W, Bailey M 2003 Radical lymph node dissection for melanoma. Australian and New Zealand Journal of Surgery 73: 294–299

Shaw J H F, Rumball E M 1990 Complications and local recurrence following lymphadenectomy. British Journal of Surgery 77: 760–764

Sitzia J, Sobrido L 1997 Measurement of health-related quality of life of patients receiving conservative treatment for limb lymphoedema using the Nottingham Health Profile. Quality of Life Research 6: 373–384

Stanton A 2000 How does tissue swelling occur? The physiology and pathophysiology of interstitial fluid formation. In: Twycross R, Jenns K, Todd J (eds) Lymphoedema. Radcliffe Medical Press, Oxford, ch 2

Stanton A W B, Badger C, Sitzia J 2000 Non-invasive assessment of the lymphoedematous limb. Lymphology 33: 122–135

Svensson W E, Mortimer P S, Tohno E, Cosgrove D O 1994 Increased arterial flow demonstrated by Doppler ultrasound in arm swelling following breast cancer treatment. European Journal of Cancer 30: 661–664

Tiwari A, Cheng K S, Button M et al 2003 differential diagnosis, investigation, and current treatment of lower limb lymphedema. Archives of Surgery 138: 152–161

Todd M, Key M R, Rice M, Welsh J 2003 Does lymphoedema bandaging reduce the risk of toe ulceration? Journal of Wound Care 12: 311

Vaqas B, Ryan T J 2003 Lymphoedema: pathophysiology and management in resource-poor settings- relevance for lymphatic filariasis control programmes. Filaria Journal 2: 4. Available on line at: www.filariajournal.com/content/2/1/4

Vowden K 1998 Lipodermatosclerosis and atrophie blanche. Journal of Wound Care 7: 441–443

Werngren-Elgström M, Lidman D 1994 Lymphoedema of the lower extremities after surgery and radiotherapy for cancer of the cervix. Scandinavian Journal of Plastic and Hand Surgery 28: 289–293

Wheatley D C, Wastie M L, Whitaker S C et al 1996 Lymphoscintigraphy and colour Doppler sonography in the assessment of leg oedema of unknown cause. British Journal of Radiology 69: 1117–1124

Williams A E 2002 A condition specific quality of life tool for lymphoedema. Presentation to British Lymphology Conference, October 2002

Williams A F, Franks P J, Moffatt C J (2005) Lymphoedema: estimating the size of the problem. Palliative Medicine 19: 300–313.

Williams A F, Keller M (2005) Practical guidance on lymphoedema bandaging of the upper and lower limbs. In: EWMA. Lymphoedema bandaging in practice; Focus Document. European Wound Management Association, MEP Ltd.

Williams A F, Vadgama A, Franks P J, Mortimer P S 2002 A randomized controlled crossover study of manual lymphatic drainage therapy in women with breast cancer-related lymphoedema. European Journal of Cancer Care 11: 154–261

Williams A F, Moffatt C J, Franks P J 2004 A phenomenological study of the lived experiences of people with lymphoedema. International Journal of Palliative Nursing 10: 279–286

Woods M 1993 Patients perceptions of breast cancer-related lymphoedema. European Journal of Cancer Care 2: 125–128

Useful contacts

British Lymphology Society
P.O. Box 196
Shoreham
Sevenoaks, Kent TN13 9BF
Tel: 01959 525524
Fax: 01959 525524
Website: www.lymphoedema.org/bls/

The Lymphoedema Support Network
St Luke's Crypt

Sydney Street
London SW3 6NH
Tel: 020 7351 4480
Fax: 020 7349 9809
Website: www.lymphoedema.org/lsn/

MLD UK
PO Box 14491
Glenrothes, Fife KY6 3YE
Tel/Fax: 01592 748008
Website: www.mlduk.org.uk

Arterial ulcers: theories of causation

Alison Kite, Janet Powell

PERIPHERAL ARTERIAL DISEASE

Leg ulceration is not a disease per se but a symptom of an underlying disease in large or small blood vessels. One in five of the 65–75 year age group in the UK have evidence of peripheral arterial disease on clinical examination, although only a quarter of these will have symptoms (Burns et al 2003). In the patients who have symptoms, peripheral arterial disease can cause intermittent claudication or more severe ischaemic symptoms if left untreated.

Intermittent claudication is a cramping pain in the calf or buttocks that develops during episodes of exercise and is rapidly relieved by rest. The location of the pain indicates the area of stenosed or occluded artery within the arterial tree. Buttock pain indicates stenosed/occluded arteries in the aortic and iliac region, with calf pain suggesting stenosed/occluded arteries in the femoral and/or popliteal artery. This is usually the first sign that patients report to the family practitioner with, and is indicative of peripheral arterial disease. For patients this is a very disabling condition that can restrict their lifestyle drastically, causing some patients to retire or be signed off sick from work. Unless risk factors are managed and lifestyle adjustments made, the disease may progress further, causing the pain of intermittent claudication to develop at a shorter distance, and can render the patient housebound.

There are different stages of ischaemia, ranging from intermittent claudication through to critical limb ischaemia as the disease process advances (Table 15.1). Patients with intermittent claudication usually do not complain of rest pain, although they may experience night cramps as the disease progresses. Persistent, intense pain indicates rest pain. This generally occurs in the foot when the patient is supine. It can be relieved by keeping the foot down, i.e. hanging it over the edge of the bed. Many patients will report sleeping in a chair and needing large doses of opiates to reduce their pain. Development of rest pain or critical limb ischaemia indicates progression of the disease as the blood supply becomes more compromised, so that the skin's nutritional requirements are not met at rest. This may be the start of skin breakdown and ulcer formation (Fig. 15.1).

Acute limb ischaemia is caused by the sudden cessation of blood supply to the tissues beyond the obstruction. It does not allow time for the formation of a collateral blood supply. If blood supply is not restored within 36 hours of onset, the tissues of the limb can quickly become necrotic and amputation may be the only treatment option. Thrombi or emboli totally occluding the artery cause acute limb ischaemia. Thrombus originates from a fissure or rupture of an atherosclerotic plaque occluding the vessel at the level of rupture. Emboli originate elsewhere in the body and are associated with the following conditions: atrial fibrillation, abdominal aortic aneurysms – or indeed any arterial aneurysm – and atheromatous arteries may cause distal emboli. Additionally, invasive procedures such as arterial surgery and angiography can cause emboli.

Peripheral arterial disease is most commonly a manifestation of systematic atherosclerosis in which the arterial lumen of the lower extremities becomes progressively occluded by atherosclerotic

Table 15.1   Classification of stages of ischaemia

Intermittent claudication	Chronic limb ischaemia
Rest pain	Critical limb ischaemia
Ulceration and tissue loss	Loss of limb threatened Surgical intervention

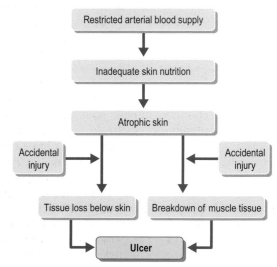

Figure 15.1   Causation of arterial ulceration

plaque causing ischaemia. The process by which arterial ulcers develop is complex but can be likened to the development of digital gangrene at high altitude or in polar and ice expeditions. Explorers of the Antarctic, including those on the Scott and Shackleton expeditions at the beginning of the 20th century, suffered losses and death from cold gangrene and more recently Sir Ranulph Fiennes, on his North Pole expedition, suffered from gangrene. In an attempt to conserve core body temperature, there is superficial vasoconstriction to divert blood away from the cold skin of the extremities into the deeper and more central circulations.

The blood supply to the skin is controlled by arteriovenous anastomoses in the dermis, where the arteriole connects directly to the venules, bypassing any capillary bed (Levick 1991). Here, the arterioles have little basal tone and are regulated primarily by sympathetic vasoconstrictor fibres (Gorgas et al 1977). Cold causes vasocon-

striction of the arterial supply and the arterioles, diverting blood into the deep venous system. Not surprisingly, there are compensatory responses, and blocking of the local sympathetic response causes paradoxical vasodilatation, causing the familiar red nose seen on cold days. If the exposure to cold persists, vasoconstriction recurs. This is followed by vasoconstriction in the deeper vessels and imposes mounting stress on already cold limbs, the loss of oxygen and nutrient supply causing the death (necrosis) of cells and tissue, initially in the skin and later in the dermis and deeper tissue. Ice crystals form in the cells and extracellular fluid (frostbite), which hastens the start of gangrene. Similarly, the tissue loss evident in arterial ulcers results from local areas of tissue being deprived of blood supply.

Commonly, arterial ulcers occur at the extremities and are the consequence of severe atherosclerosis, restricting blood supply from the major vessels supplying the limb. Exceptions can be found in patients with Buerger's syndrome or scleroderma, where digital ulcers arise from inflammation of smaller supply vessels and nerves. In diabetes, the original damage may be a result of neuropathy (insensitivity of the foot to injury) but is perpetuated by inadequate blood supply to permit healing. Unusual causes of leg ulceration include rheumatoid arthritis, infection and cancer. Arterial ulcers may be located between toes, on toe tips, on the outer ankle or where there is trauma and/or friction from walking. The classic arterial ulcer found on the lateral aspect of the shin will be the focus of this chapter.

The characteristics of arterial ulceration include:

- Pale base colour when the leg is elevated, red base colour when the legs are dependent
- Surrounding skin is shiny, taut, thin, dry and hairless
- Ulcerated area will be deep
- Even wound margins
- Minimal exudate
- Variable amounts of oedema
- Skin temperature is cold to the touch
- Granulation tissue is rarely present
- Diminished/absent peripheral pulses
- Delayed capillary refill
- Necrotic tissue or gangrene may be present
- Infection.

Arterial ulcers on the lateral or frontal aspect of the shin are found in patients with limited mobility and poor blood supply to the leg (low ankle systolic pressures and low ankle/brachial pressure index). There are several reasons why the tissue loses viability:

- Loss of arterial pressure leading to malfunction of the dermal arteriovenous anastomoses
- Loss of exercise leading to absence of the hyperaemic response in capillaries
- Inadequate development of collateral circulation between anterior tibial and peroneal arteries in the vulnerable region of the leg
- Loss of oxygen and nutrient delivery leading to tissue stress.

Once the tissue loses viability there is a vicious cycle of infection and inflammation that is not resolved unless the arterial blood supply can be improved or restored.

ARTERIAL PRESSURE AND SKIN NUTRITION

Atherosclerosis arises from alterations in endothelial cells, platelet interactions and lipid and lipoprotein metabolism. Hyperglycaemia, hyperlipidaemia, hypertension, smoking and homocysteine damage the endothelium, leading to excess endothelial production of vasoconstrictors. Macrophages and platelets aggregate in areas of damaged endothelial, releasing cytokines and growth factors, which initiate an inflammatory reaction. Low-density lipoprotein cholesterol is incorporated into the vessel wall, directly or in the form of lipid-laden foam cells, resulting in the formation of fatty streaks. Vascular smooth muscle cells migrate from the media into the intima, proliferate and form an organized atherosclerotic plaque.

Atherosclerosis in iliac, femoral or below-knee arteries occludes the lumen, resulting in loss of arterial pressure in the tibial and peroneal arteries. This results in the systolic blood pressure, as measured at the ankle, being significantly lower than the brachial artery pressure: the drop in pressure can be measured and is reported as ankle/brachial pressure index. The presence of arterial ulcers and tissue loss is categorized as critical limb ischaemia and this is likely to occur when the ankle pressure is reduced to 40 mm Hg or below (Anonymous 2000). The ulcers often are associated with pain.

The degree of atherosclerosis and occlusion (or stenosis) is not necessarily uniform. Digital subtraction angiography may show generalized 'raggedy' disease or discrete areas of severe stenosis. The latter are more likely to be successfully treated by angioplasty or bypass surgery. The risk factors for coronary artery atherosclerosis are well established. They include hypercholesterolaemia, hypertension and smoking. In contrast, the key risk factor for peripheral artery atherosclerosis is smoking, with hypertension and hyperlipidaemia playing secondary roles.

As pressure in the lower leg is reduced, the terminal branches of the tibial and peroneal arteries suffer the most extreme loss of pressure and flow into the dermal vasculature trickles to a halt. As a result, skin in the shin area becomes atrophic. Thus skin becomes the first tissue where viability is compromised by the lack of sufficient blood supply. If this skin is damaged, the normal response to trauma of hyperaemia and increased delivery of white cells, immunoglobulins and defensive elements is absent, because the dermal blood supply is absent. The shin is an area with little underlying adipose tissue and is particularly vulnerable to trauma from chairs, tables and other household furniture. Subsequently, the underlying muscle becomes vulnerable to ulceration as ischaemia progresses.

The death of cells and the accumulation of metabolites that are normally removed into the venous circulation can stimulate nociceptors, causing pain in the leg. When hands are placed into very cold water (<10°C), there is an early painful sensation (before the paradoxical vasoconstriction described above; Levick 1991). Rest pain is a pathophysiological example of where loss of blood supply to the skin causes pain.

EXERCISE AND CAPILLARY SUPPLY TO MUSCLE

The process of atherosclerosis is a gradual, degenerative process that over time may allow a collateral circulation to be established, which can bypass the occluded vessel. This may reduce the problem of deprivation of oxygen and nutrients in the tissues distal to the occlusion. However, the collateral vessels do not stop the progression of peripheral arterial disease and indeed are very small and friable vessels.

The normal metabolism of the leg muscles is adapted to cope with the increased demand on these muscles imposed by physical exercise. The blood flow in the resting phasic muscles is about 5 ml per minute for each 100 g of tissue, but this increases tenfold or more during exercise. During exercise additional nutrients (principally oxygen and glucose) must be supplied to the muscle, and waste products (such as lactate) must be removed. This is achieved by muscle extracting an increasing proportion of oxygen and nutrients from the blood and opening up capillaries to increase the blood supply. This latter is the hyperaemic response.

As atherosclerosis of the peripheral arteries limits blood flow, the pressure becomes insufficient to open fully the capillary bed in exercising muscle. This results in local lactic acidosis and the build up of lactate and other metabolites, which stimulate the nociceptors to cause pain, the pain of intermittent claudication. This pain often results in a person's reluctance to exercise and the full capillary bed is not opened up regularly. At this stage, pushing exercise through the pain threshold may

be helpful. The prolonged local hypoxia stimulates muscle tissue to synthesize and secrete a growth factor, vascular endothelial growth factor (VEGF; Fig. 15.2; Hudlicka et al 2002, Lu et al 2003). This growth factor stimulates the growth of new capillaries from existing capillaries, a mechanism that can increase local capillary flow by up to twofold. With increased capillary density, exercise tolerance may increase.

Exercise therapy has been shown to double patients' walking distance before the pain of intermittent claudication develops (Hiatt et al 1990, Regensteiner 2001). The improvement in patients' walking distances is primarily due to the development of the collateral blood supply, reducing muscle pain and assisting in improving patients' wellbeing, allowing them to return to a more active lifestyle. Smoking cessation also improves vascular function and improves walking distance.

As atherosclerosis advances and pressures fall in the branches of the tibial and peroneal arteries supplying the lower leg muscles, the capillaries supplying the muscle become closed at rest. Muscle below the atrophic, and perhaps injured, skin now becomes starved of oxygen and nutrients. The muscle cells become necrotic and release chemicals that will fuel and perpetuate the formation of an ulcer.

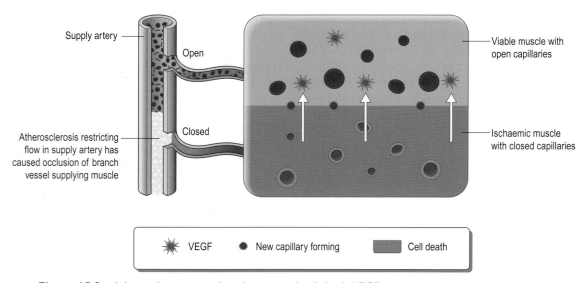

Figure 15.2   Atherosclerosis, muscle ischaemia and cell death. VEGF, vascular endothelial growth factor

INCREASING BLOOD SUPPLY IN THE LEG: PHYSIOLOGICAL BYPASS MECHANISMS

There are two pathophysiological mechanisms that can increase blood flow in regions of ischaemia: angiogenesis and arteriogenesis. Angiogenesis is the formation of new capillary networks in ischaemic muscle through endothelial sprouting. Although angiogenesis may alleviate some of the symptoms of critical limb ischaemia, it is not capable of rectifying the underlying process of limitation of arterial supply to the lower limb. The provision of new arteries is known as arteriogenesis and occurs by the conversion of an existing arteriole to an artery (Schaper & Scholz 2003).

Angiogenesis is dominated by the activity of a single growth factor, VEGF. Hypoxia or ischaemia prevents the destruction of a transcription factor (hypoxia-inducible factor, HIF), which stimulates increased production of both VEGF and its receptors on endothelial cells (Lu et al 2003). Under the influence of VEGF, the proliferation and sprouting of endothelial cells occurs from existing capillaries. Subsequently, smooth muscle cells or pericytes are recruited from adjacent tissues to support the new capillary. Inflammation of the damaged tissue will support angiogenesis. Nevertheless, the total increase in blood flow as a result of angiogenesis is modest, up to twofold (Schaper & Scholz 2003). Angiogenesis cannot replace a conducting artery, since too many capillaries would be required to generate the same lumen and flow delivery as a conducting artery.

Arteriogenesis is the moulding of a pre-existing arteriole into a collateral artery. Collateral arteries and an arteriolar network is a characteristic of the femoral arterial system in the upper leg, a site remote from the common signs and symptoms of lower limb ischaemia but a site where stenoses and occlusions are a common cause of lower limb ischaemia. The stimuli that promote arteriogenesis include shear stress. The increased fluid shear stress is sensed by the arteriolar endothelium, with pleiotropic responses including the increased expression of leukocyte adhesion molecules and cytokines such as monocyte chemoattractant protein (MCP)-1 (Schaper & Scholz 2003). Together the responses favour the recruitment of monocytes and T lymphocytes, both from the lumen and from the perivascular tissues. The paradigm of arteriogenesis is that the media of the arteriole is surrounded on both sides (lumen and adventitia) by inflammatory cells, which play a critical role in vessel remodelling (Schaper & Scholz 2003). Therefore, it is not surprising that many different growth factors and cytokines have important roles in arteriogenesis. The growth factors include fibroblast growth factor (FGF), colony stimulating factor (GM-CSF) and transforming growth factor (TGF-β). Although the process is more complex than angiogenesis, arteriogenesis is capable of increasing blood flow by an order of magnitude and hence is capable of compensating for an occluded femoral artery. There is no evidence that arteriogenesis occurs below the anastomotic circulation in the popliteal fossa, at the back of the knee. Therefore, it is possible that patients with severe stenosing lesions in the tibial and peroneal arteries are more vulnerable to the formation of arterial ulcers than patients with occlusions in the femoropopliteal or more proximal arteries. The differences between angiogenesis and arteriogenesis are summarized in Table 15.2.

In critical limb ischaemia, evidenced by arterial ulceration, arteriogenesis has not taken place. Instead the release of specific cytokines (including tumour necrosis factor (TNF-α) from the ischaemic tissue (Meldrum 1998) stimulates a spiral of further tissue destruction and interference with the normal healing process (Fig. 15.3).

LOSS OF OXYGEN AND NUTRIENTS: THE BIOCHEMISTRY OF MUSCLE CELL NECROSIS

Oxygen is required for muscle cells to synthesis the adenosine triphosphate (ATP) that is needed to support the contraction of the striated myosin rich filaments. Glucose is the normal fuel that, in the presence of oxygen, is broken down into water and carbon dioxide to generate ATP. ATP is synthesized in the mitochondria of cells and this is where the earliest signs of oxygen deprivation can be detected. The mitochondria, usually elongated organelles, round up as their membranes lose their ability to regulate ion and metabolite flux. Ischaemia has compromised the viability of the muscle cells and

Table 15.2 Arteriogenesis versus angiogenesis

	Arteriogenesis	**Angiogenesis**
Process	Conversion arteriole to artery	New capillary networks
Location	Upper leg	Lower leg
Stimuli	Shear stress inflammation	Hypoxia, ischaemia
Biological mechanism	Inflammation-dependent; multiple growth factors; vessel remodelling	VEGF-dependent; endothelial sprouting to new vessels
Compensation for occluded artery	Yes; 10–20 fold increase in blood flow	No; maximum twofold increase in blood flow

VEGF, vascular endothelial growth factor

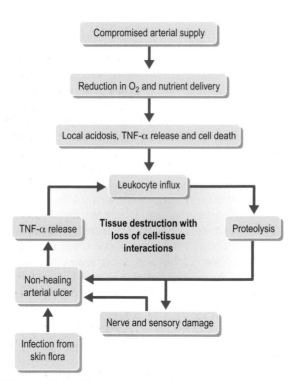

Figure 15.3 The vicious cycle that prevents healing in arterial ulcers

skeletal muscle following a similar pattern (Meldrum 1998). Proinflammatory cytokines increase their own production, stimulate the synthesis of other small inflammatory mediators such as platelet activating factor or interleukin-1β and stimulate the cellular mediators of the inflammatory response. Leukocytes are recruited into the area of tissue damage. The activated monocytes that are recruited can increase the rate of muscle apoptosis and produce TNF-α, to increase the local concentration (Meldrum 1998). Other tissue cells (fibroblasts, pericytes, etc.) die by necrosis, releasing inflammatory factors that exacerbate the local inflammatory response. The neutrophils that are recruited secrete elastase and other proteases in an attempt to clean up the area of tissue damage. In the absence of an adequate supply of oxygen and nutrients, there is no subsequent healing response, with granulation and epithelialization of the ischaemic wound. Moreover, the damaging reduction product of oxygen, hydrogen peroxide, is produced. The continued secretion of proteases by the neutrophils disrupts the proper interactions between tissue cells and their matrix, both in the developing ulcer and in the surrounding tissue. Disruption of cell-matrix interactions in the surrounding tissues leads to a third form of cell death, anoikis (Michel 2003). Colonization of the necrotic ulcer by skin bacteria perpetuates a low-grade inflammatory response at the surface of the wound.

So in an arterial ulcer cells are dying by all possible mechanisms, apoptosis, necrosis and anoikis (Table 15.3). In the absence of an adequate oxygen supply, granulation and healing of the ulcer cannot occur. Local production of TNF-α, aggravated by

alters gene expression within the cell (Temsah et al 2001, Hoppeler et al 2003). A pathway using the increased expression of caspases (proteases) leads to cell death by apoptosis, cell death without an inflammatory response. Ischaemia provokes the synthesis of TNF-α, a proinflammatory cytokine, from cardiac muscle, with synthesis of TNFα from

Table 15.3 Mechanisms of cell loss in arterial ulcers

	Stimulus	Cell changes	Effect on local tissue
Necrosis	TNF-α Inflammation	Release of cell contents including chemical toxins and messengers	Protease release Continued cell loss Inflammation with protease and TNFα release, promoting further cell death by necrosis, apoptosis and anoikis
Apoptosis	TNF-α	Shrinkage without release of cell contents	Individual cell loss Minimal external effects
Anoikis	Proteolysis, causing loss of cell matrix interactions	Cell (particularly endothelial cell) changes to round shape and detaches from matrix	Individual cell loss Minimal external effects

TNF, tumour necrosis factor

bacterial colonization, perpetuates a destructive inflammatory response. Additionally, the dead tissue at the centre of the ulcer can be slow to break down since, in the absence of blood flow, white cells cannot enter the tissue to hasten its removal. This can be observed in many arterial ulcers, where the base of the wound cannot be seen for necrotic tissue. The necrotic tissue is generally removed by surgical debridement so that the wound bed can be assessed and healing can be attempted.

DIABETES

While the standard arterial ulcer forms on the lateral aspect of the shin, in diabetes the ulcers are more commonly found between toes, on toetips, on the outer ankle or where there is trauma and/or friction from walking. The two main causes of ulcer in patients with diabetes are neuropathy and ischaemia. Neuropathic ulcers develop as a result of the loss of sensation in the feet, which means that the patient does not respond to mechanical trauma (poorly fitting shoes, penetration of a sharp object or heat from fires, radiators or hot water). In the diabetic ulcer both neuropathy and ischaemia are generally observed. Both of these features predispose to infection and tissue necrosis.

Type 2 diabetes is a potent risk factor for the development of arterial disease. The development of arterial disease in diabetic patients is the same process as in a non-diabetic, except that the disease occurs more frequently, is more diffuse and severe

and is more lethal in patients with type 2 diabetes. Diabetic patients tend to have more tibial disease than non-diabetic patients, the lesions are multiple and diffuse and they are less straightforward to bypass or dilate by angioplasty. Consequently, more amputations are performed on diabetic patients than non-diabetic patients, with the USA reporting a 15 times higher risk of lower extremity amputation for patients with diabetes than individuals without diabetes (Fylling & Knighton 1989).

Arterial disease is more severe and diffuse in type 2 diabetics than non-diabetics because of the development of the diabetic state within these patients (Wills 2001). Impaired glucose tolerance refers to a condition in which the blood sugar levels are higher than normal but not high enough to be classified as diabetes. Impaired glucose tolerance is a major risk factor for type 2 diabetes and would explain the severity of arterial disease in this patient group.

Patients presenting with an arterial ulcer or intermittent claudication should be screened for diabetes, as 20% of patients with intermittent claudication will be diabetic. However up to 50% of cases will be undiagnosed at the time of presentation (Wills 2001). In order for every patient presenting with peripheral vascular disease to receive the best medical therapy a random glucose test should be performed to establish whether the patient is diabetic. Thus measures to assist them in achieving normal glucose levels can be discussed with the patient.

CLINICAL SUMMARY

Unless the arterial oxygen supply can be improved, an arterial ulcer will not heal. Bypass or angioplasty of occluded or stenotic segments of the proximal arteries can sometimes support a dramatic improvement in blood flow, ankle pressures, oxygen and nutrient delivery, so that ulcer healing can occur. If such treatments are not possible, arterial ulcers may herald future amputation.

References

Anonymous 2000 Management of peripheral arterial disease (PAD). Transatlantic Intersociety Consensus (TASC). Section D: chronic critical limb ischaemia. European Journal of Vascular and Endovascular Surgery 19(Suppl A): 144–243

Burns P, Gough S, Bradbury A W 2003 Management of peripheral arterial disease in primary care. British Medical Journal 326: 584–587

Fylling C P, Knighton M D 1989 Amputation in the diabetic population: Incidence, causes, cost, treatment and prevention. Journal of Enterostomal Therapy 16: 247–245

Gorgas K, Bock P, Tischendorf F, Curri S B 1977 The fine structure of human digital arterio-venous anastomoses (Hoyer-Grosser's organs). Anatomy and embryology 150: 269–289

Hiatt W R, Regensteiner J G, Hargarten M E et al 1990 Benefit of exercise conditioning for patients with peripheral arterial disease. Circulation 81: 602–609

Hoppeler H, Vogt M, Weibel E R, Fluck M I 2003 Response of skeletal muscle mitochondria to hypoxia. Experimental Physiology 88: 109–119

Hudlicka O, Milkiewicz M, Cotter M A, Brown M D 2002 Hypoxia and expression of VEGF-A protein in relation to capillary growth in electrically stimulated rat and rabbit skeletal muscles. Experimental Physiology 87: 373–381

Levick J R 1991 An introduction to cardiovascular physiology. Butterworths, London

Lu E, Wagner W R, Schellenberger U et al 2003 Targeted in vivo labeling of receptors for vascular endothelium growth factor: approach to identification of ischaemic tissue. Circulation 108: 97–103

Meldrum D R 1998 Tumour necrosis factor in the heart. American Journal of Physiology 274: 577–595

Michel J B 2003 Anoikis in the cardiovascular system: known and unknown extracellular mediators. Arteriosclerosis, Thrombosis, and Vascular Biology 23: 2146–2154

Regensteiner G 2001 Review: exercise programmes increase walking times in patients with intermittent claudication. Evidence-Based Nursing 4: 21

Schaper W, Scholz D 2003 Factors regulating arteriogenesis. Arteriosclerosis, Thrombosis, and Vascular Biology 23: 1143–1151

Temsah R M, Kauabata K, Chapman D, Dhalla N S 2001 Modulation of cardiac sarcoplasmic reticulum gene expression by lack of oxygen and glucose. FASEB Journal 15: 2515–2517

Wills C 2001 Vascular risk in diabetes: defusing the time bomb. Modern Diabetes Management 2: 6–9

Ischaemic ulceration: investigation of arterial disease

Peter Vowden, Kathryn Vowden

INTRODUCTION

Ischaemia comes from the Greek *ischein haima*, 'to suppress blood', and can be defined as a 'localized deficiency of arterial blood which may be due to occlusion of the arteries due to atherosclerosis or local occlusion of "tissues" due to pressure and is often acutely painful' (Collins et al 2002). It has been stated that 'ischaemia is arguably the most significant factor contributing to human wound chronicity associated with diabetes, peripheral arterial disease, venous stasis and pressure sores, with a stronger impact on aged individuals than the young' (Mogford & Mustoe 2001).

The presence of ischaemia is not always obvious. Its occurrence can be directly related to tissue perfusion, which itself varies according to a number of pathophysiological factors, including:

- Decrease in perfusion pressure
  - ◆ 'Pump' failure
  - ◆ Hypovolaemia
- Increased resistance
  - ◆ 'Atherosclerosis'
  - ◆ Vasospasm
  - ◆ Hyperviscosity
  - ◆ External compression of vessels and the microcirculation
  - ◆ Oedema – 'tissue pressure'
  - ◆ Extrinsic pressure – 'interface pressure'.

Perfusion, ischaemia and hypoxia

Reduced perfusion does not, however, always equate to tissue or wound ischaemia, as ischaemia is functional and is permanent only when physiological reserves are exhausted. If ischaemia is prolonged and severe enough, cell death will occur and gangrene or ischaemic ulceration follows. Periods of ischaemia are tolerated differently by individual tissue types, as cellular oxygen requirements and hypoxic tolerance vary markedly between individual cells. The most common impact of ischaemia is, however, not cell death but a slowing of cell activity and division, leading to a reduction in the rate of, or a pause in, the healing process (Burns et al 2003). This is associated with:

- Parenchymal deprivation of gaseous exchange and metabolites
- Increasing vascular permeability
- Increasing intravascular white cell marginalization and trapping
- Increasing release of free radicals and proteolytic enzymes
- Stimulation of a compensatory response in capillaries.

Experimental research has established a direct relationship between oxygen tension and lactate levels and collagen deposition by fibroblasts (Herrick et al 1996, Steinbrech et al 1999, Trabold et al 2003). In animal models hypoxia results in a decrease in granulation tissue formation and collagen synthesis (Mustoe et al 1994). Hypovolaemia has also been linked to impaired wound healing (Arkilic et al 2003), as has hypothermia (Kurz et al 1996) both of which reduce skin perfusion, produce relative ischaemia and therefore increase the risk of ulceration and delayed healing.

As both clinical and laboratory data demonstrate that ischaemia is clearly an important cause of both ulcer formation and delayed ulcer healing, assessment of wound and periwound perfusion and, where necessary, the restoration of an adequate blood supply by either interventional radiology, surgical bypass or medical intervention is an essential part of all wound management strategies. For patients with extensive tissue loss, ulceration or gangrene of the foot or lower limb, restoration of pulsatile blood flow is usually required for healing. Aggressive arterial reconstruction, including bypass to foot vessels, allows extensive debridement of soft tissue and bone without amputation and may aid plastic reconstruction of the foot. Such complex management strategies are only possible when arterial disease is correctly diagnosed and assessed. Ischaemia clearly acts as the cause of arterial ulceration and gangrene but it also plays a part in the delayed healing of venous and diabetic foot ulceration and, in the case of 'mixed' venous ulcers, reduces treatment options by restricting the use of compression bandaging.

CLINICAL EVALUATION OF THE ARTERIAL SYSTEM OF THE LOWER LIMB

To evaluate lower limb perfusion and understand the impact of peripheral arterial disease on lower limb circulation it is necessary first to look at the anatomy of the arterial system and the pathophysiological processes that result in occlusive arterial disease.

Arterial anatomy

The basic anatomy is set out in Figure 16.1. The profunda femoris supplies the muscles of the hip and thigh while the superficial femoral artery, which becomes the popliteal artery at the level of the adductor hiatus, is the 'artery of conduction', carrying blood through the thigh to the knee and calf. In the calf the below-knee popliteal artery divides into the three crural vessels, the anterior and posterior tibial arteries and the peroneal artery, each of which supplies a muscle compartment within the calf and the associated structures, including the overlying skin. The anterior and posterior tibial arteries cross the ankle joint (Figure

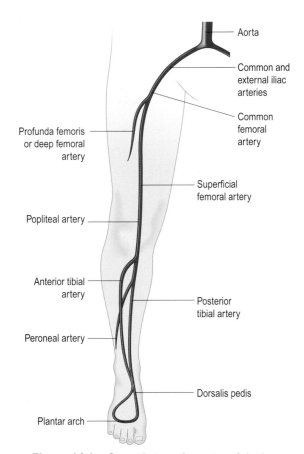

Figure 16.1   General view of arteries of the leg

16.2) while the peroneal artery, the deeper of the three calf vessels, terminates above the ankle, giving off two main terminal branches, the anterior and posterior perforating arteries. These feed, along with the terminal branches of the anterior and posterior tibial arteries, into the plantar arch, which supplies the foot, and this in turn gives rise to the digital vessels.

All other than the smallest blood vessels have walls consisting of three layers:

- The *tunica intima*, formed from the endothelium, a subendothelial supportive layer and an internal elastic membrane
- The *tunica media*, consisting mainly of an innervated smooth muscle and a thin external elastic lamina
- An outer *tunica externa or adventitia*, which in arteries consists mainly of collagen fibres.

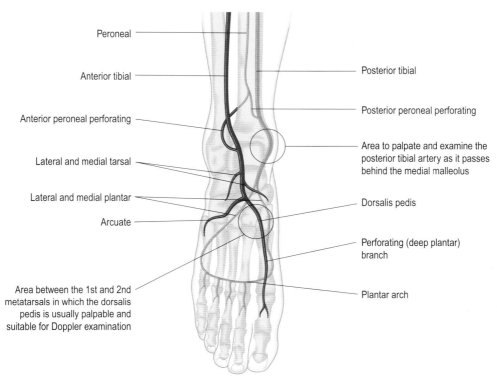

Peroneal

Anterior tibial

Anterior peroneal perforating

Lateral and medial tarsal

Lateral and medial plantar

Arcuate

Area between the 1st and 2nd metatarsals in which the dorsalis pedis is usually palpable and suitable for Doppler examination

Posterior tibial

Posterior peroneal perforating

Area to palpate and examine the posterior tibial artery as it passes behind the medial malleolus

Dorsalis pedis

Perforating (deep plantar) branch

Plantar arch

Figure 16.2 Relationship of the crural vessels at the ankle

As with all arteries, those in the lower limb are of four types:

- *Conducting (elastic) arteries*, which function mainly as low-resistance pathways, their high elastin content being responsible for sustaining forward flow in diastole
- *Distributing or muscular arteries*, which distribute blood to specific organs or muscle groups and which have, proportionally the thickest medial layer
- *Resistance arteries or arterioles*, which direct and control flow to the capillary bed by changing resistance
- *Metarterioles* (Fig. 16.3), which connect the arterial tree to the capillaries, through which flow is regulated by precapillary sphincters.

Arterial pathology as it relates to ischaemic ulceration

Vascular disease which can affect any or all of these vessel types or can involve the capillary bed or venous outflow system, may result in a deranged perfusion system and ultimately may lead to ischaemia. Investigation can be targeted to assess each part of the arterial system and can give both anatomical and functional data. Investigations are designed to answer one or both of two fundamental questions:

- What is the severity of the ischaemia?
- Where within the arterial system is the disease located?

The fundamental process in the pathogenesis of critical limb ischaemia and arterial ulceration is atherosclerosis. The process, which is initiated by the deposition of fat within the arterial wall, gradually disrupts the intima and results in progressive narrowing of the vessel lumen (Fig. 16.4), finally resulting in thrombosis and occlusion of the vessel. It mainly involves the proximal conducting arteries and reduces blood flow, perfusion pressure and pulsatility, progressively impacting on microcirculatory function. Platelets and leukocytes become activated as they pass over ulcerated atherosclerotic plaques, clot may form on the plaque and embolization can occur, further damaging the

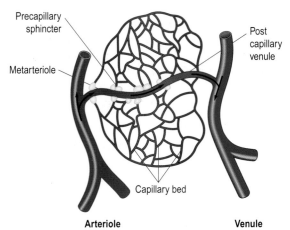

Precapillary sphincter
Post capillary venule
Metarteriole
Capillary bed
Arteriole
Venule

Figure 16.3 Arterial and venous systems linking via the capillary bed

distal circulation. Atherosclerotic plaques may become progressively calcified and the arteries rigid and non-compliant as a result of long-standing disease.

The microcirculation comprises of the arterioles, capillaries and venules. In the skin these vessels comprise thermoregulatory and nutritional capillaries, the latter carrying only 15% of total flow (Dormandy & Stock 1990). The number of capillaries and the function and morphology of the capillary bed can be affected by proximal atherosclerotic disease, venous outflow resistance, red cell morphology and deformability, blood viscosity, autoimmune disorders, such as scleroderma, which affect the capillary basement membrane, and the presence of ischaemia itself. Changes in capillary

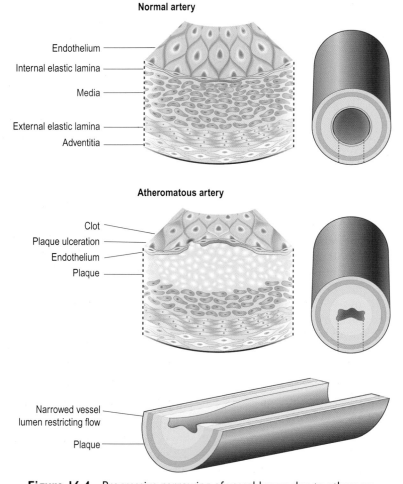

Normal artery

Endothelium
Internal elastic lamina
Media
External elastic lamina
Adventitia

Atheromatous artery

Clot
Plaque ulceration
Endothelium
Plaque

Narrowed vessel lumen restricting flow
Plaque

Figure 16.4 Progressive narrowing of vessel lumen due to atheroma

function have been observed by capillaroscopy, transcutaneous Po_2 ($tcPo_2$) measurement and laser Doppler flux measurement (Netten et al 1996, Junger et al 2000) and have been found to be similar in both ischaemic and venous ulceration (Gschwandtner et al 2001).

Evaluation of symptoms and signs

The classic symptoms of peripheral arterial disease are those of:

- *Claudication*, a pain, usually felt in the calf, brought on by exercise and relieved by rest
- *Rest pain*, severe ischaemic pain, classically felt with the limb elevated, which wakes a patient from sleep and is only relieved by lowering the limb to the floor (Marston 1992).

The European Consensus Document on Critical Limb Ischaemia (Anonymous 1992) definition of critical limb ischaemia is set out in Box 16.1 along with the Fontaine classification of peripheral arterial disease.

Claudication is frequently under reported and the true prevalence of peripheral vascular disease often goes unrecognized in primary care (Khunti 2003). Reliance on symptoms alone may therefore result in an underestimate of the contribution of peripheral arterial disease and ischaemia to ulceration and the non-healing of a chronic wound.

Arterial ulcers are frequently described as being on the foot or lateral aspect of the leg, deep, with exposure of muscle or tendon, painful and rapidly deteriorating, while venous ulcers are usually found in the medial gaiter area and are described as usually shallow, oval in shape with an irregular flat margin and associated with skin changes typical of venous disease (Morison & Moffatt 1994). These observations should not be taken as confirming or refuting the diagnosis of arterial ulceration. Many arterial and mixed ulcers occur in the gaiter area, particularly over the malleoli, and can easily be misdiagnosed if reliance is placed on symptoms and signs alone. Signs suggestive of but not specifically related to ischaemia include:

- Coldness of the limb or foot
- Pallor on elevation of the limb and a capillary return of longer than 3 seconds after blanching of the skin by pressure

---

Box 16.1 *The European Consensus Document definition of critical limb ischaemia (1992) and, for comparison, the Fontaine classification*

European Consensus Statement

Recommendation 2A

Critical limb ischaemia is defined by the following two criteria:

- Persistently recurring rest pain requiring regular analgesia for >2 weeks and/or
- Ulceration of the foot or toes plus
- Ankle systolic pressure <50 mmHg.

Calcification of the arteries in diabetes and other disease makes measurement of the ankle pressure unreliable – absent palpable pulses are sufficient for definition of critical limb ischaemia in diabetics and patients with calcified arteries.

Recommendation 2B

A more precise definition is required for published reports and for the design and reporting of clinical trials. In addition to the above definition, further evidence of ischaemia has to be obtained by angiography and/or one of the following tests:

- Toe systolic blood pressure <30 mmHg
- Transcutaneous oxygen pressure of the ischaemic area <10 mmHg and does not increase with the inhalation of oxygen
- Absence of arterial pulsation in the big toe (measured with strain gauge or photoplethysmography after vasodilatation)
- Marked structural or functional changes of the skin capillaries in the affected area.

Fontaine's classification of peripheral arterial occlusive disease

Stage 1	Asymptomatic
Stage 2	Intermittent claudication
Stage 3	Rest pain
Stage 4	Development of ulceration and/or gangrene.

- Dependent rubor (sunset foot)
- Atrophic, shiny skin
- Trophic changes in the nails
- Loss of hair over the foot or lower limb
- Ischaemic tissue, including dry or wet gangrene
- Abnormal or absent pedal pulses.

Careful palpation of pedal pulses, although of value as part of the initial assessment of a patient presenting with lower limb ulceration, is, in general, an unreliable method of assessing arterial disease and should not be relied upon as the sole method of assessment, particularly if compression is to be applied to the limb (Moffatt et al 1994, Moffatt and O'Hare 1995). When used, the presence or absence, strength and nature of the pulse should be recorded, along with information on the arterial wall such as rigidity or aneurysmal dilatation.

IMAGING AND PHYSIOLOGICAL MEASUREMENT TECHNIQUES

It is important to select the appropriate investigation(s) to provide the correct type and level of information required in each clinical situation, particularly as some investigations are invasive and potentially hazardous. Investigations of the peripheral arterial circulation can provide both anatomical and functional information. Visual information, such as that provided by arteriography, shows where the arterial disease is but may give little information on its functional significance. Other investigations, such as pressure measurements like the ankle systolic blood pressure and the ratio derived from it, the ankle brachial pressure index (ABPI), indicate that arterial disease is present but do not necessarily identify its location. Some investigations, such as duplex colour flow ultrasonography, have the advantage of being non-invasive and safe and provide both anatomical and functional information. This makes this form of investigation ideal for initial screening.

Functional investigations

Functional investigations are designed to give an indication of the severity of the peripheral vascular disease. The modality chosen to provide the information is often dependent on local availability of equipment and technical skill and individual clinical preference.

The simplest and perhaps the most commonly performed functional assessment of the peripheral circulation is a measurement of blood pressure. While this is easy to perform in the upper arm with a sphygmomanometer, stethoscope and blood pressure cuff, and forms a routine part of patient monitoring (Beevers et al 2001), it is not, however, easy to use this equipment to perform pressure measurements in the lower limb, although the technique has been used to measure ankle blood pressure (Hocken 1967). The method has therefore been adapted to utilize other equipment, such as the hand-held Doppler or a pulse oximeter to detect flow (Yao et al 1969, Whiteley et al 1998).

An alternative to non-invasive pressure measurement is to use direct arterial puncture. This technique is frequently used when monitoring patients during anaesthesia and can be combined with arteriography, when it allows quantification of the effect of an arterial stenosis on both the absolute intra-arterial pressure and the arterial pulse waveform (Macpherson et al 1984, Baker et al 1987). The effectiveness of this method of assessment can be enhanced by combining the measurements with the administration of a vasodilator (Vowden 1997). Hamilton et al (1936, cited in Hocken 1967) established the link between invasive and non-invasive blood pressure measurement. Using non-invasive and invasive techniques it was noted that arm systolic pressure usually differed from ankle systolic pressure (Winsor 1950), the latter being on average 20 mmHg higher (Hocken 1967).

Doppler

Doppler ultrasound relies on the principle that the frequency of a sound reflected by a moving object (in this case red blood cells) is shifted in proportion to its velocity. This non-invasive method for measuring peripheral blood flow in humans was first described in 1959 (Satomura 1959, cited in Yao 1970) and the technique was shown to be a reliable method of measuring ankle systolic pressure (Yao et al 1969).

A simple Doppler probe consists of a transmitting crystal emitting ultrasound and a receiving

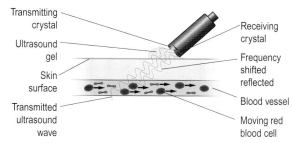

Figure 16.5 Continuous wave handheld Doppler. Ultrasound waves reflected from a moving object (red blood cells) undergo a frequency shift. This is dependent upon the speed of movement of the red cells and the angle of the probe (which should be 45°)

crystal that picks up both reflected ultrasound at the emitting frequency and frequency-shifted ultrasound (Fig. 16.5). Most hand-held Dopplers work in the frequency range 1–10 MHz. At this frequency the shift produced is in the audible range, giving a characteristic 'whooshing' sound (Beard & Scott 1991). Doppler probes in the range 6–10 MHz are used to assess vessels close to the skin, such as those at the ankle, for which an 8 MHz probe is usually used, while probes in the range 1–5 MHz are used to assess deeper vessels (Williams et al 1993). A 5 or 6 MHz probe may be needed to gain an adequate signal from a large or lymphoedematous leg. As the Doppler probe will register red cell movement in the underlying vessel, it is possible to use the system to detect systolic blood pressure by incorporating a sphygmomanometer and blood pressure cuff into the system.

Ankle brachial pressure index

Absolute ankle systolic pressure can be a useful indicator of the likelihood of healing of ischaemic ulceration (Takolander & Rauwerda 1995); absolute pressure is, however, subject to day-to-day variation. It is therefore often more useful to use a ratio, the ABPI, which is defined as the ratio of the highest brachial systolic pressure, taken as an estimate of the true systolic pressure, and the highest pressure obtained from one of the three ankle vessels (the anterior tibial, posterior tibial or peroneal). A separate ratio is defined for each leg.

The technique for Doppler ABPI assessment is well described (Vowden et al 1996, Vowden &

Vowden 2001) and is summarized in Box 16.2. A normal ABPI is usually taken as being 0.92 or more (Sumner 1989). An ABPI of less than this is usually taken to indicate the presence of peripheral arterial disease, but this may not be symptomatic. Those with ABPI values of 0.5 or less are usually symptomatic and may go on to develop, or may already have developed, rest pain, ulceration or gangrene (Beard & Scott 1991). In general, an ABPI of less than 0.8, taken together with symptoms of peripheral arterial disease such as claudication, is an indication for referral to a vascular surgeon for further assessment (Cornwall 1991, Williams et al 1993). An ABPI of less than 0.8 is also taken as the cut-off point for the safe use of high-compression bandages (Royal College of Nursing 1998). The value of an ABPI is that it can be repeated frequently and allows the progress of individual patients to be followed over time. A fall of more than 0.15 in the ABPI is considered significant and usually suggests worsening arterial disease (Sumner 1989). Falls of this magnitude indicate the need for caution if using compression therapy, even if the ABPI is still above 0.8.

Although the calculation of the ABPI uses only the highest systolic pressure recorded, it is important to remember that the data from the other vessels may be useful in gauging the severity of peripheral arterial disease. A pressure difference of more than 15 mmHg between individual vessels at the ankle indicates significant disease in the vessel with the lower pressure at some point between its origin and the point of measurement (Sumner 1989).

Faint signals are easily missed, particularly if the pressure of the probe on the skin is too high. Signals may be easier to identify with the feet dependent (Beard & Scott 1991), but pressures recorded in this position should not be used to calculate an ABPI. Similarly, in patients with extensive ulceration at the ankle, although it may seem more appropriate to position the blood pressure cuff higher on the leg, this should be avoided, as the pressures recorded no longer reflect the ankle pressure and should therefore not be used to calculate the ABPI (Vowden & Vowden 2001). When ever possible, the ulcerated area should be protected (we find it useful to use cling film for this) and readings should be taken with the cuff at malleolar level (Fig. 16.6).

Box 16.2 *Measurement of systolic pressure with the hand-held Doppler and calculation of the ankle brachial pressure index*

With the subject lying flat rested and comfortable with no pressure on the proximal vessels.

1. **Measure the brachial blood pressure**
   - Place an appropriately sized cuff around the upper arm and locate the brachial pulse, applying ultrasound contact gel over the pulse
   - Using the gel for contact angle the Doppler probe at 45° and move the probe to obtain the best signal
   - Inflate the cuff until the signal is abolished then deflate the cuff slowly and record the pressure at which the signal returns, being careful not to move the probe from the line of the artery while doing this
   - Repeat the procedure for the other arm
   - Use the highest of the two arm systolic pressures in the calculation of the ABPI

2. **Measure the ankle systolic pressure**
   - Place an appropriately sized cuff around the ankle immediately above the malleoli, having first protected any ulcer that may be present
   - Examine the foot, locating the dorsalis pedis(DP) or anterior tibial (AT) pulse and apply contact gel
   - Continue as for the brachial pressure, recording this pressure in the same way
   - Repeat this for the posterior tibial (PT) and peroneal arteries, using the highest reading obtained to calculate the ABPI for that leg using the formula below
   - Repeat for the other leg

$$\text{For each leg ABPI} = \frac{\text{Highest ankle pressure (AT/PT/DP/peroneal) for that leg}}{\text{Highest of the brachial systolic pressures for each arm}}$$

Problems and errors may arise if:

- The cuff is repeatedly inflated or inflated for long periods: this can cause the ankle pressure to fall
- The cuff is not placed at the ankle: ankle systolic pressure is not measured and pressure recorded is usually higher than ankle pressure
- The pulse is irregular or the cuff is deflated too rapidly: the true systolic pressure may be missed
- The vessels are calcified (diabetics), the legs are large, fatty or oedematous, the cuff size is too small, or the legs are dependent: an inappropriately high reading will be obtained.

A defined range for normal and abnormal ABPI has been established and the deficiencies of the technique have been noted (Vowden & Vowden, 2001)

Carter (1969) emphasizes that meticulous attention to detail is necessary to obtain valid measurements and a lack of awareness of the limitations of the ABPI leads to conflicting results and misinterpretation of data. The use of the hand-held Doppler to measure systolic blood pressure and calculation of the ABPI is safe and reliable and has been accepted as a routine part of clinical practice. Providing its limitations are remembered it is an effective method to both diagnose and monitor arterial disease.

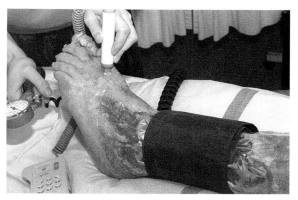

Figure 16.6 Measuring systolic pressure in the dorsalis pedis with the cuff overlying a large bimalleolar ulcer

Segmental and toe pressures

The same principles that apply to the derivation of ankle systolic blood pressure may be applied elsewhere in the limb. By so doing, a pressure profile can be derived down the limb and this can be used to identify areas of stenosis. When carrying out segmental pressures the thigh pressure is typically 30–40 mmHg higher than the brachial pressure (Hirai & Shionoya 1978). A difference of more than 30 mmHg between sites on the same leg or more than 20 mmHg between the same sites on the two legs is taken as an indication of significant arterial disease (Sumner 1989).

Although more difficult to measure the same principles can be applied to the measurement of toe systolic pressure (Carter 1993, Sumner 1993; Fig. 16.7). This can be of great value in assessing the peripheral circulation in individuals with diabetes, in whom medial sclerosis and vessel calcification can compromise the measurement of ankle systolic pressure. Brooks et al (2001) have suggested that this investigation should be reserved for patients with overt evidence of vascular calcification, such as an ABPI of 1.3 or more. A toe pressure index (TBPI) can be calculated in a similar way to the ABPI. Commercially available equipment is available that automates the process of toe pressure measurement (Fig. 16.8). Absolute toe systolic pressure and the TBPI can be related directly to diabetic and non-diabetic foot ulcer healing (Carter 1993; Table 16.1), patients with rest pain generally having a toe pressure of less than 30 mmHg

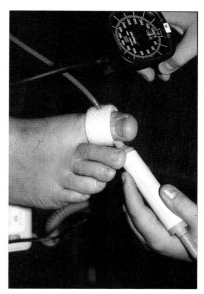

Figure 16.7 Measuring toe pressure with the hand-held Doppler: note the neonatal blood pressure cuff on the great toe

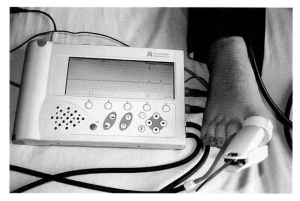

Figure 16.8 Automated measurement of toe pressures using the Assist (Courtesy of Huntleigh Diagnostics)

(Sumner 1989). Normally, toe pressure is lower than ankle and brachial pressures, a normal TBPI is more than 0.7 and a value of less than 0.65 would indicate arterial disease (Carter 1993, Baker & Rayman 1999).

The information obtained from simple Doppler systolic pressure measurements can be further enhanced by combining the test with limb elevation as in the Pole test (Smith et al 1994) and by including exercise or ischaemic stress (hyperaemic

Table 16.1   Relationship between ankle pressure, toe pressure and transcutaneous PO_2 and healing

	Absolute pressure (mmHg)	Diabetic patients (% healed)	Non-diabetics (% healed)
Ankle pressure	≤55	–	–
	55–90	45	85
	≥90	90	100
Toe pressure	≤30	45	70
	30–50	75	100
Transcutaneous PO_2	≥55	95	100
	<20	Healing unlikely	
	≥40	Healing likely	

testing) in the test protocol. The conventional method for exercise testing is to place the patient on a treadmill at a speed of 4 km/h and a gradient of 10% (Beard & Scott 1991). The test may take several forms, a standardized 1 minute walking test (Laing & Greenhalgh 1980, 1986) can be applied or the maximum walking distance can be recorded by continuing the exercise to the time that the patient was stopped by pain (Sumner 1989). It is also useful to record the recovery time (the time it takes for the ankle systolic pressure and ABPI to return to pre-exercise levels), as this also gives an indication of the severity of any arterial disease and the impact it will have on the patient's quality of life. Other medical conditions, such as angina and shortness of breath, place limits on the number of patients able to perform an acceptable exercise test. An alternative is to use single-leg ankle exercise testing (Beard & Scott 1991). The fall in ankle systolic pressure (and ABPI) with exercise can be used to reveal occult arterial disease (Laing & Greenhalgh 1983) or to assess the severity of symptomatic arterial disease.

Alternative methods of measuring perfusion pressure

Although the Doppler technique described above is the most commonly used method of assessing peripheral perfusion pressure, alternative methods of measuring systolic pressure exist. These include:

- Pulse oximetry (Samuelsson et al 1996, Bianchi et al 2000), in which changes in capillary oxygen levels with restoration of arterial flow on release of a blood pressure cuff are used to indicate systolic pressure
- Laser Doppler (Fagrell & Nilsson 1995), in which red cell movement is used
- Strain gauge, volumetric and impedance plethysmography, which detects circumference or volume changes within a limb or part of a limb with blood flow, or the change in electrical impedance of a limb with influx of blood, which is a good conductor
- Photoplethysmography, which detects changes in reflectivity of the skin as the volume of blood within it changes (Sumner 1989, 1993).

Of these methods only pulse oximetry has been suggested as a realistic alternative to Doppler ABPI (Bianchi et al 2000) and systolic pressure measurement in the general assessment and monitoring of patients with lower limb ulceration however the information obtained is a poor substitute for the information available from Doppler.

Doppler: spectral and waveform analysis and the pulsatility index

In most normal peripheral arteries the arterial pressure wave is triphasic; there is strong forward flow in systole, transient reverse flow in early diastole and weak forward flow in late diastole. This is modified progressively with increasing arterial disease and loss of elasticity, finally becoming a slow, prolonged, monophasic flow pattern with a slow systolic rise, reduced peak velocity, loss of early diastolic flow reversal and the progressive development of a more 'rounded', damped waveform.

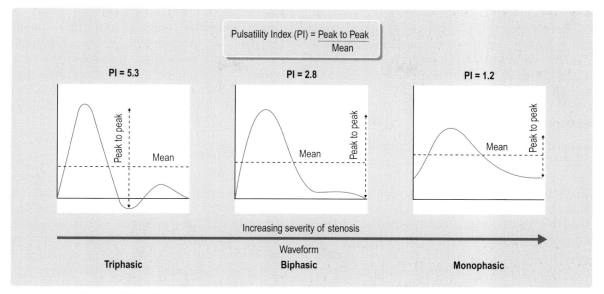

Figure 16.9   Relationship of degree of arterial stenosis to waveform and pulsatility index

These flow changes are reflected in the audible Doppler signal, the spectral output and the Doppler waveform. This output can be analysed and provides a method of quantifying the degree of stenosis and its impact on the distal circulation. One such method of analysis is used to derive the pulsatility index (PI; Fig. 16.9): the lower the PI the greater the degree of proximal stenosis (Burns 1993). Spectral analysis of the Doppler signal allows the mixture of frequency shifts related to the variable red-cell velocity to be displayed. A stenosis produces a high peak velocity within the narrowing and turbulence with a wide range of velocities (spectral broadening) beyond (Giddens & Kitney 1985). Such analysis is of great value when combined with the anatomical information provided by colour flow duplex ultrasonography and is used regularly when assessing carotid disease and monitoring vein grafts for stenosis (Strandness 1996). The combination of spectral analysis and colour flow duplex ultrasonography can be used as the primary diagnostic tests in assessing peripheral vascular disease (Pemberton et al 1996).

Plethysmography

In venous occlusion plethysmography, originally described by Brodie and Russell in 1905 (Cheatle et al 1991), has in the past been widely used to assess limb blood flow. A number of different methods can be applied. These include gravimetric, capacitance and strain gauge plethysmography. The technique can be used in the same way as the hand-held Doppler to measure systolic pressure and is a very effective method for measuring toe pressure (Sumner 1989).

An adaptation of this technique, photoplethysmography, can be used to measure skin blood flow (Fagrell & Nilsson 1995) and it has been suggested as an alternative to the hand-held Doppler in measuring ABPI (Whiteley et al 1998). Both this and laser Doppler can be used to examine skin perfusion in the areas around skin ulcers (Guillot et al 1988). They are also useful methods of assessing perfusion when planning skin flaps for amputation or evaluating flaps following vascular and plastic surgery.

Laser Doppler

The major drawback of this technique is that it requires a good optical path between the probe and the sample area. Having said that, the accuracy and resolution in optimal conditions are far greater than in Doppler ultrasound instruments (Giddens & Kitney 1985). The technique, which uses low-intensity laser light, relies on the frequency shift in the light caused by reflection from moving objects such as red blood cells and provides a method of assessing the skin microcirculation. The technique is of value in assessing skin perfusion and healing in both venous and arterial ulcers (Gschwandtner et al 2001) and in patients with diabetes, particularly after revascularization (Arora et al 2002).

Isotope techniques

Isotope clearance rates, usually using xenon-133, can also be related to local perfusion and have been used to define the likely viability of amputation flaps (Silberstein et al 1983). Similar techniques have also been used in an attempt to quantify limb blood flow but these have never gained widespread acceptance as a standard investigation for peripheral vascular disease (Cheatle et al 1991). A technique has been described, using hyperaemic blood flow, to measure limb perfusion, the technique providing an answer in millilitres of blood per 100 ml of tissue per minute (Wilkinson et al 1987b, 1990).

Thermography

Although not widely used, thermography can be used to evaluate skin perfusion and may be used to inform amputation level (Chant 1992). Limb temperature and cooling rates are directly related to blood flow but are subject to local climatic varia-

tion. Despite this, by carrying out investigations in an environmentally controlled room, the technique has been used successfully to determine amputation level and to evaluate digital vasospasm in Raynaud's phenomenon and vibration white finger disease (Wilkinson et al 1987a). It has been used to look at skin ulcer perfusion and healing (Armstrong & Lavery 1996).

Transcutaneous oximetry

This technique, which measures oxygen tension in the skin, can, when combined with the stress tests, be used to evaluate both the severity of limb ischaemia and the presence of ischaemia around an ulcer. The technique is, however, difficult and time-consuming and is not widely practised. As with other techniques that examine local perfusion, it has been shown to be of value in selecting amputation level and results correlate well with subsequent healing of both amputation wounds and ulcers (Karanfilian et al 1986, van Urk & Feenstra 1988).

Anatomical Investigations

Although arteries are not generally visible on plain radiography they can be visualized if the arterial wall contains significant amounts of calcium (Fig. 16.10).

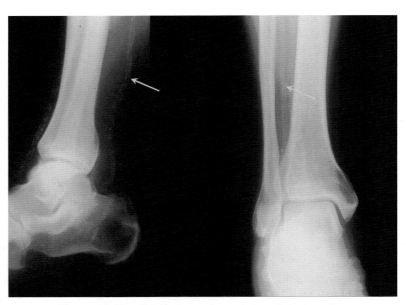

Figure 16.10 Calcified crural vessels in a diabetic patient

In general, however, contrast imaging techniques such as conventional and digital subtraction angiography are still often required to visualize the peripheral arterial tree. There are a number of newer diagnostic imaging procedures for the evaluation of lower limb atherosclerosis. In particular, multislice computed tomography (CT) and magnetic resonance angiography (MRA) are rapidly developing, and the latter may soon replace angiography as the investigation of choice for some patients with peripheral arterial disease (Cotroneo et al 1997). However, their role in clinical practice is still to be fully defined and arteriography is still regarded as the gold standard against which other modalities are judged (Beard & Scott 1991).

Contrast imaging techniques

The use of some, but not all types of contrast can be contraindicated in situations such as contrast allergy (Goss et al 1995), the presence of significant renal failure and some drug therapies such as the use of metformin (Thomsen & Morcos 1999). It may compromise renal function in some patients, particularly if the patient is dehydrated, on high-dose diuretic therapy and non-steroidal anti-inflammatory drugs, or has pre-existing renal impairment. In such situations alternative imaging modalities such as ultrasound or magnetic resonance imaging (MRI) may be appropriate, or alternative contrast agents such as CO_2 may be used (Kessel et al 2002).

Arteriography

Despite recent advances in ultrasound, MRI and CT, conventional and digital subtraction angiography remains the primary investigation for diagnosis of peripheral arterial disease. The technique, which is invasive, is performed by injecting contrast, usually via an artery, often the common femoral artery. Because of this the technique carries with it the risks of contrast-related anaphylaxis, and may also be complicated by haemorrhage, embolization, damage to the artery, haematoma formation and false aneurysm formation (Hessel et al 1981). In general, a Seldinger technique (Doby 1984) is used to position the catheter tip some distance from the puncture site. For lower limb arteriograms the catheter is placed in the aorta and images of both

limbs are obtained. The technique also allows selective catheterization of individual vessels.

Digital subtraction angiography produces an image that is stored on computer and can be manipulated. By summing serial images and subtracting the stationary background, an enhanced image can be obtained showing just the arterial tree. The technique has advantages over conventional arteriography in that a lower dose of contrast material is required, which can be administered through a smaller-gauge catheter. In addition, lower limb arteriography can, in some situations, be performed via an intravenous injection. The technique is of significant advantage to the interventional radiologist when carrying out angioplasty, as the technique allows 'road-mapping', which guides catheter placement (Cumberland 1992). This form of angiography can be also carried out using mobile equipment in an operating theatre and is of value in checking anastomoses and evaluating run-off (Mills et al 1992).

Scoring systems have been developed based on the number of patent crural vessels and the nature of the pedal arch, which can help predict preoperatively the success or failure of bypass surgery (Scott et al 1990) or wound healing (Gentile et al 1998), although intraoperative peripheral resistance measurements are probably a better guide (Bergqvist & Lundell 1993).

Magnetic resonance imaging

Recent years have seen an increasing use of MRI in diagnostic medicine, as the imaging technique avoids the use of ionizing radiation. The imaging relies upon the realignment of protons, and in particular ^1H, which return to their equilibrium state, emitting radiofrequency waves at the resonance frequency and proportional to the strength of the magnetic field when the electromagnetic pulse ceases. MRA is an extension of this technique which, with contrast enhancement, allows excellent visualization of the aorta and iliac vessels and can produce good visualization of vessels to the popliteal artery (Fig. 16.11). Continual development of the supporting software and hardware means that this technique is, along with colour flow duplex ultrasonography, progressively taking over from angiography as the investigation of choice

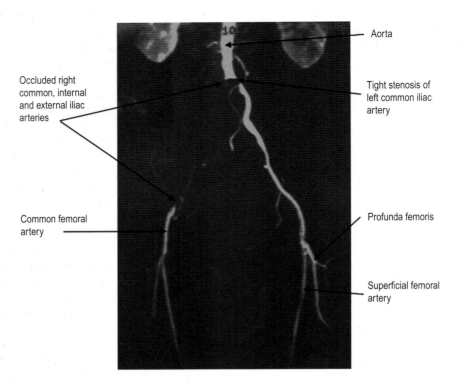

Aorta

Occluded right
common, internal
and external iliac
arteries

Tight stenosis of
left common iliac
artery

Common femoral
artery

Profunda femoris

Superficial femoral
artery

Figure 16.11   Magnetic resonance angiography of a patient with lower limb ulceration, claudication and absent femoral pulses

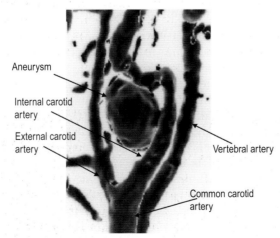

Aneurysm

Internal carotid
artery

External carotid
artery

Vertebral artery

Common carotid
artery

Figure 16.12   An example of three-dimensional imaging, in this case of a true aneurysm of the internal carotid artery, obtained with magnetic resonance angiography

for some patients with peripheral arterial disease. With appropriate software, three-dimensional images can be obtained (Fig. 16.12). Problems do remain, however: some patients find the procedure very claustrophobic and the presence of metal implants, surgical clips and cardiac pacemakers may prevent MRI examination.

Computed tomography

Computed tomography uses a rotating X-ray source and a series of detectors to collect data that, in effect, give images consisting of a slice through the area examined. The introduction of spiral CT, in which the patient also moves through the X-ray beam, has allowed faster and more detailed scans. The use of intravascular radio-opaque contrast provides an arteriogram from which a three-dimensional reconstruction can be obtained. The method is of great value in assessing abdominal aortic aneurysms and is being developed for more peripheral studies (Heuschmid et al 2003); this group found, however, that the technique was limited to routine diagnostic purposes because of severe calcifications, which created artefacts, and time-consuming reconstruction procedures.

Colour flow duplex ultrasonography

Ultrasound imaging depends on two factors:

- The penetration of tissue by ultrasound
- The reflectivity of different tissues.

When an ultrasound beam encounters a boundary or interface between two different structures, some of the ultrasound is reflected back towards the transducer. The strength of the reflected beam depends on differences in reflective properties of the two or more tissues forming the boundary. An ultrasound image is formed by plotting the strength of the reflected beam, the strongest being the brightest. This form of imaging is known as B-mode (brightness mode) imaging (Merritt 1993) and produces a greyscale image (Fig. 16.13). Increasing resolution has allowed the vessel wall to be studied in greater detail and atheromatous plaque morphology to be analysed.

Duplex ultrasound adds Doppler to the B-mode image and in so doing provides both anatomical data (B-mode) and functional data (Doppler). This can be further enhanced by representing the frequency shift as a colour scale, which allows both the direction of flow to be visualized and the velocity of flow to be calculated (Zwiebel 1992). In colour mapping, the colour Doppler image that represents moving blood cells is superimposed on the anatomical greyscale image. This aids visualization of vascular structures and highlights areas of stenosis. By focusing the Doppler beam and 'sampling' within a vessel, spectrum analysis can be undertaken and the degree of stenosis calculated. If the vessel diameter and the angle of the probe are also known, then a measure of blood flow can be derived (Zwiebel 1992).

The increasing sensitivity and non-invasive nature of this form of investigation mean that it is now the investigation of choice for screening arterial bypass grafts (Harris & Moody 1992) and carotid disease (Farmilo et al 1990), and it is becoming the initial investigation after functional assessment for people with peripheral vascular disease that warrants either surgical or intervention radiological treatment (Pemberton et al 1996, Varty et al 1996, Sensier et al 1998, McCarthy et al 1999). Increasing sensitivity continues to expand the role of colour duplex assessment as both crural and pedal vessels can now be examined (Karacagil et al 1996). Additional data may also be acquired by using ultrasound contrast materials (Karacagil et al 2003) and by intravascular ultrasound (Cwikiel et al 2002). Duplex ultrasound examination is both time-consuming and operator-dependent; it can, however, provide both functional and anatomical information and it is quite rightly now used as the primary investigation in patients with lower limb arterial disease, particularly for those in whom significant aortoiliac disease is not suspected. The modality can provide three-dimensional vascular images and may be used for intravascular imaging (White 1996).

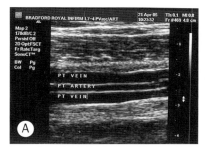 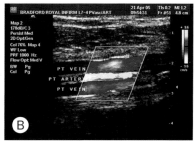 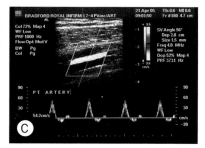

Figure 16.13 Duplex ultrasound of posterior tibial vascular bundle. (**A**) Grey-scale image. (**B**) Image enhanced with colour flow data; colours reflect the direction and velocity of flow and have been arranged to show the veins in blue. (**C**) Doppler data showing triphasic waveform from the artery

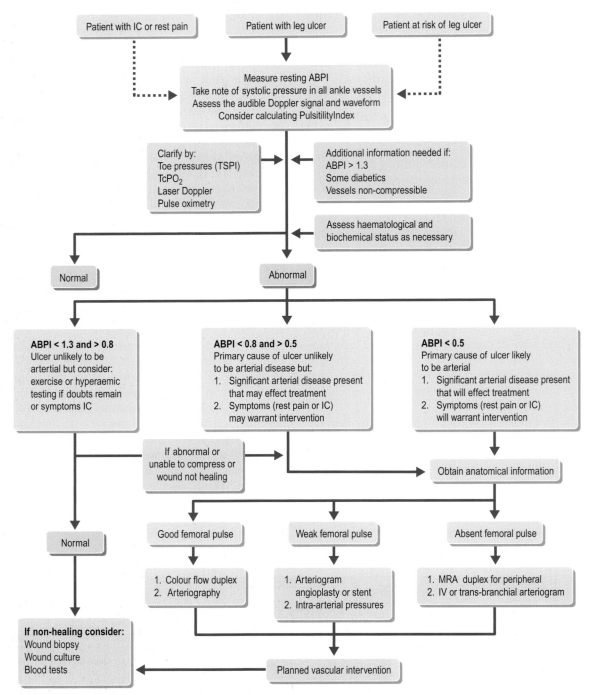

Figure 16.14 Management pathway for patient presenting with possible ischaemic lower limb ulceration or gangrene. ABPI, ankle brachial pressure index; IC, intermittent claudication; IV, intravenous; MRA, magnetic resonance angiography

Other investigations

A number of other investigations may be relevant when assessing a patient presenting with an apparently ischaemic ulcer, as they may assist in defining the underlying cause for ulceration and allow effective management of conditions such as hypertension, diabetes mellitus, hyperlipidaemia and polycythaemia, all of which may contribute to wound ischaemia. These include:

- Urine testing
- Routine haematology and biochemistry
- Erythrocyte sedimentation rate (ESR) or plasma viscosity
- Blood glucose and haemoglobin $A1_c$
- Lipid profile
- Inflammatory markers and autoantibody screen (ANS, ANCA, RhF, anticardiolipin antibody)
- Thrombophilia screen and homocystine levels
- Cryoglobinins.

When a vasculitis is suspected as the cause of the ulceration, wound and vascular biopsy should be considered in addition to the measurement of the above haematological and biochemical markers.

Wound cultures should be obtained when indicated by the clinical status of the wound, and if possible the bacterial load should be reduced prior to undertaking vascular reconstructive surgery, particularly if synthetic graft material is to be used for bypass.

Conclusion

Ischaemia is both a recognized cause of lower limb ulceration and a major factor in delayed wound healing. All wounds require careful and detailed assessment prior to treatment so that both the aetiology of the wound and factors that may delay healing can be identified. Modern wound care is quite correctly based on the principles of moist wound healing, yet there are situations, such as when non-reconstructable arterial disease is present, in which best practice would suggest that the maintenance of dry gangrene or hard eschar may prevent amputation. Such treatment decisions are based on an integrated team approach to wound care and an understanding of the pathophysiology of arterial disease, its investigation and treatment.

A suggested management pathway for a patient either with symptoms suggestive of peripheral arterial disease or who is considered to be at risk of, or has, overt lower limb ulceration is given in Figure 16.14. This pathway attempts to bring together the areas discussed in this chapter and to provide health-care professionals managing potentially ischaemic lower limb wounds with a method of integrating simple, non-invasive function investigations and invasive anatomical investigations into an overall treatment plan.

References

Anonymous 1992 Second European Consensus Document on chronic critical leg ischemia. European Journal of Vascular Surgery 6(Suppl A): 1–32

Arkilic C F, Taguchi A, Sharma N et al 2003 Supplemental perioperative fluid administration increases tissue oxygen pressure. Surgery 133: 49–55

Armstrong D G, Lavery L A 1996 Monitoring neuropathic ulcer healing with infrared dermal thermometry. Journal of Foot and Ankle Surgery 35: 335–338; discussion 372–373

Arora S, Pomposelli F, LoGerfo F W, Veves A 2002 Cutaneous microcirculation in the neuropathic diabetic foot improves significantly but not completely after successful lower extremity revascularization. 50 35: 501–5

Baker N, Rayman G 1999 Clinical evaluation of Doppler signals. Diabetic Foot 2: 22–25

Baker A R, Macpherson D S, Evans D H, Bell P R 1987 Pressure studies in arterial surgery. European Journal of Vascular Surgery 1: 273–283

Beard J D, Scott D J 1991 Investigation of chronic limb ischaemia. Hospital Update 17: 496–506

Beevers G, Lip G Y H, O'Brien E 2001 ABC of hypertension: Blood pressure measurement Part 1 – Sphygmomanometry: factors common to all techniques. British Medical Journal 322: 981–985

Bergqvist D, Lundell A 1993 Prediction of early graft occlusion in femoropopliteal and femorodistal reconstruction by measurement of volume flow with a transit time flowmeter and calculation of peripheral resistance. European Journal of Vascular Surgery 7: 704–708

Bianchi J, Douglas W S, Dawe R S et al 2000 Pulse oximetry: a new tool to assess patients with leg ulcers. Journal of Wound Care 9: 109–112

Brooks B, Dean R, Patel S et al 2001 TBI or not TBI: that is the question. Is it better to measure toe pressure than ankle pressure in diabetic patients? Diabetic Medicine 18: 528–532

Burns P N 1993 Principles of deep Doppler ultrasonography. In: Bernstein E F(ed.) Vascular diagnosis. Mosby, St Louis, MO, pp 249–268

Burns J L, Mancoll J S, Phillips L G 2003 Impairments to wound healing. Clinics in Plastic Surgery 30: 47–56

Carter S A 1969 Clinical measurement of systolic pressures in limbs with arterial occlusive disease. Journal of the American Medical Association 207: 1869–1874

Carter S A 1993 Role of pressure measurement. In: Bernstein E F(ed.) Vascular diagnosis. Mosby, St Louis, MO, pp 486–512

Chant A D B 1992 Amputations. In: Bell P R F, Jamieson C W, Ruckley C V (eds) Surgical management of vascular disease. W B Saunders, London, pp 597–607

Cheatle T R, Coleridge Smith P D, Scurr J H 1991 The investigation of peripheral vascular disease: a historical perspective. Vascular Medicine Review 2

Collins F, Hampton S, White R 2002 A–Z Dictionary of Wound Care. Quay Books, Dinton, Wiltshire

Cornwall J 1991 Managing venous leg ulcers. Community Outlook May: 36–38

Cotroneo A R, Manfredi R, Settecasi C et al 1997 Angiography and MR-angiography in the diagnosis of peripheral arterial occlusive disease in diabetic patients. Rays 22: 579–590

Cumberland D C 1992 Techniques in angioplasty. In: Bell P R F, Jamieson C W, Ruckley C V (eds) Surgical management of vascular disease. W B Saunders, London, pp 491–500

Cwikiel W, Midia M, Williams D 2002 Non-traumatic vascular emergencies: imaging and intervention in acute arterial conditions. European Radiology 12: 2619–2626

Doby T 1984 A tribute to Sven-Ivar Seldinger. American Journal of Roentgenology 142: 1–4

Dormandy J A, Stock G (eds) 1990 Critical leg ischaemia: its pathophysiology and management. Springer-Verlag, Berlin

Fagrell B, Nilsson G 1995 Advantages and limitations of one-point laser Doppler perfusion monitoring in clinical practice. Vascular Medicine Review 6: 97–101

Farmilo R W, Scott D J, Cole S E et al 1990 Role of duplex scanning in the selection of patients for carotid endarterectomy. British Journal of Surgery 77: 388–390

Gentile A T, Berman S S, Reinke K R et al 1998 A regional pedal ischemia scoring system for decision analysis in patients with heel ulceration. American Journal of Surgery 176: 109–114

Giddens D P, Kitney R I 1985 Blood flow disturbances and spectral analysis. In: Bernstein E F(ed.) Vascular diagnosis. Mosby, St Louis, MO, pp 58–68

Goss J E, Chambers C E, Heupler F A Jr 1995 Systemic anaphylactoid reactions to iodinated contrast media during cardiac catheterization procedures: guidelines for prevention, diagnosis, and treatment. Laboratory Performance Standards Committee of the Society for Cardiac Angiography and Interventions. Catheterization and Cardiovascular Diagnosis 34: 99–104

Gschwandtner M E, Ambrozy E, Maric S et al 2001 Microcirculation is similar in ischemic and venous ulcers. Microvascular Research 62: 226–235

Guillot B, Dandurand M, Guilhou J J 1988 Skin perfusion pressure in leg ulcers assessed by photoplethysmography. International Angiology 7: 33–34

Hamilton W F, Woodbury R A, Harper H J 1936 Physiologic relationships between intrathoracic, intraspinal and arterial pressures. Journal of the American Medical Association 107: 853–856

Harris P L, Moody P 1992 Postoperative surveillance of saphenous vein graft. In: Bell P R F, Jamieson C W, Ruckley C V (eds) Surgical management of vascular disease. W B Saunders, London, pp 587–596

Herrick S E, Ireland G W, Simon D et al 1996 Venous ulcer fibroblasts compared with normal fibroblasts show differences in collagen but not fibronectin production under both normal and hypoxic conditions. Journal of Investigative Dermatology 106: 187–193

Hessel S J, Adams D F, Abrams H L 1981 Complications of angiography. Radiology 138: 273–281

Heuschmid M, Krieger A, Beierlein W et al 2003 Assessment of peripheral arterial occlusive disease: comparison of multislice-CT angiography (MS-CTA) and intraarterial digital subtraction angiography (IA-DSA). European Journal of Medical Research 8: 389–396

Hirai M, Shionoya S 1978 Segmental blood pressure of the leg and its clinical use. Japanese Journal of Surgery 8: 102–110

Hocken A G 1967 Measurement of blood-pressure in the leg. Lancet 1: 466–8

Junger M, Steins A, Hahn M, Hafner H M 2000 Microcirculatory dysfunction in chronic venous insufficiency (CVI). Microcirculation 7: S3–S12

Karacagil S, Lofberg A M, Granbo A et al 1996 Value of duplex scanning in evaluation of crural and foot arteries in limbs with severe lower limb ischaemia–a prospective comparison with angiography. European Journal of Vascular and Endovascular Surgery 12: 300–333

Karacagil J P, Hansen M A, Jensen F et al 2003 Ultrasound contrast-agent improves imaging of lower limb occlusive disease. European Journal of Vascular and Endovascular Surgery 25: 23–28

Karanfilian R G, Lynch T G, Zirul V T et al 1986 The value of laser Doppler velocimetry and transcutaneous oxygen tension determination in predicting healing of ischemic forefoot ulcerations and amputations in diabetic and nondiabetic patients. Journal of Vascular Surgery 4: 511–516

Kessel D O, Robertson I, Patel J T et al 2002 Carbon-dioxide-guided vascular interventions: technique and pitfalls. Cardiovascular and Interventional Radiology 25: 476–483

Khunti K 2003 Screening for asymptomatic peripheral vascular disease in primary care. British Journal of Cardiology 10: 315–317

Kurz A, Sessler D I, Lenhardt R 1996 Perioperative normothermia to reduce the incidence of surgical-wound infection and shorten hospitalization. Study of Wound Infection and Temperature Group. New England Journal of Medicine 334: 1209–1215

Laing S P, Greenhalgh R M 1980 Standard exercise test to assess peripheral arterial disease. British Medical Journal 280: 13–16

Laing S, Greenhalgh R 1983 The detection and progression of asymptomatic peripheral arterial disease. British Journal of Surgery 70: 628–630

Laing S, Greenhalgh R M 1986 Treadmill testing in the assessment of peripheral arterial disease. International Angiology 5: 249–252

McCarthy M J, Nydahl S, Hartshorne T et al 1999 Colour-coded duplex imaging and dependent Doppler ultrasonography in the assessment of cruropedal vessels. British Journal of Surgery 86: 33–37

Macpherson D S, Evans D H, Bell P R 1984 Common femoral artery Doppler wave-forms: a comparison of three methods of objective analysis with direct pressure measurements. British Journal of Surgery 71: 46–49

Marston A 1992 Clinical evaluation of the patient with atheroma. In: Bell P R F, Jamieson C W, Ruckley C V (eds) Surgical management of vascular disease. W B Saunders, London, pp 119–130

Merritt C R B 1993 Vascular imaging. In: Bernstein E F (ed.) Vascular diagnosis. Mosby, St Louis, MO, pp 235–240

Mills J L, Fujitani R M, Taylor S M 1992 Contribution of routine intraoperative completion arteriography to early infrainguinal bypass patency. American Journal of Surgery 164: 506–510

Moffatt C, O'Hare L 1995 Ankle pulses are not sufficient to detect impaired arterial circulation in patients with leg ulcers. Journal of Wound Care 4: 134–138

Moffatt C J, Oldroyd M I, Greenhalgh R M, Franks P J 1994 Palpating ankle pulses is insufficient in detecting arterial insufficiency in patients with leg ulceration. Phlebology 9: 170–172

Mogford J E, Mustoe T A 2001 Experimental models of wound healing. In: Falanga V (ed.) Cutaneous wound healing. Martin Dunitz, London, pp 109–122

Morison M, Moffatt C 1994 A colour guide to the assessment and management of leg ulcers. Wolfe Publishing, London

Mustoe T A, Ahn S T, Tartley J E, Pierce F G 1994 Role of hypoxia in growth factor responses: differential effect of basic fibroblast growth factor and platelet-derived growth factor in an ischaemia wound model. Wound Repair and Regeneration 2: 277–283

Netten P M, Wollersheim H, Thien T, Lutterman J A 1996 Skin microcirculation of the foot in diabetic neuropathy. Clinical Science (Colchester) 91: 559–565

Pemberton M, Nydahl S, Hartshorne T et al 1996 Colour-coded duplex imaging can safely replace diagnostic arteriography in patients with lower-limb arterial disease. British Journal of Surgery 83: 1725–1728

Royal College of Nursing 1998 The management of patients with venous leg ulcers. Royal College of Nursing Institute, York

Samuelsson P, Blohme G, Fowelin J, Eriksson J W 1996 A new non-invasive method using pulse oximetry for the assessment of arterial toe pressure. Clinics in Physiology 16: 463–467

Satomura S 1959 Study of the flow patterns in peripheral arteries by ultrasonics. Journal of the Acoustic Society of Japan 15: 151

Scott D J, Vowden P, Beard J D, Horrocks M 1990 Non-invasive estimation of peripheral resistance using Pulse Generated Runoff before femorodistal bypass. British Journal of Surgery 77: 391–395

Sensier Y, Fishwick G, Owen R et al 1998 A comparison between colour duplex ultrasonography and arteriography for imaging infrapopliteal arterial lesions. European Journal of Vascular and Endovascular Surgery 15: 44–50

Silberstein E B, Thomas S, Cline J et al 1983 Predictive value of intracutaneous xenon clearance for healing of amputation and cutaneous ulcer sites. Radiology 147: 227–229

Smith F C, Shearman C P, Simms M H, Gwynn B R 1994 Falsely elevated ankle pressures in severe leg ischaemia: the pole test – an alternative approach. European Journal of Vascular Surgery 8: 408–412

Steinbrech D S, Longaker M T, Mehrara B J et al 1999 Fibroblast response to hypoxia: the relationship between angiogenesis and matrix regulation. Journal of Surgical Research 84: 127–133

Strandness D E Jr 1996 Arterial and venous haemodynamics. In: Ouriel K (ed.) Lower extremity vascular disease. W B Saunders, Philadelphia, PA, pp 3–12

Sumner D S 1989 Non-invasive assessment of peripheral arterial occlusive disease. In: Rutherford K S (ed.) Vascular surgery, vol 1. W B Saunders, Philadelphia, PA, pp 61–111

Sumner D S 1993 Mercury stain-gauge plethysmography. In: Bernstein E F(ed.) Vascular diagnosis. Mosby, St Louis, MO, pp 205–223

Takolander R, Rauwerda J A 1995 The use of non-invasive vascular assessment in diabetic patients with foot lesions. Diabetic Medicine 13: S39-S42

Thomsen H S, Morcos S K 1999 Contrast media and metformin: guidelines to diminish the risk of lactic acidosis in non-insulin-dependent diabetics after administration of contrast media. ESUR Contrast Media Safety Committee. European Radiology 9: 738–40

Trabold O, Wagner S, Wicke C et al 2003 Lactate and oxygen constitute a fundamental regulatory mechanism in wound healing. Wound Repair and Regeneration 11: 504–509

Van Urk H, Feenstra W A 1988 What can transcutaneous oxygen measurements tell us? In: Greenhalgh D G, Jamieson C W, Nicholaides A N (eds) Limb salvage and amputation for vascular disease. W B Saunders, Philadelphia, PA, pp 75–83

Varty K, Nydahl S, Butterworth P et al 1996 Changes in the management of critical limb ischaemia. British Journal of Surgery 83: 953–956

Vowden P 1997 Peripheral arterial disease. 2: Anatomical investigations. Journal of Wound Care 6: 129–132

Vowden P, Vowden K R 2001 Doppler assessment and ABPI: interpretation in the management of leg ulceration. Internet Journal: World Wide Wounds. Available on line at www.worldwidewounds.com

Vowden K R, Goulding V, Vowden P 1996 Hand-held Doppler assessment for peripheral arterial disease. Journal of Wound Care 5: 125–128

White R A 1996 Endovascular imaging techniques. In: Ouriel K (ed.) Lower extremity vascular disease. W B Saunders, Philadelphia, PA, pp 223–241

Whiteley M S, Fox A D, Horrocks M 1998 Photoplethysmography can replace hand-held Doppler in the measurement of ankle/brachial indices. Annals of the Royal College of Surgeons of England 80: 96–98

Wilkinson D, Vowden P, Kester R C 1987a The use of thermography in the assessment of Raynaud's syndrome and Vibration White Finger Disease. In: Price R, Evans J A (eds) Blood flow '87. Blood flow measurement in clinical diagnosis, vol 4. Biological Engineering Society, Leeds, pp 20–26

Wilkinson D, Vowden P, Parkin A, Wiggins P 1987b The value of isotope limb blood flow measurement in the assessment of peripheral vascular disease. In: Price R, Evans J A (eds) Blood flow '87. Blood flow measurement in clinical diagnosis, vol 4. Biological Engineering Society, Leeds, pp 44–50

Wilkinson D, Parkin A, Vowden P et al 1990 Application of a new method of limb blood flow measurement using a radioactive isotope and a gamma camera. Angiology 41: 297–304

Williams I M, Picton A J, McCollum C N 1993 The use of Doppler ultrasound: 1. Arterial disease. Wound Management 4: 9–12

Winsor T 1950 Influence of arterial disease on the systolic pressure gradients of the extremities. American Journal of Medical Science 220: 117

Yao S T 1970 In: Gillespie J A (ed.) Modern trends in vascular surgery 1. Butterworth, London, pp 281–309

Yao S T, Hobbs J T, Irvine W T 1969 Experience with the Doppler ultrasound flow velocity meter in peripheral vascular disease. Ankle systolic pressure measurements in arterial disease affecting the lower extremities. British Journal of Surgery 56: 676–9

Zwiebel W J (ed.) 1992 Introduction to vascular ultrasound. W B Saunders, Philadelphia

Leg ulcers associated with arterial insufficiency: treatment

William A. Marston

INTRODUCTION

Patients with non-healing leg ulcers and significant arterial insufficiency are at increased risk for limb loss. It is generally believed that arterial revascularization, by percutaneous or surgical techniques, is required to improve the chances of limb salvage in this group of patients. However, some patients are poor candidates for these procedures because of anatomical difficulties or patient comorbidities. Arterial reconstruction by surgical means involves a significant risk of major complications, which may be life-threatening, particularly in patients with coronary artery disease, pulmonary disease or renal insufficiency. Therefore, in high-risk patients and in those in whom revascularization has failed, treatments employing non-invasive techniques are preferable if these techniques can improve the chances of limb salvage.

The treatment of patients with chronic non-healing leg ulcers associated with arterial insufficiency involves a critical assessment of the patient's suitability for invasive procedures and the potential risk of limb loss based on ulcer characteristics. In this chapter we will review the currently available pharmacological, physical and interventional treatments for these patients (Box 17.1).

Risk of limb loss based on ulcer characteristics

Although there is a large body of information in the literature reviewing the rate of limb salvage for patients with leg ulcers and arterial insufficiency who undergo revascularization, there is only limited information on the outcome in all patients who present with this problem. The clinician is faced with a variety of presentations, from the patient with a superficial Wagner grade 1 wound (Fig. 17.1) to a deep, complicated leg ulcer involving tendon or bone (Fig. 17.2), to varying amounts of pedal gangrene. Many clinicians believe that these patients will require different treatment plans but there is limited information stratifying outcome on the basis of wound characteristics.

In a recent study of 302 patients presenting with chronic limb ulcers and arterial insufficiency, a protocol was reviewed in which patients were treated initially with conservative wound care, including debridement, pressure offloading and moist wound healing, in a multispecialty wound centre (Mendes et al 2004). If the wound became larger, or did not improve with extended treatment, revascularization was performed if possible. This review attempted to include all patients presenting with arterial ulcers, not just those that might be candidates for revascularization. The only patients excluded were those in whom the initial evaluation concluded that the only reasonable option, because of the severity of tissue loss, was amputation.

A total of 45% of all limbs were treated without revascularization, and limb salvage was achieved in 78% of these patients. It was found that patients with diabetes were at mildly increased risk for limb loss (relative risk, RR = 1.2), and those with renal insufficiency were at major increased risk for limb loss (RR 3.8). Wound grade was also a positive predictor of outcome, with wound grades 1 and 2 having a significantly better chance of healing

Box 17.1 *Treatments for arterial ulcers*

Pharmacological
- Pentoxifylline
- Cilostazol
- Heparinoids
- Prostaglandins
    - Prostaglandin E_2 (PGE_2)
    - Prostacyclin (PGI_2)
- Growth factors
    - Platelet-derived growth factor (PDGF)
    - Vascular endothelial growth factor (VEGF)
    - Fibroblast growth factor type 1 (FGF)

Physical modalities
- Epidural spinal cord stimulation
- Direct electrical stimulation
- Intermittent pneumatic compression

Hyperbaric oxygen

Revascularization
- Percutaneous endovascular techniques
- Surgical bypass

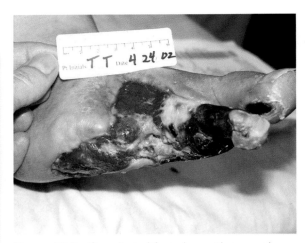

Figure 17.2 Complicated foot ulcer with exposed tendon and bone

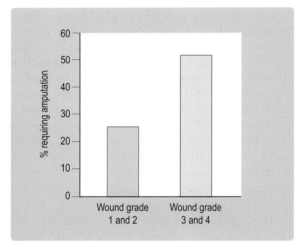

Figure 17.3 Comparison of rate of healing in patients with arterial insufficiency between Wagner grade 1 and 2 wounds and Wagner grade 3 and 4 wounds (p <0.03)

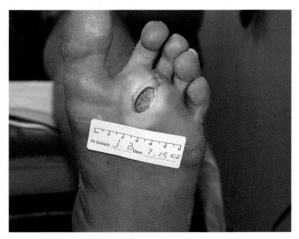

Figure 17.1 Wagner grade 1 foot ulcer involving only subcutaneous tissue

without revascularization than grades 3 and 4 (Fig. 17.3). From this review, the authors recommended that patients with limited wounds could be reasonably treated without revascularization and many would experience limb salvage. Revascularization should be considered in those who do not improve after a trial of non-invasive treatment. However, in more severe wound grades, including patients with pedal gangrene, revascularization should be considered early to improve the chances of limb salvage.

Initial evaluation of ulcers suspected to be associated with arterial insufficiency

It is important to remember that many limb ulcers are multifactorial in origin. 15% of patients with venous insufficiency and leg ulcers also exhibit significant arterial insufficiency (Marston et al 1999). A larger percentage of diabetic foot ulcers are complicated by arterial insufficiency. Other, less common causes of leg ulcers, such as rheumatological diseases, are also frequently complicated by poor arterial supply. Therefore, in each limb ulcer, a search must be made for each of the aetiological factors commonly associated with leg ulcers: diabetic neuropathy, chronic venous insufficiency, arterial insufficiency and inflammatory diseases. Once the aetiology is known, appropriate wound management can be selected.

Non-invasive methods to predict potential for healing

Patients with limb ulcers and associated arterial insufficiency should undergo some form of diagnostic evaluation to attempt to predict whether the ulcer is able to heal without revascularization. Potential studies include the ankle/brachial index, toe pressures, transcutaneous Po_2 and laser Doppler. These have been reviewed in detail in Chapter 16.

Local management of wounds in patients with arterial insufficiency

In general, principles of management are similar to those for diabetic foot ulcers, including pressure offloading, debridement of non-viable tissue, infection control and moist wound healing. Close attention to the principles of wound bed preparation will provide some potential for healing, despite arterial insufficiency (Schultz et al 2003).

In wounds caused solely by arterial insufficiency, the location typically differs from diabetic foot ulcer involving the toes, dorsum of the foot, heel or bony prominence of the ankle. The plantar foot is a less common site. Total contact casting is not advised given the increased risk of complications with arterial insufficiency. Pressure offloading methods must be individualized based on the specific location of the wound.

Sharp surgical debridement of non-viable or infected tissue should be performed as often as needed to maintain a clean wound bed. The primary exception involves adherent eschar or dry gangrene. We recommend leaving this material in place (unless infected) until after revascularization is performed (Fig. 17.4).

The principles of moist wound healing are also followed. Wounds primarily of arterial origin are typically dry, with little tissue oedema or drainage. Hydrogels or similar hydrating agents should be applied to prevent desiccation of exposed layers after debridement is performed. We typically reserve expensive modalities such as growth factors or living human tissue substitutes for use after revascularization is performed.

The need for revascularization is assessed using several variables. If the patient has severe rest pain and is a good candidate for revascularization, this should be performed electively as soon as possible. Most patients with diabetes and arterial insufficiency have little rest pain, probably because of neuropathy, so they rarely complain of significant rest pain. Wound size, depth and character are all important measures. A small, grade 1 ulcer on the dorsum of the foot is much more likely to heal without revascularization than a large, complicated, deep wound on the plantar surface of the foot. The

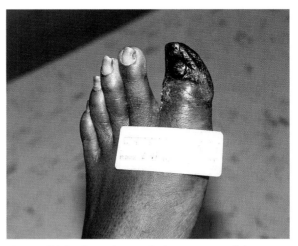

Figure 17.4 Foot ulcer with dry gangrene of digit. Debridement or amputation is recommended several days after revascularization is performed as long as no infection develops

potential for healing based on non-invasive tests must be balanced with the potential risk of complications associated with the required intervention for revascularization. In patients in whom the risk/benefit assessment does not favour revascularization, we optimize potential for healing with standard wound care along with the modalities described below.

Pain control in patients with severe arterial insufficiency may be difficult. Those without diabetic neuropathy may experience severe, debilitating pain that affects sleep patterns, activity level and healing potential. Those with neuropathy are more affected by burning pain and numbness, which may be just as debilitating. Determining the aetiology of the pain is important, as treatment modalities differ. Available options include non-steroidal anti-inflammatory medicines, and opioids of various strengths and addictive potential.

In a recent review article, Freedman et al (2004) recommended the use of analgesics based on the guidelines of the World Health Organization analgesic ladder. However, for significant ischaemic pain, non-steroidal anti-inflammatory medications are usually inadequate, and some opiate analgesia is required. They have found tricyclic antidepressants such as nortriptyline to assist in reducing narcotic requirements in many patients. Long-acting opioids are preferable for ischaemic pain, either using transdermal systems such as the fentanyl patch or long-acting oral agents like OxyContin.

PHARMACOLOGICAL THERAPIES FOR ARTERIAL ULCERS:

Pentoxifylline

Pentoxifylline is a methylxanthine that is classified as a haemorrheological agent. It increases phosphorylation of the proteins of the red blood cell membrane resulting in an increase in adenosine triphosphate in the membrane (Dettelbach & Aviado 1985). This allows an increase in cell flexibility and a reduction of blood viscosity. Another effect of pentoxifylline is inhibition of platelet aggregation. It was initially studied in claudication and was found to significantly increase walking distance in these patients (Porter et al 1982).

Pentoxifylline has been studied in several randomized trials for the healing of leg ulcers associated with venous insufficiency, and most have identified a positive result (Falanga et al 1999). A recent review by the Cochrane database found that pentoxifylline appears to be an effective adjunct to compression bandaging for treating venous leg ulcers (Jull et al 2002).

Unfortunately, no studies have been conducted on the use of pentoxifylline for arterial leg ulcers that would support its use for this indication.

Cilostazol

Cilostazol is a selective inhibitor of phosphodiesterase-III with vasodilating and antiplatelet properties. It also exhibits antiproliferative effects on smooth muscle cells (Dawson et al 1998). It has been extensively tested and is approved for the treatment of intermittent claudication. In a prospective randomized study comparing cilostazol to pentoxifylline and placebo for claudicants, cilostazol was found to produce a significantly higher improvement in walking distance than either pentoxifylline or placebo (Dawson et al 2000). This appears to occur primarily through its vasodilatory effect. The primary side effect of cilostazol has been headaches, which occurred in 34% of treated patients compared to 14% taking placebo. It is not recommended in patients with congestive heart failure, due to the potential for exacerbation of this condition with vasodilation.

Cilostazol has also undergone limited study for patients with ulcers. In a case series of 21 patients with non-healing leg ulcers and arterial insufficiency, 100 mg of cilostazol was administered twice daily because patients were not candidates for or refused revascularization. A variety of conditions, including inflammatory disorders and vasculitis, were included. Improvement was seen at 2 weeks in pressure pain, numbness, pain at rest and erythema. Subjects with diabetic ulcer showed the greatest improvement. Overall, 48% showed marked improvement of symptoms, 24% showed improvement, 10% showed slight improvement and 19% worsened. The authors concluded that cilostazol might be useful in the treatment of skin ulcer secondary to vascular disorders (Arakawa & Arada, 1993).

Based on these results and others from similar studies, a prospective randomized trial was initiated to determine the benefit of cilostazol in healing ischaemic leg ulcers. This trial is currently enrolling patients, with results expected in 12–24 months.

At this time, cilostazol cannot be strongly recommended for the treatment of ischaemic leg ulcers. However, the risk of use is low, and it is not unreasonable to add this agent as an adjunct to standard therapies in patients who can tolerate the medication.

Heparinoids

The use of heparin has been proposed to assist in healing of ischaemic leg ulcers, particularly in patients with diabetes, because of its anti-inflammatory and anticoagulant properties. A small case series was performed using a low-molecular-weight heparin administered subcutaneously (Jorneskog et al 1993). The results suggested a positive effect on ulcer healing, which was believed to be due to improved skin microcirculation.

Based on these results, a prospective randomized study was designed to determine whether a low-molecular-weight heparin, dalteparin, could influence healing rate in diabetic patients with significant arterial occlusive disease. 87 patients with an ankle-to-brachial pressure index (ABPI) of less than 0.6 were randomized to dalteparin or placebo along with standard wound therapy in both groups (Kalani et al 2003). Although there were some trends towards improved outcomes in the dalteparin group, they did not reach statistical significance in this limited study. Amputation occurred in eight of 42 patients in the placebo group and two of 43 in the dalteparin group. 14 patients healed in the dalteparin group, compared to nine in the placebo group ($p = NS$).

In summary, despite encouraging initial results, there is no strong evidence to support the use of low-molecular-weight heparins for ischaemic ulcers at this time. Larger prospective randomized studies are needed to determine whether any benefit can be expected from the use of anticoagulants in this patient population.

Prostaglandins

A wide variety of vasodilating agents have been evaluated in the treatment of ischaemic leg ulcers. Most of these agents were found to have little effect on improving the circulatory status of truly ischaemic limbs. The concept therefore developed that the ischaemic limb was already maximally dilated, and the use of vasodilating medications would add little to tissue perfusion. However, extensive study of various prostaglandins has yielded positive results. It is possible that these compounds have effects other than potent vasodilation that allow an improvement in ischaemic leg ulcers (Lowe 1990). Further study of the microcirculation in patients with occlusive arterial disease has evaluated the distribution of flow in the peripheral capillaries. It appears that, in some cases, the microcirculation abnormally vasoconstricts in the periphery, shunting blood away from the skin capillaries. Also, ischaemic tissue is associated with activation of the complement system with recruitment of white blood cells and platelets. These may release vasoactive mediators, which increase capillary permeability and tissue oedema, and cause significant tissue inflammation. Agents with the potential to ameliorate these effects of PAD may result in improvement in some patients.

Prostaglandins, and in particular prostaglandin $(PG)E_2$ and prostacyclin (PGI_2), have been found, in addition to their potent vasodilatory effect, to prevent leukocyte activation and platelet aggregation. In some studies, treatment has resulted in significant improvement in patients with critical limb ischaemia (CLI; Telles et al, 1984, Altstaedt et al 1993). However, a number of problems with the use of prostaglandins have impacted on their widespread use. Most are intravenous medications with short half-lives, requiring intravenous infusions for administration. Also, troubling side effects at clinically relevant doses, including headaches and dizziness, have been frequent.

PGI_2 is the most often studied of the prostanoids. Initial evaluations of PGI_2 were with intravenous infusions of various doses and lengths. Some studies achieved encouraging results. Staben & Albring (1996) reported a multicentre retrospective review of 853 patients with rest pain or ischaemic ulcers receiving intravenous PGI_2 for at least 6 hours per day for up to 42 days. Improvement was reported in 66% of patients with rest pain and in 42% of patients with ulceration. However, only 12% of patients with leg ulcers were able to achieve complete healing of the ulcer. Limb salvage was encouraging, with 83% limb salvage at 12 months for the ulcerated group. Adverse events were frequent, including headache, nausea and dizziness, requiring dose modification or drug discontinuation in approximately 25% of patients.

The UK Severe Limb Ischaemia Study Group reported on a multicentre randomized study of intravenous iloprost (a PGI_2 analogue) compared to placebo in 151 patients with non-healing ulcers or gangrene (Anonymous 1991a). Intravenous infusions continued for 14–28 days. One month after randomization, 45% of patients in the iloprost group showed evidence of improvement in clinical status, compared to 29% in the placebo group (p<0.05). Six months after enrolment, 42% of the iloprost group continued to demonstrate improvement in clinical status compared to 26% in the control group (p <0.01). Major amputation was required in significantly fewer patients treated with iloprost (31%) than in control patients (45%, p <0.05).

Conversely, in a prospective randomized study of another prostacyclin analogue (ciprostene), equivocal results were obtained (Anonymous 1991b). Although 211 patients with ischaemic leg ulcers were randomized, only 45% of ciprostene-treated patients and 55% of controls were able to complete the trial. There was no difference between the groups in the incidence of amputation or the need for bypass surgery. There was no significant difference in the percentage of patients achieving complete ulcer healing. Four months after enrolment, a significantly higher number of ciprostene-treated patients achieved more than 50% healing of the leg ulcer compared to control (p = 0.005), but at the price of a significantly higher incidence of adverse events.

Several additional randomized studies of the use of various intravenous prostaglandins have been performed, some finding a positive benefit for their use in CLI, and some failing to confirm this benefit. Selected prospective randomized studies including patients with non-healing leg ulcers are summarized in Table 17.1. A consistent finding has been the frequency of adverse side effects and the high cost of treatment due to the need for intravenous infusion. Efforts were therefore directed in the evaluation of alternate forms of administration of prostaglandin therapy.

An oral form of iloprost has been evaluated in several prospective trials. A multicentre prospective study of 178 patients randomized patients to placebo, low-dose iloprost or high-dose iloprost for 5 months (Anonymous 2000). Approximately 45% of patients were able to complete the iloprost protocol. The percentage of patients who survived without amputation, with healed ulcers and no rest pain was higher in the iloprost groups (28% for high-dose, 19% for low-dose) than in placebo-

Table 17.1 Summary of prospective trials of prostanoids for ischaemic leg ulcers

Study	n	Comparison	Length of follow-up	Endpoint	Result
Ciprostene study (Anonymous 1991b)	211	PGEI vs placebo	4 months	Ulcer size reduction >50%	Better in PGE group, p <0.005
Trubestein et al 1989	70	PGEI vs pentoxifylline	6 months	Reduction in ulcer size	Greater in PGE group, p <0.05
Diehm et al 1989	101	Iloprost vs placebo	28 days	Reduction in ulcer size	Greater in iloprost group, p <0.05
Norgren et al 1990	103	Iloprost vs placebo	6 months	Reduction in ulcer size	No significant difference
Brock et al 1990	109	Iloprost vs placebo	28 days	Reduction in ulcer size	Greater in iloprost group, p <0.05
UK Ulcer Study Group (Anonymous 1991b)	151	Iloprost vs placebo	6 months	Ulcer healing	Greater in iloprost group, p <0.01

treated patients (11%, $p = 0.04$). Subsequently, a larger confirmatory study was performed in 624 patients treated for a year with low- or high-dose oral iloprost compared to placebo (Trubestein et al 1989). No benefit was found in this study for treatment with iloprost in reducing amputations or rest pain. The only significant benefit to oral iloprost was found by pooling endpoints such that the number of patients surviving with no ulcers, rest pain or need for analgesia was higher in the iloprost groups (23% low-dose, 26% high-dose) than in placebo (18%, $p < 0.05$).

After reviewing the evidence concerning prostaglandin treatment for CLI, the TransAtlantic Inter-Society Consensus Group recommended in 2000 that prostanoids be considered only in patients with a viable limb who cannot undergo revascularization or in whom revascularization has failed (Dormandy & Rutherford 2000a). Overall the benefit appears to be modest, with few major side effects but frequent minor side effects. Further study is necessary to better select patients who are likely to benefit from prostanoid therapy. Given the modest benefit with these agents, many countries have not approved prostanoids for use in patients with CLI.

Growth factors

The only clinically available growth factor for topical application, becaplermin (PDGFβ, Ortho-McNeill Pharmaceuticals), has been studied in several randomized trials for the treatment of diabetic foot ulcers (Smiell et al 1999). Patients with arterial insufficiency were excluded from these trials, and few data exist on the potential benefit of this treatment in ischaemic ulcers. One small retrospective study reported a healing rate of 67% in small, uncomplicated ulcers treated with becaplermin in patients with ischaemic ulcers (McCulloch et al 2003). However, with no placebo group for control, the results cannot be interpreted as implying a benefit for becaplermin in this indication. Platelet releasates have also been reported for the treatment of chronic ulcers but no significant studies have addressed their efficacy in the treatment of ischaemic ulcers. In summary, given the relative safety and ease of use of becaplermin, it is not unreasonable to consider its use in patients

with ischaemic leg ulcers as an adjunctive measure. But the significant cost (US$450 per tube) and lack of known benefit argue against its routine use.

Since the discovery of vascular endothelial growth factor (VEGF) and techniques that allow it to be delivered to target tissue, there has been great enthusiasm for this therapeutic modality. Using numerous animal models, transfer of VEGF to localized target tissues has resulted in angiogenesis, with proliferation of blood vessels and increased tissue perfusion (Gowdak et al 2000). The transfer of this powerful technology to patient treatment has been a long, arduous process due to the concern of adverse unintended effects, such as the concern of tumour induction with promotion of occult malignancies resulting in accelerated growth and metastatic potential.

Local gene transfer to facilitate therapeutic angiogenesis has the theoretic advantage of producing protracted growth factor expression when compared to single doses or applications of a growth factor. Adenovirus-mediated transfer of the *VEGF* gene attempts to transfer the *VEGF* gene to target cells, which then manufacture and secrete more VEGF, allowing amplification of the signal to increase response. This method of VEGF induction was studied in 105 subjects with claudication in a phase II randomized double-blind study (Rajagopalan et al 2003). Despite improvements in endothelial function (Rajagopalan et al 2001), a single injection of adenovirus containing an isoform of VEGF did not result in significant improvement in walking distance. Studies of this method of gene transfer have not yet been published for CLI. In several small studies of patients with CLI and no options for revascularization, intramuscular injections of VEGF were found to improve collateral flow to the calf muscle and reduce the symptoms of CLI (Vale et al 2001).

Another growth factor, fibroblast growth factor (FGF) type 1, has also been evaluated in patients with CLI. Using naked plasmid DNA encoding, FGF is transferred via intramuscular injection. In a phase I study of 51 patients, one or two doses of FGF were administered in a dosing and safety study (Comerota et al 2002). No serious adverse events related to FGF administration were reported. In a subset of 15 patients for whom 6 months of follow-up was completed, a significant increase in ABPI and tcP_{O_2} were reported, as were a significant decrease in ulcer size and limb pain. This promising agent is reportedly under study in a phase II clinical trial.

Clearly, much work remains to be performed on problems related to gene transfer therapy for CLI. Reliable transfection and protein expression from a sufficient number of cells to affect a response are significant problems, and dosing issues must be evaluated. Safety remains a significant concern, though recent phase I and II studies have reported acceptable safety profiles. Although no VEGF or FGF preparations are currently available for general clinical use, several clinical trials have been or are planning patient enrolment and may be options for appropriate patients with non-reconstructible vascular disease and CLI.

EPIDURAL SPINAL CORD STIMULATION

In patients with arterial insufficiency and critical limb ischaemia who are not candidates for revascularization procedures, epidural spinal cord stimulation (ESCS) has been advocated to improve limb salvage, heal ulcers and reduce rest pain. The technique requires implantation of a permanent epidural stimulator (Medtronic) by a surgical procedure and thus is invasive and may be associated with potential complications. Implantation is performed through an incision overlying the spinal cord, allowing insertion of leads in the epidural space. The leads are tunnelled subcutaneously to the lumbar area, where the control unit is implanted in a subcutaneous space, similarly to a pacemaker procedure. The procedure is typically performed under local anaesthesia and requires approximately 1.5 hours to complete.

Operative success and perioperative complications

In a review of 60 patients, implantation was successful in 51. Loss of stimulation due to lead displacement was the most common complication, occurring in 22% of cases. Local infection at the implantation site occurred in 5% and premature battery depletion (<2 years) occurred in 5% (Spincemaille et al 2000).

The theoretical mechanism of benefit with ESCS involves improvement in microcirculatory blood flow, resulting in increased perfusion of the skin to assist with wound healing and reduce rest pain. This mechanism has been evaluated in several studies using tcP_{O_2} (Claeys 1997) and capillary microscopy (Ubbink et al 1999) as measures of skin perfusion. In a study of 177 patients with non-reconstructible arterial insufficiency and rest pain, ECSC was initiated and limb ABPI and tcP_{O_2} were measured repeatedly (Horsch & Claeys 1994). No changes were noted in ABPI after initiation of ESCS, but tcP_{O_2} increased significantly in Fontaine class III (rest pain) patients from 24.2 to 48.1 mmHg (p <0.02) and in Fontaine class IV (tissue loss) patients from 16.4 to 37.2 mmHg (p <0.03). An increase in tcP_{O_2} of more than 50% within 3 months of initiating ECSC was predictive of clinical success.

Results of ECSC treatment for non-healing limb ulcers have been variable in several clinical trials but are generally favourable. Claeys & Horsch (1996) randomized 86 patients with ankle pressures less than 50 mmHg and non-healing ulcers to a regimen of PGE_1 with or without ECSC. There was no significant difference in the incidence of limb loss, at 16% and 20% respectively. However, in those remaining limbs, 69% healed in the ECSC group compared to 17% in the group without ECSC.(p <0.001). ECSC was again found to produce a prolonged increase in tcP_{O_2} that was not seen in the control group.

In another prospective randomized study, Ubbink et al (1999) reported that ECSC did not result in a higher incidence of limb salvage versus control. However, in a subset of patients with intermediate microcirculatory perfusion at baseline, there was a trend towards improved limb salvage with ECSC (Fig. 17.5).

In a metaanalysis, the Cochrane Library reviewed the use of ECSC for non-reconstructible critical limb ischaemia (Fontaine III and IV; Ubbink & Vermeulen 2003). They located six randomized clinical trials of generally good design. Overall, the results indicated a beneficial effect for ECSC in improving limb salvage and pain relief for patients with CLI.

Unfortunately, ECSC is not currently available or reimbursed in all countries. Also, it is more expen-

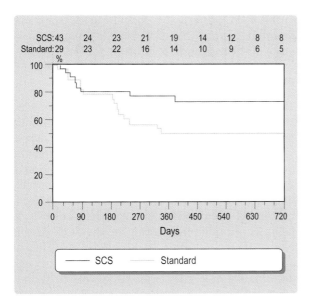

Figure 17.5 Percentage of limbs salvaged in patients with intermediate microcirculatory perfusion at baseline treated with or without epidural spinal cord stimulation (SCS). *p* value between the groups was 0.08

sive than standard treatment. In a cost comparison, ESCS was reported to cost €36 500 for 2 years of treatment compared to €28 600 for standard treatment. However, when available, it appears to be a useful modality that may improve the chances of limb salvage in selected cases, particularly those that cannot undergo revascularization.

LUMBAR SYMPATHECTOMY

Another method of producing prolonged vasodilation as a strategy for treating CLI has been lumbar sympathectomy, by chemical or surgical means. The second and third ganglia of the lumbar sympathetic chain are typically targeted. Surgical sympathectomy may be performed using laparoscopic techniques, with relatively low morbidity. Chemical sympathectomy has been performed using a variety of agents. In some cases, a temporary block is performed using an anaesthetic agent to determine whether sympathectomy will be useful in treating the patient's symptoms. For patients who experience a good temporary result, permanent surgical sympathectomy is recommended. In other cases, agents such as phenol are

injected to permanently ablate the ganglia. In a non-randomized comparison of chemical and surgical sympathectomy 76 limbs were treated (Holiday et al 1999). The short-term success rate was better with surgical sympathectomy (44%) than with chemical (18%). However, the 1-year limb salvage rates were the same (61% and 58% respectively). There was no difference in the rate of procedural complications.

In a retrospective review of 66 cases with rest pain or gangrene, Repelaer van Driel et al (1988) reported good results, with ulcer healing and resolution of rest pain in 48%. Patients with rest pain fared better than those with tissue loss. Patients with diabetes mellitus and those with an ABPI of less than 0.3 fared poorly. Although the authors concluded that lumbar sympathectomy was a useful treatment in selected patients, it was only advocated in patients without gangrenous limb lesions.

Persson et al (1985) reported a 78% limb salvage rate in 22 patients with tissue loss treated with lumbar sympathectomy, but others have reported amputation rates of 27–38% in small case series (Fulton & Blakeley 1968). To date, no prospective randomized studies have compared lumbar sympathectomy to conservative treatment or any other treatment protocols for CLI. After reviewing the above studies, the TransAtlantic Inter-Society Consensus Group recommended that there was insufficient evidence to determine which patients would benefit from lumbar sympathectomy (Dormandy & Rutherford 2000b). If considered, patients with an ABPI greater than 0.3 with limited superficial tissue loss and relief of rest pain after temporary lumbar blockade appear more likely to respond.

DIRECT ELECTRICAL STIMULATION

The use of electrical stimulation has been described as an adjunctive therapy for wound healing, most often used for chronic pressure ulcers. The most commonly described format for wound electrotherapy has been high-voltage pulsed current (HVPC). Its use in wounds associated with arterial insufficiency has been limited, and no randomized studies of significant size have examined the potential benefit of HVPC for this indication in comparison to a control group.

Goldman et al (2003) reported that $tcPo_2$ was found to increase during HVPC application to ischaemic wounds. They reported that 90% of ischaemic wounds treated with HVPC were healed at 1 year after initiating therapy. Peters and colleagues (1998) reported an evaluation of the effect of electrotherapy on microcirculatory status in diabetic patients with and without documented arterial insufficiency. In patients with normal vascular supply, no improvement in local circulation was found with electrotherapy, either during or after therapy. However, in the group with significant arterial insufficiency, electrotherapy did appear to result in an increase in $tcPo_2$, although this was a transient increase that was only present during treatment.

At this time, there is inadequate information available to determine whether electrotherapy added to a regimen of standard wound care will result in an improved incidence of limb salvage. However, this is a modality that offers little risk to the patient and is able to be easily combined with other treatment modalities. It is hoped that further research will soon assist in determining the utility of this technique in improving limb salvage for patients with ischaemic limb wounds.

INTERMITTENT PNEUMATIC COMPRESSION

The use of alternating external pressure and suction was described by several authors in the 1930s as a conservative form of therapy for atherosclerotic peripheral vascular disease. Although interest in this type of therapy waned, the use of intermittent pneumatic compression (IPC) to reduce the risk of deep venous thrombosis in immobilized patients has been extensively studied and validated. Gaskell & Parrott (1978) reported that an external foot pump applying intermittent compression could increase circulation to the feet, as measured by subcutaneous xenon-133 clearance. In the subsequent 25 years, many investigators have studied this mode of treatment in patients with claudication and CLI. Despite some encouraging results, the use of IPC has not become widely used for this indication. There are little data overall on its use for healing ischaemic limb ulcers, but numerous studies have documented the ability of various forms of IPC to increase blood flow in the ischaemic limb, suggesting that this modality may have a place in the treatment algorithm for CLI.

Methodology

There are two general types of IPC that have been studied in CLI. Both employ mechanical pneumatic pumps connected to sleeves designed to fit over a variable portion of the lower limb. Sleeves may be placed on the foot, calf, thigh or any combination of the segments of the leg (Fig. 17.6). The primary difference in the types of IPC concerns the synchronization of pneumatic inflation to the cardiac cycle using continuous monitoring of the ECG. In this type of IPC (synch-IPC) 55–80 mmHg is applied at end-diastole to maximize venous emptying. Pump decompression occurs prior to systole to reduce afterload and limit compression-related competition with systolic inflow to the limb (Vella et al 2000).

Non-synchronized IPC (n-IPC) has been described in numerous protocols, including varying pressures, inflation durations and deflation durations. Typical protocols involve the use of an inflation pressure of 120–180 mmHg, inflation duration of 3–5 seconds, and deflation times of 15–20 seconds. When multiple pump bladders are utilized, foot inflation occurs prior to more proximal inflation.

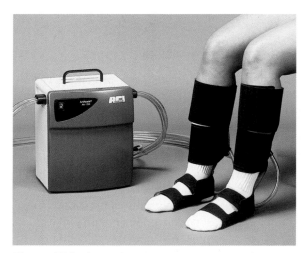

Figure 17.6 Intermittent pneumatic compression device designed specifically for augmentation of arterial flow with lower leg compression bladders (Courtesy of ACI Medical, Inc.)

IPC is recommended for 2–4 hours daily to the affected limb(s).

There have been no direct comparisons of the beneficial effect of synch-IPC compared to n-IPC. N-IPC is generally less expensive and is more amenable to home use, making it more attractive given the length of therapy required for in patients with CLI. In one study, patients required an average of 40 daily visits to a vascular centre for synch-IPC treatments (Vella et al 2000).

Mechanism of action

The aetiology of improvement with IPC is not fully defined but the following hypotheses have some support from available studies:

- IPC reduces oedema formation, which often occurs in patients with CLI. This, combined with improved venous emptying during IPC, may result in an increase in the arteriovenous pressure gradient in the limb. With less resistance to inflow, blood flow may increase, resulting in increased tissue perfusion, relief of rest pain and improved ulcer healing.
- In studies of both deep vein thrombosis and CLI, IPC has been found to increase the concentration of prostacyclin and nitric oxide. These are strong peripheral vasodilators and may stimulate improved tissue perfusion, despite the presence of large-vessel occlusive disease.

Haemodynamic studies of intermittent pneumatic compression

Several investigators have evaluated the haemodynamic effect of IPC on lower extremity blood flow. The velocity of blood flow in the popliteal artery has been reproducibly found to increase after the initiation of IPC (Labropoulos et al 1998, Morris et al 2002). This increase was also noted in patients with significant arterial insufficiency (Fig. 17.7; Delis et al 2001). IPC could be performed on the foot, calf, thigh or any combination of the above, resulting in an increase in popliteal flow. The most beneficial combination appeared to be IPC of the foot and calf together. Delis et al (2000a) reported that this combination resulted in a 174% increase in popliteal artery flow, compared to a 132% increase for calf compression alone and a 58%

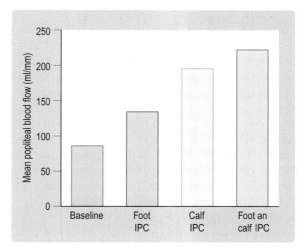

Figure 17.7 Mean popliteal artery blood flow in claudicants at baseline compared to claudicants using intermittent pneumatic compression (IPC) of various types. Each type of IPC resulted in significantly higher flows than baseline (p <0.001)

increase for foot compression alone. Labropoulos et al (1988) reported a significant increase in popliteal artery flow using foot and calf compression in each of 40 limbs studied, averaging 2.4 times over baseline. There was no persistent increase in blood flow after IPC cessation. The increase in blood flow was believed to occur due to a decrease in peripheral vascular resistance, supporting the existence of an increased arteriovenous gradient during the use of IPC.

Although an increase in popliteal artery blood flow probably improves perfusion of the calf muscle, and may alleviate claudication, patients with lower extremity ulcers and arterial insufficiency typically require increased tissue perfusion to the foot to improve their potential for healing. Many arterial insufficiency patients with ulcers have extensive tibial artery disease, particularly those with diabetes, and an increase in popliteal artery flow may not translate as improved pedal perfusion. In this group of patients, tissue oxygenation and laser Doppler studies are more relevant than popliteal flow studies.

Abu-Own and colleagues (1993) evaluated the effect of IPC on microcirculatory function of the foot in 15 patients with arterial insufficiency. They found that laser Doppler flux increased 57% with

IPC, and tcPo_2 increased 8% during use, both significant changes. These findings have been corroborated by van Bemmelen et al (2000; laser Doppler flux) and Rooke & Osmundson (1988; tcPo_2 using synch-IPC). Van Bemmelen's study was conducted specifically in patients with infrapopliteal arterial disease. In summary, it appears clear that both synch-IPC and n-IPC can increase tissue perfusion to the foot in patients with symptomatic arterial insufficiency, at least during the time period when IPC is engaged. The question remains whether this improvement is sufficient to impact on wound healing, or whether IPC leads to any longer-term improvement in limb circulation.

Louridas et al (2002) studied 33 limbs with CLI following failed bypass surgery and non-reconstructible disease on angiography. They treated these patients with n-IPC and reported that toe pressures measured 3 months after initiation of n-IPC were significantly higher than baseline. A single case of angiographic follow-up after n-IPC was reported by van Bemmelen and colleagues (2003). The patient was initially denied arterial revascularization because all three tibial vessels were obliterated. There was heavy disease and sluggish flow noted in the posterior tibial artery. After 4 months of IPC, arteriography was repeated, revealing marked improvement in the posterior tibial artery and an improved network of collateral vessels below the knee. Delis et al (2000b) studied 25 patients with claudication treated with n-IPC of the foot and calf, compared to 12 claudicants treated with an unsupervised exercise program. After 3 months of treatment, the IPC group was found to have significant improvements in claudication distance, ABPI and mean popliteal artery blood flow. Control patients demonstrated no significant improvements. Of interest, 12 months after cessation of IPC, these authors reported that the IPC group continued to demonstrate significant improvements over baseline in walking distance and ABPI.

The above information is encouraging, providing a physiological basis for a positive effect of IPC in patients with arterial insufficiency and non-healing ulcers. There is strong evidence for an increase in popliteal and pedal blood flow, and a suggestion of longer-term benefit to the use of IPC in this patient group. The question remains, however, whether the improvement in supply generated by this technique is sufficient to make a difference in the ability of the patient to heal wounds. Unfortunately, there are few clinical data to assist in this question. No prospective randomized studies of the use of IPC for ulcer healing have been performed. Several case series can be found but most are small and anecdotal.

Using synch-IPC, Vella and colleagues (2000) reported on the treatment of 98 limbs with arterial-insufficiency-related ulcers. These limbs were not candidates for revascularization, because of either inadequate outflow vessels or medical comorbidities. Treatment with the circulator boot resulted in healing in 25 limbs, improvement in 24 and no change in 7. 15 major amputations were required. If the initial tcPo_2 was less than 20 mmHg, ulcer improvement or healing was obtained in 19 of 29 limbs (65%), and when the initial tcPo_2 was more than 20 mmHg, 54 of 62 limbs (87%) healed or improved. From these data, the authors concluded that the circulator boot was useful in a subset of patients with arterial insufficiency and non-healing ulcers.

Case series of the clinical use of non-gated IPC have also been published. Louridas et al (2002) reported on the use of the ArtAssist device (ACI Medical) in 33 limbs with CLI, including 23 with non-healing ulcers. Limb salvage was attained in 58% and complete healing occurred in 26%. Chronic renal failure (CRF) was a significant negative risk factor, with limb salvage attained in 86% of patients without CRF. Van Bemmelen et al (2001) reported on the use of IPC in 13 patients with non-reconstructible arterial insufficiency and rest pain with ulceration. After 3 months of treatment nine of the 13 limbs demonstrated improved tissue perfusion by pulsed volume recordings (PVRs). All nine limbs were salvaged. Of the four remaining limbs that did not demonstrate improved PVRs after 3 months of therapy, three required amputation.

Cost and availability

Equipment rental for home use of n-IPC typically costs US$300–600 per month and varies between manufacturers. Reimbursement varies in different countries and is generally poor in the USA, where most insurers do not routinely provide coverage.

Summary

IPC has been promoted as a non-invasive modality for the treatment of CLI, most often for patients who have failed or are poor candidates for revascularization procedures. It has been shown to improve blood flow to the limb in patients with arterial occlusive disease, and studies suggest that this improvement may persist long after the cessation of therapy. Randomized trials are required to determine the efficacy of this modality in healing leg ulcers and to define its cost efficacy. Routine use of IPC is limited by the requirement for clinic treatment for synch-IPC and the high cost of home IPC, which is usually not reimbursed by insurers. If available, this appears to be a modality worth considering in selected patients with CLI.

HYPERBARIC OXYGEN

Hyperbaric oxygen therapy (HBO) involves the treatment of a patient with 100% oxygen at elevated atmospheric pressures. Beneficial aspects of increasing the partial pressure of oxygen in the tissues may include improved oxygen supply, reduction of inflammation and oedema, and inhibition of infection. HBO has been useful in the treatment of a number of wound problems, including osteomyelitis, necrotizing fasciitis and the healing of tissue flaps. Typical treatment protocols for leg ulcers involve one to two treatments daily for a total of 20–40 treatments.

HBO has long been considered as a potential treatment modality for ischaemic ulcers. Oxygen has been reported to stimulate angiogenesis, enhance fibroblast and leukocyte function, and normalize cutaneous microvascular reflexes (Knighton et al 1981, Abidia et al 2001). Clinically, HBO has been demonstrated to improve transcutaneous Po_2 in the limbs of some patients with ischaemic ulcers.

However, the use of HBO in ischaemic leg ulcers remains controversial. In a review article published in 2000, Wunderlich et al found very limited data to support the benefit of HBO in this situation. Only two prospective randomized trials were found, the larger of which enrolled only 68 patients. This study reported a benefit for HBO treatment only in the subset of patients with Wagner stage IV ulcers. Wunderlich et al (2000) concluded that further studies were necessary to determine the benefit of HBO and allow appropriate patient selection.

The difficulties raised by this review are important given the expense and potential for complications with HBO. Although reported protocols for treatment of ischaemic limb ulcers vary significantly, most involve 20–40 treatment sessions with a total cost of US$10 000–20 000. Significant side effects of treatment are uncommon but may be severe, including barotraumatic otitis, hyperoxic seizures and pneumothorax.

Since the publication of this review, several studies have focused on the use of transcutaneous oxygen tension ($tcPo_2$) as a predictive modality in selecting patients for HBO treatment. Grolman et al (2001) measured $tcPo_2$ in the ischaemic limb of 36 patients breathing room air, followed by 100% O_2. They found an increase of $tcPo_2$ in the ischaemic foot of more than 10 torr was associated with a healing rate of 70% compared to 11% in those with an increase of less than 10 torr. Others have reported that the improvement in foot $tcPo_2$ obtained during a trial session of HBO is also predictive of wound healing. In a larger study of ischaemic and non-ischaemic diabetic foot ulcers, Fife et al (2002) reported on the use of $tcPo_2$ in 1144 patients. Unfortunately, predictive values were relatively poor, with some patients healing despite low initial and in-chamber $tcPo_2$.

Currently, HBO should be an option available to the specialist caring for ischaemic diabetic foot ulcers. However, in practice, it is sometimes difficult for patients, particularly those in rural areas, to arrange daily transport to the HBO facility and comply with treatment protocols. Until larger randomized studies are performed, it cannot be recommended as a primary treatment for this patient group. But in selected cases, HBO may provide significant improvement, allowing healing of an ischaemic ulcer that appeared destined for amputation.

REVASCULARIZATION TECHNIQUES AND PATIENT ELIGIBILITY

Patient selection

When considering revascularization of the lower extremity, the patient may be considered for percutaneous endovascular techniques, including angioplasty or stent insertion, or surgical bypass procedures. Percutaneous techniques offer a less invasive method of improving blood supply when compared to surgery, but these techniques may be limited by extensive arterial disease, particularly in patients with diabetes and infrapopliteal involvement. Long-term patency is generally inferior to surgical reconstruction but, in many patients with limb ulcers, limited patency may allow temporary wound healing and limb salvage.

Conversely, surgical bypass procedures involve reconstruction of flow to the limb using autogenous vein or prosthetic materials. When possible, bypass offers the greatest potential for improvement in haemodynamic perfusion to the limb and intuitively should also offer the best chance for limb salvage. However, significant risks are involved in patients with comorbid conditions, including coronary artery disease and renal insufficiency. Therefore, surgical bypass should be offered only when necessary, and only to those patients healthy enough to benefit from this procedure.

Percutaneous endovascular revascularization

Once appropriate studies are performed, the sites of arterial obstruction are identified and revascularization can be considered. The most common sites of obstruction in non-diabetic patients are the iliac and femoral arteries, with less frequent involvement of the tibial vessels. In patients with diabetes mellitus, the iliac arteries are rarely involved, the femoral arteries more commonly, but the most common site of significant obstruction is in the tibial arteries. The pedal arteries are usually preserved and can function as recipients for bypass grafts in most cases (Fig. 17.8).

Percutaneous endovascular procedures usually employ angioplasty and stent insertion as minimally invasive methods of revascularization. In general, these techniques are better suited to larger arteries and areas of limited obstruction. An ideal arterial lesion for endovascular treatment, a short segment stenosis, is illustrated in Figure 17.9. The technical performance of endovascular revascularization requires guidewire-mediated recanalization of the lesion, usually performed percutaneously. Once the diseased artery is successfully crossed with a guidewire, treatment of the lesion can be performed using balloon angioplasty and stent insertion if

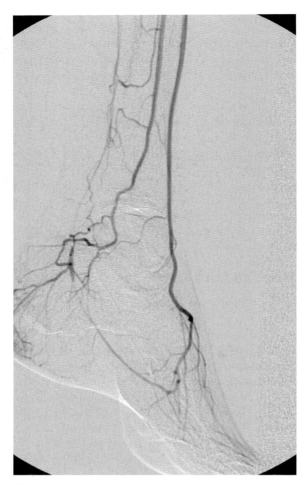

Figure 17.8 Percutaneous angiogram revealing detail of tibial and pedal arteries

required. After stent deployment, the reopened artery can be visualized with no residual stenosis. Most interventionists measure a pressure gradient across the lesion prior to treatment. A significant stenosis should result in a drop of pressure of greater than 5 mmHg below the lesion. Administration of vasodilating agents such as nitroglycerine or papaverine can assist in gradient identification. Successful treatment should result in resolution of the pressure gradient.

In longer segment lesions, or arterial occlusions (Fig. 17.10), it may be more difficult to gain guidewire access across the lesion to perform percutaneous revascularization. However, recanalization of these lesions using catheter directed hydrophilic guidewires and similar techniques has been reported, with 80–90% success rates (Gupta et al 1993).

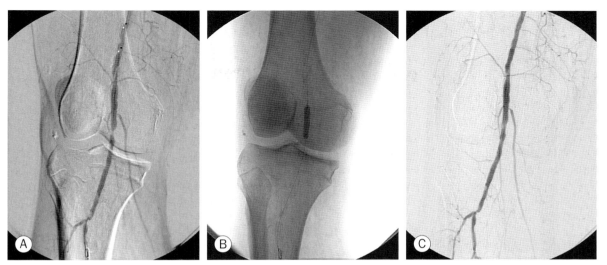

Figure 17.9 **A**. Arteriogram of arteries at the level of the knee revealing short-segment near-occlusive stenosis of the popliteal artery. **B**. Percutaneous balloon angioplasty catheter inflated in stenotic segment of popliteal artery. **C**. Postangioplasty popliteal artery arteriogram revealing improved calibre of arterial lumen

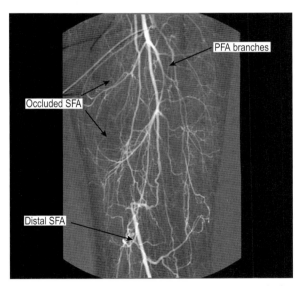

Figure 17.10 Arteriogram of femoral arteries in thigh reveals long-segment occlusion of superficial femoral artery. Large collaterals from deep femoral artery are seen supplying thigh muscle and reconstituting the popliteal artery

In a study of over 184 patients with iliac artery lesions, Henry et al (1995) reported 86% 3-year asymptomatic patency after iliac artery stent insertion. Patients who develop recurrent arterial stenosis can often undergo repeat intervention rather than requiring surgical revascularization. Other studies have reported similar or better results for percutaneous iliac artery revascularization. In some studies, external iliac lesions and longer-segment lesions had less favourable outcomes than common iliac and short-segment lesions (Johnston et al 1987). A low incidence of complications has been experienced with these procedures, mostly related to the percutaneous access site. Careful consideration of contrast nephropathy is required in patients with renal insufficiency. Given these results, endovascular procedures have become the treatment of choice for most patients with aortoiliac occlusive disease. An exception would be the younger patient with extensive disease, who may be better treated with an aortofemoral bypass procedure given the excellent long-term results with this procedure (80–90% 10-year graft patency).

In the femoral and popliteal arteries, angioplasty and stenting procedures may be performed, and have demonstrated reasonably good results for patients with stenotic lesions or short segment occlusions (<10 cm in length). Most interventionists have avoided treating the common femoral artery because of the aversion to placing stents in this vessel. The benefits of this method of revascularization for superficial femoral and popliteal lesions

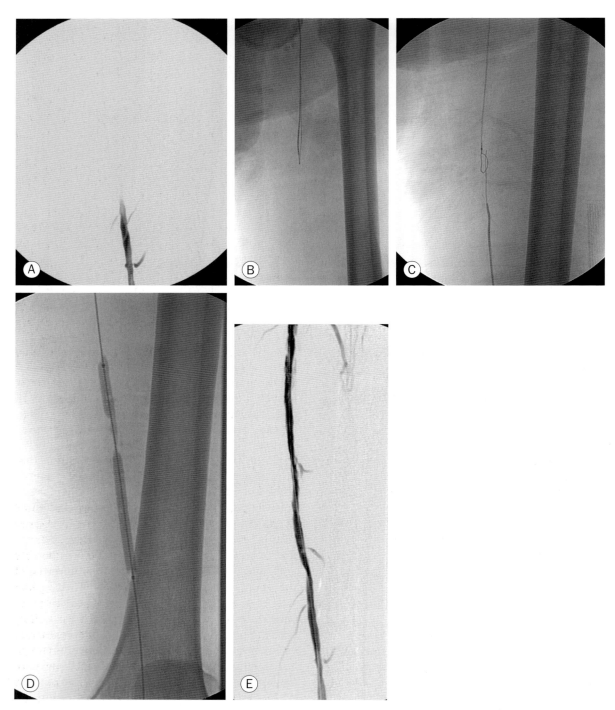

Figure 17.11   Percutaneous technique of subintimal recanalization of occluded arteries. **A.** Preprocedure angiogram of left femoral vessels revealing patent profunda femoral artery and occluded superficial femoral artery (SFA). **B.** Guidewire passage down subintimal layer of occluded SFA. **C.** Guidewire passage proximally from patent popliteal to midpoint of occluded SFA, allowing snare to grasp guidewire and complete recanalization of occluded SFA. **D.** Balloon angioplasty of recanalized SFA. **E.** Completion angiogram revealing reopened SFA after balloon angioplasty of entire artery.

compared to surgical bypass include low procedural risk and rapid resumption of activity after the procedure.

Karch et al (2000) reported an interesting review of 85 cases of femoropopliteal PTA in which the clinical outcome was correlated with anatomic outcome. The anatomic patency (ability of the treated artery segment to remain open without restenosis) was 74% at 1 year and 52% at 4 years. However, clinical success was somewhat lower, 69% at 1 year and 40% at 4 years, primarily as a result of progression of disease in untreated segments.

Although these results are somewhat less favourable than the results of surgical bypass, the reduced morbidity and ability to retreat many of the recurrent lesions percutaneously argues for an endovascular approach as the initial form of treatment in the femoropopliteal segments.

In patients with tibial artery disease, percutaneous revascularization has generally been discouraged because of poor results with angioplasty and stenting techniques. Mlekusch and colleagues reported a 52% arterial occlusion rate at 12 months (Mlekusch et al 2002). Also, in these vessels, disease is typically diffuse, extending through the majority of the length of the artery. More recently, techniques have been developed to address these lesions, particularly in patients poorly suited to surgical bypass because of severe medical comorbidity or when insufficient autogenous material (saphenous or arm vein) is available to perform surgical bypass. Numerous investigators have reported on revascularization of long-segment arterial occlusions using subintimal recanalization and subsequent angioplasty (Ingle et al 2002, Lipsitz et al 2003). This is employed when standard guidewire techniques are not able to cross an occluded artery. The subintimal space is then preferentially accessed with a directional catheter and guidewire, the lesion is crossed in this space and then the guidewire must be redirected to re-enter the lumen of the artery (Fig. 17.11). The artery can then be treated with angioplasty and stenting if recoil occurs after angioplasty. This technique is described in detail elsewhere.

Subintimal recanalization and angioplasty of infrainguinal arterial occlusions was reported in 39 patients by Lipsitz et al (2003). Subintimal recanalization was successful in 87% of cases.

Patency at 1 year in successfully treated cases was 74%. Significant haemodynamic improvement was documented, with the average ABPI increasing by 0.34. Complications occurred in two of 39 cases, both distal embolic events. Their conclusion was that these results merited an increasing role for subintimal recanalization and angioplasty in the treatment of limb threatening lower extremity ischaemia.

In another evaluation of percutaneous techniques of infrainguinal revascularization, Faglia et al reported on 221 patients with ischaemic limb ulcers (Faglia et al 2002). Percutaneous revascularization was performed in 85% of cases. Both ABPI and $tcPo_2$ were improved on average after intervention ($p < 0.0001$), and only 5.2% of patients required major amputation.

As experience increased with subintimal recanalization and other forms of percutaneous revascularization for distal arterial lesions, comparative analysis to surgical bypass will be more feasible. At this time, it appears that this technique is useful for patients who are poor candidates for surgical bypass but, in the absence of long term results, the treatment of choice for good candidates with adequate autogenous vein should remain surgical bypass for distal arterial disease.

Surgical revascularization

Surgical revascularization is optimally performed for patients who are reasonable medical candidates with lesions not amenable to percutaneous treatment. For patients with diabetes and ischaemic limb ulcers, lesions involve diffuse severe disease of the tibial vessels with reconstitution of the pedal arteries (Fig. 17.12). Despite advances in percutaneous treatment, including subintimal recanalization, many of these patients cannot be treated adequately, or will experience limited long-term patency from these procedures. The development of long leg bypasses to the pedal arteries has resulted in significant improvement in limb salvage in the diabetic population.

The treatment of extensive aortoiliac disease can be performed using aortofemoral bypass via a number of techniques. Femorofemoral bypass and axillofemoral bypass can be considered in

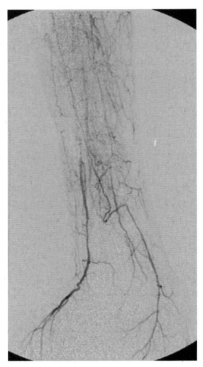

Figure 17.12 Typical angiogram of patient with diabetes and peripheral vascular disease revealing obstructed tibial arteries with preserved pedal arteries reconstituting at the ankle

Patients with lower extremity ischaemic ulcers typically have extensive disease, requiring bypass to tibial or pedal bypass. Although prosthetic bypass can be performed in these cases, results are inferior to autogenous vein bypass, so a search for the appropriate vein is performed carefully to find the best conduit. The great saphenous vein is the conduit of choice, and most surgeons will accept a vein that is no smaller than 3 mm throughout its length. Smaller veins may be inadequate and other veins are typically examined in this case, including the short saphenous and arm veins.

Once an appropriate conduit is located, the vein may be removed and reversed, to disable the valves, and sewn to a normal segment of artery above and below the obstructed limb artery. Alternatively, the vein may be left in situ, with the proximal and distal ends anastomosed to the recipient artery after disruption of the valves to allow flow distally in the vein (Fig. 17.13). Both techniques have

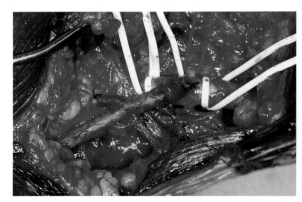

Figure 17.13 Proximal anastomosis of surgical vein graft bypass using the greater saphenous vein, which is connected to the common femoral artery in the groin.

higher-risk patients. Reported patency rates and complication rates for these procedures are listed in Table 17.2. In the majority of cases, percutaneous revascularization is preferred when possible, with surgical bypass reserved for failures and for young, otherwise healthy patients with a long life expectancy who will benefit from the excellent long-term patency of aorta-based bypass.

Table 17.2 Result ranges with surgical revascularization procedures for aortoiliac occlusive disease

Procedure	Peri-procedural mortality (%)	5-year patency (%)	10-year patency (%)	10-year survival (%)
Aortofemoral	2–3	85–90	70–75	40–50
Thoracofemoral	3.6	78	NA	NA
Femorofemoral	1–2	50–70	NA	NA
Axillofemoral	1–2	40–80	NA	NA

been reported to have good success rates, with no significant difference between the two. The risk of complications with lower extremity surgical bypass has been well documented. Perioperative myocardial infarction has been reported in 2–5% of cases, with mortality occurring in 1–3% of cases within 30 days of the procedure. More common, but less severe complications include wound healing problems, haematomas and nerve paraesthesias.

Surgical reconstruction to the tibial arteries has been documented to result in excellent graft patency and limb salvage rates. As outlined in Table 17.3, a variety of studies reported 5-year primary patency rates of 60–75% and limb salvage rates of 80–90%. The poor clinical status of this group of patients is reflected by the 5-year survival of 28–66% in this group of studies. Clearly, patients with sufficient peripheral vascular disease requiring revascularization require medical management to reduce their risk for myocardial infarction and death as a fundamental component of their treatment plan.

Prior to 1980, few patients with disease extending to the pedal arteries were offered surgical revascularization. For the diabetic patient with diabetes mellitus, the technique of pedal revascularization has significantly improved the potential for limb salvage. If arterial inflow is patent to the popliteal artery, a shorter bypass can be performed from the popliteal to pedal artery, requiring a shorter segment of quality vein. Brown et al found that progression of disease in the non-stenotic femoral artery proximal to the popliteal anastomosis rarely resulted in graft failure (Brown et al 1994).

Pomposelli and colleagues at the Beth Israel Deaconess Medical Center in Boston have published numerous studies on the performance and results of pedal artery bypass. In a recent review of over 1032 cases (92% with diabetes mellitus), the excellent outcomes with this procedure were detailed (Pomposelli et al 2003). All procedures were performed for rest pain or tissue loss, and autogenous vein was the conduit in all but two cases. Perioperative death occurred in 0.9% of cases, and 42 grafts failed within 1 month. Long-term graft patency was 57% at 5 years and 38% at 10 years. With graft salvage procedures, secondary graft patency was 63% at 5 years and 42% at 10 years. Limb salvage occurred in 78% of patients at 5 years and 58% at 10 years. Only 24% of patients undergoing pedal bypass were alive 10 years after surgery, attesting to the severe comorbid conditions present in this patient population. The authors concluded that these results justify the routine use of pedal arterial reconstruction for patients with CLI.

In cases requiring surgical bypass where quality autogenous vein is unavailable, other options may be considered, including prosthetic vein and cryopreserved saphenous vein. Although results with these conduits are significantly inferior to those obtained with autogenous vein, these conduits may allow sufficient patency for the ulcer to heal. Later graft occlusion may not result in recurrent ulceration, with careful foot care and protective footwear.

Once revascularization has been performed, through either endovascular techniques or surgical bypass, the limb should be evaluated again with Doppler ultrasound and ABPI. It is important that

Table 17.3 Results of selected reports of tibial and pedal revascularization for infrageniculate arterial occlusive disease

Study	No. limbs	Conduit	Primary patency at 4–5 years (%)	Limb salvage at 4–5 years (%)
Andros et al 1998	224	Vein	40	71
Klamer et al 1990	68	Vein	81	95
Shah et al 1992	270	Vein	61	89
Harrington et al 1992	73	Vein	50	74
Quinones-Baldrich et al 1992	28	PTFE	22	NA
Veith et al 1986	98	PTFE	12	NA

the ABPI, toe pressure or transcutaneous Po_2 in the foot improves after revascularization, indicating that the procedure has been a haemodynamic success. The ABPI should improve by at least 0.15, and the toe pressure or $tcPo_2$ by 20 mmHg to be considered a significant haemodynamic improvement. If no improvement is seen, the graft or angioplasty site should be examined with an imaging study to determine if a problem can be corrected to improve vascular supply. Alternately, another revascularization can be considered, such as a bypass procedure if angioplasty has been unsuccessful.

Surveillance of patients undergoing limb revascularization

After bypass procedures for limb salvage, it is critically important to perform routine graft surveillance with Duplex ultrasound. Numerous studies have found that graft surveillance allows identification of graft problems prior to thrombosis. These graft problems, usually stenosis at a valve cusp or an anastomosis, to be corrected with angioplasty or limited surgery, markedly improving long-term patency and limb salvage. Grafts that thrombose have significantly lower long-term patency, even if graft salvage is possible. A typical graft surveillance protocol calls for Duplex examination every 3 months for the first year, then at 6 month intervals for 2 years, then yearly if the graft has no problems. Graft velocities are measured throughout the graft, looking for focal increases in velocity, indicative of an area of narrowing. Most surgeons consider a focal graft velocity increase of greater than 3.5 times to be associated with a significant risk of graft thrombosis, and would recommend intervention for correction (Mills et al 2001). Also, unusually low graft velocities would indicate a potential problem requiring further investigation. Using these criteria, Westerband and colleagues (1997) were able to significantly reduce their incidence of graft thrombosis in patients who were compliant with graft surveillance, resulting in high graft patency and limb salvage rates.

Some interventionists performing angioplasty, stenting, and other endovascular procedures for lower limb revascularization have also recommended Duplex surveillance for follow-up. However the criteria for re-intervention, and outcomes have been less well-researched for surveillance in these procedures.

Wound management after intervention

Management of the ischaemic limb ulcer after revascularization is critical, because of changes in the local environment that occur with new blood supply. Limb oedema after surgical bypass is common and may be severe, resulting in breakdown of surgical incisions and worsening of ulcerated areas. Many vascular surgeons have been reluctant to apply compression to limbs soon after bypass procedures, fearing that the compression may increase the risk for acute graft thrombosis. Numerous options exist in this situation. While limb elevation may provide some improvement, this is often impractical and limits the patient's postoperative recovery, increasing the risk for inactivity-related complications such as pneumonia and venous thrombosis.

IPC devices are very useful for limiting limb oedema in the early postoperative period. For patients with bypass grafts ending at the popliteal level, below-knee IPC for several hours a day will reduce oedema significantly. When the distal anastomosis extends to the lower leg and ankle, a pedal compression boot can be used, with reasonably good results. Application of moderate-strength compression bandaging is not unreasonable after the first few days, as it is unlikely that 20–30 mmHg of external compression will hinder a graft that is otherwise normal. There have been few studies examining this area, so the ultimate goal should be to control oedema with the minimum amount of compression necessary for each patient.

Patients with dry gangrene of digits, or eschar over the heel or other ulcerated areas, must be followed closely after revascularization. When blood supply is successfully restored, these areas tend to begin to heal under the eschar, and the eschar begins to separate at the interface between healing and necrotic tissue. Unfortunately, this is a favourable environment for infection, and it is common for these to develop an increased bacterial load and frank infection if frequent debridement and careful wound management are not continued. We recommend aggressive surgical debridement as often as necessary to remove separating eschar and non-viable material. Enzymatic topicals are less useful in this situation because of the time required for their effect. Topical antibiotic dressings such as silver eluting dressings are often good choices for these wounds. Many surgeons prefer to perform amputation of necrotic digits and wide debridement of eschar a few days after arterial supply is improved, to prevent further infection. After debridement, the remaining healthy tissue should be able to granulate, responding to standard wound healing techniques.

SUMMARY

Patients with significant arterial insufficiency and chronic lower extremity ulcers are at high risk of limb loss. Although it is generally recommended that revascularization be performed to stimulate healing, many patients will heal with meticulous wound care even when revascularization cannot be performed. Percutaneous procedures are gaining an increasing importance as techniques such as subintimal recanalization are allowing revascularization of smaller popliteal and tibial arteries with improving results. Surgical bypass remains the optimal long-term method of limb revascularization and has been associated with excellent limb salvage rates.

Numerous adjunctive modalities have been developed to assist in the healing of ischaemic wounds. Most have few randomized data supporting their use. Cilostazol and several growth factor preparations are currently being tested in clinical trials to determine whether they can stimulate healing in ischaemic leg ulcers. Intermittent pneumatic compression and HBO also appear to be promising modalities and both require further randomized testing to firmly document their benefit in wound healing and limb salvage.

References

Abidia A, Kuhan G, Bahia H et al 2001. Microvascular reflexes are influenced by oxygen in diabetic patients with peripheral arterial disease. British Journal of Surgery 88: 749

Abu-Own A, Cheatle T, Scurr J H et al 1993. Effects of intermittent pneumatic compression of the foot on the microcirculatory function in arterial disease. European Journal of Vascular Surgery 7: 488–492

Altstaedt H O, Berzewski B, Breddin H K et al 1993 Treatment of patients with peripheral arterial occlusive disease Fontaine stage IV with intravenous iloprost and PGE1: a randomized open controlled study. Prostaglandins Leukotrienes and Essential Fatty Acids 49: 573–578

Andros G, Harris R W, Salles-Cunyha S X et al 1998 Bypass grafts to the ankle and foot. Journal of Vascular Surgery 7: 785–794

Anonymous 1991a Treatment of limb threatening ischaemia with intravenous iloprost: a randomized double-blind placebo controlled study. UK Severe Limb Ischaemia Study Group. European Journal of Vascular Surgery 5: 511–516

Anonymous 1991b The effect of ciprostene in patients with peripheral vascular disease (PVD) characterized by ischemic ulcers. The Ciprostene Study Group. Journal of Clinical Pharmacology 31: 81–8

Anonymous 2000 Two randomized and placebo-controlled studies of an oral prostacyclin analog (Iloprost) in severe leg ischaemia. The Oral Iloprost in Severe Leg Ischaemia Study Group. European Journal of Vascular and Endovascular Surgery 20: 358–362

Arakawa K, Arada J 1993 Clinical analysis of Pletal for intractable skin ulcer based on vascular damage and cutis symptom. Shinyaku to Rinsho (Journal of New Remedies and Clinics) 42: 60–68

Brock F E, Abri O, Baitsch G et al 1990 Iloprost in the treatment of ischemic tissue lesions in diabetics: results of a placebo-controlled multicenter with a stable prostacyclin derivative. Schweizerische Medizinische Wochenschrift 120: 1477–1482

Brown P S Jr, McCarthy W J, Yao J S et al 1994 The popliteal artery as inflow for distal bypass grafting. Archives of Surgery 129: 596–602

Claeys L G 1997 Improvement of microcirculatory blood flow under epidural spinal cord stimulation in patients with nonreconstructible peripheral arterial occlusive disease. Artificial Organs 21: 201–206

Claeys L G, Horsch S 1996. Transcutaneous oxygen pressure as predictive parameter for ulcer healing in endstage vascular patients treated with spinal cord stimulation. International Angiology 15: 344–349

Comerota A J, Throm R C, Miller K A et al 2002 Naked plasmid DNA encoding fibroblast growth factor type 1 for the treatment of end-stage unreconstructible lower extremity ischemia: preliminary results of a phase 1 trial. Journal of Vascular Surgery 35: 930–936

Dawson D L, Cutler B S, Meissner M H et al 1998 Cilostazol has beneficial effects in treatment of intermittent claudication: results from a multicenter, randomized, prospective, double-blind trial. Circulation 98: 678–686

Dawson D L, Cutler B S, Hiatt W R et al 2000 A comparison of cilostazol and pentoxifylline for treating intermittent claudication. American Journal of Medicine 109: 523–530

Delis K T, Nicolaides A N, Labropoulos N et al 2000a The acute effects of intermittent pneumatic foot versus calf versus simultaneous foot and calf compression on popliteal artery hemodynamics: a comparative study. Journal of Vascular Surgery 32: 284–292

Delis K T, Nicolaides A N, Wolfe J H et al 2000b Improving walking ability and ankle brachial pressure indices in symptomatic peripheral vascular disease with intermittent pneumatic foot compression: a prospective controlled study with one-year follow-up. Journal of Vascular Surgery 31: 650–661

Delis K T, Husmann M W, Cheshire N J et al 2001 Effects of intermittent pneumatic compression of the calf and thigh on arterial calf inflow: a study of normals, claudicants, and grafted arteriopaths. Surgery 129: 188–195

Dettelbach H R, Aviado D M 1985 Clinical pharmacology of pentoxifylline with special reference to its hemorheologic effect for the treatment of intermittent claudication. Journal of Clinical Pharmacology 25: 8–26

Diehm C, Abri O, Baitsch G et al 1989 Iloprost, a stable prostacyclin derivative in stage 4 arterial occlusive disease. A placebo-controlled multicenter study. Deutsche Medizinische Wochenschrift 114: 783–788

Dormandy J A, Rutherford R B (chairmen) 2000a TransAtlantic Inter-Society Consensus, management of peripheral arterial disease. Journal of Vascular Surgery 31: S265–S266

Dormandy J A, Rutherford R B (chairmen) 2000b TransAtlantic Inter-Society consensus, management of peripheral arterial disease. Journal of Vascular Surgery 31: S197–S199

Faglia E, Mantero M, Caminiti M et al 2002 Extensive use of peripheral angioplasty, particularly infrapopliteal, in the treatment of ischaemic diabetic foot ulcers: clinical results of a multicentric study of 221 consecutive diabetic subjects. Journal of Internal Medicine 225–232

Falanga V, Fujitani R M, Diaz C et al 1999 Systemic treatment of venous leg ulcers with high doses of pentoxifylline: efficacy in a randomized, placebo-controlled trial. Wound Repair and Regeneration 7: 208–213

Fife C E, Buyukcakir C, Otto G H et al 2002 The predictive value of transcutaneous oxygen tension measurement in diabetic lower extremity ulcers treated with hyperbaric oxygen therapy: a retrospective analysis of 1144 patients. Wound Repair and Regeneration 10: 198–207

Freedman G, Entero H, Brem 2004 H Practical treatment of pain in patients with chronic wounds: pathogenesis-guided management. American Journal of Surgery 1A(Suppl): 31–35

Fulton R L, Blakeley W R 1968 Lumbar sympathectomy: a procedure of questionable value in the treatment of arteriosclerosis obliterans of the legs. American Journal of Surgery 116: 735–744

Gaskell P, Parrott J C V 1978 The effect of a mechanical venous pump on the circulation of the feet in the presence of arterial obstruction. Journal of Surgery, Gynecology and Obstetrics 16: 538–592

Goldman R, Brewley B, Zhou L et al 2003 Electrotherapy reverses inframalleolar ischemia: a retrospective, observational study. Advances in Skin and Wound Care 16: 79–89

Gowdak L H, Poliakova L, Li Z et al 2000 Induction of angiogenesis by cationic lipid-mediated VEGF165 gene transfer in the rabbit ischemic hindlimb model. Journal of Vascular Surgery 32: 343–352

Grolman R E, Wilkerson D K, Taylor J et al 2001 Transcutaneous oxygen measurements predict a beneficial response to hyperbaric oxygen therapy in patients with nonhealing wounds and critical limb ischemia. American Surgeon 67: 1072–1080

Gupta A K, Ravimandalam K, Rao V R et al 1993 Total occlusion of iliac arteries: results of balloon angioplasty. Cardiovascular and Interventional Radiology 16: 165–177

Harrington E B, Harrington M E, Schanzer H et al 1992 The dorsalis pedis bypass – moderate success in difficult situations. Journal of Vascular Surgery 15: 409–414; discussion 415–416

Henry M, Amor M, Ethevenot G et al 1995 Palmaz stent placement in iliac and femoropopliteal arteries: primary and secondary patency in 310 patients with 2–4-year follow-up. Radiology 197: 167–174

Holiday F A, Barendregt W B, Slappendel R, Crul B J et al 1999 Lumbar sympathectomy in critical limb ischaemia: surgical, chemical or not at all? Cardiovascular Surgery 7: 2002

Horsch S, Claeys L 1994 Epidural spinal cord stimulation in the treatment of severe peripheral arterial occlusive disease. Annals of Vascular Surgery 8: 468–474

Ingle H, Nasim A, Fishwick G et al 2002 Subintimal angioplasty of isolated infragenicular vessels in lower limb ischemia: long-term results. Journal of Endovascular Therapy 9: 411–416

Johnston K W, Rae M, Hogg-Johnston S A et al 1987 5-year results of a prospective study of percutaneous transluminal angioplasty. Annals of Surgery 206: 403–413

Jorneskog G, Brismar K, Fagrell B 1993 Low molecular weight heparin seems to improve local capillary circulation and healing of chronic foot ulcers in diabetic patients. Vasa 2: 137–142

Jull A B, Waters J, Arroll B 2002 Pentoxifylline for treating venous leg ulcers. In: Cochrane Database of Systatic Reviews: CD001733. Update Software, Oxford

Kalani M, Apelqvist J, Blomback M et al 2003 Effect of dalteparin on healing of chronic foot ulcers in diabetic patients with peripheral arterial occlusive disease. A prospective, randomized, double-blind, placebo-controlled study. Diabetes Care 26: 2575–2580

Karch L A, Mattos M A, Henretta J P et al 2000 Clinical failure after percutaneous transluminal angioplasty of the superficial femoral and popliteal arteries. Journal of Vascular Surgery 31: 880–887

Klamer T W, Lambert G E Jr, Richardson J D et al 1990 Utility of inframalleolar arterial bypass grafting. Journal of Vascular Surgery 11: 164–169; discussion 169–170

Knighton D R, Silver I A, Hunt T K 1981 Regulation of wound-healing angiogenesis: effect of oxygen gradients and inspired oxygen concentration. Surgery 90: 262–270

Labropoulos N, Watson W C, Mansour M A et al 1998 Acute effects of intermittent pneumatic compression on popliteal artery blood flow. Archives of Surgery 133: 1072–1075

Lipsitz E C, Ohki T, Veith F J et al 2003 Does subintimal angioplasty have a role in the treatment of severe lower extremity ischemia? Journal of Vascular Surgery 37: 386–391

Louridas G, Sadia R, Spelay J et al 2002 The ArtAssist device in chronic lower limb ischemia. A pilot study. International Angiology 21: 28–35

Lowe G D O 1990 Pathophysiology of critical limb ischemia. In: Dormandy J, Stock G (eds) Critical leg ischemia: its pathophysiology and management. Springer Verlag, Berlin, pp 17–38

McCulloch S V, Marston W A, Farber M A et al 2003 Healing potential of lower-extremity ulcers in patients with arterial insufficiency with and without revascularization. Wounds 15: 390–394

Marston W A, Carlin R E, Passman M A et al 1999 Healing rates and cost efficacy of outpatient compression treatment for leg ulcers associated with venous insufficiency. Journal of Vascular Surgery 30: 491–498

Mendes R R, Marston W A, Fulton J J 2004 Outcome of conservative treatment of lower extremity ulcers associated with arterial insufficiency: when is revascularization necessary? Abstract presented at 2nd World Union of Wound Healing Societies Meeting, Paris, France

Mills J L Sr, Wixon C L, James D C et al 2001 The natural history of intermediate and critical vein graft stenosis: recommendations for continued surveillance or repair. Journal of Vascular Surgery 33: 273–278

Mlekusch W, Schillinger M, Sabeti S et al 2002 Clinical outcome and prognostic factors for ischaemic ulcers treated with PTA in lower limbs. European Journal of Vascular and Endovascular Surgery 24: 176–181

Morris R J, Woodcock J P 2002 Effects of supine intermittent compression on arterial inflow to the lower limb. Archives of Surgery 137: 1269–1273

Norgren L, Alwmark A, Angqvist K A et al 1990 A stable prostacyclin analogue (iloprost) in the treatment of ischaemic ulcers of the lower limb. A Scandinavian–Polish placebo controlled, randomized multicenter study. European Journal of Vascular Surgery 4: 463–467

Persson A V, Anderson L A, Padberg F T 1985 Selection of patients for lumbar sympathectomy. Surgical Clinics of North America 65: 393–403

Peters E J, Armstrong D G, Wunderlich R P et al 1998 The benefit of electrical stimulation to enhance perfusion in persons with diabetes mellitus. Journal of Foot and Ankle Surgery 37: 396–400

Pomposelli F B, Kansal N, Hamdan A D et al 2003 A decade of experience with dorsalis pedis artery bypass: analysis of outcome in more than 1000 cases. Journal of Vascular Surgery 37: 307–315

Porter J M, Cutler B S, Lee B Y et al 1982 Pentoxifylline efficacy in the treatment of intermittent claudication: multicenter controlled double-blind trial with objective assessment of chronic occlusive arterial disease patients. American Heart Journal 104: 66–72

Quinones-Baldrich W J, Prego A A, Ucelay-Gomez R et al 1992 Long-term results of infrainguinal revascularization with polytetrafluoroethylene: a ten-year experience. Journal of Vascular Surgery 16: 207–217

Rajagopalan S, Shah M, Luciano A et al 2001 Adenovirus-mediated gene transfer of $VEGF_{121}$ improves lower extremity endothelial function and flow reserve. Circulation 104: 753–755

Rajagopalan S, Mohler E R, Lederman R J et al 2003 Regional angiogenesis with vascular endothelial growth factor in peripheral arterial disease. A phase II randomized, double-blind, controlled study of adenoviral delivery of vascular endothelial growth factor 121 in patients with disabling intermittent claudication. Circulation 108: 1933–1938

Repelaer van Driel O J, van Bockel J H, van Schilfgaarde R 1988 Lumbar sympathectomy for severe lower limb ischaemia: results and analysis of factors influencing the outcome. Journal of Cardiovascular Surgery (Torino) 29: 310–314

Rooke T W, Osmundson P J 1988 Effect of intermittent venous occlusion on transcutaneous oxygen tension in lower limbs with severe arterial occlusive disease. International Journal of Cardiology 21: 76–78

Schultz G S, Sibbald R G, Falanga V, Ayello E A, Dowsett C et al 2003 Wound bed preparation: a systematic approach to wound management. Wound Repair and Regeneration 11(Suppl 1): S1–S28

Shah DM, Darling RC III, Chang BB et al 1992 Is long vein bypass from groin to ankle a durable procedure? An analysis of a ten-year experience. Journal of Vascular Surgery 15: 402–408

Smiell J M, Wieman T J, Steed D L et al 1999 Efficacy and safety of becaplermin (recombinant human platelet-derived growth factor-BB) in patients with non healing, lower extremity diabetic ulcers: a combined analysis of four randomized studies. Wound Repair and Regeneration 7: 335–346

Spincemaille G H, Klomp H M, Steyerberg E W et al 2000 Technical data and complications of spinal cord stimulation: data from a randomized trial on critical limb ischemia. Stereotactic and Functional Neurosurgery 74: 63–72

Staben P, Albring M 1996 Treatment of patients with peripheral arterial occlusive disease Fontaine stage III and IV with intravenous iloprost: an open study in 900 patients. Prostaglandins, Leukotrienes and Essential Fatty Acids 54: 327–333

Telles G S, Campbell W B, Wood R F et al 1984 Prostaglandin E1 in severe lower limb ischaemia: a double-blind controlled trial. British Journal of Surgery 71: 506–508

Trubestein G, von Bary S, Breddin K et al 1989 Intravenous prostaglandin E1 versus pentoxifylline therapy in chronic arterial occlusive disease: a controlled randomized multicenter study. Vasa Supplementum 28: 44–49

Ubbink D T, Vermeulen H 2003 Spinal cord stimulation for non-reconstructable chronic critical leg ischaemia (Cochrane Methodology Review). In: The Cochrane Library. John Wiley & Sons, Chichester

Ubbink D T, Spincemaille G H, Prins M H et al 1999 Microcirculatory investigations to determine the effect of spinal cord stimulation for critical leg ischemia: the Dutch multicenter randomized controlled trial. Journal of Vascular Surgery 30: 236–244

Vale P R, Isner J M, Rosenfield K 2001 Therapeutic angiogenesis in critical limb and myocardial ischemia. Journal of Interventional Cardiology 14: 511–528

Van Bemmelen P S, Weiss-Olmanni J, Ricotta J J 2000 Rapid intermittent compression increases skin circulation in chronically ischemic legs with infra-popliteal arterial obstruction. Vasa 29: 47–52

Van Bemmelen P S, Gitlitz D B, Faruqi R M et al 2001 Limb salvage using high-pressure intermittent compression arterial assist device in cases unsuitable for surgical revascularization. Archives of Surgery 136: 1280–1285

Van Bemmelen P, Char D, Giron F et al 2003 Angiographic improvement after rapid intermittent compression treatment (ArtAssist) for small vessel obstruction. Annals of Vascular Surgery 17: 224–228

Veith F J, Gupta S K, Ascer E et al 1986 Six-year prospective multicenter randomized comparison of autologous saphenous vein and expanded polytetrafluoroethylene grafts in infrainguinal arterial reconstructions. Journal of Vascular Surgery 3: 104–114

Vella A, Carlson L, Blier B et al 2000 Circulator boot therapy alters the natural history of ischemic limb ulceration. Vascular Medicine 5: 21–25

Westerband A, Mills J L, Kistler S et al 1997 Prospective validation of threshold criteria for intervention in infrainguinal vein grafts undergoing duplex surveillance. Annals of Vascular Surgery 11: 44–48

Wunderlich R P, Peters E J, Lavery L A 2000 Systemic hyperbaric oxygen therapy: lower-extremity wound healing and the diabetic foot. Diabetes Care 23: 1551–1555

The diabetic foot

Mike Edmonds

INTRODUCTION

Over the last 20 years there has been considerable progress in the care of the diabetic foot. There is an increased limb survival rate in patients attending multidisciplinary clinics. This has resulted from advances in the care of the neuropathic foot and of the neuroischaemic foot and also from advances in the management of infection.

There has been increased interest in the diabetic foot resulting in guidelines (Pinzur et al 1999) and consensus development (International Working Group on the Diabetic Foot 2003, American Diabetes Association 1999). These reports have stressed the importance of early recognition of the at risk foot, the prompt institution of preventive measures and the provision of rapid and intensive treatment of foot infection in multidisciplinary foot clinics. Such measures can reduce the number of amputations in diabetic patients. Reports from Sweden (Larson et al 1995), Denmark (Holstein et al 2000), Italy (Faglia et al 1998) and the UK (Edmonds & Foster 2001) have shown a reduction in major amputations.

This chapter outlines a simple classification of the diabetic foot into the neuropathic and neuroischaemic foot and then describes a simple staging system of the natural history of the diabetic foot and a treatment plan for each stage, within a multidisciplinary framework (Edmonds & Foster 2000). Successful management of the diabetic foot needs the expertise of a multidisciplinary team, which should include physician, podiatrist, nurse, orthotist, radiologist and surgeon working closely together, within the focus of a diabetic foot clinic.

CLASSIFICATION

An important prelude to proper management of the diabetic foot is the correct diagnosis of its two main syndromes: the neuropathic foot, in which neuropathy predominates but the major arterial supply to the foot is intact, and the neuroischaemic foot, where both neuropathy and ischaemia resulting from a reduced arterial supply, contribute to the clinical presentation (Edmonds & Foster 1994; Fig. 18.1).

The significance of structural abnormalities of the skin microcirculation is not fully understood, although there are numerous functional abnormalities that may be important. These include increased blood flow, widespread vascular dilation, increased vascular permeability, impaired vascular activity and limitation of hyperaemia (Flynn 1999).

Infection is rarely a sole factor but often complicates neuropathy and ischaemia and is responsible for considerable tissue necrosis in the diabetic patient. In diabetes, deficiencies in neutrophil chemotaxis, phagocytosis, superoxide production, respiratory burst activity and intracellular killing have all been described (Johnston 1997).

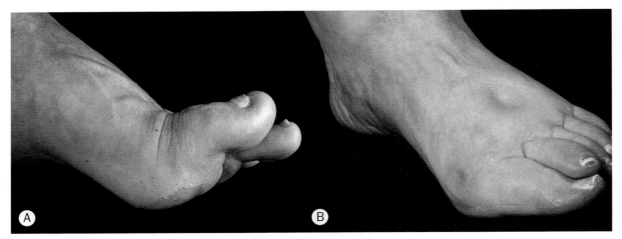

Figure 18.1 (**A**) Neuropathic foot (**B**) Neuroischaemic foot

Neuropathic foot

This is a warm, well perfused foot with sensory deficit and autonomic dysfunction leading to arteriovenous shunting and distended dorsal veins. Peripheral autosympathectomy damages the neurogenic control mechanisms that regulate capillary and arteriovenous shunt flow and loss of precapillary vasoconstriction (Flynn 1999). The pulses are palpable. Sweating is diminished and the skin may be dry and prone to fissuring. Motor neuropathy also plays a role, with paralysis of the small muscles contributing to structural deformities such as a high arch and claw toes. This leads to prominence of the metatarsal heads. It has two main complications, the neuropathic ulcer and the neuropathic (Charcot) foot.

Neuroischaemic foot

This is a cool, pulseless foot with poor perfusion. It also has neuropathy. Ischaemia results from atherosclerosis of the leg vessels. This is often bilateral, multisegmental and distal, involving arteries below the knee. Intermittent claudication and rest pain may be absent because of coexisting neuropathy and the distal distribution of the arterial disease to the leg. Ulcers in the neuroischaemic foot develop on margins of the foot at sites made vulnerable by underlying ischaemia to moderate but continuous pressure, often from poorly fitting shoes.

THE NATURAL HISTORY OF THE DIABETIC FOOT

The natural history of the diabetic foot can be divided into six stages (Edmonds & Foster 2000):

1. *The foot is normal and not at risk*: Patients do not have the risk factors that render them vulnerable to foot ulcers – these are neuropathy, ischaemia, deformity, callus and oedema.
2. *High risk foot*: The patient has developed one or more of the risk factors for ulceration of the foot.
3. *Foot with ulcer*: Ulceration is on the plantar surface in the neuropathic foot and on the margin in the neuroischaemic foot (Fig. 18.2).
4. *Foot with cellulitis*: The ulcer has developed infection with the presence of cellulitis, which can complicate both the neuropathic and the neuroischaemic foot (Fig. 18.3a).
5. *Foot with necrosis*: In the neuropathic foot, infection is usually the cause. In the neuroischaemic foot, infection is still the most common reason, although severe ischaemia can directly lead to necrosis (Fig. 18.3b).
6. *The foot cannot be saved and will need a major amputation.*

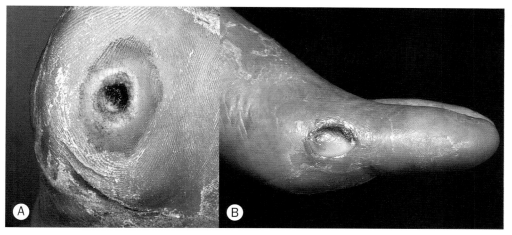

Figure 18.2 (**A**) Neuropathic ulcer (**B**) Neuroischaemic ulcer

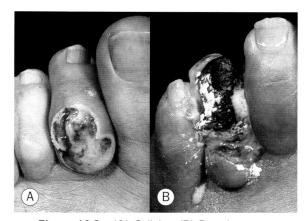

Figure 18.3 (**A**) Cellulitis (**B**) Digital necrosis

Every diabetic patient can be placed into one of these stages and the appropriate management then carried out, as described below. In stages 1 and 2, the emphasis is on prevention of ulceration. In stage 3 the presentation and management of foot ulceration is discussed. Finally, stages 4 and 5 address complications of foot ulceration, notably cellulitis and necrosis.

THE PRESENTATION, ASSESSMENT AND MANAGEMENT OF THE DIABETIC FOOT, STAGE BY STAGE

At each of the six stages described above it is necessary to take 'control' to prevent further progression of diabetic foot disease and management is considered under the following headings:

- Wound control
- Microbiological control
- Mechanical control
- Vascular control
- Metabolic control
- Educational control.

Metabolic control is important at every stage. Tight control of blood glucose, blood pressure and blood cholesterol and triglycerides should be followed to preserve neurological and cardiovascular function. Advice should be given to stop smoking. In stages 4 and 5, considerable metabolic decompensation may occur in the presence of infection, and full metabolic resuscitation is often required (Edmonds & Foster 2000).

STAGE 1: THE NORMAL FOOT

Presentation and assessment

By definition, the foot does not have the risk factors for foot ulcers: neuropathy, ischaemia, deformity, callus and swelling, and the diagnosis of stage 1 is made by screening patients and excluding these five risk factors.

Neuropathy

A simple technique for detecting patients with loss of protective pain sensation is to use a nylon monofilament, which, when applied perpendicular to the foot, buckles at a given force of 10 g. The filament should be pressed against several sites, including the plantar aspect of the first toe, the first, third and fifth metatarsal heads, the plantar surface of the heel and the dorsum of the foot. The filament should not be applied at any site until callus has been removed. If the patient cannot feel the filament at any of these tested areas, then significant neuropathy is present and protective pain sensation is lost (Rith-Najarian et al 1992).

Ischaemia
The most important manoeuvre to detect ischaemia is the palpation of the foot pulses – the dorsalis pedis pulse and the posterior tibial pulse. If either of these foot pulses can be felt then it is highly unlikely that there is significant ischaemia. A small hand-held Doppler can be used to confirm the presence of pulses and to calculate the pressure index, which is the ratio of ankle systolic pressure to brachial systolic pressure. In normal subjects, the pressure index is usually more than 1 but in the presence of ischaemia it is less than 1. Thus, absence of pulses and a pressure index of less than 1 confirms ischaemia. Conversely, the presence of pulses and a pressure index of more than 1 rules out ischaemia and further vascular investigations are not necessary. However, many diabetic patients have medial arterial calcification, giving an artificially elevated systolic pressure even in the presence of ischaemia. It is thus difficult to assess the diabetic foot when the pulses are not palpable but the pressure index is more than 1. It is then necessary to use other methods to assess flow in the arteries of the foot, such as examining the pattern of the Doppler arterial waveform or measuring transcutaneous oxygen tension or toe systolic pressures (Hurley et al 1993).

Deformity
Deformity often leads to bony prominences, which are associated with high mechanical pressures on the overlying skin. This leads to ulceration, particularly in the absence of protective pain sensation and when shoes are unsuitable. Common deformities are claw toes, pes cavus, hallux valgus, hallux rigidus, hammer toe and nail deformities, and Charcot foot (see below).

Callus
This is a thickened areas of epidermis that develops at sites of high pressure and friction. It should not be allowed to become excessive as this can be a forerunner of ulceration in the presence of neuropathy.

Oedema
Oedema is a major factor predisposing to ulceration by reducing skin oxygenation. It often exacerbates a tight fit inside poorly fitting shoes.

Management
This stage, by definition does not have any evidence of skin breakdown or ischaemia. However, mechanical and educational control are important to prevent development of ulceration.

Mechanical control
Mechanical control is based upon wearing sensible footwear. Shoes should have broad, rounded or square toes, adequate toe depth, low heels to avoid excessive toe pressure on the forefoot and lace up, Velcro or buckle straps to prevent movement within the shoe (Tovey 1984).

Educational control
Advice on basic foot care, including nail-cutting techniques, the treatment of minor injuries and the purchase of shoes, should be given. Educational programmes involving behavioural contracts and organizational intervention for health-care providers have shown a significant reduction in foot ulceration at 1-year follow-up (Litzelman et al 1993).

STAGE 2: THE HIGH RISK FOOT
Presentation and assessment
The foot has developed one or more of the risk factors for ulceration: neuropathy, ischaemia, deformity, callus and oedema. It is important to detect these by a regular screening examination. Referral of such patients at risk to a multidisciplinary programme of care has been shown to reduce amputations (McCabe et al 1998).

Management
Mechanical, vascular and educational control are important.

Mechanical control

Deformity must be accommodated and callus, dry skin, fissures and oedema must be treated.

Deformities   Deformities in the neuropathic foot tend to render the plantar surface vulnerable to ulcers, requiring special insoles, whereas, in the neuroischaemic foot, the margins need protection and appropriately wide shoes should therefore be advised.

  Footwear can be divided into three broad types: sensible shoes (from high street shops) for patients with minimal sensory loss, ready-made stock (off the shelf) shoes for neuroischaemic feet that need protection along the margins of the foot but are not greatly deformed, and customized or bespoke (made to measure) shoes containing cradled, cushioned insoles. These are necessary to redistribute the high pressures on the plantar surface of the neuropathic foot.

Callus   Patients should never cut their callus off or use callus removers. It should be removed regularly by sharp debridement.

Dry skin and fissures   Dry skin should be treated with an emollient such as E45 cream or Calmurid cream.

Oedema   Oedema may complicate both the neuropathic and the neuroischaemic foot. Its main cause will be impaired cardiac and renal function, which should be treated accordingly. Oedema may rarely be secondary to neuropathy. It responds to ephedrine, starting at a dose of 10 mg three times daily and increasing up to 30–60 mg three times daily.

Vascular control

Patients with absent foot pulses should have the pressure index measured to confirm ischaemia and to provide a baseline, so that subsequent deterioration can be detected. If the patient has rest pain, disabling claudication or a pressure index below 0.5, then they already have severe ischaemia and should be referred for a vascular opinion. All diabetic patients with evidence of peripheral vascular disease may benefit from antiplatelet agents: 75 mg aspirin daily or, if this cannot be tolerated, clopidogrel 75 mg daily.

Educational control

Patients have lost protective pain sensation and therefore need advice to protect their feet from mechanical, thermal and chemical trauma. They should establish a habit of regular inspection of the feet so that problems can be detected quickly and they seek help early.

Charcot foot

The term Charcot foot refers to bone and joint destruction that occurs in the neuropathic foot (Sanders & Frykberg 1991). It can be divided into three phases:

1. Acute onset
2. Bony destruction/deformity
3. Stabilization.

Acute onset
The foot presents with unilateral erythema, warmth and oedema. There may be a history of minor trauma. About 30% of patients complain of pain or discomfort. X-ray at this time may be normal. However, a technetium-99m diphosphonate bone scan will detect early evidence of bony destruction. Cellulitis, gout and deep vein thrombosis may masquerade as a Charcot foot. Initially the foot is immobilized in a non-weight-bearing cast to prevent deformity. After a month, a total contact cast is applied and the patient may mobilize for brief periods. An alternative is the Aircast, but a cradled moulded insole should protect the sole. Such treatment, if given early, should help to prevent the second phase, that of bony destruction and deformity. Bisphosphonates may be helpful in the initial treatment of the Charcot foot (Jude et al 2001).

Bony destruction
Clinical signs are swelling, warmth and deformities, which include the rocker bottom deformity and the medial convexity. X-ray reveals fragmentation, fracture, new bone formation, subluxation and dislocation. The aim of treatment is immobilization until there is no longer evidence on X-ray of continuing bone destruction and the foot temperature is within 2°C of the contralateral foot. Deformity in a Charcot foot can predispose to ulceration, which may become infected and lead to osteomyelitis. This

may be difficult to distinguish from neuropathic bone and joint changes, as, on X-ray, bone scan or magnetic resonance imaging, appearances may be similar. However, if the ulcer can be probed to bone, osteomyelitis is the more likely diagnosis.

Stabilization

The foot is no longer warm and red. There may still be oedema but the difference in skin temperature between the feet is less than 2°C. X-ray shows fracture healing, sclerosis and bone remodelling.

The patient can now progress from a total contact or Aircast to an orthotic walker, fitted with cradled, moulded insoles. However, too rapid mobilization can be disastrous, resulting in further bone destruction. Extremely careful rehabilitation should be the rule. Finally, the patient may progress to bespoke footwear with moulded insoles.

The rocker bottom Charcot foot with plantar bony prominence is a site of very high pressure. Regular reduction of callus can prevent ulceration. If ulceration does occur, an exostectomy may be needed. The most serious complication of a Charcot foot is instability of the hind foot and ankle joint. This can lead to a flail ankle on which it is impossible to walk. Reconstructive surgery and arthrodesis, with a long-term ankle–foot orthosis, has resulted in high levels of limb salvage (Papa et al 1993).

STAGE 3: THE ULCERATED FOOT

Presentation and assessment

It is essential to differentiate between ulceration in the neuropathic foot and that in the neuroischaemic foot.

Neuropathic ulcer

Neuropathic ulcers result from mechanical, thermal or chemical injuries that are unperceived by the patient because of loss of pain sensation. The classical position is under the metatarsal heads, but it is more frequently found on the plantar aspects of the toes. Direct mechanical injuries may result from treading on sharp objects but the most frequent cause of ulceration is the repetitive mechanical forces of gait, which result in callosity formation, inflammatory autolysis and subkeratotic haematomas. Tissue necrosis occurs below the plaque of callus, resulting in a small cavity filled with serous fluid, which eventually breaks through to the surface, with ulcer formation.

Neuroischaemic ulcer

Ulceration in the neuroischaemic foot usually occurs on the margins of the foot and the first sign of ischaemic ulceration is a red mark, which blisters and then develops into a shallow ulcer with a base of sparse, pale granulations or yellowish, closely adherent slough. Although ulcers occur on the medial surface of the first metatarsophalangeal joint and over the lateral aspect of the fifth metatarsal phalangeal joint, the commonest sites are the apices of the toes.

Management

Mechanical, wound, microbiological, vascular and educational control are important.

Mechanical control

In the neuropathic foot the aim is to redistribute plantar pressures, while in the neuroischaemic foot it is to protect the vulnerable margins of the foot.

Neuropathic foot The most efficient way to redistribute plantar pressure is by the immediate application of some form of cast (Armstrong & Lavery 1998). Various casts are available and include the Aircast total contact cast and Scotchcast boot.

The Aircast (Kalish et al 1987) is a removable, bivalved cast and the halves are joined together with Velcro strapping. It is lined with four air cells, which can be inflated with a hand pump through four valves to ensure a close fit. The total contact cast should be reserved for plantar ulcers that have not responded to other casting treatments. It is a close fitting plaster of Paris and fibreglass cast applied over minimum padding. The Scotchcast boot (Burde et al 1983) is a simple removable boot made of stockinette, felt and fibreglass tape, which is effective in redistributing plantar pressure. If casting techniques are not available, temporary ready-made shoes with a Plastazote insole, such as a Drushoe, can offload the site of ulceration.

The 5-year cumulative rate of ulcer recurrence is 66% (Apelqvist et al 1993). In the long term, cradled or moulded insoles are designed to redistribute weight-bearing away from the vulnerable pressure areas and prevent recurrence. In a controlled trial of therapeutic shoes compared with patient's own shoes, the risk of ulcer recurrence at 1 year was 27% in the intervention group and 58% in the control group (Uccioli et al 1995). However, in a recent study of persons without severe foot deformity but with a history of foot ulcer, custom footwear conferred no significant ulcer reduction compared with control footwear (Reiber et al 2002).

Neuroischaemic feet   Ulcers in neuroischaemic feet are often associated with tight shoes, which lead to frictional forces on the vulnerable margins of the foot. A high street shoe that is sufficiently long, broad and deep and fastens with a lace or strap high on the foot may be sufficient. Alternatively, a ready-made stock shoe that is wide-fitting may be suitable.

Wound control

Wound control consists of three parts: debridement, dressings and stimulation of wound healing.

Debridement   Debridement is the most important part of wound control and is best carried out with a scalpel. It allows removal of callus and devitalized tissue and enables the true dimensions of the ulcer to be perceived. It reduces the bacterial load of the ulcer even in the absence of overt infection, restores chronic wounds to acute wounds and releases growth factors to aid the healing process (Edmonds & Foster 2000). It also enables tissue and/or a deep swab to be taken for culture. The larvae of the greenbottle fly are sometimes used to debride ulcers, especially in the neuroischaemic foot.

Dressings   Sterile, non-adherent dressings should cover all ulcers to protect them from trauma, absorb exudate, reduce infection and promote healing. There is no evidence to support a particular dressing (American Diabetes Association 1999). The following dressing properties are essential for the diabetic foot: ease and speed of lifting, ability to be walked on without disintegrating and good exudate control. Dressings should be lifted every day to ensure that problems or complications are detected quickly, especially in patients who lack protective pain sensation.

Stimulation of wound healing   Techniques to stimulate wound healing include Regranex (platelet-derived growth factor), Dermagraft, Apligraf, Hyaff, Promogran and vacuum-assisted closure.

Platelet-derived growth factor (Regranex) stimulates chemotaxis and mitogenesis of neutrophils, fibroblasts and monocytes. It is used in the form of a gel and several trials have shown improved healing rates compared with controls (Steed 1995, Wieman et al 1998).

Dermagraft is a bioengineered living human dermis, which is delivered frozen but needs to be thawed warmed and rinsed prior to application. Controlled trials have shown significant improvement in neuropathic ulcers treated with Dermagraft (Marston et al 2003).

Apligraf is a bioengineered, bilayered skin substitute consisting of human fibroblasts embedded in bovine collagen and covered by human keratinocytes. It is stored in an incubator. Controlled studies have shown significantly increased healing rates in neuropathic ulcers (Veves et al 2001).

Protease inhibitors such as Promogran consist of oxidized regenerated cellulose and collagen. Promogran inhibits proteases in the wound and protects endogenous growth factor. In a 12-week study of 184 patients, 37% of Promogran-treated patients healed compared with 28% of saline-gauze-treated patients, a non-significant difference (Veves et al 2002).

Hyaluronic acid ester (Hyaff) is a fibrous ester of hyaluronic acid, which is a polysaccharide that is integral to the extracellular matrix and controls hydration and osmoregulation. When Hyaff is applied to the wound, hyaluronic acid is released. It is useful in treating neuropathic ulcers complicated by sinuses (Foster et al 1999).

The vacuum-assisted closure (VAC) pump is a major advance in treating diabetic foot wounds. It is important to use the pump on wounds that have been thoroughly debrided and do not contain slough. The pump applies a continuous negative pressure of 125 mmHg to the ulcer through a tube and foam sponge, which are applied to the ulcer and sealed in place with a plastic film to create a vacuum. The sponge is replaced every 2–3 days. Exudate from the wound is sucked along the tube to a disposable collecting chamber. The negative pressure improves the dermal blood supply and stimulates granulation, which can form even over bone and tendon. It reduces bacterial colonization and diminishes oedema and interstitial fluid. The VAC pump is increasingly used to treat postoperative wounds in the diabetic ischaemic foot, especially when revascularization is not possible.

Microbiological control

When the skin of the foot is broken, the patient is at great risk of infection, as there is a clear portal of entry for invading bacteria. At every patient visit, the foot should be examined for local signs of infection, cellulitis or osteomyelitis. If these are found, antibiotic therapy is indicated.

However, uniform agreed practice on the place of antibiotics in the clinically non-infected ulcer has not been established. In a recent investigation, 32 patients with new foot ulcers were treated with oral antibiotics and 32 patients without antibiotics (Foster et al 1998). In the group with no antibiotics, 15 patients developed clinical infection compared with none in the antibiotic group (p <0.001). Seven patients in the non-antibiotic group needed hospital admission and three patients came to amputation (one major and two minor). 17 patients healed in the non-antibiotic group compared with 27 in the antibiotic group (p <0.02). Furthermore, out of the 15 patients who became clinically infected, 11 had positive ulcer swabs at the start of the study compared with only one patient out of 17 in the non-infected group (p <0.01). Ulcer healing rate was higher in the antibiotic ischaemic group compared with the non-antibiotic group. From this study, it was concluded that diabetic patients with clean ulcers associated with peripheral vascular disease and positive ulcer swabs should be considered for early antibiotic treatment.

Thus for the neuropathic ulcer, at the first visit, if there is no cellulitis, discharge or probing to bone (indicative of osteomyelitis – see below), then debridement, cleansing with saline, application of dressing and daily inspections will suffice.

For the neuroischaemic ulcer, at the initial visit, if the ulcer is superficial, oral amoxicillin 500 mg three times daily and flucloxacillin 500 mg four times daily may be prescribed. (If the patient is penicillin allergic, prescribe erythromycin 500 mg four times daily or cefadroxil 1 g twice daily). If the ulcer is deep, extending to the subcutaneous tissue, trimethoprim 200 mg twice daily and metronidazole 400 mg four times daily may be added (Edmonds & Foster 2000).

The patient is reviewed, preferably at 1 week, together with the result of the ulcer swab. If the ulcer shows no sign of infection and the swab is negative, treatment is continued without antibiotics. However, in the cases of severe ischaemia (pressure index <0.5), antibiotics may be prescribed until the ulcer is healed. If either the neuropathic or neuroischaemic ulcer has a positive swab, the patient may be treated with the appropriate antibiotic, according to sensitivies, until the repeat swab, taken at weekly intervals, is negative.

Vascular control

If an ulcer has not responded to optimum treatment within 6 weeks and ankle brachial pressure index is less than 0.5 and the Doppler waveform is damped, or transcutaneous oxygen is less than 30 mmHg or toe pressure is less than 30 mmHg, then angiography should ideally be carried out.

This can be performed by a Duplex examination, which combines the features of Doppler waveform analysis with ultrasound imaging to produce a picture of arterial flow dynamics and morphology (Edmonds & Foster 2000). Alternatively, transfemoral angiography can be performed, together with digital subtraction angiography to assess the distal arteries.

Angioplasty is a valuable treatment to improve arterial flow in the presence of ischaemic ulcers and is indicated for the treatment of isolated or multiple stenoses as well as short-segment occlusions less than 10 cm in length (Edmonds & Walters 1995). If lesions are too widespread for angioplasty, then arterial bypass may be considered. However, this is a major, sometimes lengthy, operation, not without risk, and is more commonly reserved to treat the foot with severe tissue destruction, which cannot be managed without the restoration of pulsatile blood flow.

Educational control

Patients should be instructed on the principles of ulcer care, stressing the importance of rest, footwear, regular dressings and frequent observation for signs of infection.

STAGE 4: FOOT ULCER AND CELLULITIS

Presentation and assessment

Infection is caused by bacteria that invade the ulcer from the surrounding skin. Staphylococci and streptococci are the most common pathogens (Lipsky 1999). However, infection due to Gram-negative and anaerobic organisms occurs in approximately 50% of patients and infection is often polymicrobial (Grayson 1995). The most common manifestation is cellulitis. However, this stage covers a spectrum of presentations, ranging from local infection of the ulcer to spreading cellulitis, sloughing of soft tissue and, finally, vascular compromise of the skin, seen as a blue discoloration, when there is an inadequate supply of oxygen to the soft tissues.

Infected ulcer

Local signs that an ulcer has become infected include colour change of the base of the lesion from healthy pink granulations to yellowish or grey tissue, purulent discharge, unpleasant smell, and the development of sinuses with undermined edges or exposed bone. There may also be localized erythema, warmth and swelling. In the neuroischaemic foot, it may be difficult to differentiate between the erythema of cellulitis and the redness of ischaemia. However, the redness of ischaemia is usually cold, although not always so, and is most marked on dependency, whereas the erythema of inflammation is warm.

Cellulitis

When infection spreads there is widespread intense erythema and swelling, and lymphangitis, regional lymphadenitis, malaise, 'flu-like' symptoms, fever and rigors may develop. In the presence of neuropathy, pain and throbbing are often absent but, if present, usually indicate pus within the tissues. Palpation may reveal fluctuance, suggesting abscess formation, although discrete abscesses are relatively uncommon in the infected diabetic foot. Often there is a generalized sloughing of the ulcer and surrounding subcutaneous tissues, which liquefy and disintegrate (Fig. 18.4). Subcutaneous gas may be detected by direct palpation of the foot and the diagnosis is confirmed by the appearance of gas in the soft tissue on the radiograph. Although

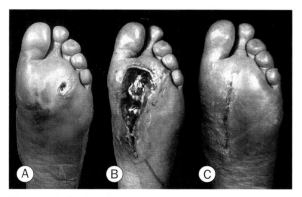

Figure 18.4 (**A**) On presentation (**B**) After surgical debridement (**C**) On healing

clostridial organisms have previously been held responsible for this presentation, non-clostridial organisms are more frequently the offending pathogens. These include *Bacteroides* sp., *Escherichia coli* and anaerobic streptococci. Only 50% of episodes of severe cellulitis will provoke a fever or leukocytosis (Armstrong et al 1996). A substantial number of patients with a deep foot infection do not have severe symptoms and signs indicating the presence of deep infection. However, when increased body temperature or leukocytosis is present, it usually indicates a substantial tissue damage (Eneroth et al 1997).

Osteomyelitis

If a sterile probe inserted into the ulcer reaches bone, this strongly suggests the diagnosis of osteomyelitis. In the initial stages, plain X-ray may be normal, and localized loss of bone density and cortical outline may not be apparent until at least 14 days later. The radionuclide bone scan using technetium-99m diphosphonate is very sensitive but not specific for osteomyelitis. Gallium or indium scans may improve specificity but magnetic resonance imaging may be most helpful in demonstrating loss of bony cortex (Longmaid & Kruskal 1995). Chronic osteomyelitis of a toe has a swollen, red, sausage-like appearance (Rajbhandari et al 2000).

Management

Infection in the diabetic foot needs full multidisciplinary treatment. It is vital to achieve microbiological, wound, vascular, mechanical and educational control, for, if infection is not controlled, it can spread with alarming rapidity, causing extensive tissue necrosis and taking the foot into stage 5 (Fig. 18.3b).

Microbiological control

General principles At initial presentation, it is impossible to predict the organisms from the clinical appearance. Thus, it is important to prescribe broad-spectrum antibiotics and to take cultures without delay in all stage 4 patients. Deep swabs or tissue should be taken from the ulcer after initial debridement and if the patient undergoes operative debridement then deep tissue should also be sent. Ulcer swabs should be taken at every follow-up visit. It is possible that bacterial species that are usually not pathogenic can cause a true infection in a diabetic foot when part of a mixed flora. As there is a poor immune response of the diabetic patient to sepsis, even bacteria regarded as skin commensals may cause severe tissue damage. These include Gram-negative organisms such as *Citrobacter*, *Serratia*, *Pseudomonas* and *Acinetobacter* spp. When Gram-negative bacteria are isolated from an ulcer swab, they should not automatically be regarded as insignificant. If there is fever and systemic toxicity, blood cultures should also be sent.

Antibiotic treatment Infection in the neuroischaemic foot is often more serious than in the neuropathic foot that has a good arterial blood supply; therefore a positive ulcer swab in a neuroischaemic foot has serious implications, and this influences antibiotic policy.

Antibiotic treatment is discussed both as initial treatment and at follow up: dosage should be determined by the level of renal function and serum levels when available. Clinical and microbiological response rates have been similar in trials of various antibiotics and no single agent or combination has emerged as most effective (American Diabetes Association 1999). Chantelau randomized patients with neuropathic ulcers (some of which had cellulitis) to oral amoxicillin plus clavulanic acid or matched placebo. At 20 days follow-up, there was no significant difference in outcome (Chantelau et al 1996). Lipsky randomized 56 patients with an infected lesion to oral clindamycin or oral cephalexin in an outpatient setting and at 2 weeks there was no difference in treatment (Lipsky et al 1990). Grayson randomized 93 patients to intravenous imipenem/cilastatin or intravenous ampicillin/sulbactam and after 5 days cure had been effected in 60% of the ampicillin/sulbactam group and 58% of the imipenem/cilastatin group (Grayson 1995).

The regime set out in Box 18.1 has been developed and is based on many years of treating the diabetic foot and significantly reducing amputations.

Wound control

Diabetic foot infections are almost always more extensive than would appear from initial examination and surface appearance.

Box 18.1 *Antibiotic treatment of stage 4 diabetic foot ulcer*

Local signs of infection in the ulcer or mild cellulitis

Initial treatment
- Give amoxicillin, flucloxacillin, metronidazole and trimethoprim orally. If the patient is allergic to penicillin, substitute erythromycin for amoxycillin and flucloxacillin.
- Cellulitis on the borderline of mild to severe can be treated with intramuscular ceftriaxone.

Follow-up plan (with reference to previous visit's swab)
- If no signs of infection and no organisms isolated, stop antibiotics but if the patient is severely ischaemic, with a pressure index below 0.5, consider continuing antibiotics until healing.
- If no signs of infection are present but organisms are isolated, focus antibiotics and review in 1 week.
- If signs of infection are present but no organisms are isolated, continue the antibiotics as above.

- If signs of infection are still present and organisms are isolated, focus antibiotic regime according to sensitivities.
- If methicillin-resistant *Staphylococcus aureus* (MRSA) is grown but there are no local or systemic signs of infection, use topical mupirocin 2% ointment (if sensitive).
- If MRSA is grown with local signs of infection, consider oral therapy with two of the following: sodium fusidate, rifampicin, trimethoprim and doxycycline, according to sensitivities, together with topical mupirocin 2% ointment.

Foot with severe cellulitis

Initial treatment

- If admission is not possible, then give ceftriaxone intramuscularly and metronidazole orally. On review as an outpatient, if cellulitis is controlled, continue ceftriaxone intramuscularly and metronidazole orally, and review 1 week later.
- If cellulitis is increasing, then admit for intravenous antibiotics. Quadruple therapy is indicated: amoxicillin, flucloxacillin, metronidazole and ceftazidime. If patient is allergic to penicillin, replace amoxicillin and flucloxacillin with erythromycin or vancomycin (with doses adjusted according to serum levels). On admission the foot should be urgently assessed as to the need for surgical debridement (see Wound control).

Follow up plan

- The infected foot should be inspected daily to gauge the initial response to antibiotic therapy.
- Appropriate antibiotics should be selected when sensitivities are available. If an infection responds well to the initial antibiotics but the swabs suggest that these antibiotics are resistant to the isolated organisms, it is best to change the antibiotics according to sensitivities, although this is not universal practice.
- If no organisms are isolated and yet the foot remains severely cellulitic, then a repeat deep swab should be taken but the quadruple antibiotic therapy, as above, should be continued.
- If MRSA is isolated, give vancomycin (dosage to be adjusted according to serum levels) or teicoplanin. These antibiotics may need to be accompanied by either sodium fusidate or rifampicin orally. Intravenous antibiotic therapy can be changed to the appropriate oral therapy when the signs of cellulitis have resolved.

Osteomyelitis

Initial treatment

- At first, antibiotics will be given for the associated infected ulcer and cellulitis as above.

Follow up plan

- On review, antibiotic selection is guided by the results of deep swabs, but it is useful to choose antibiotics with good bone penetration, such as sodium fusidate, rifampicin, clindamycin and ciprofloxacin. Antibiotics should be given for at least 12 weeks.
- Such conservative therapy is often successful and is associated with resolution of cellulitis and healing of the ulcer. However if, after 3 months treatment, the ulcer persists, with continued probing to bone, which is fragmented on X-ray, then, in the neuropathic foot, resection of the underlying bone is probably indicated.

It is wise to perform an initial debridement so that the true dimensions of the lesion can be revealed and samples obtained for culture. Often callus may overlie the ulcer and this must be removed to reveal the extent of the underlying ulcer and allow drainage of pus and removal of infected sloughy tissue.

Cellulitis should respond to intravenous antibiotics but the patient needs daily review to ensure the erythema is resolving. In severe episodes of cellulitis, the ulcer may be complicated by extensive infected subcutaneous soft tissue. At this point, the tissue is not frankly necrotic but has started to break down and liquefy. It is best for this tissue to be removed operatively. The definite indications for urgent surgical intervention are a large area of infected sloughy tissue, localized fluctuance and expression of pus, crepitus with gas in the soft tissues on X-ray and purplish discoloration of the skin, indicating subcutaneous necrosis.

The role of hyperbaric oxygen in the management of wounds is not yet established but two small, randomized, controlled trials found that systemic hyperbaric oxygen reduced the absolute risk of foot amputation in people with severely infected ulcers compared with routine care (American Diabetes Association 1999).

Vascular control
It is important to explore the possibility of revascularization in the infected neuroischaemic foot. Improvement of perfusion will not only help to control infection but will also promote healing of wounds if operative debridement is necessary.

Mechanical control
Patients should be on bed rest with heel protection with foam wedges.

Educational control
The patient should be advised of the importance of rest in severe infection. If patients have mild cellulitis and are treated at home they should understand the signs of advancing and progressing cellulitis so as to return early to clinic. Patient education provided after the management of acute foot complications decreases ulcer recurrence and major amputations (Malone et al 1989).

STAGE 5: FOOT ULCER AND NECROSIS

Presentation and assessment

This stage is characterized by the presence of necrosis (Fig. 18.5). It is classified as either wet necrosis due to infection or dry necrosis due to ischaemia. In wet necrosis, the tissues are grey or black, moist and often malodorous. Adjoining tissues are infected and pus may discharge from the ulcerated demarcation line between necrosis and viable tissue. Dry necrosis is hard, blackened, mummified tissue and there is usually a clean demarcation line between necrosis and viable tissue.

Necrosis presents in both the neuropathic and the neuroischaemic foot and the management is different in both.

Neuropathic foot
In the neuropathic foot, necrosis is invariably wet and is usually caused by infection complicating an ulcer and leading to a septic vasculitis of the digital and small arteries of the foot. The walls of these arteries are infiltrated by polymorphs, leading to occlusion of the lumen by septic thrombus.

Necrosis can involve skin, subcutaneous and fascial layers. In the skin, it is easily evident but in the subcutaneous and fascial layers it is not so

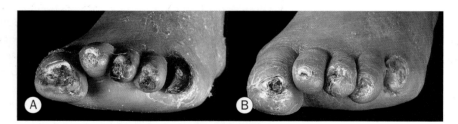

Figure 18.5 (**A**) Digital necrosis (**B**) After repeated podiatric debridement and antibiotics

apparent. Often the bluish-black discoloration of skin is the 'tip of an iceberg' of deep necrosis that occurs in subcutaneous and fascial planes, so called necrotizing fasciitis.

Neuroischaemic foot

Both wet and dry necrosis can occur in the neuroischaemic foot.

Wet necrosis is also caused by a septic vasculitis. However, reduced arterial perfusion to the foot resulting from atherosclerotic disease of the leg arteries is an important predisposing factor.

Dry necrosis is usually secondary to a severe reduction in arterial perfusion and occurs in three circumstances: severe chronic ischaemia, acute ischaemia and emboli to the toes.

Severe chronic ischaemia   A gradual but severe reduction in arterial perfusion results in vascular compromise of the skin, leading to blue toes, which usually become necrotic unless the foot is revascularized.

Acute ischaemia   Blue discoloration leading to necrosis of the toes is also seen in acute ischaemia. It presents as a sudden onset of pain in the leg, associated with pallor of the foot, quickly followed by mottling and slaty grey discoloration.

Emboli to the toes   Emboli to the digital circulation results in a bluish or purple discoloration that is quite well demarcated but quickly proceeds to necrosis. If it escapes infection, the toe will dry out and mummify. Microemboli present with painful petechial lesions in the foot that do not blanch on pressure.

Digital necrosis in the patient with renal impairment

Digital necrosis is a relatively common problem in patients with advanced diabetic nephropathy. It may result from a septic neutrophilic vasculitis but can occur in the absence of infection. It may be precipitated by trauma.

Management

Patients should be admitted for urgent investigations and multidisciplinary management. It is important to achieve wound, microbiological, vascular, mechanical and educational control.

Wound control

Neuropathic foot   Operative debridement is almost always indicated for wet gangrene. It is important to remove all necrotic tissue, down to bleeding tissue, as well as opening up all sinuses. Deep necrotic tissue should be sent for culture immediately. Although necrosis in the diabetic foot may not be associated with a definite collection of pus, the necrotic tissue still needs to be removed. In the neuropathic foot, there is good arterial circulation and the wound always heals as long as infection is controlled. Wounds should not be sutured. Skin grafting may be the best way to accelerate healing of large tissue deficits. When there is extensive loss of tissue, modern reconstructive surgical techniques have recently proved useful (Armstrong et al 1997).

Neuroischaemic foot   In the neuroischaemic foot, wet necrosis should also be removed when it is associated with severe spreading sepsis. This should be done whether pus is present or not.

In cases when the limb is not immediately threatened and the necrosis is limited to one or two toes, it may be possible to control infection with intravenous antibiotics and proceed to urgent revascularization and, at the same operation, perform digital or ray amputation. Wounds in the neuroischaemic foot may be slow to heal even after revascularization, and wound care needs to continue as an outpatient in the diabetic foot clinic but, with patience, outcomes may be surprisingly good.

If revascularization is not possible for digital necrosis, then a decision must be made to either amputate the toe in the presence of ischaemia or allow the toe, if infection is controlled, to convert to dry necrosis and autoamputate. Surgical amputation should be undertaken if the toe is painful or if the circulation is not severely impaired, i.e. pressure index above 0.5 or transcutaneous oxygen tension above 30 mmHg (Edmonds & Foster 2000).

Microbiological control

Wet necrosis   When the patient initially presents, wound swabs and tissue specimens should be sent for culture. Deep tissue taken at operative debridement must also go for culture. Intravenous antibiotic therapy (amoxicillin, flucloxacillin, metronidazole and ceftazidime) should be given. However, if the patient is allergic to penicillin, then erythromycin or vancomycin (dosage adjusted according to serum levels) may be used instead of amoxicillin and flucloxacillin. Intravenous antibiotics can be replaced with oral therapy after operative debridement and when infection is controlled. When the wound is granulating well and swabs are negative then the antibiotics may be stopped.

Dry necrosis When dry necrosis develops secondary to ischaemia, antibiotics should be prescribed if discharge is present or the wound swab is positive, and continued until there is no evidence of clinical or microbiological infection.

Vascular control

After operative debridement of wet necrosis, revascularization is often essential to heal the tissue deficit. In dry necrosis that occurs against a background of severe macrovascular disease, revascularization is necessary to maintain the viability of the limb. When dry necrosis is secondary to emboli, a possible source should be investigated.

In some patients, increased perfusion following angioplasty may be useful. However, unless there is a very significant localized stenosis in iliac or femoral arteries, angioplasty rarely restores to the foot the pulsatile blood flow that is necessary to keep the limb viable in severe ischaemia or restore considerable tissue deficits secondary to necrosis. This is best achieved by arterial bypass.

Peripheral arterial disease is common in the tibial arteries and distal bypass with autologous vein has become an established method of revascularization, in which a conduit is fashioned from either the femoral or popliteal artery down to a tibial artery in the lower leg or the dorsalis pedis artery on the dorsum of the foot. Patency rates and limb salvage rates after revascularization do not differ between diabetic patients and non-diabetic patients, and a more aggressive approach to such revascularization procedures should be promoted (Pomposelli et al 1995).

Mechanical control

During the peri- and postoperative period, bed rest is essential, with elevation of the limb to relieve oedema and afford heel protection. After operative debridement in the neuroischaemic foot, non-weight-bearing is advised until the wound is healed, especially when revascularization has not been possible. In the neuropathic foot, non-weight-bearing is advisable initially and then offloading of the healing postoperative wound may be achieved

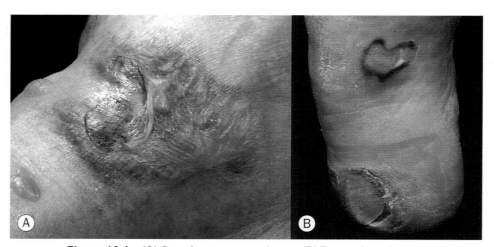

Figure 18.6 (**A**) Burn from covection heater (**B**) Trauma from foot spa

by casting techniques. If necrosis is to be treated conservatively, by autoamputation, which can take several months, then the patient needs a wide-fitting shoe to accommodate the foot and dressings.

Educational control

For patients in hospital, advice is similar to that given for severe cellulitis.

For patients undergoing autoamputation at home, it is important to rest the foot and keep it dry and covered with a dressing and bandage. Patients should be advised to return to the clinic immediately if the foot becomes swollen, painful, develops an unpleasant smell or discharges pus.

CONCLUSION

This chapter has outlined a simple classification of the diabetic foot into the neuropathic and neuro-ischaemic foot and defined six specific stages in its natural history. It has described a simple plan of management for each stage, which requires a well organized, multidisciplinary approach that provides continuity of care between primary and secondary sectors (Edmonds et al 1996). Secondary care should be focused on a diabetic foot clinic, to which rapid referrals should be possible. Such clinics have reported a reduction in amputations and should be available to all diabetic patients (Larsson et al 1995).

References

American Diabetes Association 1999 Consensus Development Conference on Diabetic Foot Wound Care. Diabetes Care 22: 1354–1360

Apelqvist J, Larsson J, Agardh C-D 1993 Long term prognosis for diabetic patients with foot ulcers. Journal of Internal Medicine 233: 485–491

Armstrong D G, Lavery L A 1998 Evidence based options for off loading diabetic wounds. Clinics in Podiatric Medicine and Surgery 15: 95–104

Armstrong D G, Lavery L A, Sariaya M, Ashry H 1996 Leukocytosis is a poor indicator of acute osteomyelitis of the foot in diabetes mellitus. Journal of Foot and Ankle Surgery 4: 280–283

Armstrong M D, Villalobos R E, Leppink D M 1997 Free tissue transfer for lower extremity reconstruction in the immunosuppressed diabetic transplant recipient. Journal of Reconstructive Microsurgery 13: 1–5

Burden A C, Jones G R, Jones R, Blandford R L 1983 Use of the 'Scotchcast boot' in treating diabetic foot ulcers. British Medical Journal 286: 1555–1557

Chantelau E, Tanudjaja T, Altenhofer F et al 1996 Antibiotic treatment for uncomplicated neuropathic forefoot ulcers in diabetes: a controlled trial. Diabetic Medicine 13: 156–159

Edmonds M E, Foster A V M 1994 Classification and management of neuropathic and neuroischaemic ulcers. In: Boulton A J M, Connor H, Cavanagh P R (eds) The foot in diabetes, 2nd edn. John Wiley & Sons, Chichester

Edmonds M E, Foster A V M 2000 Managing the diabetic foot. Blackwell Science, Oxford

Edmonds M, Foster A V M 2001 Reduction of major amputations in the diabetic ischemic foot: a strategy to 'take control' with conservative care as well as revascularisation. Vasa 58(Suppl): 6–14

Edmonds M E, Walters H 1995 Angioplasty and the diabetic foot. Vascular Medicine Reviews 6: 205–214

Edmonds M, Boulton A, Buckenham T et al 1996 Report of the diabetic foot and amputation group. Diabetic Medicine 13: S27–S42

Eneroth M, Apelqvist J, Stenstrom A 1997 Clinical characteristics and outcome in 223 diabetic patients with deep foot infections. Foot and Ankle International 18: 716–722

Faglia E, Favales F, Aldeghi A et al 1998 Change in major amputation rate in a center dedicated to diabetic foot care during the 1980s: prognostic determinants for major amputation. Journal of Diabetes Complications 12: 96–102

Flynn M D 1999 The diabetic foot. In: Tooke J E (ed.) Diabetic angiopathy. Edward Arnold, London

Foster A, McColgan M, Edmonds M 1998 Should oral antibiotics be given to clean foot ulcers with no cellulitis? Diabetic Medicine 15(Suppl 2): S10

Foster A M, Bates M, Doxford M, Edmonds M E 1999 The treatment of indolent neuropathic ulceration of the diabetic foot with Hyaff. Diabetic Medicine (Suppl): 94

Grayson M L 1995 Diabetic foot infections: antimicrobial therapy. In: Eliopoulos G M (ed.) Infectious disease clinics of North America. W B Saunders, Philadelphia, PA pp 143–162

Holstein P, Ellitsgaard N, Olsen B B, Ellitsgaard V 2000 Decreasing incidence of major amputations in people with diabetes. Diabetologia 43: 844–847

Hurley J J, Woods J J, Hershey F B 1993 Non invasive testing: practical knowledge for evaluating diabetic patients. In: Levin M F, O'Neal L W, Bowker J H (eds) The diabetic foot. Mosby Year Book, St Louis, MO, pp 321–340

International Working Group on the Diabetic Foot 2003 International Consensus on the Diabetic Foot. International Working Group on the Diabetic Foot, on line at www.iwgdf.org/

Johnston C L W 1997 Infection and diabetes mellitus. In Pickup J, Williams G (eds) Textbook of diabetes, vol 2. Blackwell Science, Oxford, pp 70.1–70.14

Jude E B, Selby P L, Burgess J et al 2001 Bisphosphonates in the treatment of Charcot neuroarthropathy: a double-blind randomised controlled trial. Diabetologia 44: 2032–2037

Kalish S R, Pelcovitz N, Zawada S et al 1987 The Aircast walking brace versus conventional casting methods. Journal of the American Podiatric Medical Association 77: 589–595

Larsson J, Apelqvist J, Agardh C D, Stenstrom A 1995 Decreasing incidence of major amputation in diabetic patients: a consequence of a multidisciplinary foot care team approach? Diabetic Medicine 12: 770–776

Lipsky B A 1999 A current approach to diabetic foot infections. Current Infectious Disease Reports 1: 253–260

Lipsky B A, Pecoraro R E, Larson S A et al 1990 Outpatient management of uncomplicated lower-extremity infections in diabetic patients. Archives of Internal Medicine 150: 790–797

Litzelman D K, Slemenda C W, Langefield CD et al 1993 Reduction of lower extremity clinical abnormalities in patients with non-insulin dependent diabetes mellitus. Annals of Internal Medicine 199: 36–41

Longmaid H E III, Kruskal J B 1995 Imaging infections in diabetic patients. In: Eliopoulos G M (ed) Infectious disease clinics of North America. W B Saunders, Philadelphia, PA pp 163–182

McCabe C J, Stevenson R C, Dolan A M 1998 Evaluation of a diabetic foot screening and protection programme. Diabetic Medicine 15: 80–84

Malone J M, Snyder M, Anderson G et al 1989 Prevention of amputation by diabetic education. American Journal of Surgery 158: 520–524

Marston W A, Hanft J, Norwood P, Pollak R 2003 The efficacy and safety of Dermagraft in improving the healing of chronic diabetic foot ulcers: results of a prospective randomized trial. Diabetes Care 26: 1701–1705

Papa J, Myerson M S, Girard P 1993 Salvage with arthrodesis in intractable diabetic neuropathic arthropathy of the foot and ankle. Journal of Bone and Joint Surgery 75A: 1056–1066

Pinzur M S, Slovenkai M P, Trepman E 1999 Guidelines for diabetic foot care. Foot and Ankle International 20: 695–702

Pomposelli F B, Marcaccio E J, Gibbons G W et al 1995 Dorsalis pedis arterial bypass: durable limb salvage for foot ischaemia in patients with diabetes mellitus. Journal of Vascular Surgery 21: 375–384

Rajbhandari S, Sutton M, Davies C et al 2000 Sausage toe: a reliable sign of underlying osteomyelitis. Diabetic Medicine 17: 74–77

Reiber G E, Smith D G, Wallace C et al 2002 Effect of therapeutic footwear on foot reulceration in patients with diabetes: a randomized controlled trial. Journal of the American Medical Association 287: 2552–2558

Rith-Najarian S J, Stolusky T, Godhes D M 1992 Identifying diabetic patients at risk for lower extremity amputation in a primary healthcare setting. Diabetes Care 15: 1386–1389

Sanders L J, Frykberg R G 1991 Diabetic neuropathic osteoarthropathy: the Charcot foot. In: Frykberg R G (ed.) The high risk foot in diabetes. Churchill Livingstone, New York pp 227–238

Steed D L 1995 Clinical evaluation of recombinant human platelet-derived growth factor for the treatment of lower extremity diabetic ulcers, the Diabetic Ulcer Study Group. Journal of Vascular Surgery 21: 71–81

Tovey F I 1984 The manufacture of diabetic footwear. Diabetic Medicine 1: 69–71

Uccioli L, Aldeghi A, Faglia E et al 1995 Manufactured shoes in the prevention of diabetic foot ulcers. Diabetes Care 18: 1376–1378

Veves A, Falanga V, Armstrong D G, Sabolinski M L 2001 Apligraf Diabetic Foot Ulcer Study. Graftskin, a human skin equivalent, is effective in the management of noninfected neuropathic diabetic foot ulcers: a prospective randomized multicenter clinical trial. Diabetes Care 24: 290–295

Veves A, Sheehan P, Pham H T 2002 A randomized, controlled trial of Promogran (a collagen/oxidized regenerated cellulose dressing) vs standard treatment in the management of diabetic foot ulcers. Archives of Surgery 137: 822–827

Wieman T J, Smiell J M, Su Y 1998 Efficacy and safety of a topical gel formulation of recombinant human platelet derived growth factor – BB (Becaplermin) in patients with non healing diabetic ulcers: a phase III, randomized, placebo-controlled, double-blind study. Diabetes Care 21: 822–827

Malignancy, including surgical treatment

Baldur T. Baldursson

HISTORY AND NOMENCLATURE

In 1828 Marjolin, a French surgeon, wrote the chapter on ulcers in a medical dictionary and included carcinomatous ulcers (Marjolin 1828). A century later, Knox reviewed cancer in venous ulcers and cited a number of publications from the period 1885–1925 (Knox 1925). From Knox's excellent review it can be concluded that, in the last decades of the 18th century, physicians had the knowledge to use the cause–effect relationship inherent in the concept of chronic ulcers as a cause of squamous cell carcinoma (SCC). As for the cause of the cancer, the theories mirror the opinions of each era, as for instance the so called 'irritation theory' does in Knox's article and the discussion appended to it (Varmus & Weinberg 1993). Today our ignorance of the causes of SCC in chronic ulcers is in sharp contrast to the abundance of knowledge on SCC of the skin, where the mechanisms are reasonably well known. This, of course, reflects the burden of disease: if basal cell carcinoma is not counted, SCC of the skin is the most prevalent human cancer (Marks 1996).

The term Marjolin's ulcer has often been advocated as an eponym for the condition of squamous cell carcinoma in chronic ulcers. Since this term is also used to describe malignancy in burn scars and malignancy in chronic osteomyelitis, we suggest that the most practical name for this neoplasm is squamous cell carcinoma (SCC) in chronic leg ulcers.

PRACTICAL APPROACH AND EPIDEMIOLOGY

The approach of most clinicians to rare complications such as SCC in chronic ulcers is to ask colleagues and do a literature survey. Most senior dermatologists remember one or more cases, which most often have not been reported. On the other hand, an abundance of cases can be found in the literature. A literature review carried out by myself amassed a total of 157 cases, most often collected retrospectively from the diagnostic registries of one or more clinics. Interestingly, many specialities address this issue – departments of radiology, pathology, surgery and dermatology are represented (Tenopyr & Silverman 1932, Black 1952, Cruickshank et al 1963). From the number of cases reported and the fact that busy clinicians seldom report their interesting cases despite wishful thinking in that direction, it can be inferred that the incidence of SCC in chronic ulcers is much higher than reported and that they should not be considered to be rare (Baldursson et al 1993). Constant vigilance is therefore necessary in order not to miss this complication where timely diagnosis is essential.

My colleagues and I have investigated SCC in venous ulcers in an epidemiological study where the cases were taken from a known population. This allows comparison of the group with disease with the whole population at risk and it is therefore possible to calculate statistically the risk for patients with chronic leg ulcers to get cancer in their wounds and see whether it is increased. The results from the study show that this risk is indeed greatly increased. There is therefore no doubt that SCC is a complication of chronic ulcers, which allows scientists to study it as a specific complication instead of it being considered as a coincidental occurrence of SCC at or near a chronic leg ulcer. In the study the cases were found by matching the data of 10 913 patients with a diagnosis of venous leg ulcers from the Swedish Inpatient Registry with reported cases of SCC on the lower limb in the Swedish Cancer Registry.

In short, the study showed that the risk of developing SCC in a chronic leg ulcer is at least 5.8 times more than the risk of getting skin cancer on the lower limb in a comparable population (Baldursson et al 1995). Of the 25 cases found, 11 were well differentiated, 10 moderately and four poorly differentiated. All patients with poorly differentiated SCC died within a year from diagnosis. In these and six more with moderately differentiated tumour, the SCC was the cause of death (Baldursson et al 1999).

An SCC on the skin is normally an infiltrated hyperkeratotic nodule, often associated with pain. It is not associated with high mortality, unless the diagnosis is late and the tumour is allowed to metastasize. This is precisely why the diagnosis of SCC in a leg ulcer is important since the appearance of the tumour in a pre-existing ulcer might delay the correct diagnosis until the cancer has spread too widely. Another concern is that a tumour can dedifferentiate and become more aggressive with time. In other words, patients with SCC in their leg ulcer might be at higher risk of dying from their tumour than 'ordinary' patients who develop SCC, because the diagnosis might be delayed. We wanted to see whether the mortality of leg ulcer patients was increased compared to other patients who developed SCC on their legs. We therefore constituted a comparison group from the Swedish Cancer Registry where all the patients had a diagnosis of SCC on lower limb without ulcer and found that the survival was much poorer in patients who got SCC in an ulcer compared to this control group. The grade of the tumour was not different, however. The increased mortality of the ulcer patient is a fact, and might be a result of late diagnosis (Baldursson et al 1999).

This further underlines the fact that it is important to diagnose SCC in leg ulcers early and treat it assertively.

CLINICAL APPEARANCE

The most usual reason for suspecting a diagnosis of SCC in a chronic leg ulcer is a sudden change in the appearance of the ulcer. These changes are commonly divided into three categories: an exophytic mass; irregularities in the ulcer bed; or a thickening, a 'rolling up', of the edge of the ulcer. In the authors series there was exophytic growth in 12 cases, thickened ulcer margin in five cases, irregular ulcer bed in four cases and non healing ulcer in four cases (Baldursson et al 1999). Any of these, but especially the exophytic changes, can show what dermatologists call a vegetative appearance – a fungus-like growth in the ulcer bed. This is probably due to keratin production in the tumour, which, when saturated with wound fluid, swells and takes on a lighter hue than the rest of the wound. Apart from seeing abnormal growth or any other of the changes outlined above, non-healing of the ulcer or an inappropriate increase in its size should prompt the clinician to consider the diagnosis of tumour. In reality, the time non-healing is allowed before deciding to take a biopsy depends on the clinical status of the ulcer. An uncomplicated venous ulcer that deteriorates without obvious explanation would be biopsied sooner than an ulcer where the assumed course is unfavourable; both should be biopsied!

OTHER TYPES OF CANCER

Many reports of basal cell carcinoma in leg ulcers have been published. This tumour is not unusual and can be difficult, since its appearance in the ulcer can be quite undramatic (Phillips et al 1991). It is not at all rare to be consulted for a non-healing shallow ulcer that on closer inspection proves to be a basal cell carcinoma. A nodular basal cell carcinoma can imitate a granulating wound quite convincingly. The signs to look for are a shallow ulcer not showing any tendency to heal, the absence of other signs of venous disease and a peculiar localization of the 'ulcer'. For example an ulcer on the proximal two-thirds of the lower leg should always be submitted to close scrutiny. A close look will often reveal the classic signs of basal cell carcinoma, such as the pearly edge and a telangiectatic surface; these often show themselves after a week

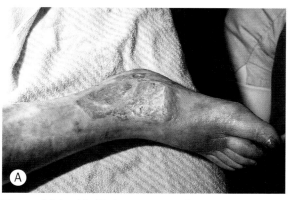

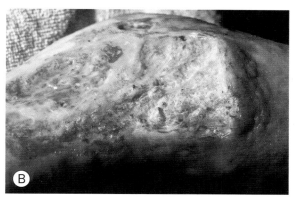

Figure 19.1   (**A, B**) A squamous cell carcinoma on the medial aspect of the lower leg. The distal edge of the ulcer is thickened

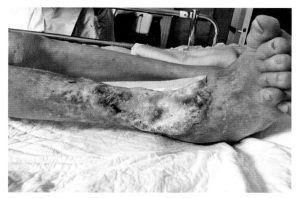

Figure 19.2   A squamous cell carcinoma on a chronic ulcer. In this case the carcinoma has almost filled up the ulcer (Courtesy of Dr Nicolas Foureur, Paris)

increasing thickness the prognosis becomes less favourable. An ulcerated melanoma is therefore an ominous sign, since its thickness is probably considerably more than the millimetre that defines 'thin melanomas'. The tumour should be excised and local recurrences likewise. An oncologist is the appropriate person to refer to. Any discussion of tumours caused by solar radiation should remind us that the lower legs of females have probably received more solar radiation than most other body parts, because of fashion trends, and that elderly females are the prototype of the chronic leg ulcer patient; therefore the wound care professional should be alert to skin changes on the legs they see every day (Figs 19.1, 19.2).

DIAGNOSIS

The biopsy is the diagnostic procedure that gives us the most important information on the SCC. For those clinicians with less experience of ulcer treatment, the infliction of a wound necessary to obtain a biopsy is unsettling. It is, however, my experience and that of colleagues that biopsy wounds heal well, given that the ulcer itself is treated correctly. Pathologists are fond of large biopsies, preferably taken with a scalpel. These would be taken at the edge of the ulcer at right angles to the ulcer margin, comprising both the skin at the margin and a part of the ulcer. The resulting wound is then closed with one or two sutures. Punch biopsies are an option if they are sufficiently large and the locality is well chosen. There must then be several

or two of correct wound treatment. These caveats apply to other differential diagnoses of venous leg ulcers, such as pyoderma gangrenosum.

There are even some reports of sarcomas. Sarcomas are rapidly growing and metastasizing tumours. Smith et al found three in their study of 21 cancers in chronic leg wounds, all of which proved fatal (Smith et al 2001).

Very rarely, an atypical ulcer is diagnosed as a malignant melanoma. It is either an amelanotic melanoma that has grown into a nodule and then ulcerated, or a pigmented melanoma that has been neglected. The most important staging of a melanoma, and thereby the prognosis of the patient, is decided by the thickness of the tumour and designated as Breslow or Clarke stages. With

of them. It is practical to suture the biopsy wound to avoid bleeding. Fungating masses are cut tangentially and bleeding is stopped with pressure or a ligature. A healthy approach, apart from including SCC in one's differential diagnosis directory, is to take a biopsy every time a surgical procedure such as sharp revision is planned on the ulcer.

HISTOPATHOLOGIC LABORATORY ANALYSIS

Histological examination of SCC of the skin shows masses of epidermal cells that invade the dermis (Fig. 19.3). The level of differentiation of the tumour is estimated by considering its similarity or dissimilarity to normal epidermis. A benign histopathological condition called pseudoepitheliomatous hyperplasia is sometimes seen at the edges of chronic ulcers and in proliferating skin diseases. Heaping up of epidermal cells makes this condition a differential diagnosis with SCC in chronic ulcers when the tumour is well differentiated. The histopathological diagnosis of pseudoepitheliomatous hyperplasia cannot be taken as an answer to a single punch biopsy. A new biopsy has to be performed, either a biopsy taken with a scalpel as described above or several deep punch biopsies. The site of the biopsy or biopsies is crucial. If the answer is still pseudoepitheliomatous hyper-

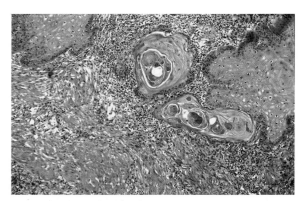

Figure 19.3 A photomicrograph of the squamous cell carcinoma in Figure 19.1, showing sheets of carcinomatous growth to the right and above, and rests of dermis to the left and below. The keratin production and nests of keratin (bright pink) indicate that the tumour is well differentiated

plasia, the patient should be followed closely. A non-healing ulcer with a diagnosis of pseudoepitheliomatous hyperplasia merits consideration of treatment by excision of the wound. It can then be treated with a split-skin graft or conservative treatment. This, of course, will give excellent material for the pathologist.

Even a histopathological diagnosis of SCC demands further biopsies to map the extent of the SCC and to see whether a poorer degree of differentiation is present. The grade of the tumour is very important with regard to the choice of treatment. In any case, a discussion with the pathologist is a crucial part of the evaluation of the findings.

FURTHER INVESTIGATIONS

Palpation of the lymph node glands must be done and subsequent extirpation if an enlarged node is found, both for diagnostic and treatment purposes. An X-ray of the leg is a simple way of seeing whether the lesion reaches the bone.

A standard malignancy workup is important. This can be done in cooperation with an oncologist. A chest X-ray and a CT scan of the pelvis, abdomen and brain is one example of the alternatives.

TREATMENT

This of course is the main concern, once the problem has been assessed. There are no prospective studies on treatment. There are, however, several large case series that, with the case reports, give an indication of the treatment options. Again, these series come from different specialities and regions of the globe. In our series from Sweden, four patients were treated with excision and six with amputation as the first and only treatment. Another five were amputated after other treatments such as radiation or excision. Three excisions were followed by re-excision and node dissection. Five patients received no treatment.

Two recent reports reflect the differences in material and methods seen in the literature. One is a report from a plastic surgery unit in Turkey on a group of patients where 26 patients with SCC in burn scars were included (Copcu et al 2003). All the patients were treated with excision and transplantation. Pathological lymph nodes were found in four out of six patients with enlarged nodes. All patients seemed to have fared well, but the follow-up period was short. The other report is from a radiology department in Brazil where 18 patients with SCC in leg ulcerations of different aetiologies were investigated. All patients had radiological signs of bone involvement and all were amputated (Smith et al 2001).

If lymph nodes are enlarged, they should be excised, both for treatment and for staging purposes. Even though follow-up is short in some reports, this seems sound practice.

By considering the case reports at hand, the treatment of choice for well differentiated SCC seems to be a wide excision down to fascia or deeper. A split-skin transplant can be performed directly, or conservative treatment, depending on the status of the wound. Recurrences are common, hence the wide excision.

A poorly differentiated tumour has to be approached quite differently. In our above-mentioned study of 25 cases, all four patients with poorly differentiated SCC in their leg ulcer died within a year of diagnosis. Therefore, a radical procedure such as an amputation has to be considered. The in-between histopathological diagnosis – moderately differentiated SCC – calls for careful scrutiny of the clinical and histopathological aggressiveness of the tumour, since some of these tumours killed the patients while others seemed to run a similar course to well differentiated SCCs. Perineural invasion, the size of the tumour and invasion beyond the subcutaneous fat are negative prognostic factors in large SCCs (Clayman et al 2005). Exact staging of the tumour requires a large biopsy. A large aggressive tumour favours amputation, while a small, better defined one favours wide excision.

Because of frequent local recurrences both in the material cited and reported in the literature, thorough mapping with biopsies and a careful follow up are important (Figs. 19.4, 19.5).

What about other treatment modalities such as radiation treatment and chemotherapy? Radiation can be excluded in these circumstances. It might eradicate the carcinoma cells but the ulcer will become a therapeutic problem, leading to excision and transplantation or amputation, which is an unacceptable increase in the morbidity of the patient. Black had this to say: 'Operation was forced

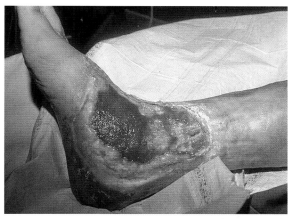

Figure 19.4   The case in Figure 19.1 some time after excision. Note nice healing and, alas, recurrence (arrow)

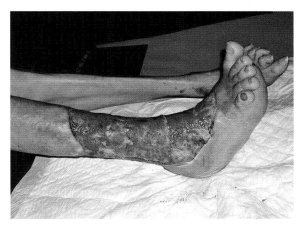

Figure 19.5   The patient in Figure 19.2 after excision of the tumour (Courtesy of Dr Nicolas Foureur, Paris)

upon us by the fact that, although the malignant disease had been eradicated by radiotherapy, the patients were still made utterly miserable by a large, weeping, painful and foul-smelling ulcer' (Black 1952). Having said that, palliative treatment with radiation, given the quality of the dressings of today, is an option. Cancer metastases are often treated by radiation.

Chemotherapy is not considered to be a feasible alternative treatment for SCC; however, this is a constantly evolving science and an opinion should be obtained from the oncologist, especially if there is suspicion of spread to or beyond local lymph nodes.

The surgeon will probably not have seen a case like this, so collaboration at all stages of the treatment process is important, as well as sharing of the available data.

In spite of the relatively clear algorithm outlined above, there will always be a group of patients who for some reason will not accept or tolerate the surgical intervention suggested. For these, palliative treatment must be a possibility. Even though the malignant wounds of metastatic carcinoma are not the immediate subject of this chapter, the considerations pertaining to the malodorous exudative wound apply to them.

In the malignant wound there is uncontrolled production of tissue, often in excess of vascular supply, which leads to necrosis. In moderately and well differentiated SCCs there is keratin formation. These circumstances, along with exuberant wound fluid, often lead to a terrible odour, which is socially disastrous for the patient, leading to isolation (Grocott 2000). The cornerstone of therapy for this is superabsorbent dressings with an airtight backing membrane. Further ammunition includes silver dressings, activated charcoal dressing and, metronidazole gel (other local antibiotics: clindamycin, bacitracin, etc. are also worth trying). Larval therapy has been suggested, as well as yoghurt. In exceedingly weeping ulcers, application of an improvised ostomy with pouch can be tried.

A reduction of the tumour burden by simple tangential excision under local anaesthesia with vasoconstrictors is conceivable, with or without local application of cytostatics or radiation, if this makes the patient's life more bearable. The key aims are: less pain and embarrassment, less health-care contact, more of own life.

PATHOGENESIS

The vast majority of SCCs in the world arise on skin and are caused by the ultraviolet rays of the sun. SCC of the cervix uteri is another form of cancer in squamous epithelium; the primary carcinogen here is probably the human papillomavirus (HPV). In SCC of the oral cavity, airways and lungs the main carcinogens are the chemicals in tobacco and tobacco smoke. In SCC in chronic leg ulcers, however, the carcinogen is not known. There is no clear premalignant phase such as can be seen in ultraviolet-induced SCCs of the skin. HPV has been looked for but not found; indeed, not even in the epidermis at the margin of ordinary venous leg ulcers was HPV to be found (Baldursson et al 2000a). In tumour biology the various proteins involved in the cancer defences of the body are studied in different cancers. Brief descriptions of some of these are given below. These proteins have effects on different phases of the cell cycle and influence whether the cell is allowed to divide and multiply. Cancer is, of course, cells that multiply without control.

p53 is probably the single most important tumour defence of the body. When the cell is challenged by DNA-damaging agents such as radiation, the activity of this 'guardian of the genome' is increased. This seemingly has the function of stopping the cell cycle in order to repair the DNA or launch automatic cell death – apoptosis.

Bcl-2: Programmed cell death, apoptosis, is a well regulated cellular pathway that makes it possible to get rid of cells that are unnecessary or dangerous, such as cells with dysregulated proliferative behaviour, i.e. cancer cells. Thus the cancer defences order the cell to commit suicide. Bcl-2 halts this command and is one way in which cancer cells evade the body's defences.

p21 is a downstream product in the p53 pathway of cell cycle control. Upregulation of p21 brings the cell cycle to a halt before DNA production starts, to prepare for cell division, in the same way as the police stop a car before asking to see the driver's licence.

PCNA and *ki-67* are both proliferation markers that show which cells are within an active cell cycle preparing for division and which are not. Cancer cells are continuously proliferating and should therefore express these markers (King 1996).

Studies of p53, p21, ki67, PCNA, bcl-2 and other tumour markers have been carried out for SCC in leg ulcers. In solar SCC, considerable expression of mutant p53 can be found, whereas perilesionally in SCC in leg ulcers no such expression is to be found. Other markers of malignancy have been positive and might serve to distinguish between pseudoepitheliomatous hyperplasia and well differentiated SCC but do not give an explanation of the carcinogenesis (Baldursson et al 2000b). The plausible cause of SCC in chronic ulcers is the paradox that the chronic wound represents. The three tenets of tissue repair – inflammation, proliferation and remodelling – are disintegrated. At some stage the healing process halts, while on the molecular level proliferation is enhanced (Galkowska et al 2003). There is constant pressure to proliferate, yet the ulcer does not heal.

A theory to explain how deranged wound healing leads to cancer, within the frame of multi-step carcinogenesis (Weinberg 1989), must take into account the abnormal situation in the wound. Chronically elevated proliferation is a well known risk factor for neoplasia (Moore & Tsuda 1998) and studies of acute wounds have shown downregulation of p53 during the proliferative phase and upregulation during the remodelling phase (Hausman et al 1998, Nagata et al 1999). The downregulation of p53 is probably necessary to allow the proliferation inherent in wound repair. If an ulcer is seen as a wound with a chronic stimulation to proliferate, perhaps including prolonged downregulation of p53, this is a conceivable carcinogenic situation, especially when a relative growth advantage is present in the form of the stimulators of proliferation inherent in wound healing called growth factors (Alexander et al 1965, Abramovitch et al 1999). If a mutation is introduced into this situation it might not be removed by the cell's tumour defences because of the diminished inhibition of proliferation inherent in wound healing mentioned above. This mutation could be caused by neutrophil free radicals, therapeutical chemicals or spontaneous occurrence. The mutated cells proliferate, building a clone of cells that have a growth advance over the normal cells in the neighbourhood – ergo: cancer.

A proto-oncogene is a gene, often with a key role in control of proliferation, that, if mutated, can turn into a perpetual proliferation stimulant. This is the Achilles heel of the powerful cancer defences of the body. The question is whether some specific proto-oncogene is vulnerable to the circumstances in the chronic wound, so that a majority of squamous cell carcinoma in chronic ulcers could be tracked to a specific mutation. p53 would be the logical culprit but we did not find increased activity of p53 in samples of SCC in leg ulcers. Ouahes et al compared the expression of the proto-oncogenes c-*fos* and c-Ha-*ras* in acute and chronic wounds, and found that they were upregulated (Ouahes et al

1998) in the chronic wounds. Obviously, the molecular studies up until now have barely scratched the surface of the riddle of the cause of cancer in chronic ulcers.

FUTURE PERSPECTIVES

The duration of leg ulcers before development of SCC is extremely long. It is not unusual to see a patient with a leg ulcer with a remitting relapsing course over decades. Many of the patients we see today have had their ulcers for many years. Often, they got them as a result of a venous insufficiency after venous thrombosis complicating childbirth or a surgical operation. Today, the understanding of the importance of thrombosis prophylaxis and early mobilization should have decimated this cause of ulceration. Even better treatment of leg ulcers should lead to less morbidity. The counter-effect is that the numbers of elderly people are steadily increasing and thus we still see people with ulcers many decades old; the only difference is that the patients are older.

Thus the future is hard to predict, as usual, and the only thing clinicians can do is to be on their guard, since population statistics apply to populations and our duty is to the individual patient.

Because SCC in chronic ulcers is not common, future studies on the subject of this chapter are not likely to amount to heavy expenditure. However, the obscurity of the cause of SCC in venous leg ulcers should warrant some curiosity and encourage scientists to explore this field, since the answer to other questions might lie therein.

CONTROVERSIES

There are some controversies that have been discussed in this chapter. The problem of SCC is discussed in Case Study 10. The seemingly different, yet unknown cause of SCC in venous leg ulcers versus the well known factors behind sun-induced SCC of the skin is another. The use of different active treatment modalities must proceed with a certain caution in circumstances in which carcinogenesis seems enhanced and I would like to touch upon this.

The evolution towards use of growth factors in chronic wounds should induce awareness of the potential risks. One conceivable initiating mechanism is that potential oncogenes from the cell cultures used for production of growth factors might transfect the cells of the ulcer, leading to uncontrolled proliferation and finally to cancer. This is speculative. It is, however, well established that platelet-derived growth factor enhances the growth of cancer cells when transformation has occurred (Dabrow et al 1998, Skobe & Fusenig 1998) and that wound fluid and wound-derived growth factors have well known tumour enhancing properties (Alexander et al 1965, Abramovitch et al 1999). Further, it has been shown that overexpression of transforming growth factor α bypasses the need for Ha-*ras* mutation in experimental mouse skin tumorigenesis (Vassar et al 1992). The proliferation associated with wound healing is in itself a tumour promoter (Alberts et al 1994, Cannon et al 1997) comparable to phorbol esters, a well known potent experimental carcinogen. In other words, there is a carcinogenic situation in the wound and further induction should be carried out with caution.

SUMMARY OF PRINCIPLES OF BEST PRACTICE

- Squamous cell carcinoma is a complication of venous leg ulcers.
- The important thing is to always have the possibility of a malignant change in mind. The diagnosis should be made with the help of biopsies. Every effort should be made to map the grade of the tumour and how widespread it is. A commendable attitude is to make a biopsy every time a surgical procedure is done under any type of anaesthesia on a chronic ulcer.
- The treatment is surgical, either a wide excision or amputation depending on the grade and spread of the tumour. Especially with excision, careful follow-up is important to detect local recurrence.

References

Abramovitch R, Marikovsky M, Meir G, Neeman M 1999 Stimulation of tumour growth by wound-derived growth factors. British Journal of Cancer 79: 1392–1398

Alberts B, Bray D, Lewis J et al 1994 The cell. Garland Publishing, New York

Alexander J W, Shucart W A; Altemeier W A 1965 Enhancement of tumor growth by growth promoting factor from injured tissues. Surgical Forum 16: 111–113

Baldursson B, Sigurgeirsson B, Lindelöf B 1993 Leg ulcers and squamous cell carcinoma: An epidemiological study and a review of the literature. Acta Dermato-Verereologica (Stockholm) 73: 171–174

Baldursson B, Sigurgeirsson B, Lindelöf B 1995 Venous leg ulcers and squamous cell carcinoma: a large scale epidemiological study. British Journal of Dermatology 133: 571–574

Baldursson B, Hedblad M-A, Beitner H, Lindelöf B 1999 Squamous cell carcinoma complicating venous leg ulceration: a study of the histopathology, course and survival in 25 patients. British Journal of Dermatology 140: 1148–1152

Baldursson B, Beitner H, Syrjänen S 2000a Human papillomavirus in venous ulcers with and without squamous cell carcinoma. Archives of Dermatological Research 292: 275–278

Baldursson B, Syrjänen S, Beitner H 2000b Expression of p21$^{WAF/CIP1}$, p53, Bcl-2 and Ki-67 in venous leg ulcers with and without squamous cell carcinoma. Acta Dermato-Verereologica 80: 251–255

Black W 1952 Neoplastic disease occurring in varicose ulcers or eczema: a report of six cases. British Journal of Cancer 6: 120–126

Cannon R E, Spalding J W, Trempus C S et al 1997 Kinetics of wound-induced v-Ha-*ras* transgene expression and papilloma development in transgenic Tg.AC mice. Molecular Carcinogenesis 20: 108–114

Clayman G L, Lee J J, Holsinger F C et al 2005 Mortality risk from squamous cell skin cancer. Journal of Clinical Oncology 23: 759–765

Copcu E, Aktas A, Sisman N, Oztan Y 2003 Thirty one cases of Marjolin's ulcer. Clinical and Experimental Dermatology 28: 138–141

Cruickshank A H, Mavis E, McConnell, Miller G 1963 Malignancy in scars, chronic ulcers and sinuses. Journal of Clinical Pathology 16: 573–580

Dabrow M B, Francesco M R, McBrearty F X, Caradonna S 1998 The effects of platelet-derived growth factor and receptor on normal and neoplastic human ovarian surface epithelium. Gynecologic Oncology 1998; 71: 29–37

Galkowska H, Olszewsk W L, Wojewodzka U et al 2003 Expression of apoptosis and cell cycle related proteins

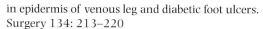
in epidermis of venous leg and diabetic foot ulcers. Surgery 134: 213–220

Grocott P 2000 The palliative management of fungating malignant wounds. Journal of Wound Care 9: 4–9

Hausmann R, Nerlich A, Betz P 1998 The time-related expression of p53 protein in human skin wounds –a quantitative immunohistochemical analysis. International Journal of Legal Medicine 111: 169–172

King R J B 1996 Cancer biology. Longman, Singapore

Knox L C 1925 Epithelioma and the chronic varicose ulcer. Journal of the American Medical Association 85: 1046–1048

Marjolin J N 1828 Ulcers. Dictionnaire de medecine. Bèchet Jeune, Paris, vol 21, pp 31–50

Marks R 1996 Squamous cell carcinoma. Lancet 347: 735–738

Moore M A, Tsuda H 1998 Chronically elevated proliferation as a risk factor for neoplasia. European Journal of Cancer Prevention 7: 353–385

Nagata M, Takenaka H, Shibagaki T, Kishimoto S 1999 Apoptosis and p53 protein expression increase in the process of burn wound healing in guinea-pig skin. British Journal of Dermatology 140: 829–838

Ouahes N, Phillips T, Hee-Young P 1998 Expression of c-*fos* and c-Ha-*ras* proto-oncogenes is induced in human chronic wounds. Dermatologic Surgery 24: 1354–1358

Phillips T J, Salman S M, Rogers G S 1991 Nonhealing leg ulcers: a manifestation of basal cell carcinoma. Journal of the American Academy of Dermatology 25 : 47–49

Skobe M, Fusenig N E 1998 Tumorigenic conversion of immortal human keratinocytes through stromal cell activation. Proceedings of the National Academy of Sciences of the USA 95: 1050–1055

Smith J, Mello L F B, Nogueira Neto N C et al 2001 Malignancy in chronic ulcers and scars of the leg (Marjolin's ulcer): a study of 21 patients. Skeletal Radiology 30: 331–337

Tenopyr J, Silverman I 1932 The relation of chronic varicose ulcer to epithelioma. Annals of Surgery 95: 734–748

Varmus H, Weinberg RA 1993 Genes and the biology of cancer. Scientific American Library, New York, p 48

Vassar R, Hutton M E, Fuchs E 1992 Transgenic overexpression of transforming growth factor alpha bypasses the need for c-Ha-*ras* mutations in mouse skin tumorigenesis. Molecular and Cellular Biology 12: 4643–4653

Weinberg R 1989 Oncogenes, antioncogenes and the molecular bases of multistep carcinogenesis. Cancer Research 49: 3713–3721

Inflammatory ulcers

Vincent Falanga

CHAPTER

20

INTRODUCTION

Inflammatory ulcers constitute a category of ulceration that is becoming increasingly important in terms of its recognition and treatment. This group of ulcers is generally underestimated in terms of its medical and economic significance, and such wounds are frequently difficult to diagnose and manage. While ulcers due to vascular insufficiency, such as venous and arterial ulcers, are generally easily recognized, inflammatory ulcers often present a very serious challenge in clinical practice (Falabella & Falanga 1998, Falanga 2000a).

Many inflammatory ulcers are related to collagen vascular (connective tissue) diseases and immunological conditions. These conditions include rheumatoid arthritis, systemic lupus erythematosus, scleroderma, dermatomyositis, polyarteritis nodosa and leukocytoclastic vasculitis. However, other types of inflammatory ulceration are not associated with collagen vascular diseases. Box 20.1 provides a partial list of these ulcers, their distinctive systemic and localized features, and clues that are helpful in diagnosis and management. Because of space limitations and practical issues, it is not possible to provide a complete list and discussion here of all possible ulcers (Helfman & Falanga 1995, Falanga 2000a, 2001). However, I have listed the main ulcers one is likely to encounter in this field.

Some of the ulcers listed in Box 20.1 are accompanied by arthralgia, arthritis, myalgia and myositis. Other types of ulcer are associated with cryoglobulinaemia (particularly related to hepatitis C), cryofibrinogenaemia, serum sickness, drug reactions and vasculitis (Kerdel 1993, Falanga 2000a). Also part of the spectrum are inflammatory ulcers related to immunosuppressed states and those due to immunobullous disorders (pemphigus) and accompanying immunological abnormalities affecting the joints, muscles and gastrointestinal tract. Among the most common of these ulcers are those associated with rheumatoid arthritis and other systemic conditions, including inflammatory bowel disease. However, there are also ulcers due to coagulation abnormalities, such as the antiphospholipid syndrome or those in which the blood vessels are affected by excessive deposition of calcium (calcinosis as in scleroderma and dermatomyositis, calciphylaxis; Kalaaji et al 1998, Essary & Wick 2000). The question is where one draws the line regarding the classification of 'inflammatory' ulcers. Do we call them inflammatory because they are caused primarily by inflammation rather than secondarily? The answer is no, as shown by my inclusion of ulcers where the primary defect is occlusion of small blood vessels (antiphospholipid syndrome, calciphylaxis, etc.; Table 20.1) with minimal inflammatory changes. Moreover, many of the typical vascular ulcers, especially venous ulcers, are characterized by intense inflammation. It seems to me that the field has evolved, correctly or incorrectly, to label as inflammatory ulcers those that are not primarily vascular or neuropathic in aetiology (venous, arterial, diabetic, pressure or decubitus ulcers) and are associated with local or systemic inflammatory conditions (Box 20.1).

Box 20.1 *Management of inflammatory ulcers*

1. **Partial list of inflammatory ulcers**
   - Pyoderma gangrenosum
   - Rheumatoid arthritis (often with high rheumatoid factor)
   - Vasculitis (superficial angiitis, medium-sized vessel)
   - Necrobiosis lipoidica diabeticorum (strongly associated with diabetes)
   - Panniculitis (lupus, pancreatic cancer, others)
   - Cryoglobulinaemia (strongly associated with hepatitis C)
   - Cryofibrinogenaemia
   - Arising from Raynaud's phenomenon
   - Scleroderma (systemic sclerosis, and mostly digital ulcers)
   - Fasciitis (from scleroderma, eosinophilic fasciitis)
   - Antiphospholipid syndrome (with lupus anticoagulant)
   - Chronic use of immunosuppression
   - Calcinosis (calciphylaxis, scleroderma, dermatomyositis)

2. **Distinctive clues away from the ulcer**

Clinical clues	Conditions
Hard fingers, face	Scleroderma
Facial butterfly rash	Lupus erythematosus
Muscle weakness, eyelid rash	Dermatomyositis
Ear redness with sparing of ear lobe	Relapsing polychondritis
Livedo reticularis or micro-livedo	Occlusion of small blood vessels, from vasculitis, coagulopathy, cryoglobulin, cryofibrinogen
Rheumatoid hands	Pyoderma gangrenosum, rheumatoid ulcers
Swelling of face, posterior neck	Cushingoid appearance (steroids)

3. **Consideration of inflammatory aetiology/pathogenesis**

When these signs are present	When these signs are absent
Livedo reticularis or microlivedo	No definite signs of venous insufficiency: lipodermatosclerosis, hyperpigmentation
Purple edges	Good arterial pulses
Undermined or undulating borders	No evidence of a neuropathy to explain the ulcer
Unusual location, not consistent with a vascular ulcer	Ulcer not in an area subject to trauma

4. **Cutaneous microthrombotic ulcers**

Clinical features	Severe pain, atrophie blanche, livedo reticularis, microlivedo, dark eschar within ulcer bed or at the edges
Aetiology	Cryofibrinogenaemia, antiphospholipid syndrome, coagulopathies, thrombocytosis, idiopathic livedoid vasculitis
Laboratory findings	Dermal vessel microthrombi, plasma cryofibrinogen, lupus anticoagulant, anticardiolipin antibodies, thrombocytosis, coagulopathies
Treatment	Anticoagulants, antiplatelet agents, high doses of pentoxifylline, anabolic steroids

Table 20.1 Classification of different types of vasculitis that can cause cutaneous ulceration

Medium-sized-vessel vasculitis	Small-vessel vasculitis
Polyarteritis nodosa. Necrotizing inflammation of medium-sized or small arteries. Biopsy of deep subcutaneous tissues may be required to identify an affected vessel	*Wegener's granulomatosis.* Granulomatous inflammation, also involving the respiratory tract, kidney. Cutaneous ulcerations are uncommon
Kawasaki disease. More commonly seen in children. Larger vessels may also be involved. Ulceration is rare	*Churg–Strauss syndrome.* Granulomatous inflammation with tissue and often peripheral blood eosinophilia *Microscopic polyangiitis.* Necrotizing vasculitis with only rare immune deposits. It may affect also medium-sized blood vessels. Systemic involvement frequent *Henoch–Schönlein purpura.* Vasculitis of small vessels with IgA deposits. Often associated with abdominal pain and bleeding, arthritis *Essential cryoglobulinaemic vasculitis.* Vasculitis and cryoglobulin deposits. Kidney involvement common, in addition to skin *Leukocytoclastic vasculitis.* Cutaneous small-vessel vasculitis, with destruction of blood vessels, nuclear dust, restricted to skin

In this review, I will discuss the major inflammatory ulcers and ways to approach this difficult problem both diagnostically and therapeutically. It will become quite obvious that the approach needs to be an all-encompassing one. One cannot simply examine the ulcer itself but has to take into consideration the systemic condition causing or associated with the ulceration, as well as identifying the hidden systemic diseases that led to the ulceration in the first place (Falanga & Eaglstein 1995).

OVERALL ASSESSMENT OF ULCERATION

Box 20.1 reminds us of the fact that the diagnostic approach to inflammatory ulcers begins when we first enter the examining room. I have emphasized the importance of this thorough approach in previous publications (Falanga & Eaglstein 1995, Falabella & Falanga 1998, Falanga 2000a, 2001). There may be distinctive clues that are present in other parts of the body or become evident upon physical examination. Involvement of the fingers and face with skin induration would lead one to suspect the diagnosis of systemic sclerosis (scleroderma; Falanga 2000a, Korn et al 2004). Similarly,

the presence of an erythematous butterfly rash on the face and photosensitivity will lead us to think of systemic lupus erythematosus (Falabella & Falanga 1998, Falanga 2000a). A purple-to-violaceous rash on the eyelids would be very suggestive of dermatomyositis. Involvement of the ear with redness and sparing of the earlobe (lacking cartilage) would suggest the rare condition of relapsing polychondritis, which is associated with severe joint involvement as well as life-threatening conditions of the larynx and the heart. The fact that a patient has neuropathy and diabetes would lead us to look for the yellow-orange discoloration of the skin on the legs (occasionally with ulceration) that is typical of necrobiosis lipoidica diabeticorum; these patients either have diabetes, will develop diabetes or have a strong family history of diabetes (Noz et al 1993, Handfield-Jones et al 1998, Evans & Atherton 2002).

Therefore, simply walking into the room, shaking the patient's hand and looking at the patient's face has important consequences for properly diagnosing unusual ulcerations of the extremities. A case in point is the appearance of the hands. Much has been written about the appearance of the hands in different rheumatic conditions

(Schorn & Anderson 1975, Kim & Collins 1981, Alarcon-Segovia et al 1983). Here, one would definitely pay attention to the ulnar deviation and the deformities of the hands that are associated with rheumatoid arthritis. Identifying rheumatoid arthritis would lead one to think that the ulceration might possibly represent pyoderma gangrenosum. Inflammatory lesions on the fingers can be important in distinguishing dermatomyositis from systemic lupus erythematosus. In dermatomyositis, purple papules or nodules occur over the finger joints, while the lesions of systemic lupus erythematosus are between the knuckles. These subtleties can be critical when first approaching the patient (Falanga 2000a).

The legs themselves, where the ulcers are commonly located, can be a vast source of clues. Not infrequently, patients present with ill-defined red streaks, often reticulated, on the lower extremities. Although these may represent the full-blown expression of livedo reticularis, one is frequently looking at what has been called microlivedo. The presence of this physical finding points to micro-occlusive disease, which may cause cutaneous ischaemia and subsequent ulceration (Falanga et al 1991, Helfman & Falanga 1995). Even the possibility that the ulcers may be due to medication or associated with certain systemic therapeutic agents can often be ascertained by simply examining the patient in an overall fashion. For example, bulging of the posterior portion of the neck may make us think of Cushing's syndrome or the cushingoid appearance resulting from the use of systemic corticosteroids.

Figure 20.1 shows several examples of inflammatory ulcers and illustrates several situations in which one has to look for particular physical findings peculiar to the ulceration. Pyoderma gangrenosum ulcers can be quite heterogeneous in their appearance. The textbook description is of an undermined ulcer with purple edges, often beginning as a blister. However, clinical practice indicates that pyoderma gangrenosum ulcers can be quite difficult to diagnose. Figure 20.1A–D gives an example of this heterogeneity.

Box 20.1 summarizes some physical findings and how they can be interpreted in terms of considering inflammatory ulcers. The presence of livedo, purple or undermined ulcer edges and unusual ulcer location are important clues that one may be dealing with nonvascular ulcers. The four cardinal clues shown in Box 20.1 (section 3) are very much critical to the diagnosis of inflammatory ulcers. For example, the presence of livedo is an important clue to the possibility of cryofibrinogenaemia, cryoglobulinaemia, hypercoagulable states and the antiphospholipid syndrome. Purple or undermined edges strongly suggest the possibility of pyoderma gangrenosum. Rheumatoid ulcers tend to have an undulating border, which is a very distinctive sign. Important in all this, in addition to satisfying ourselves that venous and arterial insufficiency do not play a prominent role in the pathogenesis of the ulceration, is also the assessment that the ulcers are not due to pressure. In many cases, pressure-induced ulcers are quite obvious, for example when the ulcers are on the solar surface or on the patient's lower back. However, the possibility of pressure can sometimes be more subtle. For example, a patient with kyphosis may have thoracic vertebral bodies that are quite prominent and create enough pressure to lead to ulceration.

GENERAL MEASURES

The fact that we are dealing with inflammatory ulcers does not mean that the basic fundamentals of wound care are not important or applicable. In this regard, wound bed preparation is critical. We were the first to propose this concept of wound bed preparation, aimed at maximizing the endogenous process of wound healing (Falanga 2000b). The wound bed preparation approach dictates that all aspects of wound care are properly adhered to. These aspects include the proper formation of wound bed granulation tissue, decreasing the bacterial burden, downregulating the inflammatory process and decreasing the amount of exudate so as to maintain proper and appropriate moisture balance (Falanga 2000b, 2004). Only then can we hope that the other therapeutic approaches I am going to discuss can heal inflammatory ulcers. The use of autolytic debridement with occlusive dressings and the amelioration of pain with dressings are also important (Helfman et al 1994, Ovington 1999). For example, some conditions that are intensely painful, such as cryoglobulinaemia and

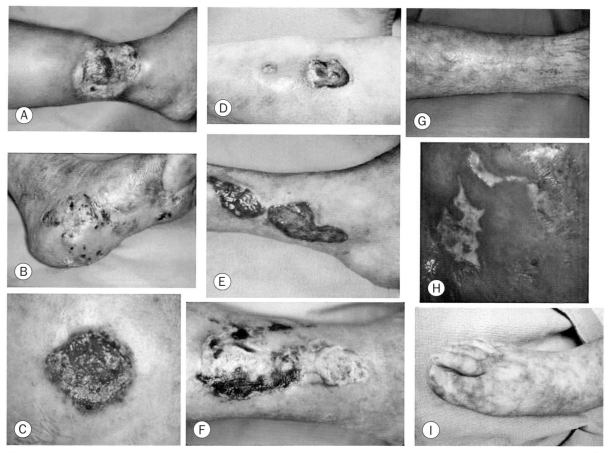

Figure 20.1   Examples of some inflammatory ulcers. (**A**) Pyoderma gangrenosum in a patient with rheumatoid arthritis. (**B**) The more 'granulomatous' appearance of pyoderma gangrenosum. (**C**) Typical pyoderma gangrenosum with purple edges. (**D**) Undermined ulcer of pyoderma gangrenosum. (**E**) The undulating borders of a rheumatoid ulcer. (**F**) Eschar in an ulcer due to polyarteritis nodosa. (**G**) Same patient shown in (F), after successful use of immunosuppressants. (**H**) The 'angular' ulcers seen in patients with collagen vascular diseases, often mimicking factitial ulcers. (**I**) Livedo reticularis and small ulcers in a patient with cholesterol embolization. Copyright, V Falanga, 2005.

vasculitis, can be improved, in terms of pain control, by the use of moisture-retentive dressings. Also, and I will discuss this later, the use of bio-engineered skin or even autologous split-thickness grafts for coverage of difficult and painful inflammatory wounds can be very important in terms of controlling pain and stimulating the process of epithelialization (De Imus et al 2001).

Having discussed in general terms some of the approaches we use in diagnosing inflammatory ulcers, I will now go into more detail about individual types of inflammatory ulcer, their diagnostic pitfalls and the therapeutic approach.

PYODERMA GANGRENOSUM

Pyoderma gangrenosum is a well known inflammatory ulceration associated classically with rheumatoid arthritis, inflammatory bowel disease and, more rarely, monoclonal gammopathies (usually IgA; Falabella & Falanga 1998, Riahi et al 2001). Patients with other immunological disorders, such as relapsing polychondritis, may also develop pyoderma gangrenosum (Fig. 20.2). Sometimes, surgery to the particular skin site can be the initiating event, but often pyoderma gangrenosum develops without a defined initiating event. Textbooks

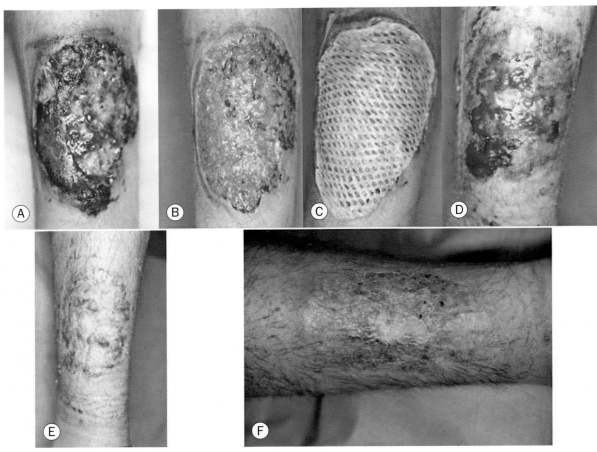

Figure 20.2. Sequence of clinical presentation and outcome in a patient with pyoderma gangrenosum. (**A**) Pyoderma gangrenosum of the tibial surface in a 26-year-old woman. (**B**) Appearance of wound a few days after pulse steroid therapy and the use of cyclosporin. (**C**) Application of a bioengineered bilayered skin equivalent to expedite healing and avoid creating a split-thickness donor site. (**D**) 2 weeks after wound coverage. (**E**) 6 weeks later. (**F**) Several months later. Copyright, V Falanga, 2005.

commonly state that pyoderma gangrenosum starts as blisters or pustules, which shortly thereafter ulcerate and lead to ulcers with a necrotic ulcer bed with undermined ulcer edges (Fig. 20.1D). A purple edge to the ulcer is also said to be typical for this condition (Fig. 20.1C). Although this classical presentation does occur, in my general experience the condition is very heterogeneous. For example, concomitant leukocytoclastic vasculitis is a rather frequent finding (Riahi et al 2001). Not uncommonly, pyoderma gangrenosum may develop without prior blister formation. The typical undermining may not always be present, and the purple edges are not always easily identifiable (Fig. 20.1B).

One distinctive feature of pyoderma gangrenosum is pathergy, which refers to the propensity for this type of ulceration to develop, rapidly deteriorate or enlarge upon trauma or biopsy. Pathergy is a true phenomenon, but I feel it has often been overplayed, even to the extent of not removing obviously infected or heavily colonized necrotic tissue (Gudi et al 2000).

The typical history of pyoderma gangrenosum is of a necrotic ulceration referred for surgical debridement, with the outcome being that the ulcer vastly enlarges within days of the procedure. Clearly, this does occur. However, one cannot stand idle and do nothing about an ulcer bed characterized by necrotic tissue that needs to be removed. Therefore, the clinician has to walk a very fine line in terms of removing obviously necrotic and infected tissue and yet not injuring viable tissue that could easily ulcerate because of pathergy. Figures 20.1 and 20.2 show a spectrum of ulcerations that are highly suggestive of pyoderma gangrenosum. Figure 20.3A shows a pyoderma gangrenosum ulcer that was associated with relapsing polychondritis. The association of these two conditions has been reported before, especially in the setting of a myelodysplastic syndrome (Hedayati et al 1993, Tsanadis et al 2002). This

was a typical example of how careful examination of the patient gives clues about the aetiology of the ulcer. We first noted the involvement of his ears, with sparing of the earlobe, which is classical for relapsing polychondritis (Fig. 20.3B). This important finding made the diagnosis of the leg ulcer and arthropathy so much easier. Occasionally, pyoderma gangrenosum has a clinically 'granulomatous' appearance (Fig. 20.1B), and this can also be seen on histology (Riahi et al 2001). These are difficult cases because one might be led astray by the possibility of fungal infections and other conditions that would not normally be treated with

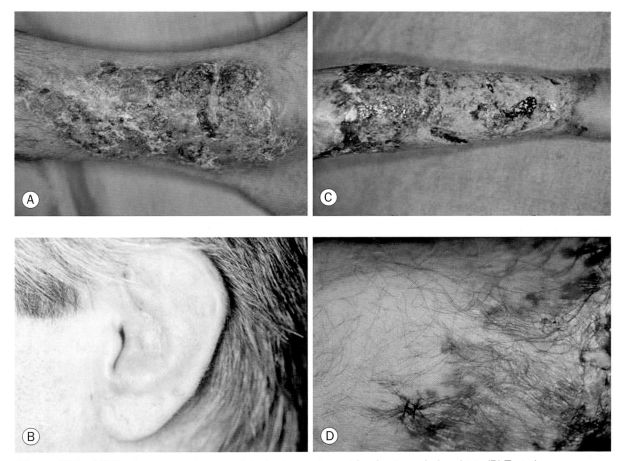

Figure 20.3 (**A**) Pyoderma gangrenosum of the leg in a patient with relapsing polychondritis. (**B**) Typical ear appearance in a patient with relapsing polychondritis whose ulcer is shown in (A). The cartilage-bearing portion of the ear shows erythema, while the earlobe is spared. (**C**) Extensive leukocytoclastic vasculitis in a patient who was hospitalized several times with a diagnosis of cellulitis. The wound on the lower leg is the result of a large excisional biopsy that failed to reveal the correct diagnosis. (**D**) Close-up of the upper margin of the vasculitis shown in (C). Proper diagnosis was established after a biopsy was taken of the advancing margin of the vasculitis. Copyright, V Falanga, 2005.

immunosuppressive therapy, which is the common therapy for pyoderma gangrenosum (Falanga 2000a).

For pyoderma gangrenosum, an ample biopsy is required, not so much to confirm the diagnosis of pyoderma gangrenosum but more for exclusion of other conditions. In fact, it should be made clear that there is no perfect histological or diagnostic picture of pyoderma gangrenosum. Classically, one sees rather extensive infiltration of neutrophils in the ulcer bed. However, there can be 'granulomatous' histological findings in pyoderma gangrenosum, and this is to be borne in mind when the clinical picture is very much consistent with that diagnosis and fungal aetiologies have been excluded by both special histological stains and by culture (Falabella & Falanga 1998, Riahi et al 2001). Nevertheless, the biopsy is important because of the necessity to exclude easily treatable ulcers that may respond to antituberculous or antifungal therapy. In some cases, clinicians have advocated the necessity for a bone marrow biopsy to exclude an underlying lymphoma or other types of haematological malignancies. If this becomes necessary, it is important to perform the bone marrow aspiration or biopsy on the iliac crest and not the sternum. I say this because, were the diagnosis truly pyoderma gangrenosum, the patient might develop massive ulceration involving the sternal area and even extending to the thoracic cavity.

The mainstay of therapy for pyoderma gangrenosum has always been the use of systemic corticosteroids (Gettler et al 2003). We often see patients referred to us who have been diagnosed as pyoderma gangrenosum and have been treated with short tapering courses of systemic corticosteroids. This is ineffective treatment. If the diagnosis is truly pyoderma gangrenosum, one needs to treat with relatively high doses (60 mg or greater) of prednisolone for many weeks or months. Only then can one can obtain a sustained therapeutic response. Because systemic corticosteroids are associated with substantial side effects, including infection, hypertension/congestive heart failure, avascular hip necrosis and cataracts, the diagnosis has to be clear before embarking on such therapy. Yet, in other cases where the diagnosis is unclear and the presence of other infectious causes has been excluded, one often is left with a therapeutic

trial of systemic steroids that may give us clues that this is indeed pyoderma gangrenosum or an immunological condition that is steroid-responsive. In such situations, we prefer the use of intravenous pulse therapy with methylprednisolone (Johnson et al 1982, Prystowsky et al 1989, Gettler et al 2003). Patients are often hospitalized for this therapy and, if there is any question of arrhythmias or other cardiac conditions, telemetry may be necessary during the period of steroid infusion. Indeed, concomitant therapy with diuretic agents represents a relative contraindication to the use of intravenous pulse steroid therapy because of the definite possibilities of disturbances in potassium levels and the occurrence of sometimes fatal arrhythmias. In the usual case, patients are hospitalized under telemetry and given 1 g of methylprednisolone intravenously every day for 3–5 days. When discharged, hopefully at a time when the ulcers have readily shown response to the steroids, one needs to keep in mind that the patient has to be kept on either steroid therapy or some alternative immunosuppressive agents (see below).

Over the last few years, cyclosporin seems to have replaced corticosteroid therapy in the treatment of pyoderma gangrenosum (Matis et al 1992). The usual dose of cyclosporin for this condition is 2.5–5 mg/kg a day. Needless to say, one needs to keep in mind the potentially life-threatening side effects of cyclosporin. The patient's blood pressure needs to be monitored closely and one needs to follow the usual recommendations for the use of cyclosporin to avoid renal deterioration. It has been stated that pyoderma gangrenosum responds readily to the use of cyclosporin. In our experience, this is not the case. I do feel that cyclosporin is effective in this condition but I also believe that it takes several weeks for an appropriate response to the therapy. Therefore, in the first few weeks of treatment, we are very much satisfied that the ulcer is not deteriorating any further. This good sign is then followed by the development of good granulation tissue and eventual re-epithelialization of the ulcer. Other immunosuppressive agents have been used for pyoderma gangrenosum. These include cyclophosphamide and, more recently, mycophenolic acid (Liu & Mackool 2003). The latter, in our experience, is not as effective as initially reported. The use of cyclophosphamide is associated with haemorrhagic bladder problems, and this must be kept in mind in terms of providing the patient with appropriate hydration during the course of therapy. Azathioprine is also an effective agent but is relatively slow in inducing a remission. Our current experience indicates that therapy directed against the action of tumour necrosis factor (TNF)α may be ideal when confronting difficult cases (McGowan et al 2004).

In one recent report, we have suggested that an effective approach to pyoderma gangrenosum may involve the use of pulse steroid therapy, the concomitant use of cyclosporin, and the relatively immediate placement of bioengineered skin as a means to achieve rapid healing (Fig. 20.2; de Imus et al 2001). Bioengineered skin circumvents the pathergy problem associated with harvesting autologous skin grafts. As stated, the use of new biological agents, such as those that interfere with the action of TNFα, appears to be quite effective. Therefore, the combination of these new biological agents and bioengineered skin may prove to be ideal.

In summary, pyoderma gangrenosum represents a challenge both diagnostically and therapeutically. However, this condition is important to recognize because of the pathergy associated with too aggressive a debridement approach and also for the response to immunosuppressive agents and new therapeutic approaches.

RHEUMATOID ULCERS

These ulcers are often associated with high levels of rheumatoid factor and severe arthritis. However, they may also be seen in patients with a rather stable course of rheumatoid arthritis (Helfman & Falanga 1995, Falanga 2000a). The appearance of these ulcerations is quite distinctive, as shown in Figure 20.1E. Rheumatoid ulcers tend to have a scalloped, undulating border. This physical finding may be quite subtle and one has to get close to the ulcer to appreciate the undulating appearance of the borders. Rheumatoid ulcers should not be mistaken for pyoderma gangrenosum. They do not have the purple edges associated with pyoderma gangrenosum, nor the undermining border, and they generally do not have the necrotic or truly eschar-like ulcer base we see in pyoderma gan-

grenosum. Also, rheumatoid ulcers are peculiarly resistant to many of the treatments we use for pyoderma gangrenosum. The ulcers are generally restricted to the lower extremities, whereas ulcers of pyoderma gangrenosum may be located on other parts of the body. In our experience, it is not uncommon for rheumatoid ulcers to have a component of vascular or venous insufficiency, which often makes the condition more difficult to diagnose.

One would think that histology would be very helpful in this condition. Indeed, biopsy is required in this situation because of the necessity to exclude other aetiologies, particularly those due to infection or malignancy. However, one does not often see evidence of vasculitis histologically, and even direct immunofluorescence is generally negative for immunoreactants. It has been stated that the immune complexes may be destroyed by the inflammatory process, and that is the reason for the negative immunofluorescence findings. The main conclusion seems to be that rheumatoid ulcers are probably multifactorial in aetiology (Oien et al 2001).

Treatment of rheumatoid ulcers is very disappointing. In our experience, immunosuppressive agents are not very effective or at least not as effective as we find them to be in pyoderma gangrenosum and other immunological ulcerations. Interestingly, perhaps because of the associated venous insufficiency that we have mentioned earlier, compression therapy may be of some value in addition to some immunosuppressive therapy. Also, split-thickness autografts can be helpful in this condition if one can get to the point that the ulcers are graftable (Oien et al 2001). In this context, we would like to mention that, indeed, autografts can be quite helpful in situations of inflammatory ulcers. One would not predict this to be the case. However, this therapeutic approach may be justified when everything else has failed. Anti-TNFα treatment may prove helpful in some patients with rheumatoid ulcers. Indeed, thalidomide may be effective because of its ability to decrease TNFα (Combe 2001).

SCLERODERMA ULCERS

Scleroderma ulcers represent a spectrum of conditions manifested by skin breakdown and associated systemic sclerosis (scleroderma). This spectrum is quite large, as it can involve ulcerations of the fingers as a result of ischaemia as well as ulcerations due to associated abnormalities in coagulation and tissue calcium deposition. Not to be forgotten is the development of ulceration purely due to indurated, tense tissues resulting from fibrosis.

More than 90% of patients have Raynaud's phenomenon. Classically, Raynaud's phenomenon presents with a triad of colour changes in the fingers and toes secondary to cold exposure or stress. Typically, there is pallor of the skin, which is followed by cyanosis, and then finally by reactive hyperaemia; the latter presents as intense redness. Some or all of the fingers and toes can be involved. A certain degree of numbness may accompany Raynaud's phenomenon. Actually, the classical presentation of Raynaud's phenomenon we have just described is quite uncommon. More often, partial symptoms or findings are present. For example, patients may only complain of intense numbness of one or more fingers on exposure to cold. The colour changes may not be as classically described (Falanga 2000a).

In the spectrum of sclerodermal ulcers, the ulcerations may be due to infection, occlusive large vessel thrombosis, ischaemia of the digits, vasculitis, as well as hypercoagulable states and calcinosis. The most common form of ulcerations in systemic sclerosis, generally called scleroderma ulcers, are those that present on the fingers (Korn et al 2004). Therefore, we should devote some discussion to that situation. Finger ulcerations can occur on the knuckles as well as the distal parts of the digits (Fig. 20.4). This distinction is important. Ulcers that develop on the proximal interphalangeal joints are generally due to trauma in the setting of intensely fibrotic skin. These ulcerations can be avoided by protecting the fingers from trauma (see below). Ulcers at the digital tip are typically due to ischaemia. In fact, the digital vessels in systemic sclerosis are narrowed and sometimes obliterated very early during the course of the disease. There is extensive intimal thickening, which leads to poor blood flow and therefore skin ulceration (Korn et al 2004). This is extremely important to recognize, because agents that are mainly directed against vasospasm are not always effective in digital ulcers associated with systemic sclerosis. The reason for

this is that the narrowing of the digital vessels is often fixed, and the degree of vasospasm is not as marked as in other patients with Raynaud's disease who do not have systemic sclerosis or may have some other type of collagen vascular disease.

A clue to the presence of systemic sclerosis in the setting of digital ulceration is the presence of abnormalities upon nailfold capillaroscopy (Nagy & Czirjak 2004, Anderson et al 2005). Capillaroscopy can be ascertained with very sophisticated imaging techniques. However, a simple way of observing the nailfold is to simply take the ocular piece of a microscope and hold it an inch or two above the nailfold while shining light transversely. In patients with systemic sclerosis, the normal filiform pattern of capillaries perpendicular to the nailfold is replaced by areas of capillary dropout and tortuous blood vessels.

Not much is known about the histology of digital ulcers in systemic sclerosis except from autopsy specimens. This is because one is always reluctant to biopsy small areas of the digital tip that are necrotic and ischaemic. However, as mentioned earlier, we do know that the small vessels are often occluded because of intimal thickening, and we also know that areas of calcinosis are commonly present (Medsger 2003). The areas of calcinosis can be extensive (Fig. 20.4D–E), and they may involve large areas of the lower extremities or other areas of the skin. These calcium deposits are often extruded spontaneously, but they do present a special problem in terms of ulceration because they are associated with pain and failure to epithelialize.

We feel that sometimes the treatment of ulcerations in systemic sclerosis proves inadequate because clinicians may not proceed aggressively in terms of their therapeutic approach. For example, the digital ulcers, whether present at the fingertips or over the interphalangeal joints, are not to be taken lightly. Immediately, one should ascertain whether underlying osteomyelitis or even septic arthritis is present. Therefore, the use of radiological tests, including magnetic resonance imaging, is important in excluding infection. Debridement of the ulcerations is a controversial topic. In general, we have the notion that areas of eschars or deep necrosis should not be debrided unless one has the means to revascularize the area. Thus, removal of an eschar without attention to revascularization

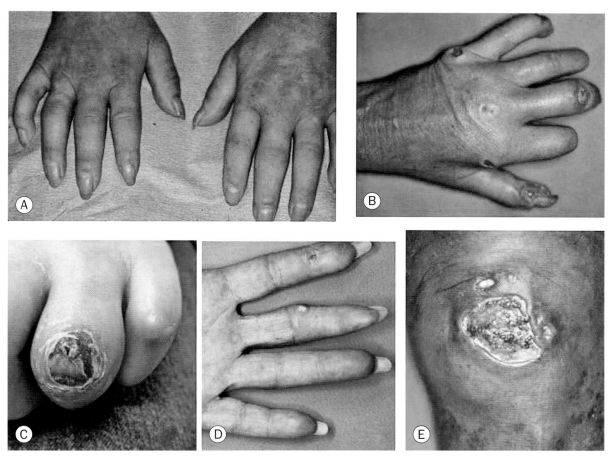

Figure 20.4 Systemic sclerosis (scleroderma). (**A**) Typical sclerodactyly, with intensely fibrotic skin. (**B**) Ulcerations and autoamputated distal portions of the digits in addition to ulcers in the knuckles. (**C**) Example of an ulcer with underlying osteomyelitis and visible underlying bone. (**D**) Areas of calcinosis on the digits. (**E**) Extensive calcinosis over the knee joint. Copyright, V Falanga, 2005.

can render the ulcer unstable. Therefore, aggressive debridement can destabilize the situation. Clinicians have advocated the use of occlusive dressings for stimulating moist wound healing and the formation of granulation tissue in these patients. Our approach has been to use occlusion and moist wound healing rather delicately. If we do use it, it is for a very short period of time, perhaps a few days to 2 weeks. This is enough to induce some gentle autolytic debridement without running into problems with maceration of the surrounding and underlying tissues.

The use of collagenase is another approach that seems to be promising in terms of allowing gentle debridement of the ulceration. Systemic vasodila-

tors have to be used also with caution. For example, nifedipine works much better in patients with Raynaud's disease without systemic sclerosis because those patients do not have the micro-occlusive disease that is so marked in systemic sclerosis (Meyrick Thomas et al 1997, Thompson et al 2001). Also, one has to be certain that the vasodilators will not cause a drop in the systemic blood pressure, to a degree that might also decrease skin perfusion. A recently published randomized controlled trial failed to show a beneficial therapeutic response of scleroderma digital ulcers to an endothelin receptor oral antagonist, although the occurrence of new ulcers seemed to decrease (Korn et al 2004).

Several questions need to be answered with scleroderma digital ulcers. Among them is whether infection is present and whether a sudden or subacute ischaemic event has occurred that requires immediate surgical intervention. The ulcers over the interphalangeal joints do not respond readily to vasodilators because they are not necessarily ischaemic, but rather secondary to trauma. One needs to look for a treatable inflammatory process such as a vasculitis or cryofibrinogenaemia. Another question is whether calcinosis complicates the management. Calcinosis is very common in the skin of patients with systemic sclerosis; sometimes deposits are clearly visible to the naked eye (Fig. 20.4E). It may be necessary to remove some of the calcium deposits surgically. Another approach, not supported by strong evidence but still promising, is the use of low-dose warfarin (Cukierman et al 2004). We use this therapy to decrease the pain and the inflammation associated with these ulcers. The dosage is generally in the 2.5 mg range and the prothrombin time needs to be monitored so as to not run into problems with coagulation; the possible mechanism of action remains unknown. Sometimes, angular-looking ulcers occur in the fibrotic skin of patients with systemic sclerosis, and indeed other connective tissue disorders such as dermatomyositis. This is shown in Figure 20.1H. Because of the odd shape of these ulcers, it is important not to conclude that they are self-induced. It is our impression that such ulcers occur in the setting of abnormal microvasculature and in fibrotic skin. Some of them respond quite readily to the use of topical vitamin A or tretinoin, which we have previously reported to improve the formation of granulation tissue in chronic ulceration (Paquette et al 2001, Paquette & Falanga 2002).

VASCULITIS

The types of vasculitis that affect the skin and cause ulceration are generally those due to either small or medium vessel involvement (Gibson & Su 1995, Csernok & Gross 2000). Table 20.1 summarizes the various types of vasculitis, specifying whether the process involves either small or medium-sized vessels or, in some cases, both. Vasculitis of large vessels, which is not really applicable to cutaneous ulceration, is not listed in Table 20.1. Leukocytoclastic vasculitis is the most common type of vasculitis that affects the skin and leads to ulceration. Polyarteritis nodosa destroys medium-sized vessels and can also cause ulcers that are very painful and difficult to treat. Figure 20.1F & G illustrates the case of a patient with cutaneous polyarteritis nodosa who responded well to treatment with cyclosporin.

At first, Table 20.1 and the diagnostic considerations listed may appear rather daunting. However, in practical terms, one is interested in determining whether the patient has a small-vessel vasculitis and ensuring that the biopsy specimen and its sectioning make it possible to diagnose involvement of a larger blood vessel, as in polyarteritis nodosa. There are clinical findings, too. The diagnosis of vasculitis is suggested clinically by the presence of areas of necrosis and redness and the presence of palpable purpura. The shape of the areas of involvement is important in trying to determine, at least clinically, the size of blood vessels that are involved. For example, leukocytoclastic vasculitis tends to lead to very regular lesions and ulcers in the skin. On the other hand, certain types of vasculitis, such as polyarteritis nodosa or those involving larger blood vessels, lead to areas of skin involvement and purpura that are irregular in appearance because of the chance of anastomosing vessels modifying the level of ischaemia at the skin surface (Braverman 1983). These considerations are illustrated in Figure 20.5. The presence of microlivedo or even full-blown livedo reticularis are other important clues to the presence of vasculitis (Falanga 2000a, Paquette & Falanga 2002). Generally, the lower extremities are involved. Blistering can occur, often with haemorrhage. The areas can be extremely painful, and the underlying joints may be swollen. Henoch Schönlein purpura is commonly associated with arthritis (Table 20.1; Gibson & Su 1995). As in other aspects of inflammatory ulcers, it is important to take into account the entire clinical picture so as not to miss associated systemic conditions. Leukocytoclastic vasculitis can often be idiopathic but may be secondary to a number of drugs or systemic diseases such as lupus erythematosus, serum sickness, dermatomyositis and rheumatoid arthritis.

As mentioned earlier, the biopsy is critical in determining and proving that the patient has a

Small vessel vasculitis Medium vessel vasculitis

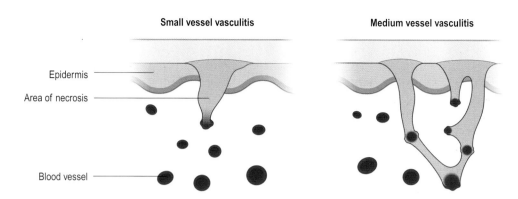

Figure 20.5 Diagrammatic representation of the difference in small versus medium-sized (deeper) vessel vasculitis and the impact on skin findings. A superficial vasculitis (left side of diagram) leads to a wedge-shaped area of necrosis and, thus, a well defined and regular skin purpura or necrosis. Conversely, occlusion of a deep vessel (right side of diagram) leaves open the chance for anastomosing vessels to alter the effect at the skin surface. As a result, the areas of purpura and necrosis tend to be irregular in shape. Copyright, V Falanga, 2005.

vasculitis. In leukocytoclastic vasculitis, one looks for the presence of superficial blood vessels in the dermis that have been destroyed by the inflammatory process, which is generally made up of neutrophils. Nuclear dust, a result of neutrophil fragmentation, is present histologically. A proper histological specimen generally requires an excision rather than a punch biopsy. This is because one is always looking for the possibility of a medium-sized vasculitis, and an excisional biopsy is more likely to show whether deeper blood vessels are involved. The site of the biopsy is also critical. One does not want to biopsy obviously necrotic areas, which have already undergone too much damage to the tissue and, therefore, are unlikely to show the primary process. Rather, one should biopsy the areas of skin that are red and at the edge of the ulceration (Fig. 20.3C & D). It should be noted that the histological picture can change dramatically with treatment. Therefore, one should be very careful in the interpretation of the biopsy results when patients have already begun treatment. In such cases, there is often a shift from a neutrophilic to a lymphocytic infiltrate. In other partially treated cases, all one can observe is a mild neutrophilic infiltration around the dermal blood vessels.

Treatment of vasculitis is very much dependent on the use of immunosuppressive or immunomodulatory agents. However, one must first exclude the possibility that a systemic medication may be the culprit. This is not easily proved, but the advice is to remove all medicines that are not totally necessary. In mild cases, colchicine, with or without the use of high doses of pentoxifylline (800 mg three times a day), can be an effective treatment. Similarly, dapsone has been a useful drug in leukocytoclastic vasculitis. The use of systemic corticosteroids in the range of 30–60 mg a day for several weeks can improve more dramatic cases of leukocytoclastic vasculitis. Other immunosuppressives, such as azathioprine or cyclosporin, can be helpful when corticosteroids are contraindicated or not effective. In the case of polyarteritis nodosa, cyclosporin has been helpful. As with other immunological disorders manifesting as skin breakdown, the newer class of biological agents, such anti-TNF drugs, can be quite effective.

CUTANEOUS MICROTHROMBOTIC ULCERS

Under this heading, one can place a host of cutaneous ulcers whose pathogenesis is characterized by occlusion of small dermal blood vessels (Box 20.1, section 4; Paquette & Falanga 2002). Clinically, these ulcers present with severe pain, atrophie blanche, livedo reticularis or microlivedo, and dark necrosis within the ulcer bed or at the edges (Fig. 20.6). The aetiologies include cryofibrino-

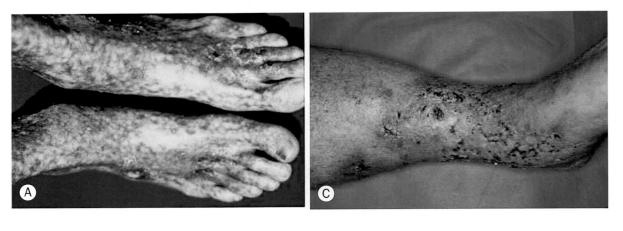

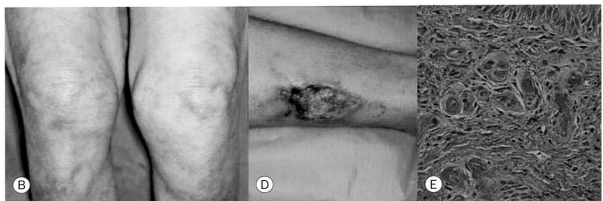

Figure 20.6 (**A**) Full-blown livedo reticularis involving the lower extremities. (**B**) Areas of microlivedo around the knee. (**C**) Necrotic skin areas in a patient with cryofibrinogenaemia, mimicking vasculitis clinically. (**D**) Ulceration of the lower leg, with necrotic edges and surrounding microlivedo, in a patient with cryofibrinogenaemia. (**E**) Histological photomicrograph of dermal blood vessels occluded by microthrombi in a patient with cryofibrinogenaemia. Copyright, V Falanga, 2005.

genaemia, the antiphospholipid syndrome, coagulopathies, thrombocytosis and idiopathic vasculitis. Histologically, one sees dermal vessels that are occluded either by microthrombi (Fig. 20.6E) or by the presence of opaque material, which may represent cryoglobulins. The patient needs to be worked up for the presence of cryofibrinogen, cryoglobulins and the lupus anticoagulant. A high platelet count as well as other types of coagulopathy can lead to the same clinical picture. In particular, many of these patients have a clinical picture of atrophie blanche (Milstone et al 1983, Paquette & Falanga 2002). It is of interest that patients on hydroxyurea, which is commonly used in the treatment of haematological malignancies, specifically poly-

cythaemia vera, can also present with ulcerations; the ulcer tends to improve or heal after the drug is discontinued (Best et al 1998).

Treatment of these types of ulcer includes anticoagulants, antiplatelet agents, high doses of pentoxifylline (800 mg three times a day) and anabolic steroids. The high-dose regimen of pentoxifylline has proved to be effective in patients with venous ulcers (Falanga et al 1999) and is now being used in other types of ulceration. Anabolic steroids have been particularly helpful in the treatment of cryofibrinogenaemia. In recent years, we described the use of stanozolol as a very promising treatment of cryofibrinogenaemia. This is an anabolic steroid, which can be very effective in the treatment of

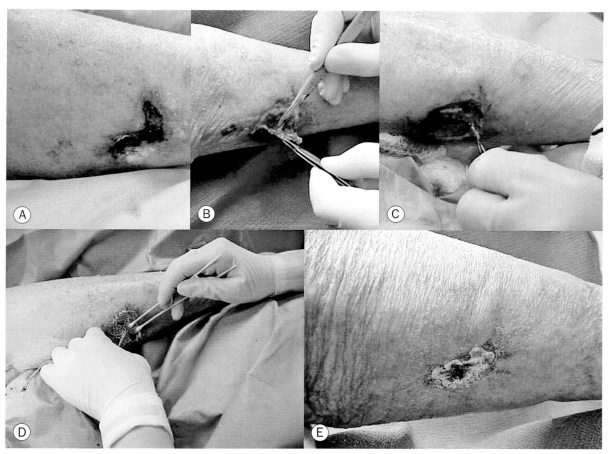

Figure 20.7 Sequence of treatment in a patient with calciphylaxis and end-stage renal failure. (**A**) Necrotic ulcer bed with surrounding microlivedo. (**B, C**) Debridement of the ulcer and calcium deposits, including a calcified blood vessel seen in C. (**D**) Application of a bilayered skin substitute after debridement. (**E**) Complete wound closure with residual crusting 5 weeks later. Copyright, V Falanga, 2005.

cryofibrinogenaemia at 2 mg twice a day. If effective, the improvement occurs within 3–4 weeks. However, recently, the drug has become unavailable even in countries in which it had remained on the market. The use of stanozolol by athletes has done a lot of damage to the reputation of the drug and has made it unavailable for patients. It seems that danazol may be an effective alternative; other anabolic steroids can also be tried. It is important to distinguish cryofibrinogenaemia from cryoglobulinaemia, in that cryofibrinogenaemia is detected in plasma whereas cryoglobulinaemia is in serum (Falanga et al 1991).

Calciphylaxis is a very-difficult-to-treat condition in which calcium is responsible for the occlusion of blood vessels (Essary & Wick 2000, Fine & Zacharias 2002, Milas et al 2003). This condition is often associated with severe renal disease and hyperparathyroidism. The ulcers are characterized by a necrotic wound bed with eschar and areas of microlivedo. Debridement of the areas of calcified blood vessels may be required in addition to grafting. That has been our approach, whenever possible. More recently, we have used bioengineered skin to relieve the pain and facilitate healing after thorough debridement (Fig. 20.7). Cholesterol embolization is caused by embolization of small (<100 μm) crystals from atherosclerotic plaques. It occurs in patients with severe atherosclerosis and can be precipitated by angiography, other vascular procedures and even the initial use of anticoagulants. Clinical features include livedo reticularis, CNS symptoms and, peculiarly, normal blood pressure. Renal failure may be a concomitant finding. Skin biopsy shows cholesterol crystals within the dermis and subcutaneous tissues. Serial subsectioning of the biopsy may be necessary to find these areas of cholesterol clefts (Fine et al 1987, Donohue et al 2003).

CONCLUSION

Inflammatory ulcers represent a group of ulcers associated with systemic complications, immunological abnormalities and joint and muscle involvement. The diagnosis stresses careful attention to the ulcer itself, surrounding skin, and physical findings away from the ulcer area. These ulcers are challenging, both diagnostically and from the therapeutic standpoint. Management needs to focus on pain relief, optimal wound care and systemic intervention. Urgency is required in many cases to improve the pain quickly and to arrive at the appropriate diagnosis and management.

References

Alarcon-Segovia D, Laffon A, Alcocer-Varela J 1983 Probable depiction of juvenile arthritis by Sandro Botticelli. Arthritis and Rheumatism 26: 1266–1268

Anderson M E, Allen P D, Moore T et al 2005 Computerized nailfold video capillaroscopy–a new tool for assessment of Raynaud's phenomenon. Journal of Rheumatology 32: 841–848

Best P J, Daoud M S, Pittelkow M R, Petitt R M 1998 Hydroxyurea-induced leg ulceration in 14 patients. Annals of Internal Medicine 128: 29–32

Braverman I M 1983 The role of blood vessels and lymphatics in cutaneous inflammatory processes: an overview. British Journal of Dermatology 109(Suppl 25): 89–98

Combe B 2001 Thalidomide: new indications? Joint, Bone, Spine 68: 582–587

Csernok E, Gross W L 2000 Primary vasculitides and vasculitis confined to skin: clinical features and new pathogenic aspects. Archives of Dermatological Research 292: 427–436

Cukierman T, Elinav E, Korem M, Chajek-Shaul T 2004 Low dose warfarin treatment for calcinosis in patients with systemic sclerosis. Annals of the Rheumatic Diseases 63: 1341–1343

De Imus G, Golomb C, Wilkel C et al 2001 Accelerated healing of pyoderma gangrenosum treated with bioengineered skin and concomitant immunosuppression. Journal of the American Academy of Dermatology 44: 61–66

Donohue K G, Saap L, Falanga V 2003 Cholesterol crystal embolization: an atherosclerotic disease with frequent and varied cutaneous manifestations. Journal of the European Academy of Dermatology and Venereology 17: 504–511

Essary L R, Wick M R 2000 Cutaneous calciphylaxis. An underrecognized clinicopathologic entity. American Journal of Clinical Pathology 113: 280–287

Evans A V, Atherton D J 2002 Recalcitrant ulcers in necrobiosis lipoidica diabeticorum healed by topical granulocyte-macrophage colony-stimulating factor. British Journal of Dermatology 147: 1023–1025

Falabella A, Falanga V 1998 Uncommon causes of ulcers. Clinics in Plastic Surgery 25: 467–479

Falanga V 2000a Text atlas of wound management. Martin Dunitz, London

Falanga V 2000b Classifications for wound bed preparation and stimulation of chronic wounds. Wound Repair and Regeneration 8: 347–352

Falanga V 2001 Cutaneous wound healing. Martin Dunitz, London

Falanga V 2004 The chronic wound: impaired healing and solutions in the context of wound bed preparation. Blood Cells, Molecules and Diseases 32: 88–94

Falanga V, Eaglstein W H 1995 Leg and foot ulcers: a clinician's guide. Martin Dunitz, London

Falanga V, Kirsner R S, Eaglstein W H et al 1991 Stanozolol in treatment of leg ulcers due to cryofibrinogenaemia. Lancet 338: 347–348

Falanga V, Fujitani R M, Diaz C et al 1999 Systemic treatment of venous leg ulcers with high doses of pentoxifylline: efficacy in a randomized, placebo-controlled trial. Wound Repair and Regeneration 7: 208–213

Fine A, Zacharias J 2002 Calciphylaxis is usually non-ulcerating: risk factors, outcome and therapy. Kidney International 61: 2210–2217

Fine M J, Kapoor W, Falanga V 1987 Cholesterol crystal embolization: a review of 221 cases in the English literature. Angiology 38: 769–784

Gettler S, Rothe M, Grin C, Grant-Kels J 2003 Optimal treatment of pyoderma gangrenosum. American Journal of Clinical Dermatology 4: 597–608

Gibson L E, Su W P 1995 Cutaneous vasculitis. Rheumatic Diseases Clinics of North America 21: 1097–1113

Gudi V S, Julian C, Bowers P W 2000 Pyoderma gangrenosum complicating bilateral mammaplasty. British Journal of Plastic Surgery 53: 440–441

Handfield-Jones S, Jones S, Peachey R 1988 High dose nicotinamide in the treatment of necrobiosis lipoidica. British Journal of Dermatology 118: 693–696

Hedayati H, Zuzga J J Jr, Faber D B 1993 Rheumatoid arthritis, relapsing polychondritis, and pyoderma gangrenosum evolving into non-Hodgkin's lymphoma. Journal of the American Osteopathy Association 93: 240–242, 6–8

Helfman T, Falanga V 1995 Stanozolol as a novel therapeutic agent in dermatology. Journal of the American Academy of Dermatology 33: 254–258

Helfman T, Ovington L, Falanga V 1994 Occlusive dressings and wound healing. Clinics in Dermatology 12: 121–127

Johnson R B, Lazarus G S 1982 Pulse therapy. Therapeutic efficacy in the treatment of pyoderma gangrenosum. Archives of Dermatology 118: 76–84

Kalaaji A N, Douglass M C, Chaffins M, Lowe L 1998 Calciphylaxis: a cause of necrotic ulcers in renal failure. Journal of Cutaneous Medicine and Surgery 2: 242–244

Kerdel F A 1993 Inflammatory ulcers. Journal of Dermatologic Surgery and Oncology 19: 772–778

Kim R C, Collins G H 1981 The neuropathology of rheumatoid disease. Human Pathology 12: 5–15

Korn J H, Mayes M, Matucci Cerinic M et al 2004 Digital ulcers in systemic sclerosis: prevention by treatment with bosentan, an oral endothelin receptor antagonist. Arthritis and Rheumatism 50: 3985–3993

Liu V, Mackool B T 2003 Mycophenolate in dermatology. Journal of Dermatological Treatment 14: 203–11

McGowan J W IV, Johnson C A, Lynn A 2004 Treatment of pyoderma gangrenosum with etanercept. Journal of Drugs in Dermatology 3: 441–444

Matis W L, Ellis C N, Griffiths C E, Lazarus G S 1992 Treatment of pyoderma gangrenosum with cyclosporine. Archives of Dermatology 128: 1060–1064

Medsger T A Jr 2003 Natural history of systemic sclerosis and the assessment of disease activity, severity, functional status, and psychologic well-being. Rheumatic Diseases Clinics of North America 29: 255–273, vi

Meyrick Thomas R H, Rademaker M, Grimes S M et al 1987 Nifedipine in the treatment of Raynaud's phenomenon in patients with systemic sclerosis. British Journal of Dermatology 117: 237–241

Milas M, Bush R L, Lin P et al 2003 Calciphylaxis and nonhealing wounds: the role of the vascular surgeon in a multidisciplinary treatment. Journal of Vascular Surgery 37: 501–507

Milstone L M, Braverman I M, Lucky P, Fleckman P 1983 Classification and therapy of atrophie blanche. Archives of Dermatology 119: 963–969

Nagy Z, Czirjak L 2004 Nailfold digital capillaroscopy in 447 patients with connective tissue disease and Raynaud's disease. Journal of the European Academy of Dermatology and Venereology 18: 62–68

Noz K C, Korstanje M J, Vermeer B J 1993 Ulcerating necrobiosis lipoidica effectively treated with pentoxifylline. Clinical and Experimental Dermatology 18: 78–79

Oien R F, Hakansson A, Hansen B U 2001 Leg ulcers in patients with rheumatoid arthritis–a prospective study of aetiology, wound healing and pain reduction after pinch grafting. Rheumatology (Oxford) 40: 816–820

Ovington L G 1999 Dressings and adjunctive therapies: AHCPR guidelines revisited. Ostomy/Wound Management 45(Suppl): 94S–106S; quiz 7S–8S

Paquette D, Falanga V 2002 Leg ulcers. Clinics in Geriatric Medicine 18: 77–88, vi

Paquette D, Badiavas E, Falanga V 2001 Short-contact topical tretinoin therapy to stimulate granulation tissue in chronic wounds. Journal of the American Academy of Dermatology 45: 382–386

Prystowsky J H, Kahn S N, Lazarus G S 1989 Present status of pyoderma gangrenosum. Review of 21 cases. Archives of Dermatology 125: 57–64

Riahi I, Mokni M, Haouet S et al 2001 [Pyoderma gangrenosum. 15 cases]. Annales de Medecine Interne (Paris) 152: 3–9

Schorn D, Anderson I F 1975 The radiographic appearance of the rheumatoid hand. South African Medical Journal 49: 752–756

Thompson A E, Shea B, Welch V et al 2001 Calcium-channel blockers for Raynaud's phenomenon in systemic sclerosis. Arthritis and Rheumatism 44: 1841–1847

Tsanadis G D, Chouliara S T, Voulgari P V et al 2002 Outcome of pregnancy in a patient with relapsing polychondritis and pyoderma gangrenosum. Clinical Rheumatology 21: 538

Tropical ulcers

Marwali Harahap

INTRODUCTION

Under the term 'tropical ulcers' a variety of skin conditions will be described. Many of these are due to microorganisms, e.g. diphtheria, mycobacteria, syphilis, yaws, pyogenic organisms, etc.

Leg ulcers result from a wide array of causes, including infections, vasculitis, trauma, burns, granulomatous diseases, skin cancers and diseases of unknown aetiology such as pyoderma gangrenosum. Both historically and worldwide, one of the commonest causes is probably a combination of trauma and infection, but in the Western world venous insufficiency is the most significant factor. All those who manage leg ulcers should nevertheless remember the possibility of other causes, because they can be encountered in every clinic. As in all branches of clinical medicine, experience is helpful, but a spot diagnosis can often be inaccurate and sensible clinicians will arrange confirmatory investigations, even when they are 90% sure of the underlying cause of the ulcer. Most leg ulcers seen in developed countries are venous or ischemic in origin. Infectious ulcers are more commonly seen in tropical countries; neoplastic ulcers are rare, but it is most important always to be aware of this possibility and there are a number of less common causes that are difficult to classify.

Whatever their original aetiology, all leg ulcers usually become infected secondarily through exposure to pathogenic bacteria on the surface of the skin and venous insufficiency and/or arterial obstruction. It must be remembered that infection may be the primary aetiological factor as well as a secondary invader. This chapter deals with all types of infection that may produce a leg ulcer.

DIPHTHERIA

Diphtheria is an acute febrile illness primarily involving the pharynx and mucous membrane of the upper respiratory tract. Rarely, the primary lesion may be located on the skin. Another type of skin involvement is that occurring in eczematous, impetiginous, vesicular or pustular lesions from which *Corynebacterium diphtheriae* may be recovered. Cutaneous bacteria are common in tropical areas.

Aetiology

The diphtheric ulcer is caused by the inoculation of *C. diphtheriae* into the skin. The organism is a Gram-positive, non-motile, non-spore-forming, club-shaped rod that exhibits metachromatic bipolar granules on staining with methylene blue. It grows well on ordinary media, although media containing potassium tellurite or coagulated serum (Loeffler's medium) promote growth.

Clinical manifestations

There are basically three types of skin involvement.

- *Primary cutaneous diphtheria* begins as a vesicle or pustule and usually breaks down and progresses to a shallow, oval, punched-out ulcer with an adherent crust of membranous base (Funt 1961). Exudate from the ulcer tends to form a yellowish or brownish-grey adherent membrane or dark crust. This ulcer does not extend below the fascia, has oedematous, rolled, bluish margins, is usually located on a lower extremity, and is most often seen in the tropics (Fig. 21.1)

- *Wound diphtheria*, as a secondary infection of a pre-existing wound, occurs in temperate as well as tropical climates and may involve any part of the body. Underlying (primary) skin lesions include those due to trauma (abrasions, lacerations, burns), chronic dermatitis (eczema, scabies, etc.) and various pyodermas. The lesion is usually partially covered with a membrane and a purulent exudate is present, with a zone of oedema and erythema surrounding the lesion
- Superinfection of eczematized skin lesions by *C. diphtheriae* forms a more superficial, membranous, tender, oedematous reaction.

Systemic manifestations are usually absent or mild in cutaneous diphtheric ulcer, but occasionally a membranous pharyngitis may accompany cutaneous diphtheria and symptoms of cranial or peripheral nerve palsies or of myocarditis may develop.

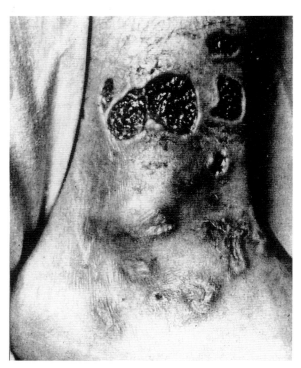

Figure 21.1 Cutaneous diphtheria begins a vesicle or pustule, and usually breaks down and progresses to a shallow, oval punched out ulcer (AFIP 76–6977).

Diphtheric ulcer occurs in the presence or absence of pharyngeal diphtheria. Usually, the site of primary infection is the nasopharynx or pharynx. However, the cutaneous lesions may serve as an important reservoir of infection from which epidemics of pharyngeal diphtheria may arise (Youmans et al 1985). The systemic consequences of the potent exotoxin are no different regardless of the site of infection.

Geographical distribution

Cutaneous diphtheria can be observed in any climate. Cutaneous diphtheria and wound diphtheria occur in tropical areas, particularly under conditions of poverty, poor hygiene and crowding. Pre-existing skin lesions create favourable circumstances for infection in unimmunized individuals. Although the disease is considered to be largely tropical, it has been observed in temperate regions. Cutaneous diphtheria in temperate areas usually presents as a secondary infection of impetigo, pyoderma, abrasion and insect bites. The course of most cases of cutaneous diphtheria is benign. A case of diphtheria was reported in the Netherlands due to an infection with *Corynebacterium ulcerans*. Physicians must consider diphtheria in the differential diagnosis of patients who present with a clinical syndrome compatible with this disease. Either *C. diphtheriae* or *C. ulcerans* could be the pathogen responsible (Van Dam et al 2003).

Laboratory findings

The organism can be isolated on appropriate media from the skin ulcer or pharyngeal membrane.

Diagnosis

A presumptive diagnosis is usually based on the findings of a shallow membrane-covered ulcer in cutaneous involvement or membranous pharyngitis in faucial diphtheria. The definitive diagnosis is based on bacteriologic studies. The finding of gram-positive Corynebacterium in smears, cultural isolation of the organism and demonstration of toxin production confirm the diagnosis.

Treatment

In ulcerative cutaneous diphtheria, combination therapy with a suitable antibiotic and specific antitoxin should be initiated on the basis of clinical suspicion without awaiting cultural confirmation, as toxin elaborated in the intervening period could lead to irreversible myocardial damage. Diphtheria antitoxin in doses of 20 000–40 000 units should be given intramuscularly, after careful testing for horse serum sensitivity. Penicillin (2–4 megaunits intramuscularly daily) is the antibiotic of choice; an alternative is erythromycin (2.0 g orally daily) administered for 7–10 days. Bed rest and prolonged observation are essential. The neurological signs and symptoms are almost always reversible.

Close contacts of a case of cutaneous diphtheria should be examined for any skin lesions (which should be cultured for *C. diphtheriae*); the pharynx should be cultured regardless of the presence of pharyngitis or a membrane. While the results of cultures are awaited, contacts should be given a dose of a diphtheria toxoid appropriate to their age if they have not completed a primary series or received a booster dose within the previous 5 years. They should receive antibiotic prophylaxis promptly with intramuscular penicillin or oral erythromycin (Brink & Hinman 1989).

SPOROTRICHOSIS

Sporotrichosis is a chronic infection of the skin and subcutaneous tissues caused by the fungus *Sporothrix schenckii*. Human infection occurs accidentally at the site of some insignificant wound and lymphatic spread may be seen.

Aetiology

S. schenckii is a dimorphic fungus that grows in a yeast form at 37°C and in a mycelial form at room temperature. It occurs in both temperate and tropical areas (Allan & Rippon 1985). *S. schenckii* is difficult to demonstrate in exudates, purulent material or tissue unless stained by a modified Schiff–McManus technique.

The fungus grows on decaying vegetable matter e.g., timbers in mines (Lynch 1971).

The organism grows slowly on Sabouraud's medium at 25°C. A moist, white colony develops within 3–7 days. The surface becomes wrinkled and folded. Later, dark mycelia may cover parts or all of the colony. Microscopically, the organism shows thin hyphae with conidia borne on very thin conidiophores, which are so delicate as to be almost invisible.

Clinical manifestations

The earliest manifestation may be a small nodule or ulcer, which may heal and disappear before the advent of further symptoms. It slightly resembles the syphilitic or tuberculous chancre (Cawley 1949). One to several weeks after the development of a primary ulcer, nodules develop along the draining lymphatics. A chain of lymphatic nodules appears. In time the overlying skin may ulcerate and may even show fistulous tracts or papillomatous vegetations. When the initial lesion occurs on an extremity, the chain of nodules arises linearly along the ascending regional lymphatics. This is the best known classic form of the disease and the commonest.

The fixed variety, where the organism remains more or less confined to the point of entry, is less common. The lesions may be verrucous, acneiform, nodular or ulcerated. An ulcer may be gummatous or covered with a thick impetiginous crust that may be surmounted by verrucous vegetations. It is thought that this type of disease reflects a higher degree of immunity of the host.

Disseminated sporotrichosis has been noted in patients with human immunodeficiency virus (HIV) infection (Lipstein-Kresch et al 1985; Bibler et al 1986).

Epidemiology

There seems to be no geographical localization to the occurrence of sporotrichosis. Sporotrichosis is found worldwide and in all age groups. Although adult men are infected most often, occupation and exposure are probably more important in acquiring the disease than are race, sex or age. Most often the primary invasion is seen as an occupational disease in gardeners, florists and labourers following injuries by thorns of plants or by straws. The usual reservoir in nature is vegetation, on which *S. schenckii* grows saprophytically, often on thorny protuberances. Sporotrichosis has been observed in horses, mules, dogs, rats, mice and cats.

Pathology

The histological changes are those of an infectious granuloma, with the formation of deep abscesses, sinuses and ulcerations. The later stage may show the arrangement of infiltrate in three zones. Toward the centre are collections of polymorphonuclears, eosinophils and macrophages. Between the central and the peripheral zones are numerous epithelioid cells and giant cells of the Langhans type, and the peripheral part is made up of lymphocytes and plasma cells.

Diagnosis

The diagnosis is established by the history of onset, the primary lesion and a chain of swollen nodules along the lymphatic drainage of the area, extending up the extremity. Biopsy with special staining and cultures, preferably from unopened lesions, clinches the diagnosis. The sporotrichin test is usually positive (Kusuhara et al 1988).

Differential diagnosis

Clinically, atypical mycobacteriosis (swimming pool granuloma), tuberculosis, syphilis, cat-scratch disease and deep fungus infections may resemble sporotrichosis, but differentiation is made without difficulty.

Treatment

The treatment of choice is a saturated solution of potassium iodide, which contains 1 g/ml of solution. Five drops are given three times a day, and the dose is increased by 5 drops each day to 30–40 drops three times a day. Because of gastrointestinal distress, the drops are usually given in juice or water. If iodides fail or are not tolerated, intravenous amphotericin B is the treatment of choice. Amphotericin B, 0.6 mg/kg of body weight per day, is given (administered intravenously in 500–1000 ml of 5% dextrose). The effectiveness of ketoconazole in the treatment of sporotrichosis appears limited (Difonzo et al 1986).

Investigators have found itraconazole at 100 mg/day to be highly effective in lymphocutaneous sporotrichosis (Restrepo et al 1986, Negroni et al 1987).

COCCIDIOIDOMYCOSIS

Coccidioidomycosis is an acute or chronic fungal disease caused by the organism *Coccidioides immitis*. This pathogenic fungus is acquired by inhalation of *C. immitis* followed by an incubation period of 10 days to several weeks, with a respiratory infection that may be mild, with occasional haematogenous dissemination to other tissues: skin, subcutaneous tissue, bone or meninges.

Aetiology

The causative organism, *C. immitis*, has been isolated from the soil and from vegetation, especially fruit. Most infections are thought to occur through inhalation of dust laden with the organisms. *C. immitis* is dimorphous and exists both in nature and on standard culture media at 25°C as hyphae, whereas in human or animal tissues it occurs as a non-budding, spherical, thick-walled structure 5–200 μm in diameter. This spherule contains numerous small endospores. At maturity the spherule ruptures, with release of the endospores.

Clinical manifestations

The lungs are almost always the initial or primary site of infection, which is usually asymptomatic but may simulate influenza. After a few weeks, some patients may develop erythema nodosum lesions over the pretibial areas or erythema multiforme, often in association with acute joint aches and fever.

Sometimes the skin is the favoured site, in which abscesses or chronic necrotic ulcers develop. After a period of months, the ulcers may undergo papillomatous changes.

Primary cutaneous coccidioidomycosis rarely occurs, since most of the lesions are attributable to dissemination from the primary lesion in the lung. The unique manifestation of primary cutaneous coccidioidomycosis is the development of the 'chancriform syndrome'. An ulcerative lesion develop at the site of cutaneous inoculation followed by lymphangitis and regional lymphadenopathy. Multiple nodules may be seen along the course of the lymphatics draining the area.

Cutaneous manifestations of disseminated coccidioidomycosis are most often verrucous granulomas, often appearing on the face.

Disseminated coccidioidomycosis was added to the surveillance definition for the acquired immunodeficiency syndrome (AIDS) in 1987 (Centers for Disease Control 1987).

An outbreak of coccidioidomycosis among 22 members of the armed forces occurred during training exercises in Coalinga, California. Ten (45%) of the 22 men had serological evidence of acute coccidioidomycosis, the highest attack rate ever reported for a military unit. Coccidioidomycosis continues to be a threat to military personnel and civilians who reside or train in areas where *C. immitis* is endemic (Cram et al 2002).

Diagnosis

A history of exposure in endemic areas or to products therefrom (Albert & Sellers 1963) might suggest the diagnosis. A definite diagnosis is made by identification of the causative fungus in sputum, smears, or biopsy specimens, or by culture of the fungus.

Treatment

In the great majority of cases the infections are self-limiting and do not require specific antifungal treatment.

In primary cutaneous coccidioidomycosis, indications for amphotericin B are the same as for the primary pulmonary form, which may heal without noticeable difficulty. A mild form does not usually require therapy.

In disseminated or progressive disease, amphotericin B given intravenously is the treatment of choice (Emmons et al 1977, Stevens 1980). Coccidioidomycosis remains a condition which is difficult to treat, and relapse is common.

An alternative to amphotericin B is ketoconazole. Although complete clearing of lesions was noted in significant numbers of patients, relapses after discontinuation were not uncommon (Galgiani 1983). Studies of doses and treatment are needed. Itraconazole showed impressive and encouraging clinical results in a series of patients (Tucker et al 1990). However, further evaluation of itraconazole is in order. Itraconazole, a new triazole currently under clinical investigation, appears very promising. It is orally administered, very well tolerated and less toxic to hepatic and endocrine function than ketoconazole (Dupont & Drouhet 1987, Lavalle et al 1987).

MYCETOMA

Mycetoma is a localized, chronic infection of the skin, subcutaneous tissues and bones, characteristically of the foot or leg but occasionally of the hands and other parts of the body. The infection occurs most frequently on the foot (Madura foot) and lower extremity.

Aetiology

Aetiologically, mycetoma is divided into two main groups (Mahgoub & Murray 1973): eumycetoma, produced by true fungi, and actinomycetoma, produced by actinomycetes. Examples of eumycetomas are those caused by *Madurella mycetomatis*, *M. grisea*, *Pyrenochaeta romeroi*, *Leptosphaeria senegalensis*, *Neotestudina rosatii*, less frequently *Exophiala jeanselmei*, *Curvularia lumata*, *Pseudallescheria boydii*, *Acremonium* sp. and *Fusarium* sp. The most common causes of actinomycetomas are *Nocardia brasiliensis*, *N. asteroides*, *Actinomadura pelletieri*, *Streptomyces somaliensis*, *A. madurae* and *Madurella mycetomatis*.

The great variety of infectious agents causing mycetoma occur as saprophytes in soil or on vegetable matter. Humans acquire the disease through penetrating injury by thorns or splinters contaminated by one of the causative infectious agents.

Clinical manifestations

Mycetoma generally begins as a rather nondescript, painless nodule. Some nodules break down and draining abscesses gradually form, usually on the foot or ankle (Fig. 21.2). The sinuses secrete microcolonies or grains of the causative organism. Partial healing brings about fibrosis and irregular contracture. Extension occurs to underlying muscles, bones and fascia, causing necrosis and depriving these structures of useful function. Most lesions are on the foot and lower leg, but any part of the body can be involved. In the lower limbs the most affected areas in order of frequency are the feet, legs, knees and thighs. The condition is comparatively painless and affected individuals manage to hobble along with their deformities for years, without obvious systemic reaction. After decades the disease, if untreated, terminates in death due to sepsis and exhaustion.

Geographical distribution

Mycetoma occurs everywhere. In the western hemisphere the incidence is highest in Mexico, followed by Venezuela and Argentina. In Africa it is found most frequently in Senegal, Sudan and Somalia.

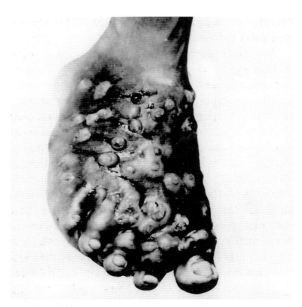

Figure 21.2 Mycetoma with painless nodules. Some nodules break down and draining abscesses gradually form (AFIP N39280).

Pathology

There is abscess formation and acute inflammatory infiltrate. Granules 0.5–2 mm in diameter are found within the abscess. The dermal inflammatory infiltrate forms microabscesses containing polymorphonuclear leukocytes with, in addition, epithelioid and multinucleated giant cells. Periodic acid–Schiff and methenamine silver stain showed septate hyphae 4–5 mm thick in the granules.

Diagnosis

There is a common clinical appearance of mycetoma: nodules and chronic sinuses, in the drainage of which the characteristic granules are found. Pus gathered from a deep sinus will show the granules when examined with the microscope. The granules are actually compact fungal or bacterial colonies. When crushed under the coverslip these will be seen to consist of dense, intertwining masses of mycelium. Cultures in appropriate medium should also be undertaken. Skin biopsy is mandatory.

Treatment

Surgical treatment should be considered in all cases of mycetoma. Localized small lesions (a few cen-timetres in diameter), which can be excised without residual disability, are best so treated. In the more advanced stages, especially of the eumycetomas, amputation is frequently necessary.

For actinomycosis (actinomycetoma) caused by *Actinomyces israelii*, penicillin is the treatment of choice. Penicillin G, 10–20 megaunits per day given intramuscularly (IM) or IV for 3–6 weeks until lesions have cleared or remain stable for 6 weeks, can be given.

The combination of streptomycin sulphate, 1 g intramuscularly daily with DDS, 100 mg twice daily with TMPS (sulfamethoxazole, 400 mg plus trimethoprim, 80 mg per tablet), two tablets every 12 h has been reported to give good result (Mahgoub 1976).

Ketoconazole 200–400 mg/day for 8–18 months may produce good results, or even complete cure, in eumycotic mycetoma (Mahgoub 1987).

SKIN TUBERCULOSIS

Tuberculosis of the skin is caused by mycobacteria of the human, bovine and, very rarely, the avian type (Christiansen 1968). In humans, *Mycobacterium tuberculosis* and *Mycobacterium bovis* cause identical skin manifestations. The skin changes caused by *M. tuberculosis/bovis* infection are polymorphous, depending upon the interplay of host immunity and bacterial virulence. Organ tuberculosis is rarely associated with cutaneous tuberculosis. Scrofuloderma and lupus vulgaris are the most frequent forms of skin tuberculosis (Kivanc-Altunay et al 2003).

The diagnostic identification of *M. tuberculosis* has remained difficult. In tuberculous skin lesions, a large number of acid-fast bacteria must be present to be detected by histopathological examination. In fact, most forms of cutaneous tuberculosis, e.g. lupus vulgaris, are paucibacillary, and acid-fast bacteria are almost never seen microscopically. Culture is currently the single most important test for the diagnosis of mycobacterial disease. However, it takes many weeks before definite results are obtained. Polymerase chain reaction using the insertion sequence IS 6110 as the target for DNA to detect *M. tuberculosis* has been studied as an additional diagnostic method (Degitz 1996, Nunez-Gussman et al 2003).

Epidemiology

With the decline of tuberculosis throughout the world through increasing affluence, advanced public health measures and the advent of effective chemotherapeutic agents, tuberculous skin lesions have become rare. The incidence of tuberculosis in the developed countries will continue to decline, although a number of problems lie concealed. In spite of the dramatic decline of tuberculosis in the developed countries from 1970, the infection has increased markedly since 1985 as a result of a number of problems. In areas with large numbers of immigrants from developing countries, tuberculosis continues to be a problem. The changing pattern of tuberculosis shows that there are problem groups in the indigenous population: middle-aged and elderly men, immunocompromised patients, drug addicts, diabetics and patients with AIDS (James & Mishra 1984). In some areas, tuberculosis has become so uncommon that it may be overlooked (McNicol 1983). In developing countries of Africa and south-east Asia, the increase of tuberculosis cases has paralleled the epidemic caused by HIV (Narain et al 1992).

Although the incidence and morbidity of tuberculosis have declined in the USA, the number of cases of tuberculosis (especially cutaneous tuberculosis) among those born outside the USA has increased. The discrepancy can be explained, in part, by the fact that cutaneous tuberculosis can have a long latency period in those individuals with a high degree of immunity against the organism (Campanelli et al 2001).

Tuberculous chancre (primary inoculation tuberculosis, primary tuberculous complex)

Primary inoculation tuberculosis consists of the cutaneous reaction at the site of inoculation of *M. tuberculosis* into a tuberculosis-free individual.

A tuberculous chancre or primary inoculation tuberculosis on the leg results from the inoculation of tubercle bacilli into the skin of a host without a naturally or artificially acquired immunity to the this organism. It occurs chiefly in children, although occasionally in adults with a prior negative tuberculin test. Most of the reported cases of inoculation cutaneous tuberculosis have been in people working in health-care professions (Rytel et al 1970, Sahn & Pierson 1974).

The inoculation may occur on the legs, which are readily injured. The site of entry may be a cut, scratch, insect bite or wound.

Not all cases of inoculation mycobacterioses involve the skin, as infection of deeper tissues may occur as a result of surgical procedures, deeply penetrating injuries or indwelling catheters (Grange et al 1988).

Clinical manifestations

The earliest lesion is a brownish red papule that develops into an indurated nodule or plaque, which may ulcerate. This is the *tuberculous chancre*. Regional lymphadenopathy occurs about 3–4 weeks or more after the development of the ulcer (Fig. 21.3). Tuberculous chancres heal by scarring, but in rare cases lupus vulgaris develops at the healed site.

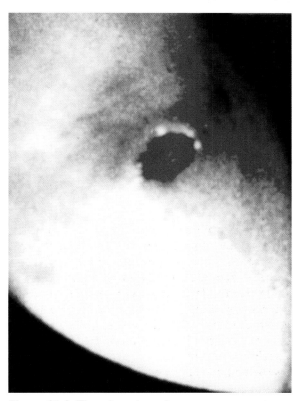

Figure 21.3 The tuberculous chancre starts as a brownish red papule, which develops into an indurated nodule or plaque that ulcerates.

A painless ulcer and unilateral regional lymphadenopathy, especially in a child, should arouse suspicion. Acid-fast bacilli can be seen in histological sections or in smears obtained from the primary ulcer and draining glands in the initial stages of the disease.

The differential diagnosis of primary inoculation tuberculosis extends over the spectrum of chancriform conditions of deep fungal or bacterial origin as coccidioidomycosis, tularaemia, primary complexes of syphilis, sporotrichosis and cat-scratch fever closely resemble tuberculous chancre. These conditions can be readily excluded by serological studies, cultures, skin biopsies, tissue smears, and historical and physical findings.

Scrofuloderma

Scrofuloderma results from the breakdown of cervical nodes, with fistula and sinus formation in the overlying skin (Fig. 21.4). It occurs most frequently over the lymph nodes but may occur over bone or about joints in children and young adults. On the legs, the inguinal lymph nodes may be involved or the lesions may accompany tuberculous disease of the phalangeal bones or joints.

The process usually begins with a deep purplish induration of the skin overlying diseased lymphatic glands, which for months have been matted together and doughy. The underlying mass suppurates and burrows to the skin surface. Ulcers and sinuses develop. Chronic discharging sinuses, soft undermined ulcers, irregular cicatricial bands and nodules together compose scrofuloderma. Excessive granulation tissue may give rise to fungating tumours.

Pathology

The tuberculous process begins in the deep dermis with caseation, necrosis and formation of a cavity filled with liquefied debris, the walls of which are formed by tuberculous granulation tissue. Collections of epithelioid cells usually surround caseation necrosis and abscess formation.

Differential diagnosis

The differential diagnosis consists of conditions that are characterized by suppurative lymphadenitis with cutaneous sinus formation, such as atypical mycobacterial infection, sporotrichosis, which yields the typical fungus when cultured, and blastomycosis, as demonstrated by the presence of *Blastomyces dermatitidis*. Lymphogranuloma venereum is ruled out by a negative LGV complement fixation test. Lymphogranuloma venereum occurs most frequently in the inguinal and perineal areas.

Other conditions that may be considered are actinomycosis and tularaemia. These can be excluded by culture.

Treatment

Incision and drainage of abscesses are not necessary. Standard multidrug therapy is indicated.

Papulonecrotic tuberculid

Papulonecrotic tuberculid is an eruption characterized by symptomless papules that appear in symmetric crops and necrose, particularly affecting the extremities. These papules may develop necrosis in the centre with ulceration and a subsequent depressed scar. The lesions appear in showers on the extensor aspects of the extremities, particularly the knees but also on the elbows, buttocks, lower trunk and sometimes the penis. New crops may continue to appear over months or years. They usually do not itch and there are no systemic symptoms.

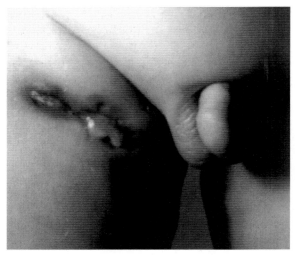

Figure 21.4 Scrofuloderma results from breakdown of lymph nodes, with fistula and sinus formation in the overlying skin.

Biopsy and tuberculin testing should be carried out in all doubtful cases. The response of this disease to antituberculous therapy supports its status as a tuberculid.

Papulonecrotic tuberculid – a cutaneous manifestation of tuberculosis – is rare even in areas where tuberculosis is endemic. Concomitant pulmonary tuberculosis is uncommon in patients with papulonecrotic tuberculid. Papulonecrotic tuberculid and simultaneous pulmonary tuberculosis has been described (Chen et al 2000).

Lupus vulgaris

Lupus vulgaris is the most common type of cutaneous tuberculosis. It is a progressive form of postprimary tuberculosis in patients with a moderate to high degree of immunity and tuberculin sensitivity. It is characterized by groups of reddish brown nodules that, when blanched by diascopic pressure, have a pale brownish yellow or apple-jelly colour. Lupus vulgaris may also appear clinically as ulcers on the leg. Ulcers may be serpiginous or arciform. Necrosis of the tissue predominates and crusts form

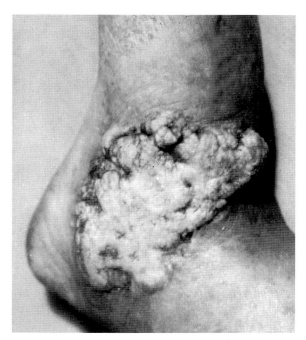

Figure 21.5 Granulations on the floor of the ulcers of lupus vulgaris lead to papillomatous, vegetating, fungoid lesions.

over areas of necrosis. Granulations at the floor of the ulcers lead to papillomatous vegetating, fungoid lesions (Fig. 21.5). On the trunk and extremities, patches of the disease may be serpiginous or form gyrate patterns, and on the hands and feet and about the genitals or buttocks may cause mutilation due to destruction, scar formation, warty thickenings and elephantiasis enlargement.

The course of lupus vulgaris is extremely slow and without treatment extends over many years or even decades. Squamous cell carcinoma, less commonly basal cell carcinoma or even sarcoma, may complicate the chronic ulcerations.

Pathology

Histological examination is mandatory. The significant histopathological changes appear in the upper corium. Acid-fast bacilli are almost never found in microscopic sections. The infiltrate, which is diffuse, is made up of epithelioid and giant cells, usually of the Langhans type, and inflammatory cells, lymphocytes, plasma cells and, occasionally, polymorphonuclear leukocytes. Caseation necrosis is only slight and may be absent within the tubercles.

Differential diagnosis

Among the conditions that may simulate the plague form of lupus vulgaris are leishmaniasis, sarcoidosis, facial granuloma and rosacea.

Treatment

Standard multidrug therapy for tuberculosis is effective. Plastic surgery, with or without chemotherapy depending on the activity of the disease, may be carried out to correct the mutilating and destructive effects of the disease. In advanced disease, the treatment of choice is systemic, and the local lesions are left alone.

Tuberculosis verrucosa cutis

Most cases are due to an exogenous reinfection in individuals with marked cutaneous hypersensitivity and good immunity. The lesions usually start as indurated, circumscribed red-brown warty plaques (Fig. 21.6). They may be single or multiple, gradually increase in number and coalesce to form nummular verrucous plaques of palm size, or even much larger. The most frequent locations are on

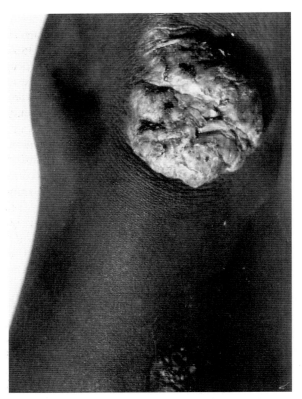

Figure 21.6 Tuberculosis verrucosa cutis usually starts as indurated, circumscribed, red-brown warty plaques that occasionally ulcerate.

the dorsal surfaces of the feet, hands, knees and buttocks. Occasionally, ulceration and sclerotic lesions or fungating granuloma are observed (Mitchell 1954).

The association of tuberculosis verrucosa cutis with visceral involvement has often been reported, the visceral lesions usually being the origin of the cutaneous lesion. It may happen, as in this case, that the visceral lesions originate from the cutaneous ones, since we are dealing with bacilliferous lesions.

The histological picture shows the usual tubercle with caseation necrosis. In addition there may be formation of new blood vessels with predominating acanthosis and hyperkeratosis. Tubercle bacilli are present.

Tuberculosis verrucosa cutis must be differentiated by culture from atypical mycobacterial granuloma (swimming pool, or balnei) due to *Mycobacterium marinum*. It must also be distin-

guished from sporotrichosis, chromomycosis, tinea profunda (Majocchi's granuloma), verrucous epidermal nevus and even verruca vulgaris.

Tuberculous gumma (metastatic tuberculous abscess)

Tuberculous gumma is the result of haematogenous dissemination of mycobacteria from a primary focus in patients who have lowered resistance. This unusual disease occurs in undernourished children of low socioeconomic status or patients who have a primary immunodeficient disorder or are secondarily and severely immunodepressed by a disease or therapy.

Clinical manifestations

Subcutaneous abscesses, which are non-tender, arise either singly or as multiples on the leg, and less often on the trunk (Fig. 21.7). Similar lesions may arise along the path of blood vessels (Ward 1971). The subcutaneous abscesses slowly soften and break down to form fistulas and ulcers. Similar lesions may arise along the course of lymphatics.

The systemic signs and symptoms of fever, chills, headache, malaise, weakness, fatigue, myalgia and night sweats are present.

On histopathological examination, tuberculous granuloma and bacilli may be seen in the discharge on special stains.

Tuberculous granuloma must be differentiated from syphilitic gumma, deep fungal infections and all forms of panniculitis.

The clinical diagnosis is confirmed by histopathology, acid-fast stains of tissue and smears, and bacterial culture.

Treatment

Multidrug therapy is indicated.

Erythema induratum

Erythema induratum (Bazin's disease, tuberculosis cutis indurativa) is a chronic benign vasculitis affecting the lower legs, characterized by painful, recurrent nodules that may progress into deep-seated indurations, ulcers and scarring. It has multifactorial causes, such as an adverse drug reaction and hypersensitivity reaction to certain infections, such as mycobacteria or streptococci. Rarely, tuber-

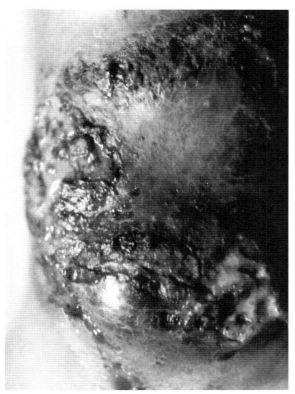

Figure 21.7 Subcutaneous abscesses of tuberculous gumma arise either singly or as multiples on the leg. The abscesses slowly break down to form fistulas and ulcers.

culosis has been diagnosed after the occurrence of erythema induratum.

Clinically, the disease appears more frequently on the legs of women and, rarely, of men. The calf is the preferred site but lesions on the shins and thighs have been described. The lesions are subcutaneous nodules or plaques, bilateral, erythematous, indolent and tender. In time, the overlying skin assumes a bluish-red colour, which frequently progresses into ulcers. The ulcers have irregular shapes and are deeply excavated, with steep or undermined edges.

The differential diagnosis includes erythema nodosum, nodular allergic vasculitis and the gummatous syphilid.

A favourable response is anticipated with antituberculous therapy (Feiwel & Munro 1965) but, in many cases, corticosteroids and bed rest are more effective.

Treatment

For tuberculous leg ulcer, standard multiple bactericidal drug therapy should be given (Harahap 1989). A 6-month regimen of chemotherapy is effective if four drugs: isoniazid (5–10 mg/kg/day up to 300 mg/day orally), rifampicin (10–20 mg/kg/day up to 600 mg/day orally), pyrazinamide (15–30 mg/kg/day up to 1 g/day intramuscularly) or ethambutol (15–25 mg/kg/day orally) are administered for 2 months and followed by an additional 4 months of isoniazid and rifampicin.

This short-course chemotherapy is now standard in drug-sensitive infections (Steele & Des Prez 1988). Plastic surgery and chemotherapy, depending on the activity of the disease, may help to repair the destructive and disfiguring effects.

Mycobacterium marinum

This infection usually starts as a small papule of indolent granuloma, located on the knees, the elbows or sometimes on the dorsum of the hands and feet. Infections have been acquired in lakes and rivers, salt water, swimming pools and aquariums or fish tanks. More infections are acquired from home aquariums than from swimming pools.

Aetiology

Mycobacterium marinum, formerly known as *M. balnei*, occurs in fresh and salt water. *M. marinum* will grow well on a standard glycerol egg media such as Löwenstein–Jensen medium. Abundant cultural growth is obtained at 30–33°C in 7–10 days. No growth occurs at 37°C (Grange 1989).

Clinical manifestations

After injury, a violaceous papule or pustule develops after 2–3 weeks at the traumatized site, usually the knees or feet. The initial lesion breaks down to form an ulcerated plaque or it may remain warty (Fig. 21.8). The lesion tends to be solitary, but occasionally lesions are multiple and ascend proximally, resembling a sporotrichoid infection. Regional lymph nodes not usually involved.

There is marked tendency to spontaneous healing within a few months to 2 years, although in an exceptional instance persistence for 17 years was reported.

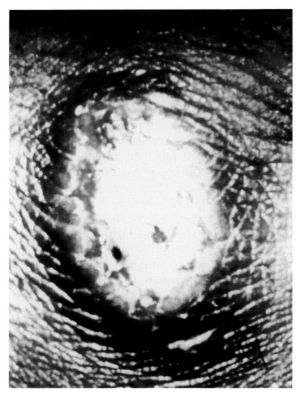

Figure 21.8 Ulcerated nodule of *Mycobacterium marinum*. A violaceous nodule develops after 2–3 weeks at the traumatized site, which later breaks down to form an ulcer.

Pathology

Histopathologically there is at first an inflammatory type of reaction with hyperkeratosis and parakeratosis. Later a more typical tuberculoid structure: epithelioid cell tubercles with Langhans giant cells are present, but true caseation is rare. Acid-fast organisms may rarely be seen, especially within the histiocytes. The organisms are longer and broader than *M. tuberculosis* may be seen intracellularly within the histiocytes (Dooley 1976).

Diagnosis

An appropriate history, supported by the demonstration of *M. marinum* in culture, provides the best means of diagnosis.

Treatment

In the absence of treatment, *M. marinum* infection usually resolves, but surgical excision, curettage, freezing and irradiation, tetracycline, minocycline and TMPS have been reported to be effective. It has been recommended tetracycline, 2 g/day, or minocycline hydrochloride 100 mg twice daily for 1–2 months (James & Mishra 1984). Rifampicin 600 mg with ethambutol 15 mg/kg for 18 months have also been used. No current recommendation for a drug of choice is available, and the clinician may choose from a number of effective options.

In vitro activities of 17 antibiotics against 53 clinical strains of *M. marinum*, were determined using the reference agar dilution method. Rifampicin and rifabutin were the most active drugs (Aubry et al 2000). Numerous options appear to exist for the contemporary therapy of *M. marinum* infections including some newer fluoroquinolones and derivatives (Rhomberg & Jones 2002).

Mycobacterium ulcerans

This is also known as Buruli ulcer and Searl's ulcer. The chronic necrotic skin ulcer due to *Mycobacterium ulcerans* was first described in Australia in 1948. Since then a similar disease was observed in Bolivia, Nigeria, Ghana, Mexico, Zaire, Uganda, Malaysia and New Guinea.

The lesions begin as solitary, hard, painless, subcutaneous nodules that subsequently ulcerate and become undermined. It is possibly inoculated into skin by injury, probably by cuts from grass. There is a predilection for the occurrence of these ulcers on the extremities.

After tuberculosis and leprosy, Buruli ulcer disease is the third most common mycobacterial disease in immunocompetent people. Countries in which the disease is endemic have been identified, predominantly in areas of tropical rain forest, the emergence of Buruli ulcer disease in West African countries over the past decade has been dramatic (Van der Werf et al 1999)

Aetiology

Mycobacterium ulcerans has been identified in this type of ulceration. It is cultured in Löwenstein–Jensen medium at 33°C and has a marked tendency to clump, especially to fibrous bundles (Tyrell et al 1975). *M. ulcerans* differs from the mammalian tubercle bacillus in its strong positive reaction to catalase test, its resistance to isoniazid and its inability to multiply in culture at temperature greater than 35°C. *M. ulcerans* produces a toxin that may be responsible for the extensive necrosis and ulceration (Krieg et al 1974).

Because of the geographical association of the disease with swamps and stagnant waters, it has been suggested that insects are the vectors.

Clinical manifestations

The incidences are mostly in children and young adults. It occurs more commonly in women than in men. The incubation period is up to 3 months. The initial lesion, usually confined to the limbs, mainly the legs, is a small painless subcutaneous nodule. A blister may appear before ulceration. The ulcer extends rapidly and irregularly with undermined hyperpigmented edges. Smears of the ulcer may reveal *M. ulcerans* with acid-fast staining, however, the organisms are always recognized histopathologically (Oluwasanmi et al 1976). The uncomplicated is painless and there is no lymphadenopathy. Unless there is secondary bacterial infection, the patients are afebrile and experience no systemic symptoms. The ulceration is chronic, may persist for months or years and then heal spontaneously with scarring (Fig. 21.9). This may lead occasionally to disabling contraction and lymphoedema.

Pathology

A non-exudative necrosis is found histopathologically that harbours colonies or individual bacilli. It initially involves the panniculus, spreads up through corium and finally causes the cutaneous ulceration. There is surprisingly little associated inflammatory reaction in the adjacent viable tissue (Cannor et al 1976).

Diagnosis

A definite diagnosis can be made on the basis of histopathology and bacterial culture from a subcutaneous node or an ulcer. Proper bacteriological examination of smears, curettage or biopsy specimen will reveal clumps of acid-fast bacilli. This organism can be cultured at a low temperature; its temperature requirements in culture are quite narrow (32–33°C).

Differential diagnosis

The differential diagnosis of the initial subcutaneous swelling includes foreign body granuloma, nodular fasciitis, phycomycetes, injection abscess, myiasis, panniculitis, inclusion cyst and appendageal tumours. The ulcerative lesions must be differentiated from aerobic and anaerobic necrotizing cellulitis, pyoderma gangrenosum, suppurative panniculitis, vasculitis with or without granuloma and gumma (syphilis, yaws).

Treatment

Simple excision of the small early lesion under local anaesthesia is curative; later, when ulceration has developed, extensive excision and subsequent skin grafting is an effective treatment.

In general, chemotherapy has not proved very successful. Local heat therapy, hyperbaric oxygen, rifampicin and trimethoprim and sulfamethoxazole (TMPS) have been reported to be of some value; as spontaneous healing may occur, this is as yet somewhat difficult to evaluate in the absence of controlled studies.

LEISHMANIASIS

Leishmaniasis is caused by an intracellular protozoal parasite of the genus *Leishmania*. The infection in humans forms a wide spectrum of clinical disease. The disease in humans is usually either cutaneous, localized to the skin without systemic involvement or systemic (visceral), known as kala-azar, involving the reticuloendothelial system. In the middle of the spectrum there are variations in disease patterns. The most important variant is the mucocutaneous infections characterized by

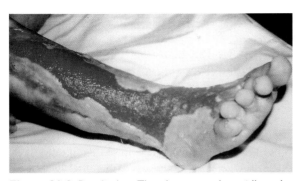

Figure 21.9 Buruli ulcer. The ulcer extends rapidly and irregularly with undermined hyperpigmented edges. The ulceration is chronic: it may persist for months or years.

cutaneous lesions and metastatic mucous membrane infection. The parasite demonstration and isolation rates are rather poor from cutaneous and mucocutaneous lesions due to low parasite load and high rate of culture contamination. Recently several recombinant proteins have been developed to accomplish accurate diagnosis. Recombinant kinesin protein of 39 kDa, called rK39, is the most promising of these molecules. The antigen used in various test formats has been proved highly sensitive and specific for visceral leishmaniasis. Molecular techniques targeting various genes of the parasite have also been reported the polymerase chain reaction being the most common molecular technique successfully used for diagnosis and for differentiation of species (Singh et al 2003).

Aetiology

The intracellular obligate parasite of leishmaniasis belongs to the genus *Leishmania* (family Trypanosomatidae). These are flagellate protozoa living in the macrophages of the skin, viscera and blood of the human host. There are two forms in which the parasite exists. The amastigote (*Leishmania* stage) form of the parasite is found in cells of the reticuloendothelial system. It is small, spherical or oval, with the flagellum retracted into the axoneme. The promastigote (*Leptomonas* stage) is found in cultures in artificial media and in the insect vector. It is spindle-shaped with a fine flagellum at one end. Some *Leishmania* isolates are difficult to maintain in culture or laboratory animals, so DNA probes, a promising new technique, have the potential for parasite characterization (Chiodini 1989).

Sand flies of the genus *Phlebotomus*, *Lutzomyia* and *Psychodopygus* are the principal vectors responsible for the continued cycle on infected animal to sandflies to healthy animal or human. There is a definite association between foci of leishmaniasis and the sandfly population, which is distributed in the tropical and subtropical regions of the eastern and western hemispheres. In most areas, leishmaniasis is a zoonosis and humans are incidental hosts. The animal reservoirs vary with the *Leishmania* species and geographical location. Monkeys and rodents have been reported to be infected in the Amazonian region of Brazil. *Leishmania major* is found in rodents in the middle East, while domestic dogs and wild foxes are reservoir of *Leishmania donovani chagasi* in South America (Morsy et al 1987).

The life cycle of the protozoan organism is initiated when the female sandfly feeds on a lesion or from the blood of an infected host. The mastigotes are ingested and lodged in the intestine of the insect, where they become flagellated and the resulting promastigotes multiply and migrate to the anterior gut. Subsequent bites of human skin release the promastigotes through the insect's proboscis.

Cutaneous leishmaniasis

Cutaneous leishmaniasis is a specific granulomatous ulceration of the skin (Old World type, Oriental sore, Bouton d'orient, Delhi boil, Aleppo boil) on the exposed parts of the body. The disease occurs in warm countries and is endemic in countries around the Mediterranean coast both in Europe and Africa, and is also seen in Asia, including China and southern Russia. Men, women and children are all susceptible. The incubation period varies from a few weeks to several months.

Clinical manifestations

The lesions appear on the unclothed parts of the body easily bitten by *Phlebotomus*. The most common lesion is an ulcerated papular or furunculoid lesion. It continues to enlarge until reaching its final size, usually 1–5 cm diameter, over weeks or months. There is no pain but there may be severe pruritus. After months or years, healing begins at the centre of the ulcer, leaving a depressed, stellate, disfiguring scar.

Diagnosis

In endemic areas, history and clinical appearance may be virtually diagnostic. Biopsy and culture permit definitive diagnosis. The leishmanin skin test is positive in 98% of cases.

The localized ulcerative lesion on the exposed parts of the body must be differentiated from ulcerative ecthymiform, chancriform lesions (syphilis, tuberculosis, nocardiosis), yaws, tropical ulcer, Buruli ulcer, sporotrichosis and chromomycosis.

Polymerase chain reaction is a useful tool in establishing the species diagnosis of leishmaniasis (Scope et al 2003).

Treatment

Glucantime (*N*-methyl-glucamine antimonate) is the most widely used treatment. It may be given in a dose of 10–20 mg/kg by intramuscular or intravenous injection daily until healing. As an alternative, sodium stibogluconate (Pentostam) 6 ml (each millilitre contains 330 mg of antimony) by intramuscular or intravenous injection daily for 15–20 days can be used (Castro 1979, Furtado 1981). Therapeutic modalities include oral ketoconazole or itraconazole, topical paromomycin sulphate, local heat or photodynamic therapy (Enk et al 2003).

Curettage and cryosurgery are methods of removing small lesions. They are painful and poorly validated.

Amphotericin B 0.5 mg/kg/day or 1.0 mg/kg on alternate days is an alternative drug for treatment in cases of antimonial failure.

Sodium stibogluconate appears to be a safe and effective treatment for *Leishmania braziliensis* infection (Scope et al 2003, Gontijo & de Carvalho 2003)

Mucocutaneous leishmaniasis

Mucocutaneous leishmaniasis (American leishmaniasis, South American leishmaniasis, espundia, pian bois, uta, Chiclero's ulcer, bush yaws, picatura de pito, etc.) is characterized by a prolonged course and deformities due to granulomatous cutaneous ulcers and, in the later stages, involves the upper respiratory tract mucosa.

Mucocutaneous leishmaniasis is found in forested country in South and Central America.

Clinical manifestations

The initial lesion develops on an exposed part at the site of the *Phlebotomus* bite as a small, erythematous, papule and gradually increases in size. In a few weeks this commonly ulcerates and is covered by a crust, but it may heal without treatment in several months. The ulcerated skin lesion continues to progress and enlarge, with a characteristic raised border. Secondary infection is common, with regional adenitis and sometimes lymphangitis. Involvement of the mucous membrane lesions tend to occur a few years later. The mucosal lesions are produced by spread through lymphatics or the blood stream and most frequently attack the nasal mucosa, nasopharynx, mouth and larynx. The

lesions become necrotic ulcers, with destruction of the nasal fossa, mucosa and cartilage. The process may progress into a fearful deformity of the nose, lips and palate.

Diagnosis

Mucocutaneous leishmaniasis must be distinguished from pyoderma, syphilis, yaws, squamous cell carcinoma, leprosy, rhinoscleroma and chromoblastomycosis.

The diagnosis is established by the isolation and identification of the causative organism in cultures of tissue or exudates from characteristic lesions. The leishmanin skin test is reliable and gives hypersensitivity reaction in 98% of cases who have or have had the disease.

Treatment

Most primary lesions of mucocutaneous leishmaniasis may be cured with glucantime or sodium stibogluconate as for cutaneous leishmaniasis. Patients with secondary involvement of mucous membranes need prolonged treatment with pentavalent antimonials. Relapsed cases of mucocutaneous leishmaniasis that have become resistant to antimonials should be treated with amphotericin B (Harman 1986). Some cases of mucocutaneous leishmaniasis may require antibiotics for secondary infection, and later reconstructive surgery.

Visceral leishmaniasis

Visceral leishmaniasis or systemic leishmaniasis, known as kala-azar, is caused by *L. donovani*. The disease is very widely distributed in tropical countries. It is present in Asia, the Mediterranean coast, Africa and some parts of South America.

The incubation period varies from 1 to 6 months or several years after inoculation of the organisms. Fever and chills are usually the initial manifestation. It may also be characterized initially by low-grade fever, weight loss and left upper quadrant pain from splenic enlargement.

Clinical manifestations

Patients with visceral leishmaniasis rarely show a primary or intercurrent skin lesion. In the Sudan, visceral leishmaniasis is characterized by the presence of a primary lesion associated with ulcerations of the skin and mucous membrane, and post-kala-azar dermal leishmaniasis (Kirk 1942). Erythematous papules or patches appear on the face and the rest of the body following successful treatment of visceral leishmaniasis in patients with post-kala-azar dermal leishmaniasis. Parasites that were previously localized in visceral reticuloendothelial tissue may come to lie in the skin. The clinical picture resembles lepromatous leprosy.

Progressive visceral leishmaniasis in patients receiving immunosuppressive therapy has been reported (Badaro et al 1986). There have also been reports of visceral leishmaniasis in patients with HIV infection (Rizzi et al 1988).

Diagnosis

Patients residing in, or who have been to, an endemic area, with fever, weight loss and splenic enlargement should be suspected. Diagnosis is established by the demonstration of *L. donovani* in smears and cultures of blood or reticuloendothelial tissue: bone marrow, splenic pulp or lymph nodes. Splenic puncture is the most sensitive diagnostic procedure but, because of potential complications, lymph node aspiration should be the primary diagnostic method (Siddig et al 1988).

Treatment

Pentavalent antimonials are the drugs of choice. In doses of 10–20 mg/kg/day, the drug is virtually non-toxic, even over periods of several months. Amphotericin B 0.5 mg/kg/day or 1.0 mg/kg on alternate days for 8 weeks has also been used effectively in cases of antimony failure and is a useful drug in resistant cases and in patients who experience unacceptable toxicity to antimonials.

TROPICAL PHAGEDENIC ULCER

Tropical phagedenic ulcer (TPU) is a painful, malodorous, necrotizing ulcer of the skin and subcutaneous tissues of the leg. *Bacillus fusiformis* and *Treponema vincentii* are usually present in the ulcer, but no one knows if they are the primary infecting agents.

Aetiology

Fusiform bacilli and spirochetes predominate in the bacterial flora. Opinions differ regarding the importance of these organisms as a cause of TPU (Loewenthal 1963). Anaerobic bacteria, mainly *Fusobacterium*, *Bacteroides* and *Veillonella* spp. and anaerobic Gram-positive cocci, have been isolated from patients with tropical phagedenic ulcers. Anaerobes, together with aerobes or facultative anaerobes, were always present, suggesting a synergistic infection (Adriaans et al 1986a).

It is likely that the combination of these organisms may be responsible for the pathogenesis of the disease (Adriaans et al 1987). Hungate tubes with pre-reduced peptone yeast broth and agar have been used for transporting specimens anaerobically from remote areas for cultural identification (Adriaans et al 1986b).

There is some evidence that PLU is transmissible. Ulcers were induced experimentally in healthy volunteers by bathing untraumatized skin in ulcer pus (McAdam 1966) but the pathogenesis remains obscure.

Clinical manifestations

Infection begins an acutely inflamed papule, which proceeds to a foul-smelling ulcer that may persist for months. Predisposing factors that produce TPU are unhygienic conditions and the added liability of trauma of the legs, where most lesions occur. Inappropriate treatment, undernutrition, poor blood supply to the pretibial area, stasis from dependency of the lower limb and excessive scarring are factors that delay or prevent healing.

TPU is limited in the leg below the knee and begins after a scratch, thorn prick or other penetrating trauma. The skin becomes red, swollen and acutely painful, following which a pustule or bleb develops. In about a week it discharges blood-stained pus and at this time may be very painful.

A small ulcer is formed, which extends in diameter and depth in a matter of days. The base has a grey fibrin cover and is foul-smelling, and, as the ulcer develops, deep structures including tendon and bone may be exposed. The putrid odour may draw flies. The ulcer margin is raised and firm, and the edges are slightly everted but not undermined (Fig. 21.10). During the acute stage, malaise and fever may develop, then subside as the acute stage passes within a few weeks.

After reaching the full extent the phagedenic process is arrested and a chronic indolent ulcer

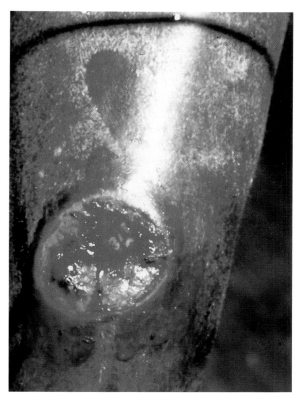

Figure 21.10 Tropical phagedenic ulcer. The ulcer margin is raised and firm, the edges are slightly everted but not undermined (AFIP 68–658).

with firm, pale, fibrotic, raised edges is left. With time, the ulcer margin becomes harder and thicker, further deepening the crater. The ulcer may continue for years. Healing may begin with spotty epithelialization extending from the periphery toward the centre. When healing eventually occurs, the site of the ulcer is marked by a scar, frequently attached to the deeper structure.

Pathology

Sections through the margin and crater of the ulcer reveal a coagulum composed of a mass of fibrin, degenerating cellular debris and masses of intermixed fusiform bacilli and spirochetes over the surface of the ulcer. Deeper, there is granulation tissue infiltrated by leukocytes. The ulcer base contains a variety of inflammatory cells, including histiocytes, eosinophils, neutrophils, plasma cells and lymphocytes. Clusters of lymphocytes, plasma cells and histiocytes are prominent around vessels in

adjacent scar tissue and occasional giant cells may also be present in the deeper layers of scar tissue.

Complications

During the acute stage, gangrene of muscle has often been recorded. Local involvement of bone – periostitis and localized bone necrosis, osteomyelitis and sequestrum formation – are frequent. Ankylosis is apt to follow deep ulcers in the neighbourhood of the knee and heel, which has led to the formation of adhesions and dense scar tissue.

Malignant degeneration in chronic, inappropriately treated TPU has been reported. Some of these may have been examples of the usual pseudoepitheliomatous hyperplasia. Routine biopsy should be done in any TPU of more than 10 years duration.

Treatment

Healing is promoted by improving the patient's general health, eliminating infection in the ulcer crater, and local cleansing and skin grafting when necessary.

Intramuscular procaine penicillin at high doses for at least 1 week is the treatment of choice. The total dose varies between 6 and 10 megaunits.

Oral tetracycline 2 g daily in divided dose or oral metronidazole 200 mg three times daily for 10 days is also effective.

Topically, wet compresses of potassium permanganate (solution 1/5000) are helpful. Immersing the lesion in 1– 2% hydrogen peroxide for an hour or longer helps to loosen the inspissated exudate.

LEPROSY

Leprosy is a chronic, infectious disease caused by *Mycobacterium leprae*. It manifests itself in the development of specific granulomatous or neurotrophic lesions that can be either self-limiting or progressive depending on the immunological status of the infected host.

There are mainly two different types of leg ulcer in leprosy patients: neuropathic ulcers and leprous or specific ulcers.

Aetiology

These two types of ulcer are caused by two separate and distinct aetiological factors. Neuropathic ulceration, particularly of the extremities, is caused by damage to one or more peripheral nerve trunks of the extremities in leprosy patients. Neuropathic ulcers are most frequently seen in the soles of the feet but they may sometimes be found in the legs and other sites. These ulcers result from repeated injuries to the denervated extremities, especially the feet, and are not directly caused by leprosy. Because the ulcer is not the result of local breakdown of leprous lesions, the discharges from these ulcers do not contain *M. leprae*.

The other type of ulcer is the leprous or specific ulcer. This type of ulcer is not very common. It can arise because of breaking down of lepromatous lesions or a group of necrotic erythema nodosum leprosum lesions or because of the intensity of the inflammatory response during reactional episodes. These ulcers are usually seen in patients with uncontrolled lepromatous leprosy.

Clinical manifestations

Neuropathic ulceration of the sole of the foot is one of the most common complications for which leprosy patients seek treatment. These ulcers, also known as 'trophic ulcers' or 'perforating ulcers', are relatively painless and very slow to heal, but quick to recur (Fig. 21.11). Most plantar ulcers occur in the soles across the forefoot under the metatarsophalangeal joints. Plantar ulcers are responsible for much suffering and disability. Another common site for this type of ulcer in the lower extremities is the region of the lateral malleolus. Occasionally, ulceration may occur at the knee. In all these sites, the skin and subcutaneous tissue gets caught between two hard objects, an underlying bone and an unyielding hard surface, such as the ground. Pressure, intermittent friction and secondary infection lead to ulcers. If neglected, infection from these ulcers may extend to the underlying bones.

Ulceration resulting from the breakdown of lepromatous nodules is sometimes seen on the leg or other non-weight-bearing areas. This leprous ulcer or specific ulcer is usually found in the centre of a heavily infiltrated area, with considerable swelling of the surrounding tissues. The ulcer is irregular in outline and shows a punched-out appearance with dirty, pale granulation. Smears from the ulcers reveal plenty of acid-fast bacilli.

Fungating masses mimicking the development of epitheliomatous changes are occasionally seen in chronic ulceration of the leg and foot in leprosy patients, but histologic examination shows the majority of these growths to be a variety of pseudoepitheliomatous hyperplasia, and not true malignant changes. However, some are definitely carcinoma (Riedel 1966, Andersen 1982, Fleury & Opromolla 1984).

Apart from the rare incidence of squamous cell carcinoma complicating chronic leg or plantar ulcer, some studies did not indicate that leprosy patients have a predisposition to malignant disease (Oleinick 1969, Purtilo & Pang 1975, Tokudome et al 1981).

Epidemiology

Estimates for 2003 indicated that there were then about 0.53 million cases of leprosy in the world, compared with 10–12 million cases in the mid-1980s and down from 1.15 million cases in 1997 (World Health Organization 2003). About 625 000 new cases of leprosy were detected in 2002.

Leprosy remains a public health problem in a number of countries but six of these, India, Brazil, Madagascar, Mozambique, Nepal and Tanzania, account for about 85% of all cases (World Health Organization 2003).

Differential diagnosis

Foot and leg ulceration in leprosy patients should be differentiated from Raynaud's disease, throm-

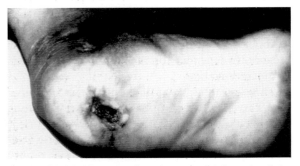

Figure 21.11 Neurotrophic ulceration of the sole of the foot in leprosy is painless and very slow to heal.

boangiitis obliterans (Buerger's disease), diabetic gangrene, syphilis and yaws.

- Raynaud's disease is usually bilateral, with acute pain and loss of sensation being confined to the gangrenous area, and the absence of thickened nerves.
- Thromboangiitis obliterans is usually unilateral, no pulsation can be felt in the dorsalis pedis or posterior tibial arteries, and the affected foot feels cooler than the unaffected foot.
- Diabetic gangrene may simulate neurotrophic ulcers of leprosy but the loss of sensation is limited to the gangrenous area. If diabetic neuropathy is also present, the loss of sensation may be of the 'glove and stocking' type. History of diabetes, signs and symptoms of the disease, and examination of urine and blood for sugar are differentiating points.
- Gummatous syphilis can be differentiated from the history of the case, absence of diagnostic signs of leprosy, and serologic tests for syphilis.
- The fissures and ulcers caused by yaws are painful. The presence of characteristic skin lesions of yaws, and absence of anaesthesia, will differentiate the ulcers from those due to leprosy.

Treatment

The principles of treatment of neuropathic ulcers are: providing rest to the ulcerated area, eradication of secondary infection and promotion of healing.

During the acute stage, immobilization, rest, antiseptic dressing, elevation of the leg and antibiotics are necessary. Persistent chronic ulcers might need a below-knee walking plaster of Paris cast for about 6 weeks (Brand & Fritschi 1985), after removal of slough and degenerate tissue, and trimming of unhealthy, overhanging edges. The application of a plaster cast to encase the leg and foot avoids interference, as well as protecting them from the stresses and strains of walking.

Local applications of adhesive zinc tape have shortened healing time in leprosy patients in India, with the advantages of being easy to apply and cheap, without the necessity for bandages (Soderberg et al 1982).

Besides the specific treatment for leprosy (McDougall 1989), prompt treatment of leprous or specific ulcer often heals it without much difficulty. Keeping the ulcer scrupulously clean and using a topical antibiotic or, if necessary, a systemic antibiotic, help healing.

TREPONEMAL INFECTIONS

Treponematosis as a cause of leg ulcer is today less frequent, because of the continued improvement of standards of living and the availability and widespread use of a large variety of potent antibiotics.

Syphilis (tertiary syphilis, gummata)

Late syphilis, also called tertiary syphilis, may occur as early as 6 months after infection but in general most often appears after 3–5 years or as long as 20 years after the primary infection (Clark & Danbolt 1964, Lamholt 1972).

Clinical manifestations

Lesions may be single or multiple, superficial or deep, and are characterized by indolence, painlessness, a tendency to ulcerate, with a punched-out appearance, and scar formation. Some may appear as a superficial nodular type on the leg. Some nodular lesions ulcerate. The ulcerations are multiple and usually deep. The destruction is usually in the centre of the nodule and is associated with healing in the centre over weeks or months, followed by progression of the lesions by peripheral extension, resulting in serpiginous plaques with arciform and scalloped borders.

Treponemas are usually not found by silver stains or dark-field examination but may be demonstrated by using a modified indirect immunofluorescent technique. Two main types are recognized, the noduloulcerative syphilid and the gumma.

In contrast to the multiple lesions of the nodular and noduloulcerative stages, gummas tend to be solitary lesions. A gumma of the skin is a mass of syphilitic granulation tissue, beginning as one or several painless subcutaneous tumours on the leg. As it increases in size and involves more superficial layers of the dermis, softening of the mass occurs and it eventually breaks down to form a punched-out ulcer. The ulcer walls are vertical and its base consists of clean, red granulations. Gummata are usually painless, even when they ulcerate. The granulomatous ulcer may extend peripherally or may heal spontaneously, leaving an atrophic scar. Only occasionally will a gumma resolve without ulceration and form a scar-like retraction of the overlying skin.

Differential diagnosis

Ulcers of the legs caused by late benign syphilis most be differentiated from scrofuloderma, atypical mycobacterial infection, sporotrichosis, blastomycosis and, occasionally, squamous cell carcinoma and basal cell carcinoma. Biopsy, culture and other appropriate diagnostic studies are indicated. A diagnosis of late benign cutaneous syphilis is usually made when the lesions are morphologically compatible and the serologic test for syphilis is reactive. An FTA-ABS test may be necessary to confirm the diagnosis.

Treatment

The World Health Organization makes the following recommendation (World Health Organization 1989): benzathine penicillin G 7.2 megaunits in total (2.4 megaunits by intramuscular injection weekly for 3 successive weeks). An alternative is aqueous procaine penicillin G 24 megaunits in total (1.2 megaunits by intramuscular injection daily for 20 days).

For penicillin-sensitive patients, tetracycline hydrochloride or erythromycin 500 mg four times a day by mouth for 30 days should be given.

Endemic syphilis

The disease occurs mainly among nomads and semi-nomads in western Asia, Pakistan, Saudi Arabia, Sudan, the sub-Saharan regions – Mali, Nigeria, Burkina Faso and Mauritania – and Australia (Luger 1988). The source of infection in such outbreaks is usually communicable lesions in venereally infected adults.

It is acquired through casual, non-venereal contact in childhood and is subsequently transmitted to adolescents and adults. It is peculiarly restricted to backward communities, in hot, dry (arid) regions, in parts of Africa and Asia. It is caused by *Treponema pallidum*.

Clinical manifestations

The presentation of endemic syphilis is similar to secondary syphilis: condylomata lata, angular cheilitis and cutaneous papular eruptions comparable to those seen in venereal syphilis are common. It is characterized by the frequent absence of a primary chancre, the presence of early mucocutaneous lesions and, after a variable latent period, gummata affecting skin and bone appear.

By the time signs and symptoms become evident, serological tests are invariably reactive.

Treatment

Endemic treponematosis is very sensitive to penicillin and other antibiotics. The drug of choice is 2.4 megaunits of benzathine penicillin given by intramuscular injection (Anthal & Cause 1985; Anonymous 1987).

Yaws

Yaws is an infectious, acute and chronic, nonvenereal, relapsing disease caused by *Treponema pertenue*. The causative agent is morphologically, bacteriologically and immunologically indistinguishable from *T. pallidum* of venereal syphilis. Yaws is not a sexually transmitted disease but a childhood infection, usually before puberty. Like syphilis, yaws progresses through four stages: a primary lesion, early secondary and relapsing secondary with periods of latency between relapses, a latent period and a late destructive stage (Manson-Bahr & Bell 1987; Luger 1988).

Aetiology

T. pertenue is identical morphologically with the *T. pallidum* of syphilis, being a slender spiral with six to 20 coils. In demonstrating *T. pertenue*, slides for dark-field examination should be prepared from the lesion after the crust has been removed.

Clinical manifestations

In areas where yaws is endemic, it appears clinically in children 2–3 years of age and older. The disease is spread through small abrasions following skin contact with an infectious lesion of a child. Like syphilis, the spirochete of yaws enters the abraded skin, multiplies and then enters the lymphatics and, from there, the general blood circula-

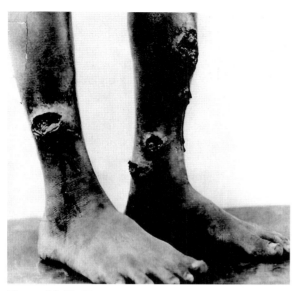

Figure 21.12 The initial papules of yaws burst open and later ulcerate, and are covered by a yellowish crust formed by the exudates (AFIP 40815).

tion. The incubation period varies from 2 weeks to 6 months. The primary lesion usually begins as a papule at the point of inoculation on the exposed area of the body, particularly the legs.

The initial lesion bursts open and later ulcerates and is covered by a yellowish crust formed by the exudates (Fig. 21.12). Over the next 2–6 months, primary lesions may persist and heal spontaneously, leaving a large, atrophic and depressed scar with a hypopigmented centre.

After the primary lesion heals, there is a period of latency of several weeks. As the eruption of secondary yaws appears, there is generalized lymphadenopathy. Secondary lesions are characterized by the appearance of small papules, which rapidly become raised, ulcerated and covered with yellow crusts. The secondary lesions disappear spontaneously after a variable period of 6 months to 3 years, sometimes leaving scars.

After 3–4 years, the disease becomes late chronic or enters the tertiary stage. Late lesions are characteristically destructive, presenting as gummata of the skin and bones, localized predominantly on the lower extremities. These include cutaneous and subcutaneous nodules that break down and ulcerate, forming superficial, spreading, serpiginous ulcers or deeper ulcers. When gummas heal, they leave atrophic, non-contractile scars.

Pathology

In the primary and secondary stages, the epidermis shows elongation and a broadening of the inter-papillary processes. The blood vessels are near the surface and predispose the lesions to bleed readily. The dermis shows a fairly dense infiltrate primarily with plasma cells, but neutrophils, eosinophils, lymphocytes, histiocytes and fibroblast are also present. Unlike syphilis, the blood vessels do not show endothelial proliferation. *T. pertenue* is usually demonstrable in the primary and secondary stages. In late yaws, ulcerative lesions are very similar to those of late syphilis except that the vascular changes are either discrete or non-existent.

Diagnosis

The diagnosis is established by the typical clinical appearance in a person living in an endemic area. This is confirmed by the demonstration by dark-field microscopy of treponemes in the exudate in primary and secondary lesions. Serologic tests (both reagin and treponemal) are positive. Diagnosis of late yaws depends upon the destructive gummatous lesions of skin and bones, the reactive serological tests and a biopsy with the histological picture of a gumma.

Late yaws must be differentiated from impetigo, tropical phagedenic ulcer, ecthyma, mycosis and syphilis, the details of which have been documented (Hackett et al 1960).

Treatment

Yaws responds to smaller doses than those used in syphilis. A single intramuscular injection of 1.2 megaunits of benzathine penicillin should be given to adults and half doses are given to children under 10 years of age. For patients allergic to penicillin, tetracycline or erythromycin 500 mg by mouth four times daily for 15 days may be used (World Health Organization 1986; Anonymous 1987).

CONCLUSION

Bed rest and good nursing in hospital, with daily dressings and appropriate antibiotics for infected ulcers, will often effect remarkable improvement, particularly in the elderly and in those on low income and in poor housing. Dressings should consist of one layer of non-adhesive dry dressing covered by absorbent cotton gauze and kept in place by a lightly applied crepe bandage.

Initial surgical debridement is usually necessary and this should be followed by full doses of appropriate antibiotics.

Clearly the ideal solution is to correct the malnutrition at the same time as undertaking simple local treatment of the ulcer.

References

Adriaans B, Drasar B, Hay R J 1986a The role of anaerobic in the pathogenesis of tropical (phagedenic) ulcer. British Journal of Dermatology 115(Suppl 30): 15–16

Adriaans B, Hay R J, Drassar B S et al 1986b Anaerobic bacteria in tropical ulcer the application of a new transport system for their isolation. Transactions of the Royal Society of Tropical Medicine and Hygiene 80: 793–794

Adriaans B, Hay R J, Drasar B S, Robinson D 1987 The infectious etiology of tropical ulcer – a study of the role of anaerobic bacteria. British Journal of Dermatology 116: 31–37

Albert B L, Sellers T F Jr 1963 Coccidioidomycosis from fomites. Archives of Internal Medicine 112: 253–261

Allan H B, Rippon J W 1985 Subcutaneous and systemic fungal infections. In: Moschella S L, Hurley H J (eds) Dermatology, 2nd edn. W B Saunders, Philadelphia, PA, pp 774–816

Andersen J G 1982 Malignant degeneration in chronic ulceration of the leg and foot in leprosy patients: Two case reports. Leprosy Review 53: 265–269

Anonymous 1987 Programme for the control of the endemic treponematoses. World Health Organization, Geneva

Anthal G M, Cause G 1985 The control of endemic treponematoses. Review of Infectious Diseases 7(Suppl 2): S220–S226

Aubry A, Jarlier V, Escolano S et al 2000 Antibiotic susceptibility pattern of *Mycobacterium marinum*. Antimicrobial Agents and Chemotherapy 44: 3133–3136

Badaro R, Carvalho E M, Rocha H et al 1986 *Leishmania donovani*: an opportunistic microbe associated with progressive disease in three immunocompromised patients. Lancet 1: 647–649

Bibler M R, Luber H J, Glueck H I et al 1986 Disseminated sporotrichosis in a patient with HIV infection after treatment for acquired factor VIII inhibitor. Journal of the American Medical Association 256: 3125–3126

Brand P W, Fritschi E P 1985 Rehabilitation in leprosy. In: Hastings RC (ed.) Leprosy. Churchill Livingstone, Edinburgh, p 301

Brink E W, Hinman A R 1989 *Corynebacterium* infections. In: Kelley W N (ed.) Textbook of internal medicine. J B Lippincott, Philadelphia, PA, pp 1514–1516

Campanelli C D, Santoro A F, Webster C G et al 2001 Symmetrically distributed orange eruption on the ears: a case of lupus vulgaris. Cutis 67: 311–314

Cannor D H, Meyers W M, Krieg R G 1976 Infection by *Mycobacterium ulcerans*. In: Binford C H, Cannor D H (eds) Pathology of tropical and extraordinary diseases. Armed Forces Institute of Pathology, Washington DC, pp 226–234

Castro R M 1979 Trotamento de leishmaniose tugementar americana. World Health Organization Report of the Workshop on Chemotherapy of Mucocutaneous Leishmaniasis, Brazil, July 10–13

Cawley E P 1949 Sporotrichosis, a protean disease: with report of a disseminated subcutaneous gummatous case of the disease. Annals of Internal Medicine 30: 1287–1294

Centers for Disease Control 1987 Revision of the CDC surveillance case definition for acquired immunodeficiency syndrome. Morbidity and Mortality Weekly Report 36(Suppl): 35–155

Chen S C, Tan H Y, Tseng H H 2000 Papulonecrotic tuberculid-a rare skin manifestation in a patient with pulmonary tuberculosis. Journal of the Formosan Medical Association 99: 857–859

Chiodini P L 1989 Parasitology. In: Reeves D S, Geddes A M (eds) Recent advances in infection. Churchill Livingstone, Edinburgh, p 242

Christiansen J V, 1968 Lupus vulgaris gigantea caused by *Mycobacterium avium*. In: Jadassohn W, Schirren C G (eds) Proceedings of the 12th International Congress of Dermatology. Springer, Berlin, vol II, pp 1319–1320

Clark E G, Danbolt I V 1964 The Oslo study of the natural course of untreated syphilis. Medical Clinics of North America 48: 613

Cram N, Lamb C, Utz G, et al 2002 Coccidioidomycosis outbreak among United States Navy SEALs training in a *Coccidioides immitis*-endemic area – Coalinga, California. Journal of Infectious Diseases 186: 865–868

Degitz K 1996 Detection of mycobacterial DNA in the skin. Etiologic insights and diagnostic perspectives. Archives of Dermatology 132: 71–75

Difonzo EM, Palleschi G M, Vanmini P et al 1986 Therapeutic experience with ketoconazole. Drugs under Experimental and Clinical Research 12: 397–403

Dooley J R 1976 Other mycobacterial diseases. In: Binford C H, Cannor D H (eds) Pathology of tropical and extraordinary diseases. Armed Forces Institute of Pathology, Washington DC, 235–237

Dupont B, Drouhet E 1987 Early experience with itraconazole in vitro and in patients. Pharmacokinetic and clinical results. Reviews of Infectious Diseases 9: 571–576

Emmons C W, Binford C H, Utz U P, Kwon-Chung K J 1977 Medical mycology, 3rd edn. Philadelphia, Lea & Febiger, p 230

Enk C D, Gardlo K, Hochberg M et al 2003 Cutaneous leishmaniasis. Hautarzt 54: 506–512

Feiwel M, Munro D D 1965 Diagnosis and treatment of erythema induratum (Bazin). British Medical Journal 1: 1109–1111

Fleury R N, Opromolla D V A 1984 Carcinoma in plantar ulcers in leprosy. Leprosy Review 55: 369–378

Funt T R 1961 Primary cutaneous diphtheria. Journal of the American Medical Association 176: 273–275

Furtado T 1981 American leishmaniasis: current status and management. In: Moschella S L (ed.) Dermatology update (1980–1981). Elsevier, New York

Galgiani J N 1983 Ketoconazole in the treatment of coccidioidomycosis. Drugs 337: 346

Gontijo B, de Carvalho M de L 2003 American cutaneous leishmaniasis. Revista da Sociedade Brasileira de Medicina Tropical 36: 71–80

Grange J 1989 Tuberculosis and environmental (atypical) mycobacterioses: bacterial, pathological and immunological aspect. In: Harahap M (ed.) Mycobacterial skin disease. Kluwer Academic, Dordrecht, pp 1–32

Grange J M, Noble W C, Yates M D et al 1988 Inoculation mycobacterioses. Clinical and Experimental Dermatology 13: 211–220

Hackett C J, Loewenthal L J A 1960 Differential diagnosis of yaws. WHO Monogram Series 45. World Health Organization, Geneva

Harahap M (ed.) 1989 Mycobacterial skin diseases. Kluwer Academic, Boston, MA, pp. 99–102

Harman R R M 1986 Parasitic worms and protozoa. In: Rook A, Wilkinson D S, Ebling F J G et al (eds) Textbook of dermatology, 4th edn. Blackwell, Oxford, vol 2, p 1025

James D G, Mishra B B 1984 The changing pattern of tuberculosis. Postgraduate Medicine 60: 92–97

Kirk R 1942 Studies in leishmaniasis in the Anglo-Egyptian Sudan: cutaneous and mucocutaneous leishmaniasis. Transactions of the Royal Society of Tropical Medicine and Hygiene 35: 257

Kivanc-Altunay I, Baysal Z, Ekmekci T R et al 2003 Incidence of cutaneous tuberculosis in patients with organ tuberculosis. International Journal of Dermatology 42: 197–200

Krieg R E, Hockmeyer W T, Connor D H 1974 Toxin of *Mycobacterium ulcerans* production and effects in guinea pig skin. Archives of Dermatology 110: 783–788

Kusuhara M, Hachisuka H, Sasai Y 1988 Statistical survey of 150 cases with sporotrichosis. Mycopathologica 102: 129–133

Lamholt G 1972 Syphilis. In: Rook A, Wilkinson D S, Ebling F J G (eds) Textbook of dermatology, 2nd edn. Blackwell, Oxford, p 634

Lavalle P, Suchel P, De Ovando F et al 1987 Itraconazole for deep mycoses. Preliminary experience in Mexico. Review of Infectious Diseases 9(Suppl 1): 564–570

Lipstein-Kresch E, Isenberg H D, Singer C et al 1985 Disseminated *Sporothrix schenckii* infection with arthritis in a patient with acquired immunodeficiency syndrome. Journal of Rheumatology 12: 805–808

Loewenthal L J A 1963 Tropical phagedenic ulcer. A review. International Review of Tropical Medicine 2: 267–291

Luger A F H 1988 Endemic treponematoses. In: Parish L C, Gschnait F (eds) Sexually transmitted diseases. A guide for clinicians. Springer, New York, pp 32–58

Lynch P J 1971 Sporotrichosis in children. American Journal of Diseases of Children 122: 325–328

McAdam I 1966 Tropical phagedenic ulcer in Uganda. Journal of the Royal College of Surgeons of Edinburgh 11: 196–205

McDougall A C 1989 Leprosy: clinical aspects. In: Harahap M (ed.) Mycobacterial skin diseases. Kluwer Academic, Boston, MA, pp. 119–136

McNicol M 1983 Trends in the epidemiology of tuberculosis – a physician's review. Journal of Clinical Pathology 36: 1087–1090

Mahgoub E I S 1976 Medical management of mycetoma. Bulletin of the World Health Organization 54: 303

Mahgoub E I S 1987 Gumba. Second International Symposium on Mycetomas, Taxco, Mexico

Mahgoub E I S, Murray L G 1973 Mycetoma. Heinemann, London

Manson-Bahr P E C, Bell D R (eds) 1987 Manson's tropical diseases, 19th edn. Baillière Tindall, London, pp 633–644

Mitchell P C 1954 Tuberculosis verrucosa cutis among Chinese in Hong Kong. British Journal of Dermatology 66: 444

Morsy T A, Shoukry A, Schnur L F et al 1987 *Gerbillus pyramidum* is a host of *Leishmania major* in the Sinai Peninsula. Annals of Tropical Medicine and Parasitology 81: 741–742

Narain J P, Raviglione M C, Koch A 1992 HIV-associated tuberculosis in developing countries: epidemiology and strategies for prevention. WHO document WHO/TB/92; 166. World Health Organization, Geneva

Negroni R, Palmieri O, Koren K et al 1987 Oral treatment of paracoccidioidomycosis and histoplasmosis with itraconazole. Review of Infectious Diseases 9(Suppl): 543–546

Nunez-Gussman J, Starke J, Correa A et al 2003 A report of cutaneous tuberculosis in siblings. Pediatric Dermatology 20: 404–407

Oleinick A 1969 Altered immunity and cancer risk: a review of the problem and analysis of the cancer mortality experience in leprosy patients. Journal of the National Cancer Institute 43: 775–781

Oluwasanmi J O, Solanke T F, Olurin E O et al 1976 *Mycobacterium ulcerans* (Buruli) skin ulceration in Nigeria. American Journal of Tropical Hygiene 25: 122–128

Purtilo D T, Pangi C 1975 Incidence of cancer in patients with leprosy. Cancer 35: 1259–1261

Restrepo A, Robledo J, Gomez I et al 1986 Itraconazole therapy in lymphangitic and cutaneous sporotrichosis. Archives of Dermatology 122: 413–417

Rhomberg P R, Jones R N 2002 In vitro activity of antimicrobial agents, including gaitfloxacin and GAR 936, tested against clinical isolates of *Mycobacterium marinum*. Diagnostic Microbiology and Infectious Disease 42: 145–147

Riedel R G 1966 An additional note on malignancy in plantar ulcers in leprosy. International Journal of Leprosy 34: 287–288

Rizzi M, Arici C, Bonacorso C et al 1988 Visceral leishmaniasis in a patient with human immunodeficiency virus. Transactions of the Royal Society of Tropical Medicine and Hygiene 82: 565

Rytel M W, Davis E S, Prebil K J 1970 Primary cutaneous inoculation tuberculosis. American Review of Respiratory Disease 102: 264–267

Sahn S A, Pierson D J 1974 Primary cutaneous inoculation drug resistant tuberculosis. American Journal of Medicine 57: 676–678

Scope A, Trau H, Anders G et al 2003 Experience with New World cutaneous leishmaniasis in travelers. Journal of the American Academy of Dermatology 49:672–678

Siddig M, Ghalib H, Shillington D C et al 1988 Visceral leishmaniasis in the Sudan: comparative parasitological methods of diagnosis. Transactions of the Royal Society of Tropical Medicine and Hygiene 82: 66–68

Singh S, Sivakumar R 2003 Recent advances in the diagnosis of leishmaniasis. Journal of Postgraduate Medicine 49: 55–60

Soderberg T, Hallmans G, Strenström S et al 1982 Treatment of leprosy wounds with adhesive zinc tape. Leprosy Review 53: 271–276

Steele M A, Des Prez R M 1988 The role of pyrazinamide in tuberculosis chemotherapy. Chest 94: 845–850

Stevens DA 1980 Coccidioidomycosis. A text. Plenum, New York, p 261

Tokudome S, Kono S, Ikeda M et al 1981 Cancer and other causes of death among leprosy patients. Journal of the National Cancer Institute 67: 285–289

Tucker R M, Denning D W, Arathoon E G et al 1990 Itraconazole therapy for non-meningeal coccidioidomycosis: clinical and laboratory observations. Journal of the American Academy of Dermatology 23: 593–601

Tyrell D A J, McLauchlan S L, Goodwin C S 1975 The growth of some mycobacteria on cultured human tissues. British Journal of Experimental Pathology 56: 99–102

Van Dam A P, Schippers E F, Visser L G et al 2003 A case of diphtheria in the Netherlands due to an infection with *Corynebacterium ulcerans*. Nederlands Tijdschrift voor Geneeskunde 147: 403–406

Van der Werf T S, van der Graaf W T, Tappero J W et al 1999 *Mycobacterium ulcerans* infection. Lancet 354: 1013–1018

Ward A S 1971 Superficial abscess formation: an unusual presenting feature of tuberculosis. British Journal of Surgery 58: 540–543

World Health Organization 1986 Expert Committee on Venereal Diseases and Treponematoses, Sixth Report.

WHO Technical Report Series. World Health Organization, Geneva, p 736

World Health Organization 1989 STD treatment strategies. WHO consultation on development of sexually transmitted diseases. WHO/VDT/89/447. World Health Organization, Geneva

World Health Organization 1998 WHO Expert Committee on Leprosy, Seventh Report. Technical report series 874. World Health Organization, Geneva

World Health Organization 2003 Leprosy elimination programme. Status report 2003. Available on line at: http://www.who.int/lep/Reports/s20042.pdf

Youmans G P 1985 Diphtheria. In: Youmans G P, Paterson P Y, Sommers H M (eds) The biologic and clinical bases of infectious diseases. W B Saunders, Philadelphia, p 224

CHAPTER

22

Leg ulcers in sickle cell disorders

Adebayo Olujohungbe, Elizabeth N. Anionwu

INTRODUCTION

Leg ulcers are part of the clinical spectrum of sickle cell disorders (Cackovic et al 1998). Case study 1 describes the history of an adult male, and highlights many of the salient features seen with this condition.

Case Study 1   *Leg ulceration in sickle cell anaemia*

P.H. is a 41-year-old man with homozygous sickle cell anaemia. He is the second child of six born to an immigrant family from Jamaica who settled in the north of England in the early 1970s. Two younger siblings also have sickle cell anaemia and both have a history of leg ulceration. P.H. was diagnosed at the age of 7 years after a severe clinical course. His steady-state haemoglobin runs between 7 and 8 g/dl, white blood count of 10.5×10^9/litre and platelets of 288×10^9/litre. He was seen in hospital 'every 2 weeks' with painful crises, lethargy and increasing jaundice during his childhood years. He suffered from nocturnal enuresis, which was extensively investigated and treated with minimal benefit. He also developed the 'hand foot' sickle cell syndrome at the age of 2 years and had major abdominal surgery for intestinal obstruction, which has left him with a wide incision scar externally. He developed pneumonia on two occasions, both episodes requiring long periods of hospitalization. As a result of his frequent absence from school, he

was sent to a special school between the ages of 7 and 16 years. He feels that he missed out on a good education because of his ill health and the inflexible nature of the education system. Nevertheless he had no difficulty in passing his 11+ exam and had psychometric testing, which he passed as well. Despite this he was not offered a place at the local grammar school as the head teacher felt 'he could not cope with the added pressure of schoolwork'.

P.H. first developed leg ulcers in 1978 at the age of 16 years. He had been a very active football player at school as well as a member of the Boys Brigade team. He had no major recall of suffering any trauma whilst playing.

The ulcer was initially on the right medial malleolus, measuring 1×2 cm in diameter. There was no associated pain but he developed severe cellulitis in the left lower leg 6 months later. He was treated with oral antibiotics, oral zinc sulphate 200 mg three times daily and regular weekly dressing. His episodes of painful crises occurred less frequently – twice a year – and have remained so to date.

In 1982 the ulcers worsened, increasing in size with severe pain and recurring three times a year, lasting 2 months on each occasion. Further ulceration would be provoked following mild trauma, such as knocking an ankle on furniture or insect bites. The ulcers were dressed with Eusol, iodine and compression bandages. P.H. was reduced to walking on 'all fours' around the house and could hardly weight-bear. He was obliged to use crutches to get around short distances. The ulcers had darkened. Swabs from the ulcer base grew *Staphylococcus aureus* on the right and skin commensals on the left. P.H. developed septicaemia, with a temperature of 38°C, and was admitted for intravenous antibiotics. He had to repeat that year of college and was eventually obliged to leave. In an attempt to minimize absence from his second college and promote healing, he had a short period of exchange blood transfusion in 1983. The ulcers were concomitantly dressed with zinc and castor oil paste and a four-layer bandage in the community ulcer clinic. P.H. asked his doctors about complementary therapy such as selenium and antioxidants, to no avail.

P.H.'s father died of a heart attack in 1991. He had been his son's role model and had supplemented his education by teaching him crafts and woodwork. P.H. became very depressed. He was passing out frequently in church and community gatherings, from pain, anaemia and repeated infections. Between 1993 and 1995 the ulcer went through phases of healing and recurrence approximately three times a year.

P.H. felt that there was a relationship between the ulcers recurring and periods when his haemoglobin was low. The ulcers seemed less frequent during transfusion therapy but this approach had been complicated by iron overload and other problems resulting in treatment interruption.

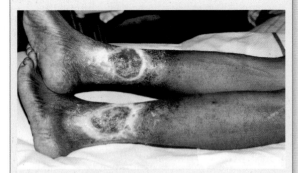

Figure 22.1 Bilateral venous leg ulcers in patient P.H.

The vascular surgery team reviewed him and arranged annual Doppler studies for monitoring. The studies showed some degree of venous incompetence within the superficial veins. P.H. had not managed to graduate by 1999 and felt that the ulcers had ruined his life. He had been dismissed twice from higher education and had to seek recourse from the Department of Education. In 2000, he belatedly underwent career counselling and a short stint of exchange transfusion to allow him to carry on with his studies. He eventually obtained his degree in 2001.

In the last year his sister, who also had sickle cell anaemia, died of acute chest syndrome and his mother died 6 months later of heart failure. P.H. lives alone and is completely cut off from society. He depends on Meals on Wheels and a home help provided by social services to assist with shopping and other domestic requirements. He feels isolated and angry. The ulcers have not healed in the last 2 years and he has been unemployed during this period. He has not had a relationship in the last 5 years. The deterrent factors are a lack of confidence, a negative self-image due to his leg ulcers, the abdominal scar and the unpredictability of his bone pain crises.

The ulcer on P.H.'s left leg is currently infected, with a bright green slough suggestive of *Pseudomonas* colonization. At present he is being treated with oral antibiotics, three-layer dressings with cytofoam antiseptic and monthly exchange transfusions. The only positive experience he can draw from his clinical illness is the support he has received from the staff in the community ulcer clinic and a sickle cell counselling centre in his locality.

DISCUSSION

The experience of P.H. has many parallels with those reported to Anionwu by 'Alesha', a 21-year-old woman with sickle cell anaemia living in London and with an 8-year history of leg ulcers (Anionwu 2002). The similarities include the following: they both experienced the onset of leg ulceration in adolescence and in each case the original ulcer went on to become bilateral and recurring. The ulcers also became infected, caused extreme pain and severe mobility problems, stigma and impacted negatively on education and family life. Both individuals experienced depression and reported difficulties in their efforts to persuade health professionals to prescribe alternative therapies to replace those that did not appear to be working.

Three significant differences emerged between these case studies. The first was that P.H. suffered several family bereavements in a very short period of time. Secondly, intervention by a sickle cell nurse specialist enabled Alesha to be referred to a multi-disciplinary leg ulcer team with an interest in sickle cell disorders. Thirdly, the ensuing comprehensive and supportive management transformed Alesha's life so that she was able to return to her studies, regain her confidence and 'thank the understanding of an excellent team. I have my life back'. In addition, she had these words for those involved with the care of individuals with sickle cell disorders and affected by leg ulcers:

> Listen to them, respect their views and understand that they have their own opinions and knowledge. Give as much support as possible, assess and refer on to appropriate professionals. Offer flexibility in treatment of ulcers, develop an understanding of sickle cell disease and of the added limitations caused by ulcers. Also try to understand the impact such a painful condition has on young people.

> Anionwu 2002, p. 57

BACKGROUND

Sickle cell disorders are a group of autosomal recessively inherited conditions affecting haemoglobin (Hb) within the red cells (Serjeant 2001, Claster & Vichinsky 2003). They arise as a result of a single amino acid substitution (glutamic acid for valine) in the β-globin chain of haemoglobin. Individuals who inherit a gene coding for normal adult HbA and a gene for sickle haemoglobin (HbS) have sickle cell trait (AS) and have little or no clinical consequences. In contrast, inheritance of a sickle gene from each parent gives rise to the

homozygous state called sickle cell anaemia (SS). Inheritance of the sickle mutation with another variant haemoglobin such as haemoglobin C or D or a β-thalassaemia mutation leads to individuals who are compound heterozygotes (e.g. SC, SD, Sβ-thalassaemia) and who have a variable clinical severity due to coexisting environmental and other genetic causes (Serjeant & Serjeant, 2001).

EPIDEMIOLOGY

The sickling disorders are prevalent in holoendemic malarial regions, notably in sub-Saharan Africa, but are also found in North America, the Indian subcontinent, South America and other parts of the world as a result of forced or voluntary migration. According to World Health Organization figures, approximately 250 000 babies are born annually worldwide with the disorders and the majority will die within the first few years of life from specific, sometimes preventable complications (Angastiniotis & Modell, 1998). It is estimated that 12 500 affected individuals currently live in the UK and the numbers are likely to increase with time (Streetly et al 1997).

PATHOPHYSIOLOGY OF SICKLING

The clinical manifestations of sickle cell disorders arise from the polymerization of deoxyhaemoglobin S within the red cell, which distorts its shape and leads to repeated sickling within the microcirculation. These changes are confounded by complex interactions with white cells, platelets and the endothelium, ultimately causing occlusion of blood within the microcirculation, haemolytic anaemia and multiple organ failure. Leg ulcers form part of that clinical spectrum and present a major therapeutic challenge for both the patient and the clinician involved.

LEG ULCERS AS A MANIFESTATION OF SICKLE CELL DISORDERS

Leg ulcers were first recognized as a specific complication of sickle cell disorders in 1940 by Cummer & LaRocco. Cackovic et al (1998) noted a 25–75% lifetime incidence of leg ulcers in affected individuals. Within the context of sickle cell disorders, their prevalence is influenced by age, genotype and geographical location and they are more common in patients with homozygous sickle cell anaemia than with other variants of sickle cell disease. Coinheritance of α-thalassaemia trait also appears to reduce the risk of occurrence (Koshy et al 1989, Steinberg 1999).

Ulcers are uncommon within the first decade of life but their prevalence rises with increasing age, with annual rates of 14.59–19.17 reported in the third decade by the Cooperative Study of Sickle Cell Disorders (Koshy et al, 1989). Patients with a past history of leg ulceration due to sickle cell disorders are more prone to chronicity and recurrence, with rates as high as 75.8 per 100 patient years.

Both 'steady state' haemoglobin and haemoglobin F levels are inversely correlated with the incidence of leg ulcers (Donaldson et al 2001). Many patients with intractable and difficult leg ulcers have a relatively benign clinical course in terms of other complications attributable to sickle cell disorders (Sawhney et al 2002). Earlier reports suggested an increased incidence of proteinuria among patients with leg ulceration but both are now recognized as specific unrelated complications of sickle cell disorders (Morgan 1982).

Geographical distribution

For hitherto unexplained reasons, leg ulcers are more frequent in Jamaican patients than in their west African, European and North American counterparts (Akinyanju & Akinsete 1979, Konotey-Ahulu, 1996, Serjeant 2001). Their prevalence in the UK is not well enough documented to allow a precise comparison to be made. Men are three times more likely to develop leg ulcers than women. This sex discrepancy is probably the result of the increased likelihood of trauma encountered by men in these countries.

AETIOLOGY

Tissue ischaemia resulting from sickling, venous congestion and lymphoedema have all been cited as contributing factors in the development of leg ulceration (Bergqvist et al 1999). The magnitude of contribution of each factor is currently unknown. The development of leg ulcers in other non-sickling haemolytic states such as hereditary spherocytosis or β-thalassaemia major suggests that sickling, however, is not the central causative factor. Lower limb chronic arterial ischaemia or digital gangrene is absent in the young group of patients usually affected by the sickling disorder, and peripheral pulses are present (Sawhney et al, 2002).

Increased venous pressure produces some of the characteristic skin changes of purpura, hyperpigmentation, liposclerosis, skin tightening and prominence of superficial vessels seen in some sickle cell patients. The function of deep leg veins is normal in most patients and varicosities are relatively uncommon in sickle cell disorders (Jones et al 1999, Mohan et al 2000, Chalchal et al 2001, Clare et al 2002, Sawhney et al 2002).

The majority of leg ulcers occur without an antecedent history of trauma. They follow on from a painful localization, skin changes, induration, necrosis within the dermis with an overlying intact epidermis, and final breakdown of skin (Serjeant & Serjeant 2001). This sequence of events suggest tissue infarction as the causative factor, and the ulcers are usually painful, of small size and heal relatively quickly.

Other leg ulcers can occur following relatively minor trauma, which then fail to heal, become infected and grow circumferentially in size. These tend to follow a chronic relapsing course over years.

Serjeant's group observed a third and rarer type of leg ulceration in the Jamaican Cohort Study, in which a blister appears and then breaks down, resulting in ulceration (Serjeant & Serjeant, 2001).

Site

Like many other haemolytic anaemias, leg ulcers have a predilection for the medial malleolus (Sawhney et al 2002), although they can affect the lateral malleoli and anterior aspect of the shin. No differences in site of affectation or the leg affected was seen in the Cooperative Study of Sickle Cell Disease (Koshy et al 1989).

Most ulcers, irrespective of aetiology, are less than 10 cm in diameter and have a punched out appearance with well defined, raised margins. Occasionally, many small ulcers coalesce to form a larger ulcer. Malignant change is not a feature of chronic leg ulcers seen in sickle cell disorders.

ASSESSMENT OF LEG ULCERS

In addition to a generic assessment of the leg ulcers (Ch. 7), a detailed documented history, including previous trauma and other sickle related complications together with transfusion history at first contact, will aid management. Conduct a thorough examination assessing the location, the size of the ulcer and the appearance of its base. In view of the vulnerability of the sickle cell patient to infections, wound swabs should be taken at this stage. This will enable speedy identification of any potential organism(s) that may delay the healing process.

The presence of infection or varicosities and the state of the surrounding skin should be recorded. A simple hand-held Doppler is sufficient for the initial assessment of the venous and arterial system. In complicated cases, referral to the appropriate medical and surgical teams in a tertiary centre may be appropriate.

INVESTIGATIONS

- Full blood count
- Haemoglobin electrophoresis and quantification of other variant haemoglobin(s), especially HbF, HbA and HbA_2.
- α-globin genotype
- Regular wound swabs
- Radiographs to exclude osteomyelitis as appropriate
- Yearly Doppler assessment – hand held Doppler ultrasonography is a non-invasive way of demonstrating flow within the superficial and deep vascular system and determines the arterial status in the limb.

GENERAL MANAGEMENT OF LEG ULCERATION

Most patients with leg ulcers due to sickle cell disease are suitable for management in the community by nurse-led clinical teams. Management principles are similar to those adopted for venous ulceration. A very small number of patients may not respond to community management and may require hospitalization for short periods to address specific issues. Multidisciplinary inputs are essential from relevant medical and surgical staff, occupational therapists and other support workers.

Medical

Leg ulcers can contribute to the chronic sickle-related pain experience. The pain may be severe, excruciating and neuropathic in origin. The characteristics may vary, resulting in physical disability and extreme frustration for the affected individual. Simple analgesia is often not powerful enough and opioid analgesia of varying potency may be required to control the pain. A recent report describes the successful application of topical opioids to relieve the pain or reduce the amount of oral analgesia required (Ballas 2002). This effect is mediated by peripheral opioid receptors rather than a systemic effect following on from drug absorption (Levine & Taiwo 1989). Amitriptyline and other neuroleptic agents such as gabapentin can be useful adjuncts to standard analgesia for the management of neuropathic pain.

Bed rest is advocated to promote healing, although it limits physical activity. The pressure on bed occupancy in many developed countries and its unavailability in countries with a large sickle-cell population make its use impractical and hardly enforceable outside the home environment. When achievable, leg elevation may improve venous drainage (Davies & Oni 1997, Ohanaka & Osarenkhoe 1999, Steinberg 1999). Prolonged periods of standing by patients should be discouraged.

Blood transfusion (simple 'top up' or exchange) has been successfully used in an uncontrolled manner to treat sickle cell leg ulcers. This effect may be directly due to relief of tissue anoxia by the corrected haemoglobin but may also operate by limiting ischaemia arising from repeated vaso-occlusion (Chernoff et al 1954; Serjeant & Serjeant 2001).

Infections

Good local hygiene is essential to prevent bacterial proliferation. Regular washing of the ulcer to remove skin scales and exudates, followed by gentle dressing with non-adherent material, is advocated. Infections should be prevented, although the role of prophylactic systemic antibiotics is controversial. In practical terms, antibiotics should be prescribed in cases with associated fever, complicating osteomyelitis or purulent discharge. Baum et al (1987) and Akinyanju & Akinsete (1979) report successful local application of non-absorbable antibiotics in cases of *Pseudomonas* colonization. Vaccination against *Clostridium tetani* should be strongly considered in developing countries.

Prevention of trauma

Once the leg ulcer has healed, measures to prevent further trauma should be encouraged. Shoes should be worn and susceptible areas of skin may be protected by a dry gauze dressing. Graded compression stockings should be worn to reduce venous hypertension.

Drug intervention

Serjeant et al (1970) reported a beneficial effect of oral zinc sulphate, 200 mg three times a day, to promote healing. Vasodilator drugs were reported in a non-randomized clinical trial (Serjeant & Howard 1977) to have no role, although further studies are warranted. Hydroxyurea is a chemotherapeutic agent that increases the level of HbF and ameliorates many of the acute manifestations of sickling. Theoretically, its sustained use may prevent many chronic sickle-cell-related complications, including leg ulceration. Anecdotally, hydroxyurea can cause leg ulcers in patients with another blood disorder, which manifests as excessive production of red cells, called polycythaemia rubra vera (Siriex et al 1999, Bader et al 2000). Reports exist in the literature of exacerbation and intractability of sickle-cell-related leg ulcers with its use, and improvement after discontinuation (de Montalembert et al 1999, Kersgard & Osswald, 2001), necessitating caution until further clarification of its role is obtained.

Surgical

Healing of leg ulcers is by secondary intent with formation of fresh granulation tissue and re-epithelialization from the margin. The process is slow and is further impaired by the cellular inflammatory nature and arteriolar changes within the ulcer bed. Slough and debris can cover the ulcer base and may require debridement. Other methods of debridement include the use of enzymatic preparation and autolytic debridement using moist wound healing. The use of potent antiseptics such as sodium hypochlorite (Eusol), as described in Case study 1, are no longer recommended because of their toxic cellular effects and severe symptoms, such as pain.

Dressings

The aim of dressing selection in managing patients with sickle-cell ulceration is to ensure non-adherence, preventing tissue trauma, moist wound healing and reduction in wound pain. Selection of dressings capable of managing large volumes of exudate may be required in those with large ulcers. Control of exudate remains an important priority, as leakage may lead to maceration and enlargement of the ulcerated area. Particular care should be taken when selecting hydrocolloids, gels or foams, as these may be associated with poor exudate management (Ch. 23). Avoid dressings that adhere to skin as they tend to de-epithelialize and blister the skin on removal.

Skin grafts

A variety of skin grafting techniques have been employed, including full-thickness grafts, pinch grafts and myocutaneous grafts, with variable success. The majority of reports in the literature cite an advantage in pinch grafting techniques resulting from their relative ease of performance and repeatability. Fewer reports exist on the use of myocutaneous grafts to allow an assessment of their efficacy. Skin grafts on their own without correction of underlying pathology have limited benefit and a higher breakdown rate.

Synthetic extracellular matrices (e.g. RGD–Peptide), usually applied topically, or human skin equivalents (Ch. 24) have been tried to provide cell anchorage into ulcer sites to accelerate the wound healing process.

Graduated compression

The role of compression bandaging in eliminating venous hypertension associated with venous leg ulcers is well established. Ensure adequate arterial perfusion before application to prevent tissue necrosis. Graduated compression may be achieved by elastic compression stockings or by multilayered bandaging. Elastic stockings have a poor patient compliance profile. Multilayered bandaging, when properly applied, may be better than single layer compression for promoting healing. The specific needs for compression in this group have not been addressed in randomized controlled trials or observational studies, although compression is clearly an integral aspect of successful treatment.

SOCIOECONOMIC BURDEN OF LEG ULCERS IN SICKLE CELL DISORDERS

Many patients with sickle leg ulcers, although reasonably free from other disabling complications of sickle cell disorders such as stroke and avascular necrosis of long bones, are not in gainful employment (Alleyne et al 1977). Some are forced to leave school prematurely or are simply dismissed from work unfairly because of the inflexibility of the educational system or employment laws. This is an additional burden for those living with sickle cell disorders (Anionwu & Atkin 2001). The patient's perceived inability to cope with schoolwork from the viewpoint of teachers or jobs from the viewpoint of work agencies may appear to the patient to be discriminatory. Absences from school due to time invested in the management of chronic recal-

---

Box 22.1   *Long term complications of leg ulcers in sickle cell disorders*

- Chronicity
- Recurrence
- Severe pain and disability
- Acute osteomyelitis, cellulitis and arthritis
- Skin fibrosis, hyperpigmentation and flexion deformities
- Emotional impact, including feeling of worthlessness and relationship problems
- Economic lack of attainment
- Septicaemia
- Tetanus infection

---

citrant ulcers may sometimes result in ineligibility to sit examinations.

Equally unappreciated is the isolation and negative self-image that these patients have because of the pain and the unsightly and offensive discharge from the ulcers (see Case study 1). They are unable to engage in age-related activities such as swimming, football, going to films, night-clubbing, formation of stable opposite- and/or same-sex or family relationships compared to sickle-cell patients without leg ulcers (Alleyne et al 1977; Box 22.1). Many siblings are also adversely affected, with breakdown of family ties arising from helplessness and inability to influence the situation (Anionwu, 2002).

CONCLUSION

The unsatisfactory nature of our understanding of the basis of leg ulceration in sickle cell disorders and the paucity of treatment modalities, most with limited success or high complication rates, identify areas of much needed research in treating this disabling, well recognized complication. There is a dearth of randomized clinical trials in this area. Such studies should include basic clinical research addressing the types of dressing or synthetic matrices available, the best surgical grafting techniques, the role of various modalities of blood transfusion (simple top-up or exchange) and of cognitive behavioural therapy in preventing long-term psychological impairment, which is currently under-recognized. Emotional trauma, negative self-image and academic underachievement minimize the potential of many individuals, many of whom are physically challenged by their underlying condition, young and from minority ethnic groups. There is a need for immediate and comprehensive education of front-line staff – teachers, health professionals and employers – to address the various aspects of care and facilitate the rightful adjustment of patients with sickle cell disorders into society.

Acknowledgement

We would like to thank Jos Joseph, Vascular Surgeon, Aintree Hospital NHS Trust, for his contribution and advice, and both individuals with sickle cell disorders who shared their experiences with us.

References

Akinyanju O, Akinsete I 1979 Leg ulceration in sickle cell disease in Nigeria. Tropical and Geographical Medicine 31: 87–91

Alleyne S I, Winter E, Serjeant G R 1977 Social effects of leg ulceration in sickle cell anemia. Southern Medical Journal 70: 213–214

Angastiniotis M, Modell B 1998 Global epidemiology of haemoglobin disorders. Annals of the New York Academy of Sciences 850: 251–269

Anionwu E N 2002 Leg ulcers and sickle cell disorders. Nursing Times 98(25): 56–57

Anionwu E N, Atkin K 2001 The politics of sickle cell disorders. Open University Press, Buckingham

Bader U, Banyai M, Boni R et al 2000 Leg ulcers in patients with myeloproliferative disorders: disease or treatment-related? Dermatology 200: 45–48

Ballas S K 2002 Treatment of painful sickle cell leg ulcers with topical opioids. Blood 99: 1096

Baum K F, MacFarlane D, Serjeant G R 1987 Topical antibiotics in chronic sickle cell leg ulcers. Transactions of the Royal Society of Tropical Medicine and Hygiene 81: 847–849

Bergqvist D, Lindhom C, Nelson O 1999 Chronic leg ulcers: the impact of venous disease. Journal of Vascular Surgery 29: 752–725

Cackovic M, Chung C, Bolton L L, Kerstein M D 1998 Leg ulceration in the sickle cell patient. Journal of the American College of Surgeons 187: 3: 307–309

Chalchal H, Rodino W, Hussain S et al 2001 Impaired venous hemodynamics in a minority of patients with chronic leg ulcers due to sickle cell anemia. Vasa 30: 277–279

Chernoff A I, Shapleigh J B, Moore C V 1954 Therapy of chronic ulceration of the legs associated with sickle cell anemia. Journal of the American Medical Association 155: 1487–1491

Clare A, FitzHenley M, Harris J et al 2002 Chronic leg ulceration in homozygous sickle cell disease: the role of venous incompetence. British Journal of Haematology 119: 567–571

Claster S, Vichinsky E P 2003 Managing sickle cell disease. British Medical Journal 327: 1151–1155

Cummer C L, LaRocco C G 1940 Ulcers of the legs in sickle cell anemia. Archives of Dermatology and Syphilology 40: 459–460

Davies S C, Oni L 1997 Management of patients with sickle cell disease. British Medical Journal 315: 656–660

De Montalembert M, Begue P, Bernaudin F et al 1999 Preliminary report of a toxicity of hydroxyurea in sickle cell disease. French Study Group on Sickle Cell Disease. Archive of Disease in Childhood 81: 437–439

Donaldson A, Thomas P, Serjeant B E, Serjeant G R 2001 Fetal haemoglobin in homozygous sickle cell disease: a study of patients with low Hb F levels. Clinical and Laboratory Haematology 23: 285–289

Jones G T, Solomon C, Moaveni A et al 1999 Venous morphology predicts class of chronic venous insufficiency. European Journal of Vascular and Endovascular Surgery 18: 349–354

Kersgard C, Osswald M B 2001 Hydroxyurea and sickle cell leg ulcers. American Journal of Hematology 68: 215–216

Konotey-Ahulu F I D 1996 The sickle cell disease patient. Tetteh-A'domeno, Accra

Koshy M, Entsuah R, Koranda A et al 1989 Leg ulcers in patients with sickle cell disease. Blood 74: 1403–1438

Levine J D, Taiwo Y O 1989 Involvement of the mu-opiate receptor in peripheral analgesia. Neuroscience 32: 571–575

Mohan J S, Vigilance J E, Marshall J M et al 2000 Abnormal venous function in patients with homozygous sickle cell (SS) disease and chronic leg ulcers. Clinical Science (London) 98: 667–672

Morgan A G 1982 Proteinuria and leg ulcers in homozygous sickle cell disease. Journal of Tropical Medicine and Hygiene 85: 205–208

Ohanaka E C, Osarenkhoe O 1999 In-patient management of leg ulcers. East African Medical Journal 76: 687–689

Sawhney H, Weedon J, Gillette P et al 2002 Predilection of hemolytic anemia-associated leg ulcers for the medial malleolus. Vasa 31: 191–139

Serjeant G R 2001 The emerging understanding of sickle cell disease. British Journal of Haematology 112: 3–18

Serjeant G R, Howard C 1977 Isoxsuprine hydrochloride in the therapy of sickle cell ulceration. West Indies Medical Journal 26: 164–166

Serjeant G R, Serjeant B E 2001 Sickle cell disorders, 3rd edn. Oxford University Press, Oxford

Serjeant G R, Galloway R E, Gueri M C 1970 Oral zinc sulphate in sickle-cell ulcers. Lancet 2: 891–893

Siriex M-E, Debure C, Baudot N et al 1999 Leg ulcers and hydroxyurea. Archives of Dermatology 135: 818–820

Steinberg M H 1999 Management of sickle cell disease. New England Journal of Medicine 340: 1021–1030

Streetly A, Maxwell K, Mejia A 1997 Sickle cell disorders in Greater London: a needs assessment of screening and care services. The Fair Shares for London Report. Department of Public Health Medicine, UMDS and St Thomas' Hospital, London

23

Wound bed preparation for venous leg ulcers

Christine J. Moffatt, Moya J. Morison, Elaine Pina

INTRODUCTION

[C]hronic wounds have a complex life of their own and … are not simply an aberration of the normal healing process. The concept of wound bed preparation allows us to dissect the different components that need to be addressed in chronic wounds, and to develop long-term strategies for the more complex issues that lead to failure to heal.

Falanga 2002, p.5.

In an era of evidence-based health care we are required to continually challenge long established practices and to determine their clinical effectiveness, based on a sound theoretical understanding of the processes that contribute to optimal healing. However, our understanding of the cascade of events involved in wound healing has largely been gained from the study of acute wounds (both in humans and in animals). Extrapolating this knowledge to chronic wounds such as leg ulcers can be overly simplistic and indeed misleading.

In this patient group the following clinical challenges are commonly encountered:

- Poor tissue perfusion and hypoxia
- Excess exudate and maceration of the wound margins
- A high bacterial load
- Necrotic tissue
- Dermatological problems of the surrounding skin, such as venous stasis eczema.

Over the last decade a number of advanced therapeutic approaches such as growth factors, gene therapy and the use of skin substitutes have become available, but their success can be challenged when the wound bed is poorly prepared. Optimizing the biological microenvironment of the wound requires that all of these issues be addressed.

For most patients with venous leg ulceration the application of high compression bandaging in combination with simple non-adherent dressings is sufficient to stimulate autolytic debridement, control moisture balance and encourage healing within 24 weeks (Effective Healthcare 1997). The challenge for effective wound bed preparation is the early detection of those ulcers unlikely to heal by simple compression therapy alone, and for which additional therapeutic interventions may accelerate or facilitate healing. This paper uses the TIME framework (Tissue management, Inflammation and infection control, Moisture balance and Epithelial (edge) advancement) to explore the concept of wound bed preparation for venous leg ulcers.

BEFORE TIME

Venous ulceration results from venous insufficiency or obstruction. Oedema occurs and it is well recognized that graduated, sustained multi-layer compression is the cornerstone of care. Wound bed preparation will not be successful unless the following management principles are taken into account, along with effective patient education and concordance with therapy (European Wound Management Association 2003):

- Correct the cause of the ulcer by managing the underlying venous disease (surgical intervention where necessary)
- Improve venous return using high-compression therapy
- Create the optimum local environment at the wound site
- Improve the wider factors that may delay healing
- Maintain ongoing assessment to identify changing aetiology
- Maintain a healed limb through a lifetime of compression therapy.

There is currently no internationally agreed standard healing rate of an uncomplicated venous ulcer: reported healing at 12 weeks ranges from 30% to over 75% (Moffatt et al 1992, Harper et al 1995). Although a number of risk factors for delayed healing are recognized (Box 23.1), there are many possible reasons why healing rates vary so widely. However, the percentage of wound reduction during the first three to four weeks of treatment can be used to predict subsequent healing, with a 44% reduction in initial area at week 3 correctly predicting healing in 77% of cases (Flanagan 2003).

Box 23.1   *Risk factors for delayed healing (European Wound Management Association 2003)*

- Ulcer duration >6 months
- Ulcer size >10 cm^2
- Reduced mobility
- Severe pain
- Psychosocial: living alone, social support, clinical depression
- Sex (male)
- Poor general health

TISSUE MANAGEMENT

Necrotic tissue

The majority of uncomplicated venous ulcers have relatively little necrotic tissue on the wound surface and do not require debridement. However, it may be beneficial for more complex ulcers, for example where severe infection, uncontrolled oedema and wound desiccation may cause tissue necrosis. In addition, ulcers of long duration may develop a chronic fibrinous base, which is pale, shiny and adherent. Removal of this layer using sharp debridement under local anaesthetic may promote healing, but care must be taken to avoid damaging deeper structures (Vowden & Vowden 1999). It should be noted that clinicians must be appropriately qualified before undertaking surgical or sharp debridement.

Ulcers lying behind the malleoli are particularly prone to slough development and heal slowly. Limited sharp debridement using forceps and scissors is often sufficient as slough is usually superficial, while simple methods of increasing local pressure on the wound, such as the use of foam shapes or firm padding cut to the contour of the area, can stimulate healing (Moffatt & Harper 1997). Adapting the method of compression can also be helpful; for example, an extra layer of bandaging will increase pressure on this area, although care should be taken to ensure there is adequate padding for the dorsum of the foot.

For more adherent slough, debridement using enzymatic preparations may be considered as a practical alternative (Westerhof et al 1990). Larval therapy can also be considered as an alternative to sharp debridement, although application under compression may be associated with practical challenges. Autolytic debridement using dressings with a high water content, such as hydrogels and hydrocolloids, is slow and clinical experience suggests that this is not an effective form of debridement under compression. Although maintenance debridement is recommended for wound bed preparation, this is rarely indicated for venous leg ulcers (Schultz et al 2003).

Surrounding skin

Surrounding skin problems, such as callus formation and hyperkeratosis, may interfere with healing. The development of hard callus or scabs, for example, may become a source of pressure beneath compression and require careful removal using fine forceps, avoiding trauma to the vulnerable underlying epithelium. Clinical experience suggests that soaking in warm water with emollient for more than 10 minutes can facilitate tissue removal. Bleeding after debridement may be resolved by the application of a haemostat such as an alginate, and compression.

INFLAMMATION AND INFECTION CONTROL

Bacteria may stimulate a persisting inflammation leading to the production of inflammatory mediators and proteolytic enzymes. Among many other effects this causes extracellular matrix (ECM) degradation and inhibition of re-epithelialization (Fray et al 2003). Bacterial burden must therefore be controlled to facilitate healing or to maximize the effectiveness of newer therapeutic techniques such as bioengineered skin or growth factors.

The diagnosis of wound infection is a clinical skill based on careful history taking and clinical observation. Infection in venous ulcers is usually localized and there may be cellulitis. On rare occasions, particularly where the patient is immunocompromised, systemic infection may develop. Leukocytosis and acute-phase reactants such as erythrocyte sedimentation rate and C-reactive protein are not reliable since these patients are constantly challenged by minor illnesses and peripheral lesions that may elevate these indices. It is therefore necessary to be aware of other signs often presenting in these wounds, such as an increase in the intensity or change in the character of pain (Box 23.2; Cutting & Harding 1994, Thomson & Smith 1994, Gardner et al 2001).

Microbiological diagnosis should be limited to situations where there is a clear indication that the bacterial load is implicated in delayed healing. Quantification of bacteria by wound biopsy has been considered the gold standard but surface sampling is easier and less costly, and it is increasingly suggested that bacterial synergistic interaction is more important than the precise number, as a greater diversity (i.e. more than four species) is associated with non-healing (Trengove et al 1996, Bowler 2002). Anaerobic organisms are considered

> **Box 23.2 Indicators of infection in venous ulcers (Cutting & Harding 1994, Gardner et al 2001)**
>
> - Increased intensity and/or change in character of pain
> - Discoloured or friable granulation tissue
> - Odour
> - Wound breakdown
> - Delayed healing
>
> Note: The classical signs and symptoms of infection (pain, erythema, heat and purulence) may be reduced (Thomson & Smith 1994) or masked by dermatological problems

to have at least as great a negative impact on healing as aerobes (Bowler 2002). *Staphylococcus aureus* and *Pseudomonas aeruginosa* are the bacteria most commonly isolated in infected leg ulcers but are also found in non-infected wounds. Haemolytic streptococci are not commonly found in leg ulcers but can be a particular cause for concern and can lead to massive tissue damage if not recognized and treated effectively and promptly (Thomson & Smith 1994). It is, however, difficult to define the role of individual species in polymicrobial infections (Trengove et al 1996, Bowler 2002). Other organisms such as mycobacteria, fungi and viruses, as well as parasites such as *Leishmania* spp. may be implicated in a differential diagnosis (Cardenas et al 2004).

TREATMENT

It is essential to enhance host resistance by correcting the underlying vascular disease and eliminating or reducing risk factors, including smoking, heart failure, oedema, pain, malnutrition and the effects of medications such as steroids and immunosuppressive agents. While management of infection is determined by local wound characteristics, clearing devitalized tissue and foreign bodies is the first step to restoring bacterial balance. This can be achieved through exudate control, cleansing with sterile saline and sharp debridement where indicated, or other methods of debridement, including larval therapy (Beasley & Hirst 2004).

Antimicrobial treatments

In wounds that exhibit local signs of infection or fail to heal in spite of appropriate care, topical antiseptics should be considered. In addition to the choice of product, the form and system of delivery are important (Eaglstein & Falanga 1997). Antiseptic solutions are not indicated because of toxicity (Mertz et al 1984, Hansson & Faergemann 1995).

The role of antiseptics was recently reappraised (Drosou et al 2003); a number of new, sustained, slow-release formulations of iodine and silver were found to reduce bacterial burden safely and efficiently. When selecting antiseptic-containing dressings (Wright et al 2003), in addition to anti-bacterial properties, other characteristics such as moisture retention, absorption of endotoxins (Ovington 2003), reduction of inflammation (Fumal et al 2002) and pain relief (Sibbald et al 2001) should be considered.

Antiseptics are preferable because resistance is not yet a clinical problem, although concern has been raised about the possibility of selecting antimicrobial-resistant strains (Russell 2003). If no improvement is observed in 2 weeks, antiseptic treatment should cease, the wound should be reassessed and systemic antibiotics may be considered. Topical antibiotics can deliver high concentrations to the wound while minimizing the risk of systemic toxicity; however, cutaneous sensitization, inactivation, inhibition of healing and selection of resistant strains have been reported (Degreef 1998) and they are therefore not recommended. Metronidazole gel has been used to manage odour and reduce anaerobic colonization (Witkowski & Parish 1991), while fusidic acid and mupirocin are active against Gram-positive bacteria, including methicillin-resistant *Staphylococcus aureus*. Polymyxin B, neomycin and bacitracin should not be used because of allergy. Systemic antibiotics should be used when there are signs of systemic invasion or cellulitis, or when active infection cannot be managed using local therapies.

MOISTURE BALANCE

Venous leg ulcers usually produce copious exudate, which can delay healing and cause maceration of the surrounding skin (Chen & Abatangelo 1999).

Chronic exudate causes the breakdown of extracellular matrix proteins and growth factors, prolongs inflammation, inhibits cell proliferation and leads to the degradation of tissue matrix (Falanga et al 1994, Barrick et al 1999, Trengove et al 1999). Its management is therefore vital to wound bed preparation (Ennis & Meneses 2000).

The removal of oedema using sustained compression therapy is fundamental to achieving moisture balance (European Wound Management Association 2003). Compression helps to optimize local moisture balance by reducing exudate production and tissue maceration and to ensure adequate tissue perfusion by improving venous return.

Compression therapy can be achieved using a variety of methods such as bandages, hosiery and intermittent pneumatic compression (European Wound Management Association 2003). Choice of method depends on resources available, patient mobility, the size and shape of the affected leg and patient preference. If venous ulcers continue to produce copious exudate and there are signs of oedema, compression may be inadequate. Bandages may need to be changed more frequently if soiled by excessive exudate or if the limb circumference is reduced markedly, when remeasuring of the ankle circumference may be necessary.

To assist the action of compression, patients should be advised to avoid standing for long periods and to elevate their legs above heart level when sitting or lying down. These steps can make a sufficient difference to allow healing in an otherwise static ulcer.

Venous ulcers require basic moist wound healing principles, as dryness of the ulcer bed is rarely a problem. Simple measures such as washing the lower limbs and effective skin care are important.

Dressing selection should take account of a number of factors. They should minimize tissue trauma, absorb excess exudate, manage slough/necrotic tissue and be hypoallergenic. Where possible, adhesive dressings should be avoided as they increase the risk of allergic reactions or contact dermatitis (Cameron 1998). Dressing performance may be affected by compression, especially those designed to deal with high levels of exudate, as compression may affect the lateral flow of fluid within the dressing (Cutting 1999).

Box 23.3 *Preventing maceration*

- Use paraffin-based products or zinc paste as a barrier

- Select appropriately sized dressing capable of handling high exudate levels, such as foams and capillary action dressings

- Carefully position the dressing so that exudate does not run below the wound

- Silver and iodine products can be used if excess exudate is caused by infection

- Avoid hydrocolloids and films

Hydration and protection of the skin using paraffin-based products or zinc paste is a fundamental aspect of care. However, these must be removed regularly by washing or they may form a thick layer preventing removal of dead keratinocytes and promoting the development of varicose eczema and hyperkeratosis.

Maceration may occur around the margins of venous ulceration and is manifested as white, soggy tissue (Cutting 1999; Box 23.3). Areas of erythema may also be present where exudate is in contact with vulnerable skin. This can lead to the development of irritant dermatitis and new areas of ulceration (Vowden & Vowden 2003).

EPITHELIAL (EDGE) ADVANCEMENT

If the epidermal margin fails to migrate across the wound bed there are many possible reasons, including hypoxia, infection, desiccation, dressing trauma, overgrowth of hyperkeratosis and callus at the wound margin. Careful clinical observation can help to determine the cause, although this will not reveal defects in the underlying cell biology.

The presence of islands of epithelium originating from hair follicles and evidence of edge stimulation at the wound margin are useful indicators of healing. However, newly formed epithelial cells can be difficult to identify as they are partly translucent and may be hidden by slough, fibrous tissue or exudate.

ADVANCED THERAPIES

Despite adequate wound bed preparation using standard methods some wounds fail to heal or heal slowly. This may be the consequence of a disordered healing response resulting from inappropriate cytokine, growth factor, protease and reactive oxygen species production by cells within granulation tissue, which leads to non-resolving inflammation, poor angiogenesis, extracellular matrix (ECM) degradation and non-migration of epithelial cells from the wound margin. Treatment leading to reversal of these defects allows initiation of healing, as shown by modification of the ECM structure, which precedes re-epithelialization in leg ulcers (Herrick et al 1992).

Based on this knowledge a number of advanced treatment strategies have been devised that show interesting results with recalcitrant wounds (Table 23.1). They are, however, only likely to be successful if applied to a well prepared wound bed (Schultz et al 2003).

Tissue engineering

Grafting of autologous skin to a prepared wound bed has been used to stimulate healing for many years (Kantor & Margolis 2003). However, this suffers from the disadvantage of donor site pain, scarring and the possibility of infection. Recent advances in cell culture techniques allow expansion of cells in vitro, which are then used to populate biocompatible scaffolds to act as a carrier and substitute for split-thickness skin grafts. Cells may be either autologous or from allogenic donors. This treatment has the added advantage that the transplanted cells interact in the healing process by producing growth factors that may also act to stimulate healing (Martin et al 2003).

Growth factors

The growth factor networks that regulate healing may become degraded (Yager et al 1997) and disorganized in the chronic wound (Agren et al 2000). This leads to the concept that supplying exogenous growth factors to the wound microenvironment may stimulate healing. Many have been evaluated but platelet-derived growth factor is, to date, the first growth factor to be licensed for topical appli-

Table 23.1 Advanced therapies

Description	Activity	Research
Tissue-engineered products		
Engineered skin constructs (neonatal allogeneic fibroblasts/keratinocytes)	Produce growth factors and stimulate angiogenesis	More effective than conventional venous leg ulcer (VLU) therapy in a clinical trial (Fivenson & Scherschun 2003) Activity demonstrated in VLU (Roberts & Mansbridge 2002). Results of ongoing trials awaited with interest
Growth factors		
Granulocyte monocyte colony stimulating factor	Activates monocytes, stimulates proliferation and migration of keratinocytes, modulates fibroblasts	Enhanced healing rates in VLU (Da Costa et al 1999)
Keratinocyte growth factor	Stimulates proliferation of keratinocytes and migration of keratinocytes and fibroblasts	Enhanced healing rates in VLU (Robson et al 2001)
Bioactive dressings/treatments		
Esterified hyaluronic acid	Delivers multifunctional hyaluronic acid to the wound	Pilot study demonstrates initiation of healing in VLU (Colletta et al 2003)
Protease modulating matrix	Stimulates angiogenesis by inactivating excess proteases	62% of VLUs improved over 8 weeks compared to 42% in control group (Vin et al 2002)

cation, and only in diabetic ulcers (Guzman-Gardearzabal et al 2000).

Bioactive dressings/treatments

Modern wound dressings developed to maintain a moist wound environment have recently evolved into a new generation of products that interact with the wound to stimulate healing. Examples are protease modulating dressings, which claim to stimulate healing by inactivating excess proteases (Cullen et al 2002), and a range of products based on esterified hyaluronic acid, which deliver multi-functional hyaluronic acid to the wound (Chen & Abatangelo 1999).

Protease inhibitors

A novel synthetic inhibitor of protease activity has recently been described (Fray et al 2003) that inhibits ECM-degrading enzymes without affecting those proteases required for normal keratinocyte migration. This suggests it will be feasible in the future to develop highly specific pharmacological agents to treat defects of non-healing wounds.

CONCLUSION

While there is a need for further research and better understanding of the cellular and biochemical abnormalities seen in patients with chronic venous ulcers, enough is already known for the clinician to be able positively and dramatically to improve the outcome for patients when certain basic principles are consistently applied, the mainstay of treatment being compression therapy.

The general aims of wound bed preparation are as relevant to the management of venous leg ulcers as any other wound type. However, its different elements do not have equal emphasis. Debridement is rarely an issue: the main priority in the management of venous ulcers is to achieve moisture balance by improving venous return using sustained compression. Edge stimulation is intrinsically linked to moisture balance, as without optimal moisture balance epidermal migration will not occur.

In addition to problems of limited resources, it is usually unnecessary to use advanced wound care products with venous leg ulcers. The challenge in managing these wounds is to predict, perhaps as early as the fourth week of standard care, which ulcers will fail to heal rapidly, as these patients benefit the most from alternative care strategies. In addition, further longitudinal studies are needed to evaluate their efficacy and cost-effectiveness in particular clinical situations so that they can be targeted at the patients most likely to benefit from these strategies.

New roles are continually being identified for 'established' treatments. As we understand more about the ideal microenvironment for wound healing and how to create it, we will be able to target our interventions ever more intelligently.

References

Agren M S, Eaglstein W H, Ferguson M W et al 2000 Causes and effects of chronic inflammation in venous leg ulcers. Acta Dermato-Venereologica Supplementum (Stockholm) 210: 3–17

Barrick B, Campbell E J, Owen C A 1999 Leukocyte proteinases in wound healing: roles in physiologic and pathologic processes. Wound Repair and Regeneration 7: 410–422

Beasley W D, Hirst G 2004 Making a meal of MRSA: the role of biosurgery in hospital-acquired infection. Journal of Hospital Infection 56: 6–9

Bowler P G 2002 Wound pathophysiology, infection and therapeutic options. Annals of Medicine 34: 419–427

Cameron J 1998 Skin care for patients with chronic leg ulcers. Journal of Wound Care 7: 459–462

Cardenas G A, Gonzalez-Serva A, Cohen C 2004 The clinical picture: multiple leg ulcers in a traveller. Cleveland Clinical Journal of Medicine 71: 109–112

Chen W Y, Abatangelo G 1999 Functions of hyaluronan in wound repair. Wound Repair and Regeneration 7: 79–89

Colletta V, Dioguardi D, Di Lonardo A et al 2003 A trial to assess the efficacy and tolerability of Hyalofill-F in non-healing venous leg ulcers. Journal of Wound Care 12: 357–360

Cullen B, Smith R, McCulloch E et al 2002 Mechanism of action of Promogran, a protease modulating matrix, for the treatment of diabetic foot ulcers. Wound Repair and Regeneration 10: 16–25

Cutting K 1999 The causes and prevention of maceration of the skin. Journal of Wound Care 8: 200–201

Cutting K, Harding K 1994 Criteria for identifying wound infection. Journal of Wound Care 3: 198–201

Da Costa R M, Ribeiro Jesus F M, Aniceto C, Mendes M 1999 Randomised, double-blind, placebo-controlled, dose-ranging study of granulocyte-macrophage colony stimulating factor in patients with chronic venous leg ulcers. Wound Repair and Regeneration 7: 17–25

Degreef H J 1998 How to heal a wound fast. Dermatologic Clinics 16: 365–375

Drosou A, Falabella A, Kirsner R S 2003 Antiseptics on wounds: an area of controversy. Wounds 15: 149–166

Eaglstein W H, Falanga V 1997 Chronic wounds. Surgical Clinics of North America 77: 689–700

Effective Healthcare 1997 Compression therapy for venous leg ulcers. Effective Healthcare Bulletin 3

Ennis W J, Meneses P 2000 Wound healing at the local level: the stunned wound. Ostomy/Wound Management 46(Suppl): 39S–48S

European Wound Management Association (EWMA) 2003 Position document: Understanding compression therapy. MEP, London

Falanga V 2002 The clinical relevance of wound bed preparation. In: Falanga V, Harding K (eds) The clinical relevance of wound bed preparation. Springer, Berlin, pp 1–12

Falanga V, Grinnell F, Gilchrest B et al 1994 Workshop on the pathogenesis of chronic wounds. Journal of Investigative Dermatology 102: 125–127

Fivenson D, Scherschun L 2003 Clinical and economic impact of Apligraf for the treatment of non-healing venous leg ulcers. International Journal of Dermatology 42: 960–965

Flanagan M 2003 Wound measurement: can it help us to monitor progression to healing? Journal of Wound Care 12: 189–194

Fray M J, Dickinson R P, Huggins J P, Occleston N L 2003 A potent, selective inhibitor of matrix metalloproteinase-3 for the topical treatment of chronic dermal ulcers. Journal of Medical Chemistry 46: 3514–3525

Fumal I, Braham C, Paquet P et al 2002 The beneficial toxicity paradox of antimicrobials in leg ulcer healing impaired by a polymicrobial flora: a proof-of-concept study. Dermatology 204(Suppl 1): 70–74

Gardner S E, Frantz R A, Doebbeling B N 2001 The validity of the clinical signs and symptoms used to identify chronic wound infection. Wound Repair and Regeneration 9: 178–186

Guzman-Gardearzabal E, Leyva-Bohorquez G, Salas-Colin S et al 2000 Treatment of chronic ulcers in the lower extremities with topical becaplermin gel 0.01%: a multicenter open-label study. Advances in Therapy 17: 184–189

Hansson C, Faergemann J 1995 The effect of antiseptic solutions on microorganisms in venous leg ulcers. Acta Dermato-Venereologica (Stockholm) 75: 31–33

Harper D R, Nelson E A, Gibson B et al 1995 A prospective randomised trial of Class 2 and Class 3 elastic compression in the prevention of venous ulceration. Phlebology Supplement 1: 872–873

Herrick S E, Sloan P, McGurk M et al 1992 Sequential changes in histologic pattern and extracellular matrix deposition during the healing of chronic venous ulcers. American Journal of Pathology 141: 1085–1095

Kantor J, Margolis D J 2003 Management of leg ulcers. Seminars in Cutaneous Medicine and Surgery 22: 212–221

Martin T A, Hilton J, Jiang W G, Harding K 2003 Effect of human fibroblast-derived dermis on expansion of tissue from venous leg ulcers. Wound Repair and Regeneration 11: 292–296

Mertz P M, Alvarez O M, Smerbeck R V, Eaglstein W H 1984 A new in vivo model for the evaluation of topical antiseptics on superficial wounds. Archives of Dermatology 120: 58–62

Moffatt CJ, Harper P 1997 Leg ulcers: access to clinical education. Churchill Livingstone, New York

Moffatt C J, Franks P J, Oldroyd M et al 1992 Community clinics for leg ulcers and impact on healing. British Medical Journal 305: 1389–1392

Ovington L G 2003 Bacterial toxins and wound healing. Ostomy/Wound Management 49(Suppl): 8–12

Roberts C, Mansbridge J 2002 The scientific basis and differentiating features of Dermagraft. Canadian Journal of Plastic Surgery 10(Suppl A): 6A–13A

Robson M C, Phillips T J, Falanga V et al 2001 Randomised trial of topically applied Repifermin (recombinant human keratinocyte growth factor-2) to accelerate wound healing in venous ulcers. Wound Repair and Regeneration 9: 347–352

Russell A D 2003 Biocide use and antibiotic resistance: the relevance of laboratory findings to clinical and environmental situations. Lancet Infectious Diseases 3: 794

Schultz G S, Sibbald R G, Falanga V et al 2003 Wound bed preparation: a systematic approach to wound management. Wound Repair and Regeneration 11: Suppl S1–28

Sibbald R G, Torrance G W, Walker V et al 2001 Cost-effectiveness of Apligraf in the treatment of venous ulcers. Ostomy/Wound Management 47: 36–46

Thomson P D, Smith D J 1994 What is infection? American Journal of Surgery 167(Suppl 1A): 7S–11S

Trengove N J, Stacey M C, McGechie D F, Mata S 1996 Qualitative bacteriology and leg ulcer healing. Journal of Wound Care 5: 277–280

Trengove N J, Stacey M C, MacAuley S et al 1999 Analysis of the acute and chronic wound environments: the role of proteases and their inhibitors. Wound Repair and Regeneration 7: 442–452

Vin F, Teot L, Meaume S 2002 The healing properties of Promogran in venous leg ulcers. Journal of Wound Care 11: 335–341

Vowden K R, Vowden P 1999 Wound debridement, Part 2: sharp techniques. Journal of Wound Care 8: 291–294

Vowden K, Vowden P 2003 Understanding exudate management and the role of exudate in the healing process. British Journal of Nursing 12(Suppl): S4–S13

Westerhof W, van Ginkel C J, Cohen E B, Mekkes J R 1990 Prospective randomised study comparing the debriding effect of krill enzymes and a non-enzymatic treatment in venous leg ulcers. Dermatologica 181: 293–297

Witkowski J A, Parish L C 1991 Topical metronidazole gel. The bacteriology of decubitus ulcers. International Journal of Dermatology 30: 660–661

Wright J B, Lam K, Olson M E et al 2003 Is antimicrobial efficacy sufficient? A question concerning the benefits of new dressings. Wounds 15: 133–142

Yager D R, Chen S M, Ward S I et al 1997 Ability of chronic wound fluids to degrade peptide growth factors is associated with increased levels of elastase activity and diminished levels of proteinase inhibitors. Wound Repair and Regeneration 5: 23–32

Skin substitutes

*Gary Sibbald, Siobhan Ryan,
Patricia M. Coutts*

Case study 1   *A non-healing leg ulcer*

E-W is a very pleasant lady who presents with a history of obesity and frequent leg swelling, especially at the end of the day. She also has a family history of leg ulcers. She has had episodes of superficial phlebitis and recurrent leg ulceration. The first leg ulceration occurred in 1987 and she has had seven episodes of re-ulceration. She notes that her ulcerations are usually preceded by minor trauma to her lower leg. Along with the leg ulceration she has experienced episodes of cellulitis and she has been diagnosed with lymphoedema.

Other relevant medical history includes spinal stenosis, osteomyelitis of her foot following surgery to straighten her toes and removal of a bunion, bilateral knee replacements and a right shoulder replacement during which she suffered a spiral fracture of her right arm. She also has hypertension and narcolepsy.

E-W worked as a school secretary for 25 years and is now retired. She has two adult children and one grandchild. One of her adult children lives at home and suffers from gross lymphoedema. His treatment and care are of great concern to her. One of the delights in her life is to enjoy activities with her grandchild. Although her husband is very helpful with day-to-day activities, E-W does the majority of work around the house. As a hobby they operate a small stall at the local flea market, selling E-W's hand-made crafts. E-W also sings in a choir and enjoys swimming in their garden swimming pool.

Her lower leg wounds were diagnosed to be venous in aetiology and were treated with compression therapy and best-practice local wound care. Episodes of ulceration have taken anything from a few months to a few years to heal. E-W has experienced several episodes of wound infection for which she received either oral or topical antibiotic therapy. On one occasion it was necessary for her to receive intravenous antibiotics.

E-W has had problems tolerating compression therapy and short-stretch bandage was found to be the best choice for effectiveness and comfort. Each breakdown of her skin and subsequent treatment with compression bandaging has limited her daily activities, such as swimming. She considers her daily swimming exercise to be an important part of her weight reduction programme.

One episode of ulceration has been present for 14 months and is not progressing towards healing. The possibility of using a skin substitute is discussed with E-W and she agrees to try this new product.

HOLISTIC ASSESSMENT OF A NON-HEALING ULCER

As part of the preparing the wound paradigm, we need to assess the cause and review patient-centred concerns before we address the components of local wound care (Fig. 24.1). There are several ulcer aetiologies that can mimic venous disease, including inflammatory conditions (pyoderma gangrenosum, vasculitis), malignancy (basal cell carcinoma, squamous cell carcinoma), infections (bacterial, deep fungal) and arterial insufficiency.

Often more than one aetiology can act as cofactors in the cause of the ulcer, and failure to recognize and treat all factors may lead to ulcer persistence. A biopsy of the ulcer edge is mandatory to diagnose or rule out unsuspected aetiologies. Signs and symptoms of venous disease, including pitting oedema, venous varicosities and submalleolar venous flare, hyperpigmentation of medial malleolar region, woody fibrosis of the distal leg and lipodermatosclerosis, are not always present in patients with ulcers secondary to venous insufficiency. In addition, signs and symptoms of venous disease may also complicate other comorbid illnesses.

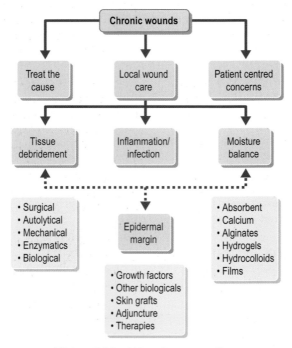

Figure 24.1 Wound care paradigm

Doppler examination is important in all patients with presumed venous ulcers. The ankle–brachial pressure index (ABPI) should be greater than 0.8; an ABPI between 0.6 and 0.8 indicates some arterial compromise. ABPIs may be falsely elevated in the elderly, particularly in patients with diabetes, because of calcification of the vessel wall. A palpable dorsalis pedis pulse is helpful and roughly represents 80 mmHg or more of pressure. A palpable pulse alone in the presence of higher brachial pressure can be present with significant compromise and may be misleading to the wound care practitioner. An ABPI measures arterial parameters and to confirm or diagnose venous disease a tourniquet test, continuous-wave Doppler studies, photoplethysmography and air plethysmography or colour duplex ultrasound scanning should be performed to demonstrate venous insufficiency and/or calf-muscle pump activity.

Re-evaluation is an essential part of the management of the non-healing ulcer and represents the first step in the approach to using skin substitutes. Postmarketing surveys demonstrated unsuccessful skin equivalent application to ulcerated skin cancers, reinforcing the concept of the necessity for comprehensive re-assessment of all non-healing ulcers.

The cornerstone of management of a venous ulcer is compression therapy (Cullum et al 2001). In individual patients it is important to assess oedema reduction on bandage removal and to make sure residual fluid is not present in the interstitial tissue of the distal leg. Your clinical tool kit should contain alternative elastic and inelastic compression bandaging systems, bolsters, additional layers and compression bandaging alternatives (pneumatic compression devices and both rigid and semirigid orthotic compression devices).

There is also a role for medical therapy in the non-healing and resistant leg ulcer. A systematic review (Jull et al 2002) has demonstrated the benefit of pentoxyphylline in the treatment of non-healing venous ulcers present for more than a year. Other practitioners have successfully used horse chestnut and rutosides (Pittler & Ernst 1998) in venous stasis ulcers. We must remember that coexisting factors must be taken into consideration. There are several previously identified regional features (Margolis et al 1999) that can delay healing, which include previous hip or knee replacement, ulcer duration greater than a year, fibrin greater than 50% of wound base, larger wound size, ABPI below 0.8 and a history of venous ligation or vein stripping.

The holistic approach is necessary. Systemic disease (rheumatoid arthritis, immunosuppression) will often increase the difficulty in healing venous ulcers. A careful medication history should pay particular attention to systemic steroids, non-steroidal anti-inflammatory drugs and chemotherapeutic agents.

Patient-centred concerns, pain, quality of life and adherence to treatment must all be evaluated. Uncorrected pain may indicate untreated cofactors of venous disease (Ryan et al 2003) and persistent pain must be addressed. Issues to consider are venous aetiologies (superficial or deep phlebitis) dermal inflammation (atrophie blanche, acute or chronic lipodermatosclerosis) and infection (local wound critical colonization, deep wound infection or surrounding cellulitis). Involving the patient in a plan of care that addresses quality of life, pain and other patient-centred issues, such as tolerance of bandaging and odour, is ideal. The patient must be the key driver in a plan of care that will meet their needs and address their concerns.

The holistic assessment has now laid the groundwork for optimizing the wound to receive a skin equivalent. The success of the skin substitute in wound healing is dependent on adequate preparation of the wound bed. The three cornerstones of local care are tissue debridement, bacterial balance and moisture balance. The necrotic debris or yellow slough on the surface of the wound bed needs to be removed, excessive exudate handled by appropriate moisture retentive dressings and increased bacterial burden treated with appropriate antimicrobial agents (Fig. 24.1).

INTRODUCTION TO SKIN SUBSTITUTES

It is the natural instinct of a wound care practitioner to want to cover a chronic wound with a layer of skin or a skin replacement that will enable a wound to close. Clinicians have placed grafts on chronic wounds to promote healing for more than 100 years. The first type of graft or skin replacement was a punch biopsy specimen of the patient's own healthy skin that was then placed in a wound

and enabled closure. The results of this technique can be beneficial, and this type of autologous grafting is still performed for a variety of problems. However, in these cases the patient is the donor, and there may not always be a donor site providing healthy tissue. Moreover, by harvesting the graft, surgeons create a new wound, which is then at risk of developing all the complications associated with healing. Other problems related to this type of grafting procedure include difficulty of the technique, as well as the cost and time of hospitalization of the patient.

In 1975, grafts composed of sheets of autologous cultured epidermal cells were available (Rheinwald & Green 1975). These were composed of the patient's own skin obtained by punch biopsy and then grown in artificial medium. Unfortunately, these cultured autologous grafts took a minimum of 2–3 weeks to grow in specialized laboratories. Nevertheless, there are benefits of this type of graft in patients with burns and chronic wounds, and autologous cultured epidermal cells remain an appropriate skin substitute, either alone or in combination with allogeneic skin replacement components.

Allografts of cultured epidermal cells from cadavers became available in 1981 and were initially used on burns (O'Connor et al 1981). The ideal source of cultured cells is neonatal, as these could be maintained longer in culture. In general, the older the cell, the more limited the life span of the cell in culture.

Allografts made up of epidermal components, dermal components or both epidermal and dermal components have been developed. In addition, there are wound care products that are acellular biologic substrates that act as scaffolding allowing cells to migrate and differentiate, subsequently leading to wound closure. Biodegradable, synthetic scaffolds are ideal as they will break down over time and can be mass-produced in laboratories and maintained for future use with a longer shelf life than most living skin equivalents. Proteoglycans, glycoproteins, glycosaminoglycans and collagen are found within these acellular matrixes, which act as a type of dermal skin substitute. The more common types of these various skin substitutes or skin replacements are listed in Table 24.1.

The nomenclature used when discussing skin substitutes, living skin equivalents (LSE) or human

Table 24.1 Common types of skin substitute

Type	Components
Epidermal	Epicel®*:cultured autologous epidermal cells
Epidermal	Epidex*: autologous epidermal cells generated from patient's hair
Epidermal	Cultured allogeneic epidermal cells – not commercially available
Dermal	Alloderm®*: allogeneic acellular dermal matrix with intact basement membrane complex
Dermal	Dermagraft®*: neonatal fibroblasts on polyglactin mesh
Dermal	TransCyte®*: a temporary skin replacement composed of extracellular matrix generated by allogeneic human neonatal fibroblasts
Acellular	Integra®*: extracellular matrix of bovine collagen and chondroitin-6-sulphate with silicone backing
Acellular	E-Z-Derm*: acellular xenogeneic (porcine) collagen matrix
Acellular	Oasis®*: porcine small intestinal submucosa: an acellular matrix
Acellular	BioBrane®*: temporary wound dressing composed of peptides derived from porcine dermal collagen bonded to nylon/silicone membrane
Combination epidermal/dermal	Apligraf®*: bovine type I collagen, allogeneic fibroblasts and neonatal epidermal cells
Combination epidermal/dermal	Orcel®*: allogeneic fibroblasts and keratinocytes seeded on opposite sides of bilayered matrix of bovine collagen
Combination epidermal/dermal	Collagen and glycosaminoglycan dermal matrix inoculated with autologous fibroblasts and keratinocytes
Combination epidermal/dermal	Composite cultured skin: collagen matrix substrate with fibroblasts and epidermal cells

* Trade names are used to differentiate products, and not meant to represent endorsement.

skin equivalents (HSE) may be confusing. Many different products are available or being studied, some living, some non-living. In some cases, composite products are being developed that combine autologous keratinocytes or epidermal cells with an allogeneic matrix or dermal components. Other products incorporate xenografts or heterologous tissue such as bovine collagen and shark cartilage in combination with allogeneic material. Tissue-engineered skin has been developed that will prepare a wound for grafting by providing an intact basement membrane. Other products are designed to generate neodermis. In each case, understanding the source of the components and the role these components play in wound healing will help to direct the most appropriate choice of skin substitute for management of a chronic wound.

Skin substitutes have a limited lifespan. After transplant in humans the cells are often undetectable. Using a specific probe for the Y chromosome present in allogeneic keratinocyte grafts from donors of the opposite sex, it was demonstrated (Brain et al 1989) that the donor cells did not persist beyond 3 weeks. The role of these products in wound repair is felt to be through the production of responsive viable cells and the stimulation of soluble mediators that in turn promote wound healing. Many of these soluble mediators are cytokines or growth factors, which are essential for the multiple and complex steps involved in wound repair. The presence of a skin substitute in a chronic wound stimulates the production of various cytokines and related substances that then play a key role in wound closure. The actual skin substitute is replaced by the host's own tissues, indicating that the role of tissue-engineered skin replacement is that of a substrate that provides viable cells and soluble mediators or promotes the stimulation of soluble factors that lead to wound healing.

WOUND HEALING AND SKIN SUBSTITUTES

Keratinocyte migration across a burn or chronic wound is an essential step in re-epithelialization. Skin substitutes can supply fibroblasts, extracellular matrix or matrix-bound growth factors that will enable this migration (Krejci-Papa et al 1999). Fibroblasts play a key role in wound healing, and cultured fibroblasts proliferate and produce collagen, glycosaminoglycans, fibronectin, growth factors and other extracellular matrix proteins. Using human skin equivalents, it has been shown (El-Ghalbzouri et al 2002) that without fibroblasts only limited epidermis will form. However, keratinocyte proliferation is stimulated by the presence of fibroblasts, which release soluble factors associated with epithelialization. The source of the fibroblasts appears to influence the degree of differentiation of the resulting skin equivalent. For example, when eyelid tissue served as the origin for cultured fibroblasts, the resulting skin equivalent was well differentiated, as compared to other adult human skin sources or lesional skin sources such as psoriatic skin and keloids (Konstantinova et al 1998). For most commercial skin substitutes, epidermal and fibroblast cell cultures are obtained from neonatal foreskin.

Wound healing is a complex process involving the interaction of specific cells of cutaneous, inflammatory and haematological origin as well as the components of the extracellular matrix (ECM) and soluble mediators. The process of wound healing is simplified into four phases:

1. Clot formation and haemostasis
2. Inflammation
3. Granulation and re-epithelialization
4. Tissue remodelling.

A review of these phases will demonstrate the role that skin substitutes play in wound repair and regeneration, with specific emphasis on inflammation and new tissue formation.

Tissue injury by any number of factors immediately leads to bleeding into the tissue, followed by blood clot formation. This clot is this first 'matrix' or temporary scaffold for cell migration. Platelets from the clot secrete wound-healing mediators, including fibronectin and platelet-derived growth factor, that lead to the activation of macrophages and fibroblasts. Other soluble mediators are generated that attract white blood cells – both leukocytes and monocytes – to the injured tissue. The monocytes become activated macrophages, which release various growth factors, including vascular endothelial growth factor, which promotes granulation tissue formation. Macrophages adhere and bind to the extracellular matrix via integrin receptors, which aids in the activity of these cells and also enables them to secrete cytokines, which promote the inflammatory process and also act as growth factors. Activated macrophages also secrete platelet-derived growth factor, which attracts fibroblasts into the wound. Macrophages play a key role in wound repair, specifically in the step from inflammation to new tissue formation.

Within hours of tissue injury, new tissue formation or re-epithelialization starts. Epidermal cells physically change so that cell migration across the wound can begin. Integrin receptors are expressed on the surface of epidermal cells allowing them to interact with ECM proteins, including fibronectin and vitronectin. Epidermal cells migrate and proliferate in response to a variety of growth factors, and at the same time basement membrane is formed.

Granulation tissue formation, angiogenesis and fibroblast migration into the wound all begins within days of the initial tissue injury. Growth factors, specifically platelet-derived growth factor and transforming growth factor, along with extracellular matrix components, play a key role in the stimulation of fibroblasts to proliferate and migrate. Fibroblasts from chronic wounds appear to be slow to respond to stimulation from growth factors, possibly by decreased expression of a growth factor receptor (Hasan et al 1997). Levels of various growth factors have also been shown to be lower in chronic wounds than in acute wounds (Cooper et al 1994), leading to much work on exogenous cytokines and promotion of wound healing.

Early extracellular matrix formation provides the scaffold for cell migration and is composed of fibrin, fibronectin and hyaluronic acid. Over time, the ECM becomes a collagenous structure and ultimately scar. Fibroblasts are responsible for formation and remodelling of the extracellular matrix, and are essential for all the various stages of the extracellular matrix.

Chronic wounds are believed to develop as a result of disruption of one or several phases of the wound healing pathway. Prolonged inflammation, often with increased matrix metalloproteinases (MMP) and decreased tissue inhibitors of matrix metalloproteinases (TIMP), impaired angiogenesis or extracellular matrix formation, inadequate collagen synthesis, abnormalities of cell migration and proliferation, and improper synthesis and secretion of growth factors are just some of the mechanisms of chronic wound formation and abnormal wound healing that have been proposed. Recently, it has been demonstrated that many components of chronic wound fluid inhibit healing. It is the role of skin substitutes to stimulate wound healing by promoting release of growth factors, by providing a scaffold for cell adhesion or migration and by promoting inflammation or granulation tissue formation. Skin substitutes appear to 'turn around' a chronic slow healing or non-healing wound, and provide a stimulus for active wound healing.

SKIN SUBSTITUTES AND DISEASE TRANSMISSION

Allogeneic grafts must undergo extensive screening to ensure that there are no genetic disorders, infections, alcohol or drug-dependency problems or recent blood transfusions in the donor. In the skin substitutes in which neonatal foreskin is used, the mother's history, physical examination and sequential blood work is essential to rule out the possibility of any transmissible condition that might be present. Testing is done for human immunodeficiency virus, hepatitis, cytomegalovirus, Epstein–Barr virus and syphilis. In addition, cultured cells are tested for human papillomavirus, human T-cell leukaemia/lymphoma, mycoplasma, other viruses and fungi. Other dermal components may include heterologous material from cows (bovine collagen) and shark cartilage. This material is tested for pathogens and contaminants. Localized

hypersensitivity to bovine collagen is a well documented, though uncommon occurrence. Patients with known sensitivity to bovine collagen should avoid these products. Moreover, clinicians should be aware that bovine collagen may theoretically contain the prions associated with bovine spongiform encephalopathy (BSE), as testing for the presence of the proteins in cultured bovine collagen is not reliable. There are no reports of transmission of BSE or variant Creutzfeldt–Jakob disease related to bovine collagen products, despite its wide use in aesthetic injectable agents, and the true risk of transmission of this disease is felt to be 'remote' (Lupi 2002). The screening of these living skin equivalents is many times more thorough than the screening procedures prior to organ transplant. Skin equivalents using human collagen have been investigated (Auger et al 1995) but are not commercially available

IMMUNOLOGICAL ASPECTS OF SKIN SUBSTITUTES

The skin acts as a primary immunological barrier to foreign antigen. It is conceivable, then, that skin substitutes of allogeneic or heterologous origin would be rejected as foreign material. However, it was found that epidermal cells maintained in culture lost the ability to express HLA-DR antigens and, for this reason, rejection of this type of allograft would not occur (Morhenn et al 1982). Living skin equivalents do not contain antigen-presenting cells such as Langerhans cells, dermal dendritic cells, endothelial cells or leukocytes. Using human skin equivalent composed of allogeneic human fibroblasts and human keratinocytes on a type 1 bovine collagen matrix, there was no clinical or laboratory evidence of rejection or sensitization (Falanga et al 1998). There was no antibody response to bovine type 1 collagen or bovine serum proteins and no anti-HLA antibodies to human dermal fibroblasts or human epidermal cells. In addition, no T-cell-specific responses were demonstrated.

Following application of a skin substitute, the host cells slowly replace the graft cells over time. This process does not appear to be a 'graft-rejection' type of phenomenon, but more of a stimulatory effect on the part of the skin replacement. This is due to the lack of specific immunological markers, or by the release of inhibitory cytokines. Biopsies of wounds following application of bilayered epidermal/dermal skin equivalents were performed and showed excess mucin production, swelling of the graft and a granulomatous reaction (Badiavas et al 2002). These histological features did not correlate with a poor outcome; however, the granulomatous reaction supports the concept that skin substitutes are replaced and not permanent structures. Because of foreign but often biodegradable components of living skin equivalents, the number of bacteria necessary for tissue damage is decreased. Clinicians need to assess the wound on a regular basis to ensure that the bacterial balance is being maintained.

TYPES OF SKIN SUBSTITUTES

Epicel® has humanitarian device approval. It consists of cultured epidermal autografts approved for use in patients with deep dermal or full-thickness burns greater than or equal to 30% body surface. The epidermal cells are cocultured with irradiated murine cells that have been screened for transmissible diseases. Genzyme Corporation maintains an Epicel® data base that contains demographic and clinical information on over 500 patients who have been managed using Epicel®. This type of graft is expensive and takes about 3 weeks to produce from the patient's own skin cells. However the cosmetic results are felt to be favourable and only a small amount of tissue is required from the patient to generate the cultured epidermal cells. Epicel® has been used in special circumstances for chronic wounds, specifically venous leg ulcers, and in patients with epidermolysis bullosa. It has also been used with success in patients who have large cutaneous defects after excision of giant congenital naevi, facilitating closure of these defects. Cultured epidermal autografts do not have a dermal component and, for this reason, wound closure may not be optimum with this skin substitute. Contraction of the scar and lack of adhesion to the underlying wound are complications of this type of grafting. However, composite grafts using either a living fibroblast layer and/or non-living matrix layer plus a cultured autologous epidermal sheet would represent a more ideal skin replacement structure.

Another source of autologous epidermal cells is the patient's own hair. Autologous cultured epidermal grafts have been derived from the outer root sheath cells of the hair follicle. Cells of the outer root sheath are an appropriate source for culture as these cells maintain a high proliferative capacity regardless of the age of the patient. This product is commercially available as EpiDex and has been successful in treating chronic leg ulcers, mainly of venous and mixed arterial/venous aetiologies (Limat et al 1996).

Cultured epidermal allografts are generated using the same techniques as epidermal autografts; however, allografts can be prepared in advance, frozen and theoretically maintained in skin banks for use when needed. Cultured epidermal allografts are used as a temporary skin cover while cultured epidermal autografts are being prepared, or for permanent wound closure. The source of epidermal cells for allografts is either cadaver skin or neonatal skin. Currently there are no widely available commercial sources of cultured epidermal allografts, although studies have shown the success of these skin replacements in burns (Hefton et al 1983), venous leg ulcers (Leigh et al 1987) and a variety of other chronic wounds.

Apligraf® (also named Graftskin®) consists of cultured neonatal fibroblasts and bovine type 1 collagen, forming a substrate for cultured neonatal keratinocytes (Anonymous 2004a). It is a living skin equivalent combining epidermal and dermal components, although it does not contain inflammatory cells, antigen-presenting cells such as Langerhans cells, or adnexal skin structures. The construct can be cut or divided to apply to multiple, smaller wounds. It can be slit to allow fluid through the surface but maintain contact with the wound base. These slits actually self-repair, with the trauma of the wounding stimulating acute healing without scarring. Apligraf® has been shown to be of benefit in patients with venous leg ulcers (Dolynchuk et al 1999), diabetic foot ulcers (Veves et al 2001), acute wounds requiring partial thickness grafts (Kirsner 1998), epidermolysis bullosa (Falabella et al 2000), burns (Waymack et al 2000) and pressure ulcers (Brem et al 2000). Additionally, Apligraf® has been reported to be of use in the management of chronic wounds in a wide variety of anecdotal cases. This product was the first combined epidermal and dermal skin equivalent that was widely used in North America, and for this reason much of the early literature involves trials and studies using Apligraf®. The product is shipped live and ready to use, but it must be applied within 5 days of leaving the lab, creating several logistical barriers.

Dermagraft® is composed of living human fibroblast cells obtained from neonatal foreskin tissue within a bioabsorbable polyglactin mesh. The mesh is biodegradable and disappears within weeks of placement in the wound bed. It is cryopreserved to maintain fibroblast viability and packaged in bovine serum. It is flexible and resistant to tearing. The fibroblasts produce dermal collagen, matrix proteins, growth factors and cytokines. Adnexal skin structures and inflammatory cells are absent (Anonymous 2004b). Dermagraft® has been shown to be of benefit in healing diabetic foot ulcers (Gentzkow et al 1996). Dermagraft® is shipped in a bioreactor and stored at −70°C. The construct must be thawed prior to clinical application but the stored product has a shelf life of 6 months.

TransCyte® is composed of allogeneic neonatal fibroblasts that are grown and embedded into a Silastic® layer. The product is then frozen without the cryopreservative, leading to non-viable fibroblasts; however, the growth factors, collagen and extracellular matrix produced by the fibroblasts in culture remain of benefit to the wound. This construct acts as a temporary or transitional covering. It is placed on a burn and after 7–14 days it is removed, when the patient's own cultured cells are available for grafting.

Alloderm®, an acellular, non-living dermal matrix, is obtained from donated human tissue. All epidermal and dermal cells are removed and the resulting product is freeze-dried (Anonymous 2004c). It has been used primarily in reconstructive and aesthetic surgical procedures (Shorr et al 2000), including repair of oral (Wagshall et al 2002), vaginal (Clemons et al 2003) and ophthalmic (Rubin et al 1999) mucous membrane. It is ideal for this type of work, as a donor site is not needed and there is limited contraction on healing. Alloderm® does not contain any adnexal structures, nor any keratinizing cells, which would be inappropriate for work on mucosal structures. It is well tolerated, non-allergenic and the cosmetic result is favourable. Cymetra is a micronized form of Alloderm® used as an injectable tissue replacement, which can also be classified as injectable scaffolding. Scaffolding or matrix than can be injected may have benefit in narrow deep wounds such as fistulae or sinuses (Kirsner 2004).

Orcel® is also a combination of epidermal and dermal components. It consists of living allogeneic epidermal cells and dermal fibroblasts – from the same source, independently cultured on a type 1 bovine collagen sponge. The epidermal cells are found on the non-porous side of the collagen matrix sponge, and the fibroblasts are on and within the porous side of the collagen matrix sponge (Anonymous 2004d).

Integra®, a dermal regeneration template, is a non-living bilayer product composed of a thin silicone film that acts as epidermis with an underlying matrix of cross-linked fibres containing bovine collagen and shark cartilage glycosaminoglycan, specifically chondroitin 6-sulfate (Anonymous 2004e). This product has been used with success in burns patients (Heimbackh et al 1988) and non-healing wounds at sites of previous radiotherapy (Gonyon & Zenn 2003). Currently in the USA, this product is approved for use as a skin replacement in patients with open wounds that require grafts, or reconstruction of scar tissue related to prior burn injuries. Integra® is applied to the burn site following debridement and left in place to act as scaffolding for wound repair and regeneration. After 2–3 weeks, the silicone layer is removed and replaced by an autologous epidermal graft. Alternative techniques using Integra® are being developed that involve seeding of autologous keratinocytes onto Integra® in order to produce a composite graft (Kremer et al 2000).

Other acellular xenografts include Oasis® and E-Z Derm®. Oasis® is a biological substrate formed from porcine small intestine submucosa (Anonymous 2004f) from which the serosa, smooth muscle and mucosa have been removed. It is an acellular matrix that contains collagen, proteoglycans, glycosaminoglycans and glycoproteins as well as transforming growth factor-β and fibroblast growth factor-2. It has been shown to be able to support the growth and differentiation of epidermal cells in culture with fibroblasts (Lindberg & Badylak 2001). A small pilot study (Brown-Etris et al 2002) indicated that Oasis® was beneficial in venous ulcers, pressure ulcers and drug induced ulcers. E-Z Derm® is a porcine derived xenograft in which the collagen has been cross-linked with aldehyde and acts as a temporary dermal matrix. In one study (Vanstraelen 1992) calcium alginate was superior to E-Z Derm® in terms of time to heal, degree of hypertrophic scarring and patient preference. As well, allergic reactions were seen to develop in this same study with E-Z Derm®. Patients with known sensitivity to porcine products must avoid these products, as well patients may choose to avoid porcine products based on their own specific cultural or religious beliefs.

BioBrane® is a temporary wound dressing composed of highly purified peptides derived from porcine dermal collagen that is bonded to a bilayer of semipermeable silicone membrane and flexible knitted trifilament nylon fabric. BioBrane-L® only has the single layer of nylon and is used with meshed autografts. BioBrane® is used for burns, as a temporary cover until an epidermal autograft is available, at which point it is removed.

PREPARATION OF THE WOUND BED

Recognizing that a wound must be in the ideal condition to receive a skin substitute is essential for successful wound closure. Preparing the wound for these products involves including the patient and their underlying disease as a vital part of wound care. Wound bed preparation was first described in 2000 by Sibbald et al (2000) and Falanga (2000). This approach to wound management stresses that successful diagnosis and treatment of patients with chronic wounds requires holistic care and a team approach. The whole patient, the underlying cause and patient-centred concerns must be considered before looking at the wound itself.

Local wound care, including tissue debridement, controlling inflammation and infection and moisture balance, must be dealt with as part of preparation of the wound bed. Along with these three factors, the wound edge must be considered, as this is the source of the epidermal cells which are required to migrate across the wound as part of wound closure. These four factors, *tissue* debridement, *inflammation/infection, *moisture* balance and wound *edge*, provide a simple mnemonic,

TIME, that can be used to remember the key factors involved in local wound care. An outline of the TIME approach is presented in Table 24.2.

The first step in managing a wound is to assess the patient for underlying causes that could be impeding healing. This is the basis of wound bed preparation. Local wound management measures are unlikely to succeed if the patient is not receiving adequate treatment for conditions that are known to impair healing, such as heart failure, uncontrolled diabetes, inadequate compression therapy or poor nutrition. Corrective measures such as pressure relief, revascularization of ischaemic tissue, control of oedema and all other relevant measures should be carried out before local wound care treatments, specifically skin substitutes are applied.

Wounds must be adequately prepared to receive a skin substitute. Infection or excess bacterial burden should be dealt with prior to any type of skin grafting.

Debridement, removal of eschar and devitalized tissue or slough, is imperative to aid in acceptance of a skin substitute. Much of the work in skin substitutes demonstrated the significance of the local wound state and how it dictates the success of specific wound care products. Preparation of the wound bed and clinically assessing the wound for signs of infection are essential prior to the addition of bioengineered skin to the management of diabetic foot ulcers (Browne et al 2001).

Much of the work using skin substitutes has been in patients with burns. It has been found that, if the wounds are not thoroughly debrided of all eschar and necrotic tissue, then the skin substitute will not cling to the wound bed. Synthetic membranes will not adhere to dead tissue, and necrotic debris under a skin replacement will increase the risk of potential infection.

The concept of the epithelial border or the edge of the wound as a key component of local wound care is emphasized by the use of skin substitutes. Wounds treated with keratinocyte sheets heal from the edge, in response to stimulation from the transplanted cells (Phillips et al 1989). The clinical status of the wound edge, as a source of these migrating keratinocytes is important to determine, prior to the addition of a skin substitute. Human skin equivalents that supply a scaffold as well as

Table 24.2   Preparation of the wound bed

Clinical observations	Molecular and cellular problems	Clinical actions	Effect of clinical actions	Clinical outcome
Non-viable **T**issue	Denatured matrix and cell debris impair healing	Debridement (episodic or continuous): autolytic, sharp surgical, enzymatic, mechanical or biological	Intact, functional extracellular matrix proteins present in wound base	Viable wound base
Infection, inflammation	**High bacteria, cause:** ↑ Inflammatory cytokines ↑ Proteases ↓ Growth factor activity ↓ Healing environment	**Topical/systemic:** Antimicrobials Anti-inflammatories Protease inhibitors Growth factors	**Low bacteria, cause** ↓ Inflammatory cytokines ↓ Proteases ↑ Growth factor activity ↑ Healing environment	Bacterial balance and reduced inflammation
Moisture imbalance	Desiccation slows epithelial cell migration Excessive fluid causes maceration of wound base/margin	Apply moisture balancing dressings	Desiccation avoided Excessive fluid controlled	Moisture balance
Edge of wound – non-advancing or undermined	Non-migrating keratinocytes Non-responsive wound cells, abnormalities in extracellular matrix or abnormal protease activity	Re-assess cause, refer or consider corrective advanced therapies: Bioengineered skin Skin grafts Vascular surgery	Responsive fibroblasts and keratinocytes present in wound	Advancing edge of wound

Source: Courtesy of International Advisory Board on Wound Bed Preparation (Sibbald et al 2003).

fibroblasts will require a healthy source of epidermal cells for keratinocyte migration. The wound edge is the source of these cells and the importance of this epithelial border must not be overlooked.

SKIN SUBSTITUTES: TECHNIQUES OF USE

Specific steps must be followed with each skin substitute in order to optimize transfer/application of the construct. All wound beds should be appropriately prepared as discussed earlier. Keeping the product secure, once it has been placed in the wound, is necessary to obtain maximum contact with the wound and to prevent friction and shear.

Examples of the procedures involved with certain types of skin substitutes follows:

Apligraf®:
1. Store in incubator at 37°C
2. Check colour indicator (pink)

3. Using sterile technique, gently lift edges from Transwell®
4. Lift with moistened gauze and gloved fingers
5. Fenestrate to form mesh, or cut if necessary
6. Apply to prepared wound bed, overlap 1–2 cm on surrounding skin
7. Apply covering consisting of silver and absorptive dressing
8. Secure to prevent friction and shear.

Dermagraft®:
1. Store in freezer at −70°C
2. Remove from freezer and place in water bath at 35–37°C for 2–3 minutes
3. Place in rinsing container and secure (may need Steri-Strips®, Mepitac®, suture or staple)
4. Open and rinse ×4 with saline to remove cryopreservative (DMSO)
5. Drain and cut to size of wound with overlap
6. Remove backing and apply to wound
7. Cover with silver and absorptive dressing
8. Secure to prevent friction and shear.

Oasis®:
1. Store in the dry (lyophilized) state at room temperature, in its sterile envelope
2. Using aseptic technique, cut the sheet to a size slightly larger than the wound bed
3. May be moistened on the wound bed, if needed, with sterile saline
4. Apply a non-adherent secondary dressing
5. Secure to prevent friction and shear
6. Portions of Oasis® that become detached and free from the wound bed with healing can be removed.
7. A second sheet can be placed in the wound if the initial piece is no longer covering the wound.

Once a clinician has become familiar with the procedure involved in transfer/application of skin substitutes, further benefits of these products as compared to autologous skin grafting can be seen – including ease of use. Additionally, these constructs can be applied quickly in an outpatient setting without anaesthesia, and do not require a donor site.

Case Study I *Final outcome*

A human skin equivalent composed of allogeneic neonatal fibroblasts and epidermal cells on a matrix of bovine collagen was chosen as the appropriate skin substitute for E-W. The skin substitute was applied, held in place with Steri-Strips® and covered with a silver-containing antibacterial layer and a non-adherent dressing. This was then covered by a compression wrap consisting of rolled gauze and a short-stretch bandage. A cohesive layer, added to prevent slippage but not significantly to increase compression, was then applied.

E-W was contacted by telephone 48 hours after the application of the skin substitute and she reported that everything was very comfortable. She was then seen in the clinic 1 week later for a follow-up assessment. Healthy granulation tissue was noted in the wound bed and at the wound periphery. No residue of the skin substitute was seen.

The wound continued to progress and was healed at 4 months after the single application. E-W continued to apply compression bandages for 2 weeks post-healing. She then wore 20–30 mmHg (CcI II 23–32 mmHg) strength compression support stockings and was able to resume all her normal activities. Ongoing use of compression support stockings has helped to prevent recurrence of ulcers.

E-W was extremely pleased with the positive outcome following the application of the skin substitute. Healing occurred in time for her and her granddaughter to enjoy the outdoor pool throughout that summer season.

SUMMARY

Skin substitutes represent a new physiological and active therapy available for the management of chronic wounds. Bioengineered skin replacements appear to enhance wound healing by a variety of mechanisms, including delivery of viable and responsive fibroblasts and epidermal cells, stimulation of growth factor production, generation of neodermis and providing scaffolding for cell migration, as well as enhancement of basement membrane formation. It is not the skin substitute itself that remains in the healed wound: the patient's own skin replaces the skin equivalent. Much has been learned about wound healing from the use of skin substitutes, and our clinical knowledge of wound care has been optimized by the results of studies of living skin equivalents and tissue repair. The concepts of wound bed preparation have been emphasized by the results of using living skin equivalents. The essential features of local wound care, including debridement, bacterial balance and moisture balance, must be followed whenever skin substitutes are chosen as part of the wound care therapy, otherwise the results may not be optimum. In addition, the long-term sequelae of the use of skin substitutes need to be examined and investigated for risks and benefits.

Other potential sources of skin substitutes are being evaluated, including embryonic stem cells, which remain controversial but may prove to be very beneficial. Lessons learned may be applied for the future to use the patient's own stem cells, which would overcome the ethical problems associated with fetal tissue donors. Studies are ongoing with numerous types of skin substitute, and the concept of introducing specific cell types into skin defects represents a form of genetic engineering. These living skin equivalents will potentially provide a platform to deliver temporary gene transfer or permanent gene therapy or replacement. The science of the laboratory is ahead of our clinical knowledge on ideal wound care, and it is with this new technology that modification and improvement of local wound care can be achieved.

References

Anonymous 2004a http: //www.apligraf.com accessed January 19, 2004

Anonymous 2004b http: //wound.smith-nephew.com/US/Product accessed January 19, 2004

Anonymous 2004c http: //www.lifecell.com/healthcare/products/alloderm/ accessed January 19, 2004

Anonymous 2004d http: //www.ortecinternational.com accessed January 21, 2004

Anonymous 2004e http: //www.skinhealing.com/5_1_aboutintegra.shtml accessed January 19, 2004

Anonymous 2004f http: //www.cooksis.com accessed January 22, 2004

Auger F A, Lopez Valle C A, Guignard R et al 1995 Skin equivalent produced with human collagen. In Vitro Cellular and Developmental Biology: Animal 31: 432–439

Badiavas E V, Paquette D, Carson P, Falanga V 2002 Human chronic wounds treated with bioengineered skin: Histologic evidence of host-graft interactions. Journal of the American Academy of Dermatology 46: 524–530

Brain A, Purkis P, Coates P et al 1989 Survival of cultured allogeneic keratinocytes transplanted to deep dermal bed assessed with probe specific for Y chromosome. British Medical Journal 298: 917–919

Brem H, Balledux J, Bloom T et al 2000 Healing of diabetic foot ulcers and pressure ulcers with human skin equivalent: a new paradigm in wound healing. Archives of Surgery 135: 627–634

Brown-Etris M, Cutshall W D, Hiles M C 2002 A new biomaterial derived from small intestine submucosa and developed into a wound matrix device, Wounds 14: 150–166

Browne A C, Vearncombe M, Sibbald R G 2001 High bacterial load in asymptomatic diabetic patients with neurotrophic ulcers retards wound healing after application of Dermagraft. Ostomy/Wound Management 47: 44–49

Clemons J L, Myers D L, Aguilar V C, Arya L A 2003 Vaginal paravaginal repair with an AlloDerm graft. American Journal of Obstetrics and Gynecology 189: 1612–1618; discussion 1618–1619

Cooper D M, Yu E Z, Hennessey P et al 1994 Determination of endogenous cytokines in chronic wounds. Annals of Surgery 219: 688–691

Cullum N, Nelson E A, Fletcher A W, Sheldon T A 2001 Compression for venous leg ulcers. Cochrane Database of Systematic Reviews, 2: CD000265. Update Software, Oxford

Dolynchuk K, Hull P, Guenther L et al 1999 The role of Apligraf in the treatment of venous leg ulcers. Ostomy/Wound Management 45: 34–43

El-Ghalbzouri A, Gibbs S, Lamme E et al 2002 Effect of fibroblasts on epidermal regeneration. Br J Dermatol 147: 230–243

Falabella A F, Valencia I C, Eaglstein W H, Schachner L A 2000 Tissue-engineered skin (Apligraf) in the healing of patients with epidermolysis bullosa wounds. Archives of Dermatology 136: 1225–1230

Falanga V 2000 Classifications for wound bed preparation and stimulation of chronic wounds. Wound Repair and Regeneration 8: 347–352

Falanga V, Margolis D, Alvarez O et al 1998 Rapid healing of venous ulcers and lack of clinical rejection with an allogeneic cultured human skin equivalent. Archives of Dermatology 134: 293–300

Gentzkow G D, Iwasaki S D, Hershon K S et al 1996 Use of Dermagraft, a cultured human dermis, to treat diabetic foot ulcers. Diabetes Care 19: 350–354

Gonyon D L Jr, Zenn M R 2003 Simple approach to the radiated scalp wound using Integra skin substitute. Annals of Plastic Surgery 50: 315–320

Hasan A, Murata H, Falabella A et al 1997 Dermal fibroblasts from venous ulcers are unresponsive to the action of transforming growth factor-beta 1. Journal of Dermatological Science 16: 59–66

Hefton J M, Madden M R, Finkelstein J L, Shires G T 1983 Grafting of burn patients with allografts of cultured epidermal cells. Lancet 2: 428–430

Heimbackh D, Luterman J A, Burke J et al 1998 Artificial dermis for major burns: a multicenter randomized clinical trial. Annals of Surgery 208: 313–320

Jull A B, Waters J, Arroll B 2002 Pentoxifylline for treating venous leg ulcers Cochrane Database of Systematic Reviews 1: CD001733. Update Software, Oxford

Kirsner R S 1998 The use of Apligraf in acute wounds. Journal of Dermatology 25: 805–811

Kirsner R 2004 Verbal communication. Symposium on Wound Healing AAD Washington DC, 7 February 2004

Konstantinova N V, Lemak N A, Duong D M et al 1998 Artificial skin equivalent differentiation depends on fibroblast donor site: use of eyelid fibroblasts. Plastic and Reconstructive Surgery 101: 385–391

Krejci-Papa N C, Hoang A, Hansbrough J F 1999 Fibroblast sheets enable epithelialization of sounds that do not support keratinocyte migration. Tissue Engineering 5: 555–562

Kremer M, Lang E, Berger A C 2000 Evaluation of dermal-epidermal skin equivalents ('composite-skin') of human keratinocytes in a collagen-glycosaminoglycan matrix (Integra artificial skin). British Journal of Plastic Surgery 53: 459–465

Leigh I M, Purkis P E, Navsaria H A, Phillips T J 1987 Treatment of chronic venous ulcers with sheets of cultured allogenic keratinocytes. British Journal of Dermatology 117: 591–597

Limat A, Mauri D, Hunziker T 1996 Successful treatment of chronic leg ulcers with epidermal equivalents generated from cultured autologous outer root sheath cells. Journal of Investigative Dermatology 107: 128–135

Lindberg K, Badylak S F 2001 Porcine small intestinal submucosa (SIS): a bioscaffold supporting in vitro primary human epidermal cell differentiation and synthesis of basement membrane proteins. Burns 27: 254–266

Lupi O 2002 Prions in dermatology. Journal of the American Academy of Dermatology 46: 790–793

Margolis D J, Berlin J A, Strom B L 1999 Risk factors associated with the failure of a venous ulcer to heal. Archives of Dermatology 135: 920–926

Morhenn V B, Benike C J, Cox A J et al 1982 Cultured human epidermal cells do not synthesize HLA-DR. Journal of Investigative Dermatology 78: 32–37

O'Connor N E, Mulliken J B, Banks-Schege et al 1981 Grafting of burns with cultured epithelium prepared from autologous epidermal cells. Lancet 8211: 75–78

Phillips T J, Kehinde O, Green H, Gilchrest B A 1989 Treatment of skin ulcers with cultured epidermal allografts. Journal of the American Academy of Dermatology 21: 191–199

Pittler M H, Ernst E 1998 Horse-chestnut seed extract for chronic venous insufficiency. A criteria-based systematic review. Archives of Dermatology 134: 1356–1360

Rheinwald J G, Green H 1975 Serial cultivation of strains of human epidermal keratinocytes: the formation of keratinizing colonies from single cells. Cell 6: 331–343

Rubin P A, Fay A M, Remulla H D, Maus M 1999 Ophthalmic plastic applications of acellular dermal allografts. Ophthalmology 106: 2091–2097

Ryan S, Eager C, Sibbald R G 2003 Venous leg ulcer pain. Ostomy/Wound Management 49(Suppl): 16–23

Shorr N, Perry J D, Goldberg R A et al 2000 The safety and applications of acellular human dermal allograft in ophthalmic plastic and reconstructive surgery: a preliminary report. Ophthalmic Plastic and Reconstructive Surgery May;16: 223–230

Sibbald R G, Williamson D, Orsted H L et al 2000 Preparing the wound bed – debridement, bacterial balance and moisture balance. Ostomy/Wound Management 46: 14–35

Sibbald R G, Orsted H, Schultz G S et al 2003 Preparing the wound bed 2003: focus on infection and inflammation. International Wound Bed Preparation Advisory Board; Canadian Chronic Wound Advisory Board. Ostomy/Wound Management 49: 23–51

Vanstraelen P 1992 Comparison of calcium sodium alginate (KALTOSTAT) and porcine xenograft (E-Z DERM) in the healing of split-thickness skin graft donor sites. Burns 18: 145–148

Veves A, Falanga V, Armstrong D G, Sabolinski M L for the Apligraf Diabetic Foot Ulcer Study 2001 Graftskin, a human skin equivalent, is effective in the management of noninfected neuropathic diabetic foot ulcers. Diabetes Care 24: 290–295

Wagshall E, Lewis Z, Babich S B et al 2002 Acellular dermal matrix allograft in the treatment of mucogingival defects in children: illustrative case report. ASDC Journal of Dentistry for Children 69: 39–43

Waymack P, Duff R G, Sabolinski M 2000 The effect of a tissue engineered bilayered living skin analog, over meshed split-thickness autografts on the healing of excised burn wounds. The Apligraf Burn Study Group. Burns 26: 609–619

Wound infection

Elaine Pina, Kátia Furtado

INTRODUCTION

Of all potential complications that can interfere with the healing process, infection of a leg ulcer is among those with the greatest impact, not only on the wound itself but also on the general condition and quality of life of the patient, as well as on the cost of care. It is therefore essential to make every effort to prevent infection through the correct identification of underlying risk factors and application of sound infection control principles.

The human body harbours an abundant flora of commensal bacteria on the skin and mucous membranes. It has been estimated that 90% of the cells in the human body are bacterial cells (Savage 1977). Under normal physiological conditions a delicate balance and mutually beneficial relation exist between the human body and this abundant indigenous flora. One important role of the host indigenous flora is to protect the underlying tissues and prevent or limit colonization by undesirable species ('colonization resistance'; Washington 1989).

The break in the epithelial barrier created by an ulcer, with exposure of subcutaneous tissue, presents an excellent habitat for microbial growth and almost all wounds contain bacteria in varying numbers and types. These bacteria can be exogenous, inoculated from the surrounding environment (via hands of carers, equipment and the environment) or endogenous, coming from the skin and mucous membranes of the host itself and building a rich and complex multispecies ecosystem. Most of these organisms remain on superficial tissue but one or more of them can invade deeper tissue, giving rise to infection.

DEFINITIONS

The role of bacteria has been defined with relation to the type of response elicited in the host (Brachman 1992). Contamination refers to microorganisms that are transiently present, without tissue invasion or physiological reaction. Colonization implies the presence of microorganisms in or on a host with growth and multiplication but without any overt clinical expression or detected immune reaction. Infection entails the deposition and multiplication of organisms in the tissues or on surfaces of the body with an associated tissue reaction. Contamination is a natural consequence of a break in the skin, and contaminating organisms are rapidly eliminated by the dynamics and pressure of the resident population of the wound. Colonization is the first step in a series of processes that can lead ultimately to infection. In some instances, in spite of the absence of host reaction, the presence of bacteria seems to be harmful to the wound, retarding healing. This has been termed critical colonization (Davis 1998). However, there are no visible clues to guide the observer in differentiating between contamination, colonization and critical colonization (Cutting 2003). Critical colonization means that, although bacteria may not yet have reached the deepest tissues, they are interfering with wound healing by enhancing their survival strategies (secretion of enzymes and toxins) to the detriment of the host. This has also been termed increased bioburden, indolent or recalcitrant wound, and covert or subclinical infection.

The significance of the number and type of microorganisms present in a chronic wound is still

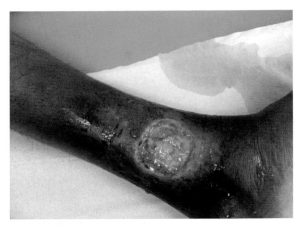

Figure 25.1 Venous leg ulcer with heavy bacterial colonization.

a matter of debate. Some researchers have shown that a small number of bacteria in the wound can be favourable to healing (De Haan et al 1974, Pollack 1984). Many investigations (Kriezek & Robson 1975, Lookingbill et al 1978, Robson 1997) have reported a correlation between heavy microbial presence and delayed wound healing. Others (Alper et al 1983, Hansson et al 1995) have found that large numbers of bacteria did not affect the healing process. Schmidt et al (2000) concluded that the effect of bacteria on wounds is different depending on the aetiology of the wound.

There is a lack of understanding, in quantitative terms, of the many factors that contribute to overt symptoms of invasive infection in any particular person. Disease production is not dependent solely on the pathogenic and virulent properties of the microorganism. The specific and non-specific defence mechanisms of a host, the general health of the individual and the various stresses to which they are subjected have a determinant role in the initiation and progression of infection. The interrelationship between host and pathogen is complex and difficult to define. Infection will result when the microorganisms overwhelm host defences and are able to proliferate unrestrained.

PATHOPHYSIOLOGY

Physiological response to the presence of pathogens varies greatly. Interactions between cells in the inflammatory process result in the production of oxygen metabolites, histamine, leukotrienes and cytokines (Thomson & Smith 1994), which in turn causes cell death and tissue necrosis, the ideal conditions for microbial growth, including fastidious anaerobes that will proliferate as residual oxygen is consumed by facultative aerobic bacteria. Microbial pathogens delay healing through persistent production of inflammatory mediators, production of metabolic wastes and toxins, maintenance of the activated state of neutrophils, which produce cytolytic enzymes and oxygen radicals, as well as through competition with host cells for oxygen and nutrients that are required for the healing process. The continued state of activation of neutrophils, in association with the presence of persistent wound microflora and their destructive enzymes, appears to be responsible for extensive matrix dissociation (Diegelmann 2003) and prevention of matrix synthesis and remodelling, which are essential for the progression of wound healing (Pierce 2001). There is also an associated impairment of epithelialization and, additionally, chronic infection can induce an adaptive down-regulation of the immune response (Dow et al 1999).

Leg ulcers are particularly prone to infection, since blood supply is often compromised and wounds will not heal below a certain arterial pressure threshold. A poorly perfused wound may not show the typical signs of inflammation even in the presence of overt infection. Ischaemia can result in

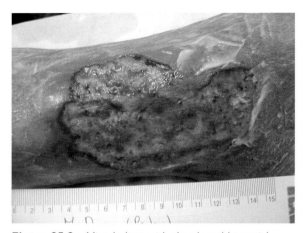

Figure 25.2 Mixed ulcer with slough and bacterial colonization, highly exudative despite compression therapy.

tissue anoxia and poor delivery of phagocytes to the wound, both of which interfere with the control of infection. Chronic leg ulcers commonly become secondarily infected, since oedema accumulation reduces lymphatic flow and increases the risk of infection.

Role of microorganisms

The measure of the ability of microorganisms to induce disease is termed pathogenicity and can be characterized by the organism's virulence and invasiveness. Virulence is related to the ability to produce toxins and other destructive enzymes, which can lead to necrosis, inhibition of local immune defences and extension of the wound. The size of the inoculum (dose) may be an important determinant of virulence and can markedly affect an organism's ability to produce infection. However, the dose necessary to cause infection varies from organism to organism and from host to host.

With prolonged presence in the wound, microorganisms change their phenotype and immune expression in order to evade detection by the body's immune system (Bowler 2002). Although laboratory studies are conducted with bacteria suspended in liquid medium (planktonic), it is increasingly being realized that, in their natural habitat, most bacteria will grow attached to surfaces (sessile). Following initial attachment to a surface, microcolonies are formed, followed by differentiation into exopolysaccharide matrix (biofilms). Living in a group gives mocroorganisms properties that they do not have as individuals and the metabolic byproducts of one species can support or limit the growth of other species. The different species communicate by quorum sensing, which has been defined as a mechanism for virulent gene regulation in bacteria so as to adjust to nutrient and waste levels and avoid outgrowing their environment's ability to support them, thus maintaining appropriate numbers within the biofilm (Greenberg 2003, Rumbaugh et al 1999).

Microorganisms in biofilms can acquire resistance through transfer of resistance plasmids and are not easily exposed to antibiotics or to the body's natural immune defence system (Donlan & Costerton 2002). Chronic wounds provide an ideal environment for development of biofilm and it has been demonstrated that they can form in wounds (Serralta et al 2001). Because the wound may have a healthy appearance and there are no overt symptoms, standard diagnostic and therapeutic strategies may not be useful. However, microorganisms detaching from biofilms can overcome the host immune system and cause infection (Ward et al 1992). Research is being directed to identify components of the body's innate defence system that can inhibit biofilm formation (Singh et al 2002) as well as methods to improve antibiotic penetration and efficacy (Costerton et al 1994, Rediske et al 2000, Wellman et al 1996). Biofilm infections constitute a problem that characterizes 65% of infections treated by physicians in the developed world (Costerton et al 1999) but the exact role of biofilm in leg ulcer infection is yet to be clarified.

DIAGNOSIS OF WOUND INFECTION

Diagnosis of infection is not an exact science but a clinical skill, requiring attention to detail that can only be acquired by experience. The key to the appropriate treatment of infection is the correct identification of both local and systemic host signs and symptoms of infection. This is achieved essentially by clinical history and observation.

Systematic evaluation of wound characteristics is critical to plan treatment strategies, appropriate adjunctive tests and referral, as well as to predict clinical outcomes. Abscess formation and cellulitis (Cutting & Harding 1994), as well as the classical

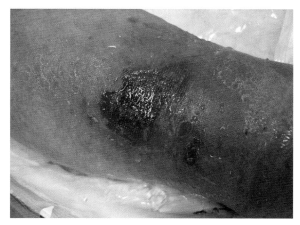

Figure 25.3 Very painful superficial arterial ulcer. Presence of erythema surrounding the ulcer.

Box 25.1 *Additional criteria for diagnosis of infection*

Delayed healing (Cutting & Harding 1994, Gardner et al 2001, Miller 2001, Sibbald et al 2001)
May be the only sign of infection. If there is no evidence of healing within 4 weeks, increased bacterial burden or infection should be suspected.

Discoloration (Cutting & Harding 1994)
Granulation tissue may appear darker or have a bright red discoloration. Discoloured tissue arises from excessive angiogenic responses caused by pathogens.

Friable granulation tissue (Cutting & Harding 1994, Gardner et al 2001, Miller 2001, Sibbald et al 2001)
Granulation tissue that bleeds easily with light pressure.

Unexpected pain/tenderness (Cutting & Harding 1994, Gardner et al 2001)
Infection may increase pain or change its pattern. Ischaemia should be ruled out by repeating measurement of the resting ankle pressure index. In the case of rheumatoid disease it must be established that the increase in pain is not an indicator of worsening disease.

Pocketing at wound base (Cutting & Harding 1994)
Caused by a lack of granulation tissue due to inhibition or digestion by bacteria.

Bridging at wound base (Cutting & Harding 1994, Miller 2001, Sibbald et al 2001)
The wound is allowed to heal in the presence of bacteria and the epithelial tissue covers the wound before the underlying tissue is fully repaired. This allows 'bridges' of epithelium to form and is likely to lead to early breakdown of the wound.

Abnormal odour (Cutting & Harding 1994, Gardner et al 2001, Miller 2001, Sibbald et al 2001)
Usually caused by Gram-negative bacilli, *Pseudomonas* spp. or anaerobic bacteria.

Wound breakdown (Cutting & Harding 1994, Gardner et al 2001, Miller 2001)
The increased inflammatory response causes the wound to increase in size or leads to satellite areas of tissue breakdown that causes adjacent ulceration

Devitalized loose yellow debris and areas of necrosis at wound base (Sibbald et al 2001)
Necrosis appearing in a previously healing wound represents infection from a localized high bioburden.

signs and symptoms of pain, erythema, oedema, heat and purulence, may be absent or diminished (Thomson & Smith 1994, Stotts & Hunt 1997) and were only observed in 33% of chronic wounds (Gardner et al 2001). Also, the presence of venous stasis, eczema and lipodermatosclerosis can mask the classical signs of infection.

Additional criteria for diagnosis of infection have been proposed and are summarized in Box 25.1. Increasing pain and wound breakdown were found to have a specificity of 100%, friable granulation tissue 82% and foul odour 80%, while inflammation and discharge have a low predictive value (Gardner et al 2001).

Fever, malaise and mental confusion can be indicative of infection. Leukocytosis and acute phase reactants such as erythrocyte sedimentation rate (ESR) or C-reactive protein (CRP) are not reliable in the compromised host since these patients are constantly challenged by minor illnesses and peripheral lesions that may elevate these indices. ESR and CRP that return to normal during the course of therapy are favourable prognostic signs.

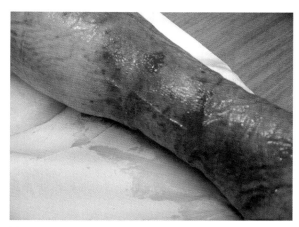

Figure 25.4 Contact irritation can be mistaken for signs of infection.

Because of the proximity of bone tissue, leg ulcers can be complicated by osteomyelitis. In contrast to hematogenous osteomyelitis, multiple bacterial organisms are usually isolated. Probing to bone is a simple technique to identify bone invasion (Grayson et al 1995). Although plain X-ray is a simple and effective examination when positive, it is usually of late presentation and, because radiographic changes (periosteal elevation, local osteolysis and sclerosis) are subtle, careful orientation is necessary to achieve diagnostic significance. Ultrasound, computed tomography and magnetic resonance imaging may be valuable in selected settings. Wound infection can be complicated by septicaemia.

MICROBIOLOGICAL ASSESSMENT

For practical purposes the diagnosis of infection is clinical but, because signs and symptoms are frequently not clear, emphasis is put on microbiological diagnosis. Microbiological information can serve to confirm the presence of infection and aid in the appropriate selection of antimicrobial therapy or assessment of its efficacy. For the contribution of the microbiological analysis of a chronic wound to be of use in clinical practice it is important to ensure the adequacy, quality and appropriateness of specimens sent for examination. Efforts must also be made to obtain appropriate specimens before the institution of antimicrobial therapy, since biopsy specimens will be affected by systemic antimicrobial therapy and swab specimens can be influenced by topical antimicrobials.

It is important to emphasize that wound sampling should be restricted to when there is a clear indication that the bacterial load is implicated in delayed healing: the presence of clinical signs of infection, deterioration in the absence of clinical signs of infection or failure to heal in spite of best clinical practice. Chesham & Platt (1987) found that potential pathogens were isolated in 82% of ulcers in the absence of infection. The practice of taking routine cultures should therefore be abandoned. Submission of inappropriate or mishandled specimens creates potentially confusing situations that could lead to institution of unnecessary therapy.

Sampling techniques

The technique for sampling and microbiological analysis is also of importance for the quality of the information. Microbiological sampling from ulcers has been described using several different quantitative, semi-quantitative and qualitative methods on wound tissue or wound fluid. Extrapolation of results from one type of wound to others has resulted in controversy compounded by confusion as to what information is required or desired, the interpretation of results and the feasibility in clinical practice of the different techniques, as well as aspects such as patient selection criteria and previous exposure to antimicrobials. There is a need to standardize methodologies in order to obtain comparable data.

Methods that involve tissue: culture of tissue obtained by biopsy has been considered the 'gold standard', the most useful and relevant method, because it allows quantitative and qualitative analysis as well as visualization of organisms invading viable tissue (Robson & Heggers 1969, Rudensky et al 1992). A detailed review of the methodology (Heggers 1998b) confirms the validity of biopsy in the diagnosis of infection, concluding that a single biopsy is considered to have more than 95% accuracy (Volenec et al 1979). However, other researchers consider that it is difficult to make conclusions from a single specimen because of variability in counts and type of microorganisms that have been described in different parts of the wound (Bowler et al 2001). Woolfrey et al (1981) found that there is a 25% chance of missing an organism due to uneven distribution within the wound bed and to the cleansing techniques used. Quantitative results varied by a factor of 100 in 27% of paired isolates. These results have been attributed to inaccuracies in methodology (Heggers 1998b). Vindenes & Bjerknes (1993) have shown that biopsy has an increased risk of transient bacteremia and fungaemia, although it was not shown to be harmful to the patient. This raises ethical concerns and the need to administer antimicrobial prophylaxis to prevent dissemination of infection, which may adversely affect biopsy culture results (Ehrenkranz et al 1990). Finally, a major drawback is that, in clinical practice, many efficient routine microbiology laboratories do not process tissue biopsies because of considerations of time, interest and cost-effectiveness.

In the presence of osteomyelitis, wound or sinus tract cultures are not reliable for predicting which organism is implicated and deep bone biopsy specimens and blood cultures are required.

Curettage of the ulcer base (Sapico et al 1984), usually performed in conjunction with surgical debridement, has been proposed and no significant differences between deep tissue and superficial curettage cultures have been found. The method of dermabrasion of the upper layers of the wound (Pallua et al 1999) using a small rotating carbon-steel disk of defined roughness also compared favourably with the biopsy technique.

Methods that use tissue fluid: It is clear that, when collected purulent fluid is present, an aspirate of the fluid is the preferred sample. Needle aspiration is normally used to culture an abscess or the ulcer margin through intact skin. Multiple samples are required to obtain a representative specimen. If used appropriately, it is reported to have a sensitivity of 100% and a specificity of 85% when compared to tissue biopsy (Lee et al 1985). It is, however, invasive and can cause discomfort. An atraumatic non-invasive procedure by gentle irrigation and aspiration of saline under the ulcer border (Ehrenkranz et al 1990) was found to have a sensitivity of 93% and specificity of 99% when compared with biopsy.

Among the non-invasive methods swabs have been the most popular. The accuracy of swab specimens has been questioned because of lack of standardization and technique variability. Cotton-tipped swabs are generally used but there can be variations in absorbency and antibacterial activity (Lawrence & Ameen 1998). Also, many studies do not refer this detail but some clearly do not clean the wound before sampling (Trengove et al 1996) while others consider it essential to remove superficial flora and tissue (Bowler 2003). Cultures performed before cleansing will collect pus and necrotic tissue and these will give information on surface contamination rather than the wound bed, although Hansson et al (1995) did not find significant differences in samples obtained before and after cleaning in wounds without infection. The other issue is the area to be sampled (whole wound to 1 cm^2) and the best option is probably to swab the part of the wound that looks most infected after cleansing. Several samples should be obtained in large wounds. A Gram stain will indicate whether the sample is appropriate (presence of neutrophils) or represents a superficial specimen or contamination from the skin of wound margins (predominant epithelial cells), which would invalidate the significance of the culture results (Miller 1996). Box 25.2 presents a method to collect swab specimens.

Box 25.2 Collection of a swab sample

Indications: Only collect swab samples if there is clinical suspicion of infection.

1. Remove superficial flora before collecting the specimen

2. Roll the swab firmly, several times (5 s), over an area of about 1 cm^2 in the advancing margin of the lesion

3. Introduce the swab into the transport medium according to the manufacturer's instructions

4. Indicate the type and anatomical site of the wound

5. Request semi-quantitative culture and anaerobic culture if indicated (deep specimen)

Specimen transport

Procedures for specimen transport must ensure the viability of pathogens as well as the limitation of contaminant growth. In deep specimens, selection of a transport medium that will support anaerobes is particularly important. Various types of transport medium are available for this purpose. Many clinical laboratories are reluctant to do anaerobic cultures on swab samples.

Interpretation of results

Results must be interpreted on the basis of the type of specimen, method of collection and also wound characteristics such as localization, duration, etc. The bacterial status of a wound changes over time. Chronic wounds are initially colonized by skin flora and have mainly Gram-positive organisms. This is also true of previously untreated infections (Lipsky et al 1990). Older wounds will also contain Gram-negatives and anaerobes. Most authors agree that superficially located bacteria play a different role from those focally infiltrating the granulating tissue underneath the ulcer surface, affecting the outcome of a chronic ulcer by releasing toxins or eliciting an immune response (Piérard-Franchimont et al 1997). However, since wound contamination almost always occurs from outside the wound, the organisms found in deep tissue will have originated from the superficial flora (Bowler 2003). Also, reduction of superficial bacteria without alteration of flora obtained by biopsy has been shown to improve healing (Sibbald et al 2001). One can conclude that, although biopsy specimens are more precise, surface sampling is easier and less costly and should suffice in everyday clinical practice.

Quantitative microbiology

A strong association exists between the number of organisms in a wound and the ability of the wound to achieve subsequent healing, with impaired healing once bacterial growth attains a quantity of 10^6 cfu/g of tissue or more (Dow 2003). This can be true for pure monomicrobial cultures, although not all microorganisms appear to conform to the required number of 10^6. Because quantitative microbiology is seen to have a role in the diagnosis of infection, and given the difficulty of obtaining biopsy specimens in clinical practice, a lot of research effort has gone into identifying quantitative methods in fluid specimens. Comparative studies (Sapico et al 1984, Bowler & Davies 1999) found a close correlation between isolation of microorganisms in superficial and deep tissue. Several studies (Levine et al 1976, Basak et al 1992, Rudensky et al 1992) have found a close correlation between tissue biopsy and swab cultures. Semi-quantitative swab culture (1+ to 4+) is a more accessible method that can be easily adopted in microbiology laboratories and has been shown to have a good sensitivity and specificity (Thomson & Smith 1994, Ratliff & Rodeheaver 2002). Sampling methods that involve rubbing can result in dispersion of clumps of bacteria to small colony-forming units (Whyte et al 1989), making it difficult to correlate numbers to the clinical situation.

Qualitative microbiology

Leg ulcer infections are frequently polymicrobial, so synergistic activity can have a significant role, making it possible to produce infection with lower numbers of bacteria of each type (Rotstein et al 1985). In polymicrobial infections, the concept of 'net pathogenic effect' is as important as the contamination level (Bowler 2003).

Although it has been suggested that specific bacteria such as *Staphylococcus aureus*, *Pseudomonas aeruginosa* and *Streptococcus pyogenes* can have a detrimental effect on healing (Madsen et al 1996), the evidence is not strong. In a review of 60 publications between 1969 and 1997, Bowler (1998) found that *S. aureus* was the single species most frequently isolated, although no correlation was found with clinical infection. *S. aureus* and *P. aeruginosa* were more frequently associated with non-infected wounds. Venous stasis ulcers are predisposed to streptococcal invasion because of their associated oedema (Heggers 1998a). *S. pyogenes* has been considered an important pathogen but is not frequently associated with infection in leg ulcers (Hansson et al 1995, Trengove et al 1996, Bowler 1998, Bowler & Davies 1999). The recognition of and importance placed on anaerobic bacteria is highly variable. In a review of nine studies it was found that 38% of non-infected and 48% of infected wounds contained anaerobic bacteria and, in 33 studies that described clinically infected wounds, *Bacteroides* spp. and *Peptostreptococcus* spp. were among the most frequently isolated (Bowler 1998). In 1995, Hansson et al concluded that there was no association between the type of bacterium and wound progress. Trengove et al (1996) investigated the bacterial profile of leg ulcers in 52 patients and concluded that the presence of one specific bacterial group did not appear to affect healing although the presence of four or more bacterial groups was associated with delayed healing. Although *S. aureus* remains the most common pathogen in chronic osteomyelitis, aerobic Gram-negative bacilli and anaerobes are frequently isolated.

More rarely, differential diagnosis may include microorganisms such as mycobacteria, fungi, viruses or parasitic organisms such as *Leishmania* spp. (Cardenas et al 2004).

TREATMENT

Host resistance is the most important determinant of wound infection. Enhancing global host defence mechanisms should be the first priority. The underlying vascular disease, whether primarily due to blood dyscrasias, venous hypertension, trauma, ischaemia or diabetes mellitus, must be treated in order to plan adequate and successful treatment. Moreover, the control of existing risk factors such as smoking, heart failure, oedema, pain, malnutrition, reduction of steroids and immunosuppressive agents is essential in order to promote normal immune function.

Key considerations related to the treatment of leg ulcer infection are listed in Box 25.3.

Individual factors that determine the presence of infection are highly complex and include non-compliance due to psychological and social limitations.

Local wound characteristics play an important role in the management of infection. These factors include wound duration, size, depth and site. For instance, location over a bony prominence and deep soft tissue destruction is highly correlated with the presence of osteomyelitis (Dow et al 1999).

Since the primary objective in wound management is to restore the bacterial balance, clearing devitalized tissue and foreign bodies is the first step in order to create the ideal local conditions to

> **Box 25.3 Key considerations related to the treatment of leg ulcers infection**
>
> - Identification and correction of inadequate blood supply
> - Control of risk factors
> - Pain control
> - Provision of good wound care:
>   - Cleansing to remove debris, foreign material and bacteria
>   - Debridement for removal of necrotic tissue
>   - Application of proper antimicrobial dressing to reduce bioburden and control exudate
> - Systemic antibiotics when necessary

prevent the progression of infection. Exudate needs to be controlled to reduce bioburden and prevent maceration in the surrounding skin. Wound cleansing will remove dead tissue and exudate. Surfactants should be avoided and antiseptic solutions should not be used for cleansing, for reasons of toxicity and inactivation (Mertz et al 1984). The best choice is sterile saline at body temperature.

When it is necessary to rapidly remove the necrotic burden, surgical or sharp debridement is indicated unless tissue perfusion status is poor (Sibbald et al 2003). Other available methods may be explored if necessary, following sharp debridement. Since they do not involve the physical removal of devitalized tissue, enzymatic and autolytic debridement are probably not as effective as surgical debridement in reducing the microbial load (Bowler et al 2001). Likewise, it has been suggested that autolytic debridement can contribute to increasing infection (Browne et al 2001).

Biosurgical debridement through larval therapy has been used in the treatment of a variety of infected chronic wounds, particularly following failure of antibiotic treatment in wounds colonized with methicillin-resistant *S. aureus* (MRSA) (Thomas et al 1998). Besides ingesting necrotic tissue, larvae also have disinfecting properties and create an ideal environment to promote healing through pH elevation and secretion of proteolytic enzymes (Beasley & Hirst 2004). Much of the existing information is related to case reports and further clinical studies are required to gain stronger evidence of the antimicrobial effects of larval therapy. Lack of widespread availability of this treatment is also an issue.

Antimicrobial treatments

In wounds that only exhibit localized signs of infection or are failing to heal in spite of appropriate clinical care (critical colonization), the first line of treatment should be topical antimicrobial agents such as antiseptics or antibiotics. Botanical extracts and antimicrobial peptides may also have a role at this stage. If no improvement is seen at the end of 2 weeks, the situation should be reassessed and systemic antibiotics should be instituted if necessary.

The clinical implications of the presence of microorganisms in leg ulcers are set out in Table 25.1.

Antiseptics

For many decades antiseptics were used without questioning their efficacy or safety. Following a number of experimental studies in vitro and in animal models showing cytotoxicity, their role has been challenged and many guidelines discourage their use, although not all studies have shown deleterious effects (Gruber et al 1975). Commonly applied antiseptics are povidone-iodine, chlorhexidine, acetic acid, silver, hydrogen peroxide and sodium hypochlorite. It is necessary to take into account the fact that many in vitro and animal studies have limited relevance to human wound healing processes (Goldenheim 1993). Beside the choice of drug, it is essential to consider the form and the system of delivery. Antiseptic solutions are ineffective because of toxicity and inactivation (Eaglstein & Falanga 1997, Mertz et al 1994). Ointments can be effective because of their associated occlusive effect and sustained delivery but are sometimes difficult to remove. Following a review of the literature, Drosou et al (2003) concluded that the position of antiseptics in wound management should be reconsidered, especially since the newer formulations (containing iodine or silver) with sustained slow release of the antiseptic appear to be safe and efficient in reducing bioburden in wounds and the advantages outweigh possible disadvantages. When choosing a dressing it is important to take into account its antimicrobial properties and mechanisms of activity but also additional properties that promote healing such as absorption of exudate, endotoxins and matrix metalloproteinases, pain relief, etc. (Sibbald et al 2001, Fumal et al 2002, Ovington 2003, Wright et al 2003).

Iodine has a broad spectrum of antimicrobial activity (McDonnell & Russell 1999). Iodophors are complexes of iodine and solubilizing agents as carriers of the active 'free' iodine. Iodophors are used in wound care in the form of solutions and

Table 25.1 Clinical implications of the presence of microorganisms in leg ulcers

	Contamination	Colonization	Critical colonization	Systemic infection
Definition	Transient presence of microorganisms	Multiplication of organisms on wound without host response	Multiplication of organisms with increased inflammatory response	Multiplication of organisms and invasion of host tissue
Clinical significance	Normal healing	Normal healing	Delayed healing	Wound deterioration with cellulitis; risk of sepsis
Interventions	No intervention required	Cleansing	Reduce bioburden with debridement and local antimicrobials	Systemic antibiotics; reduce bioburden with debridement and local antimicrobials

creams (povidone-iodine) and dressings (povidone-iodine and cadexomer-iodine). Fumal et al (2002) demonstrated the *in-vivo* efficacy of povidone-iodine solutions in the control of polymicrobial flora with additional wound healing effects. Although this is controversial, they also suggest that the toxic effects can be beneficial to control lipodermatosclerosis, since in this situation there is an excess of fibroblasts, macrophages and other cells. There are an increasing number of publications on the clinical efficacy of cadexomer-iodine, which has been found to be safe and effective while also contributing to wound healing (Mertz et al 1994, Lawrence 1997).

A range of topical silver preparations has been shown to have favourable results in chronic wounds (O'Meara et al 2001). Silver sulfadiazine is a safe broad-spectrum agent for topical use. More recently, new materials or additions to existing products have been developed for controlled release of silver. Thomas & McCubbin (2003) analysed the properties of ten silver-containing dressings and concluded that other factors besides the silver content influence performance: the distribution of silver within the dressing, the chemical or physical form and the dressing's affinity for moisture.

Although bacterial resistance to antiseptics has been shown and seems to be increasing (Russell 2002) it is not yet a clinical problem. A more recent issue is the possible effect of biocides in the selection of antibiotic-resistant bacteria (Russell 2003).

Alternative topical therapies

Many essential oils possess antimicrobial properties: for example, tea tree oil has been recognized for its efficacy against a wide range of organisms, including MRSA (Carson et al 1998). Appropriate clinical data on the efficacy of oil products and data on safety are required. Both honey and sugar paste have been used successfully in the treatment of infected wounds. Besides reducing bacterial count, they also have debriding and deodorizing properties (Knutson et al 1981, Molan 1999). Because of their osmotic effect, they will not be absorbed and are therefore suitable for diabetic patients (Booth 2004).

Topical antibiotics

Topical antibiotics have been considered as a way to deliver high concentrations to the wound while minimizing the risk of systemic toxicity. The vehicle in which the antimicrobial is formulated is an important issue to be considered. Several studies have demonstrated a good penetration of locally applied aminoglycosides (Berger et al 1981) and clindamycin (Guerrini et al 1999). However, because these are useful antibiotics for treatment of severe systemic infections and because of the increasing risk of selection of resistant strains, they should not be used topically. It is preferable to limit topical use to classes that do not need to be used parenterally. Doubts have been raised about topical formulations with regard to drug concentrations that seem to be empirical and arbitrary (Langford 1996). This can lead to excess drug delivery and consequent negative effects on tissue. Undesirable effects reported are cutaneous sensitization, inactivation of the antibiotic, inhibition of wound healing and selection of resistant strains (Degreef 1998).

Metronidazole gel has been effectively used to remove odour and reduce colonization by anaerobes (Witkowski & Parish 1991). In order to be effective the gel must be applied to all the surfaces of the wound. Fusidic acid and mupirocin exhibit a high level of activity against staphylococci (including MRSA) and streptococci and are more frequently used for skin lesions. Although polymyxin B, neomycin and bacitracin ointments can be effective, their use is not recommended because of allergy concerns.

Systemic antibiotics

Signs of invasive infection such as extending cellulitis and lymphangitis and bacteraemia, or underlying deep structure infection such as osteomyelitis, are clear indications for systemic antibiotic use.

In recent chronic wounds where flora is predominantly Gram-positive, first-line therapy should be directed at these agents. Since most chronic wounds of longer duration are characterized by polymicrobial aerobic–anaerobic flora, a broad-spectrum antimicrobial agent is indicated. Aspects such as protein binding and tissue penetration must be considered. There are few well designed trials assessing empiric antibiotic therapy. No single agent or combination has proved to be optimal. Most guidelines indicate co-amoxiclav as the single agent for first-line treatment (Nicolle et al 1996, Sanford et al 2000). Other possibly effective antimicrobial combinations include co-trimoxazole or a quinolone together with metronidazole or clindamycin. For severe infections, piperacillin/tazobactam or a third-generation cephalosporin plus clindamycin can be used. Vancomycin should be associated in the presence of MRSA. Antibiotic therapy should be adjusted according to culture results and patient response to treatment.

Because of frequent antibiotic exposure in these patients, there is a growing concern related to the emergence of resistant strains. Colsky et al (1998) compared resistance profiles between 1992 and 1998 and found a marked increase. The first vancomycin-resistant *S. aureus* in the USA was isolated in a patient with leg ulcers (Centers for Disease Control 2002). More recently, the use of quinolones has been shown to be a risk factor for the acquisition of MRSA (Weber et al 2003). This issue must be addressed in terms of choice of an antibiotic that is effective but will not contribute to resistance due to selective pressure.

The oral route is adequate for mild to moderate infections. Serious infections require hospitalization for initial parenteral therapy. Duration of treatment should be of 1–2 weeks. When osteomyelitis is present, adequate drainage, thorough debridement, obliteration of dead space, wound protection and specific antimicrobial coverage are the mainstays of therapy, which should be prolonged, from a minimum of 6 weeks up to 3 months.

Research does not support the routine use of systemic antibiotics in the absence of clinical signs of infection (Alinovi et al 1986, O'Meara et al 2001) and this practice is not recommended (American Diabetes Association 1999). Ischaemic ulcers also seldom respond to systemic antibiotics. While this has yet to be fully proved it is postulated that, since the blood supply is reduced, the antibiotic is unable to reach the site of infection in sufficient concentration to be effective.

Alternative systemic therapies

Despite the benefits of alternative therapies in the management of difficult to heal wounds, they have not yet been widely accepted because of the lack of evidence from structured randomized clinical trials involving their use in chronic wounds. Hyperbaric oxygen therapy may have a role by inhibiting anaerobic bacteria and optimizing the antimicrobial efficacy of polymorphonuclear leukocytes.

Only wounds with adequate tissue perfusion are likely to benefit (Bowler et al 2001).

CONTROL OF CROSS TRANSMISSION OF INFECTION

With increasing resistance found in bacteria in this setting, the dispersal of potentially harmful bacteria to other patients, staff and environment during wound care must be considered (Box 25.4).

Box 25.4   *Prevention of cross-transmission of infection*

- Hand-washing before and after performing dressing changes, after removing gloves or whenever hands are contaminated with blood or body fluids is essential

- Once gloved hands are contaminated with wound secretions they should not come into contact with clean dressings and other supplies

- Gloves should be removed and hands washed between patients

- When treating multiple ulcers on the same patient, the infected wound should be attended last

- Ointments and creams should not be shared between patients

- Materials should be stored in a clean, dry environment, protected from external contamination

- Only the number of dressings needed should be removed from storage containers

- Appropriate disposal of contaminated liquids is essential

- There must be containment and safe removal of soiled dressings and other used materials

- In order to contain environmental contamination, enough space with proper ventilation must be allocated for wound care, to avoid droplet contamination.

CONCLUSION

It is probable that no gold standard for diagnosis of infection in leg ulcers is going to be available in the near future. In order to be successful it will be necessary to refine clinical observation, selecting the most relevant clinical signs, standardize specimen collection methods and work closely with the microbiologists in order to improve interpretation of culture results. Treatment decisions will increasingly need to take into account the psychological aspects of the patient as well as the limitations of resources in different settings and existing professional expertise.

References

Alinovi A, Bassissi P, Pini M 1986 Systemic administration of antibiotics in the management of venous ulcers. Journal of the American Academy of Dermatology 15: 186–191

Alper J C, Welch E A, Ginsberg M et al 1983 Moist healing under a vapour permeable membrane Journal of the American Academy of Dermatology 8: 347–353

American Diabetes Association 1999 Consensus development conference on diabetic foot wound care. Diabetes Care 22: 1254–1360

Basak S, Dutta S K, Gupta S et al 1992 Bacteriology of wound infection: evaluation by surface swab and quantitative full thickness wound biopsy culture. Journal of the Indian Medical Association 90: 33–34

Beasley W D, Hirst G 2004 Making a meal of MRSA – the role of biosurgery in hospital-acquired infection. Journal of Hospital Infection 56: 6–9

Berger S A, Barza M, Haher J et al 1981 Penetration of antibiotics into decubitus ulcers. Journal of Antimicrobial Chemotherapy 7: 193–195

Booth S 2004 Are honey and sugar paste alternatives to topical antiseptics? Journal of Wound Care 13: 31–33

Bowler P G 1998 The anaerobic and aerobic microbiology of wounds: a review. Wounds 10: 170–178

Bowler P G 2002 Wound pathophysiology, infection and therapeutic options. Annals of Medicine 34: 419–427

Bowler P G 2003 The 10^5 bacterial growth guideline: reassessing its clinical relevance in wound healing. Ostomy/Wound Management 49: 44–53

Bowler P G, Davies B J 1999 The microbiology of acute and chronic wounds. Wounds 11: 72–78

Bowler P G, Duerden B I, Armstrong D G 2001 Wound microbiology and associated approaches to wound management. Clinical Microbiology Reviews 14: 244–269

Brachman P S 1992 Epidemiology of nosocomial infections. In: Bennett J, Brachman P (eds) Hospital infections, 3rd edn. Little, Brown & Company, Boston, MA

Browne A, Dow G, Sibbald R G 2001 Infected wounds: definitions and controversies. In: Falanga V (ed.) Cutaneous wound healing. Martin Dunitz, London, pp 203–220

Cardenas G A, Gonzalez-Serva, Cohen C 2004 The clinical picture. Multiple leg ulcers in a traveller. Cleveland Clinical Journal of Medicine 71: 109–112

Carson, C F, Riley, T V, Cookson, B D 1998 Efficacy and safety of tea tree oil as a topical antimicrobial agent. Journal of Hospital Infection 40: 175–178

Centers for Disease Control 2002 *Staphylococcus aureus* resistant to vancomycin – United States, 2002. Morbidity and Mortality Weekly Report 51: 565–567

Chesham J S, Platt D J 1987 Patterns of wound colonisation in patients with peripheral vascular disease. Journal of Infection 15:21–26

Colsky A S, Kirsner R S, Kerdel F A 1998 Analysis of antibiotic susceptibilities of skin wound flora in hospitalized dermatology patients. Archives of Dermatology 134: 1006–1009

Costerton J W, Ellis B, Lam K et al 1994 Mechanism of electrical enhancement of efficacy on antibiotics in killing biofilm bacteria. Antimicrobial Agents and Chemotherapy 38: 2803–2809

Costerton J W, Stewart P S, Greenberg E P 1999 Bacterial biofilms: a common cause of persistent infections. Science 284: 1318–1322

Cutting K F 2003 A dedicated follower of fashion? Topical medications and wounds. In: White R J (ed.) The silver book. Quay Books, MA Healthcare Ltd, Salisbury, p 21

Cutting K F, Harding K G 1994 Criteria for identifying infection. Journal of Wound Care 3: 198–201

Davis E 1998 Education, microbiology and chronic wounds. Journal of Wound Care 7: 272–274

De Haan B, Ellis H, Wilkes M, 1974: The role of infection in wound healing. Surgery, Gynecology, and Obstetrics 138: 693–700

Degreef H J 1998 How to heal a wound fast. Dermatologic Clinics 16: 365–375

Diegelmann R F 2003 Excessive neutrophils characterize chronic pressure ulcers. Wound Repair and Regeneration 11: 490–495

Donlan R M, Costerton J W 2002 Biofilms: survival mechanisms of clinically relevant microorganisms. Clinical Microbiology Reviews 15: 167–193

Dow G 2003 Bacterial swabs and the chronic wound: when, how, and what do they mean. Ostomy/Wound Management 49(Suppl 5A): 8–13

Dow G, Browne A, Sibbald R G 1999 Infection in chronic wounds: controversies in diagnosis and treatment. Ostomy/Wound Management; 45(8): 23–40

Drosou A, Falabella A, Kirsner R S 2003 Antiseptics on wounds: an area of controversy. Wounds 15: 149–166

Eaglstein W H, Falanga V 1997 Chronic wounds. Surgical Clinics of North America 77: 689–700

Ehrenkranz N J, Alfonso B, Nerenberg D 1990 Irrigation-aspiration for culturing draining decubitus ulcers: correlation of bacteriological findings with a clinical inflammatory scoring index. Journal of Clinical Microbiology. 28: 2389–2393

Fumal I, Braham C, Paquet P, Piérard-Franchimont C, Piérard G 2002 The beneficial toxicity paradox of antimicrobials in leg ulcers healing impaired by a polymicrobial flora: a proof of concept study. Dermatology, 204(Suppl 1):70–74

Gardner S E, Frantz R A, Doebbeling B N 2001 The validity of the clinical signs and symptoms used to identify chronic wound infection Wound Repair and Regeneration 9: 178–186

Goldenheim P D 1993 An appraisal of povidone-iodine and wound healing. Postgraduate Medical Journal 69(Suppl 3): S97–S105

Grayson M L, Gibbons G W, Balogh K et al 1995 Probing to bone in infected pedal ulcers: a clinical sign of underlying osteomyelitis in diabetic patients. Journal of the American Medical Association 273: 721–723

Greenberg E P 2003 Bacterial communication and group behavior. Journal of Clinical Investigation 112:1288–1290

Gruber R P, Vistnes L, Pardoe R 1975 The effect of commonly used antiseptics on wound healing. Plastic and Reconstructive Surgery 55: 472–476

Guerrini S, Lualdi P, Biffignandi P 1999 Treatment of venous leg ulcers with 5% amikacin gel: Phase IV trial. International Journal of Clinical Pharmacological Research 19: 35–39

Hansson C, Hoborn J, Moller A et al 1995 The microbial flora in venous leg ulcers without clinical signs of infection. Acta Dermato-Venereologica (Stockholm) 75: 24–30

Heggers J P (1998a) Defining infection in chronic wounds: does it matter? Journal of Wound Care 7: 389–392

Heggers J P (1998b) Defining infection in chronic wounds: methodology. Journal of Wound Care 7: 452–456

Knutson R A, Merbitz L A, Creekmore M A, Snipes H G 1981 Use of sugar and povidone-iodine to enhance wound healing: five years' experience. Southern Medical Journal 74: 1329–1335

Kriezek T J, Robson M C 1975 Evolution of quantitative bacteriology of wound management. American Journal of Surgery 130: 579–584

Langford J 1996 Clinical rationale for topical antimicrobial preparations. Journal of Antimicrobial Chemotherapy 37: 399–402

Lawrence J C 1997 Studies of some povidone-iodine medicated dressings using a wound healing model. Dermatology 195(Suppl 2): 158

Lawrence J C, Ameen H 1998 Swab and other sampling techniques. Journal of Wound Care 7: 232–233

Lee P C, Turnidge J, McDonald P J 1985 Fine-needle aspiration biopsy in diagnosis of soft tissue infections. Journal of Clinical Microbiology 22: 80–83

Levine N S, Lindberg R B, Mason A D et al 1976 The quantitative swab culture and smear: a quick simple method for determining the number of viable aerobic bacteria on open wounds. Journal of Trauma 16: 89–94

Lipsky B A, Pecoraro R E, Larson SA et al 1990 Outpatient management of uncomplicated lower-extremity infections in diabetic patients. Archives of Internal Medicine 150:790–797

Lookingbill D P, Miller S M, Knowles R C 1978 Bacteriology of chronic leg ulcers. Archives of Dermatology 114: 1765–1768

McDonnell G, Russell D 1999 Antiseptics and disinfectants: activity, action, and resistance. Clinical Microbiology Reviews 12: 147–179

Madsen S M, Westh H, Danielsen L et al 1996 Bacterial colonization and healing of venous leg ulcers. Acta Pathologic Microbiologica et Immunologica Scandinavica 104: 895–899

Mertz P M, Alvarez O M, Smerbeck R V, Eaglstein W H 1984 A new in vivo model for the evaluation of topical antiseptics on superficial wounds. Archives of Dermatology 120: 58–62

Mertz P M, Davis S, Brewer L, Franzen L 1994 Can antimicrobials be effective without impairing wound-healing? The evaluation of a cadexomer iodine ointment. Wounds 6: 184–193

Miller J M 1996 A guide to specimen management in clinical microbiology. ASM Press, Washington, DC

Miller M 2001 Wound infection unravelled. Journal of Community Nursing Online 15(3). Available on line at: www.jcn.co.uk (accessed 7/12/2003)

Molan P C 1999 The role of honey in the management of wounds. Journal of Wound Care 8: 415–418

Nicolle L E, Bentley D, Garibaldi R et al 1996 Antimicrobial use in long-term-care facilities. SHEA Position Paper. Infection Control and Hospital Epidemiology 17: 119–127

O'Meara S M, Cullum N A, Majid M, Sheldon T A 2001 Systematic review of antimicrobial agents used for chronic wounds. British Journal of Surgery 88: 4–21

Ovington L G 2003 Bacterial toxins and wound healing. Ostomy/Wound Management 49:(7A Suppl): 8–12

Pallua N, Fuchs P C, Hafemann B et al 1999 A new technique for quantitative bacterial assessment on burn wounds by modified dermabrasion. Journal of Hospital Infection 42: 329–337

Piérard-Franchimont, Paquet P, Arrese J E et al 1997 Healing rate and bacterial necrotizing vasculitis in venous leg ulcers. Dermatology 194: 383–387

Pierce G F 2001 Inflammation in nonhealing diabetic wounds. The space-time continuum does matter. American Journal of Pathology 159: 399–403

Pollack S 1984 The wound healing process. Clinical Dermatology 2:80

Ratliff C R, Rodeheaver G T 2002 Correlation of semi-quantitative swab cultures to quantitative swab cultures from chronic wounds. Wounds 14: 329–333

Rediske A M, Roeder B L, Nelson J L et al 2000 Pulsed ultrasound enhances the killing of *Escherichia coli* biofilms by aminoglycoside antibiotics in vivo. Antimicrobial Agents and Chemotherapy 44: 771–772.

Robson M C 1997 Wound infection. A failure of wound healing caused by an imbalance of bacteria. Surgical Clinics of North America 77: 537–650

Robson M C, Heggers J P 1969 Bacterial quantification of open wounds. Military Medicine 134: 19–24

Rotstein O D, Pruett T L, Simmons R L 1985 Mechanisms of microbial synergy in polymicrobial surgical infections. Reviews of Infectious Diseases 7: 151–170

Rudensky B, Lipschits M, Isaacsohn M et al 1992 Infected pressure sores: comparison of methods for bacterial identification. Southern Medical Journal 85: 901–903

Rumbaugh K P, Griswold J A, Iglewski B H, Hamood A N 1999 Contribution of quorum sensing to the virulence of *Pseudomonas aeruginosa* in burn wound infections. Infection and Immunity 67: 5854–5862

Russell A D 2002 Introduction of biocides into clinical practice and the impact on antibiotic-resistant bacteria. Journal of Applied Microbiology 92(Suppl):121S–135S

Russell A D 2003 Biocide use and antibiotic resistance. The relevance of laboratory findings to clinical and environmental situations. Lancet Infectious Diseases 3: 794

Sanford J P, Gilbert D N, Moellering R C Jr, Sande M A 2000 The Sanford guide to antimicrobial therapy 2000. Oregon Health Sciences University, Portland, OR

Sapico F L, Witte J L, Canawati H N et al 1984 The infected foot of the diabetic patient: quantitative microbiology and analysis of clinical features. Reviews of Infectious Diseases 6(Suppl 1): S171–S176

Savage D C 1977 Microbial ecology of the gastrointestinal tract. Annual Review of Microbiology. 31:107–133

Schmidt K, Debus E S Jessberger et al 2000 Bacterial population of chronic crural ulcers: is there a difference between diabetic, the venous, and the arterial ulcer? Vasa 29: 62–70

Serralta V W, Harrison-Balestra C, Cazzaniga L et al 2001 Lifestyle of bacteria in wounds: presence of biofilms? Wounds 1: 29–34

Sibbald G R, Browne A C, Courts P, Queen D 2001 Screening evaluation of an ionized nanocrystalline silver dressing in chronic wound care. Ostomy/Wound Management 47: 38–43

Sibbald G R, Orsted H, Schultz G S et al 2003 Preparing the wound bed 2003: focus on infection and inflammation. Ostomy/Wound Management 49: 24–51

Singh P K, Parsek M R, Greenberg E P, Welsh M J 2002 A component of innate immunity prevents bacterial biofilm development. Nature 417: 552–555

Stotts N A, Hunt T K 1997 Managing bacterial colonization and infection. Clinics in Geriatric Medicine 3: 565–573

Thomas S, McCubbin P 2003 An in vitro analysis of the antimicrobial properties of 10 silver-containing dressings. Journal of Wound Care 12: 305–308

Thomas S, Andrews A, Jones M 1998 The use of larval therapy in wound management. Journal of Wound Care 7: 521–524

Thomson P D, Smith D J 1994 What is infection? American Journal of Surgery 167(Suppl 1A): 7S–11S

Trengove N J, Stacey M C, McGechie 1996 Qualitative bacteriology and leg ulcer healing. Journal of Wound Care 5: 277–280

Vindenes H, Bjerknes R 1993 The frequency of bacteremia and fungemia following wound cleaning and excision in patients with large burns. Journal of Trauma 35: 742–749

Volenec F J, Clark G M, Mani M M et al 1979 Burn wound biopsy bacterial quantitation: a statistical analysis. American Journal of Surgery 138: 695–697

Ward K H, Olson M E, Lam K et al 1992 Mechanism of persistent infection associated with peritoneal implants. Journal of Medical Microbiology 36: 233–235

Washington J A 1989 Classification of microorganisms based on intrinsic pathogenicity. In: van Saene H F K et al (eds) Update in intensive care and emergency medicine 7. Infection control and selective decontamination. Springer, Berlin, p 8

Weber S G, Gold H S, Hooper D C et al 2003 Fluoroquinolones and the risk for methicillin-resistant Staphylococcus aureus in hospitalized patients. Emerging Infectious Diseases 9): 1415–1421

Wellman N, Fortum S M, McLeod B R 1996 Bacterial biofilms and the bioelectric effect. Antimicrobial Agents and Chemotherapy 40: 2012–2014

Whyte W, Carson W, Hambraeus A 1989 Methods for calculating the efficiency of bacterial surface sampling techniques. Journal of Hospital Infection 13: 33–41

Witkowski J A, Parish L C 1991 Topical metronidazole gel. The bacteriology of decubitus ulcers. International Journal of Dermatology 30: 660–661

Woolfrey B F, Fox J M, Quall C O 1981 An evaluation of burn wound quantitative microbiology 1. Quantitative eschar cultures. American Journal of Clinical Pathology 75: 532–537

Wright J B, Lam K, Olson M E et al 2003 Is antimicrobial efficacy sufficient? A question concerning the benefits of new dressings. Wounds 15: 133–142

CHAPTER

26

Adjuvant therapies: ultrasound, laser therapy, electrical stimulation, hyperbaric oxygen and vacuum-assisted closure therapy

Mary Dyson

INTRODUCTION

The adjuvant therapies currently available for the stimulation of healing where this is delayed include the physical modalities of ultrasound, laser therapy and other forms of photobiomodulation, electrical stimulation, hyperbaric oxygen and vacuum-assisted closure therapy. They should be used, in addition to best clinical practice in wound management, as adjuvant therapies. These modalities are described in this chapter, the emphasis being on how they work so that the practitioner has sufficient knowledge to decide which to use, for which types of leg ulcer, and how to monitor their effectiveness. Selection of the appropriate adjuvant therapy should be based on an understanding of the healing process and on the properties and mode of action of the different therapies.

ULTRASOUND

Ultrasound has been used in wound care for over 50 years. Originally only megahertz ultrasound was available but in the 1990s kilohertz devices were tested successfully. In this section the physical properties and biological effects of megahertz and kilohertz ultrasound are described, together with how they can be used in wound care. Sufficient

information is provided for the user to select the most appropriate method of treatment for leg ulcers of different types.

What is ultrasound?

Ultrasound is a mechanical vibration transmitted at a frequency above the upper limit of human hearing i.e. above 20 kHz, where 1 Hz = 1 cycle per second, 1 kHz = 1000 cycles per second and 1 MHz = 1 000 000 cycles per second. It causes the molecules of the media that can transmit it (e.g. biological tissues) to oscillate or vibrate, and can be used therapeutically to accelerate wound healing where this is delayed (Dyson 1995, 1997). Megahertz ultrasound, typically between 0.5 and 3 MHz (i.e. 0.5–3 million cycles per second) has been used for more than 50 years to stimulate healing. During the last decade, 30 kHz and 50 kHz ultrasound have also been demonstrated to have therapeutic effects (Peschen et al 1997); this new form of therapeutic ultrasound has grown rapidly in use. Diagnostic ultrasound at a centre frequency of 20 MHz allows soft tissue to be imaged at high resolution (65 μm) non-invasively. Subcutaneous and dermal injury can be detected before they are visible and repair can be monitored as it occurs.

Frequency

Many of the clinically relevant properties of ultrasound are related to its *frequency* (*f*), i.e. the number of times per second that a molecule displaced by the ultrasound completes a cycle of movement and returns to its original position (Fig. 26.1). Frequencies are expressed in hertz (i.e. cycles per second). The time (*T*) taken to complete a cycle is termed a *period*. Frequency and wavelength are inversely related: the lower the frequency the longer the wavelength. This is why kilohertz ultrasound is also known as long-wave ultrasound.

Attenuation

Attenuation is the reduction of the power of the ultrasound wave as it is transmitted through tissues and other materials. All tissues impede the passage of mechanical waves such as ultrasound. The specific impedance of a tissue is determined by its density and elasticity, which in turn affect the velocity at which the ultrasound is transmitted. Table 26.1, based on information provided by Ward (1986), compares the acoustic properties of a range of tissues to those of air, water and steel. The greater the difference in impedance at a boundary, the greater the reflection that occurs and therefore the smaller the amount of energy available for further penetration.

The tissues must absorb ultrasound for it to produce a therapeutic effect. The absorption of ultrasound is exponential, more being absorbed in the superficial tissues than in the deeper tissues. The further the ultrasound penetrates into the body, the greater the proportion of ultrasound energy that will have been absorbed and therefore the less that will be available to achieve a therapeutic effect. Lower frequencies penetrate deeper than higher frequencies because they are less readily attenuated. At higher frequencies, more of the energy is absorbed superficially so less is available to penetrate into deeper tissues.

If a wound is superficial, then 3 MHz ultrasound is effective, whereas, if it is several centimetres deep, then 1 MHz will be a more suitable choice. If bone is involved, e.g. in a type IV pressure ulcer, or if a metal implant is present, then kilohertz ultrasound may be more effective. Ultrasound is reflected from interfaces between substances differing acoustically, e.g. skin and air, collagen and tissue fluid, soft tissues and bone, soft tissues and steel, etc. Because of the reflection between skin and air, a coupling medium acoustically similar to skin has to be used between the head of the ultrasound probe and the surface of either the skin or the wound so that ultrasound can be transmitted into them. Some types of film and

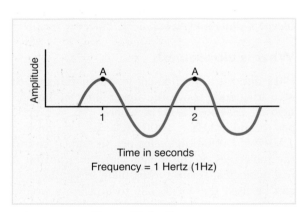

Figure 26.1 Frequency

Table 26.1 Acoustic properties of a selection of tissues and other materials (after Ward 1986)

Material	Density (kg/m³)	Velocity (m/s)	Impedance (kg/m² s⁻¹)
Adipose tissue	940	1,450	1.4×10^{6}
Muscle	1,100	1,550	1.7×10^{6}
Bone	1,800	2,800	5.1×10^{6}
Air	0.625	340	213
Water	1,000	1,500	1.5×10^{6}
Steel	8,000	5,850	47×10^{6}

hydrocolloid dressings are good coupling agents, as is warm saline.

Half-value thickness

When ultrasound is transmitted through tissue, its intensity decreases in an exponential fashion (Fig. 26.2). The half-value thickness is the depth in the tissues at which half the intensity of ultrasound (measured in W/cm^2) applied to the surface is available. The intensity available at any depth within the tissue is inversely proportional to the depth of penetration (i.e. the greater the depth, the less the remaining intensity). The half-value thickness differs according to the tissue and the frequency, as shown in Table 26.2.

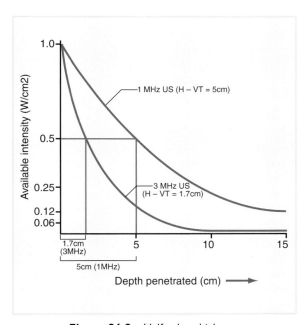

Figure 26.2 Half-value thickness

Table 26.2 Typical half value depths for 1 MHz and 3 MHz ultrasound in tissues (after Hoogland 1987)

	1 MHz (mm)	**3 MHz (mm)**
Muscle	9.0	3.0
Adipose tissue	50.0	16.5
Tendon	6.2	2.0

Absorption, which is a major cause of attenuation (e.g. loss of intensity), is frequency-dependent. The greater the frequency the shorter the wavelength. The shorter the wavelength the greater the absorption. For an ultrasound beam of 3 MHz, the wavelength is shorter than that at 1 MHz and therefore absorption occurs more readily than at 1 MHz. A frequency of 3 MHz is an efficient one to use to treat superficial regions, such as injured skin, but lower megahertz frequencies are indicated for deeper targets, such as injured muscle or bone. Kilohertz ultrasound is even more penetrative, i.e. it has a greater half-value thickness (Sussman & Dyson 1998). Applied to intact skin on the lateral aspect of a limb, kilohertz ultrasound can reach a wound on the medial aspect, so there is no need for the probe to be in contact with the wound, even through a dressing; this is clinically important if the wound is infected or if it is painful when pressure is applied to it.

Absorption varies with the composition of the tissues as well as with the wavelength, which, as described above, is inversely related to frequency. Bone is more absorptive than highly proteinaceous tissues (e.g. tendon and muscle); protein is more absorptive than fat (e.g. adipose tissue); and fat is more absorptive than water-rich materials (e.g. oedematous tissues). Because of this, the half-value thickness of bone is less than that of muscle, which is less than that of fat, which is less than that of oedematous soft connective tissue. Ultrasound can therefore penetrate skin, fat, and oedematous tissues to reach a sinus extending beyond the wound surface. Because the thickness and distribution of different tissues varies with the anatomical site and the patient, approximations of half-value thickness in soft tissue have to be made (Fig. 26.2). Ward (1986) has proposed a value of 4 cm for 1 MHz and 2 cm for 3 MHz.

Wavelength

The *wavelength* (λ) is the shortest distance, measured parallel to the direction of wave propagation, between molecules that are at equivalent points of vibration in the repeated cycle of movement that constitutes a wave. It is related to the *frequency* and *velocity* (c) of the wave by the following equation: $\lambda = c/f$. The velocity of ultrasound in water, blood, interstitial fluid and soft tissues is approximately 1500 m/s. The higher the frequency the shorter the wavelength. This is important diagnostically, because the shorter the wavelength the greater the degree of resolution. The frequency of 20 MHz, used by some high-resolution diagnostic ultrasound devices to examine skin and wounds non-invasively, produces a wavelength that is sufficiently short to allow the stratum corneum and stratum malpighii of the epidermis, the papillary and reticular layers of the dermis, the adipose hypodermis, collagen fibre bundles, necrotic tissue, oedematous tissue, granulation tissue and scar tissue to be distinguished and measured (Dyson et al 2003).

High frequencies are more readily absorbed by tissues than low frequencies and produce a greater thermal effect in them but they are more easily attenuated and therefore are less penetrative. Lower frequencies produce cavitation and the microstreaming associated with it more readily than do higher frequencies. There is evidence that many of the biological effects produced by therapeutic ultrasound are caused by cavitation and microstreaming (Dyson 1995).

The ultrasonic field

The ultrasonic pressure field generated by the transducer depends on the size and shape of the transducer and how it is mounted in the applicator. The pressure varies across the surface of the applicator and also with the distance from it. The pressure changes experienced by the tissues being treated depend in part, therefore, on their position relative to the applicator. Ultrasound is emitted from a disc-shaped transducer of the type used with megahertz therapeutic ultrasound as a beam that is at first cylindrical; this region is termed the *near field* or *Fresnel zone*, and the energy distribution in it is extremely variable. Beyond this, the beam starts to diverge and the energy distribution within it becomes more regular; this region is termed the *far field* or *Fraunhofer zone*. The distance (d) from the transducer to the beginning of the far field is related to the radius (a) of the transducer and the wavelength (λ) of the ultrasound: $d = a^2/\lambda$.

Unless the part to be treated is immersed in a water bath large enough for the target tissues to be in the far field, ultrasound therapy involves treatment of tissue in the non-uniform near field. The *beam non-uniformity ratio* (BNR) is a measure of this non-uniformity and is the ratio of the spatial peak intensity (I_{SP}) to the spatial average intensity (I_{SA}). These terms are defined below. Applicators with low BNRs give more *predictable* results and are *safer* than those with higher BNRs, since the higher spatial peak intensities of the latter are potentially damaging (Ziskin & Michlovitz, 1990).

Intensity

Intensity (I) is the amount of energy (in watts) per unit area per unit time. Applicators typically have an *effective radiating area* (ERA) of a few square centimetres. The intensity can be averaged in space over the face of the applicator (termed *spatial average*, SA) or in time (termed *temporal average*, TA). When pulsed ultrasound is used, pulse average (PA) intensity, i.e. the temporal average during the period of the pulse, should be noted, and also the temporal average during the full pulse repetition cycle. The type of intensity should be specified as either I_{SATA} if continuous or both I_{SATA} and I_{SAPA} if pulsed.

Therapeutic ultrasound equipment

The equipment used to produce therapeutic levels of megahertz ultrasound typically consists of a microcomputer-controlled high-frequency generator linked by a coaxial cable to an applicator or treatment head. The treatment head contains a disc of a piezoelectric material, such as lead zirconate titanate (PZT), which acts as a transducer changing one form of energy into another, in this case into ultrasound. When an alternating voltage is applied across such a disc, it expands and contracts at the same frequency as the oscillation, transducing electrical energy into ultrasound. A similar system is made use of for kilohertz ultrasound but the frequency of vibration is much lower and the transducers have a different composition and mode of operation. Examples of equipment for generating megahertz ultrasound, kilohertz ultrasound, and kilohertz and megahertz ultrasound are shown in Figures 26.3, 26.4 and 26.5 respectively. There is evidence that both megahertz and kilohertz ultrasound can stimulate the healing of chronic wounds, as described below.

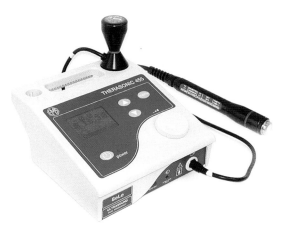

Figure 26.3 Dual frequency ultrasound therapy device producing 1 and 3 MHz ultrasound (Electro-Medical Supplies Ltd)

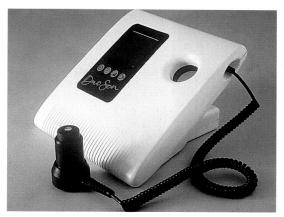

Figure 26.5 Ultrasound therapy device producing kilohertz and megahertz ultrasound either separately or simultaneously (Orthosonics Ltd)

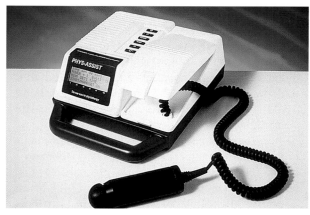

Figure 26.4 Ultrasound therapy device producing kilohertz ultrasound (Orthosonics Ltd)

Application of ultrasound to a leg ulcer

Ultrasound is reflected from the interfaces between air and skin, and between air and soft tissues, so it has to be transmitted into the tissues through a suitable coupling medium such as a gel with a high water content, a film dressing, water or saline. Open wounds should be filled with warm sterile saline and covered with either a film dressing such as Opsite (Smith & Nephew) or a hydrocolloid dressing such as Granuflex (ConvaTec), both of which transmit ultrasound from the applicator into the tissues to be treated. Putting a coupling medium such as Aquasonic 100 Gel (Parker Laboratories

Inc.) on to the ultrasound-emitting face of the applicator facilitates moving it over the skin or over the dressing covering the wound.

Treatment parameters

The following parameters should be recorded when using ultrasound to treat a wound:

- Frequency (Hz)
- Duration of treatment (min)
- Continuous or pulsed application
- If pulsed, pulse duration (ms) and space duration (ms)
- Intensity (W/cm^2):
    - as I_{SATA} for both continuous and pulsed applications and
    - either I_{SAPA} or I_{SATP} if pulsed.

A typical treatment of a leg ulcer is as follows:

- Frequency = 3 MHz
- Duration of treatment = 5 min
- Pulsed
- Pulse duration = 2 ms; space duration = 8 ms (duty cycle = 20%)
- I_{SATA} = 0.2 W/cm^2
- $I_{SAPA} = I_{SATP}$ = 1.0 W/cm^2.

Ultrasound bioeffects

The safe and effective use of ultrasound depends on an understanding of the effects it has on intact and injured living tissues. These bioeffects can be classified into:

- Thermal
- Predominantly non-thermal.

Thermal effects

Ultrasound applied to vascularized tissue in the I_{SATP} range of 1.0–2.0 W/cm^2 for between 5 and 10 minutes increases its temperature to between 40°C and 45°C which is therapeutically beneficial (Ziskin & Michlovitz 1990). This is acceptable only in adequately vascularized tissues. Temperatures above this cause *thermal necrosis* and must be avoided. Clinically beneficial thermal effects occur with both 1 MHz and 3 MHz continuous ultrasound but at different tissue depths. At a frequency of 3 MHz, energy absorption occurs mainly in superficial tissues (< 2 cm beneath the surface). At a frequency of 1 MHz, less energy is absorbed by the superficial tissues. This frequency also penetrates into deeper tissues, with effective energy levels being available up to 5 cm below the surface. Pulsing the wave, since this reduces the temporal average intensity, reduces thermal effects. Whenever ultrasound is absorbed, heat is produced but, if the temperature increases less than 1°C, this is not considered to be physiologically relevant; the therapeutic effects are then due predominantly to non-thermal mechanisms.

Predominantly non-thermal effects

Non-thermal effects of megahertz ultrasound occur at low spatial average intensities, which can be achieved by pulsing at, for example, a 20% duty cycle. They are attributed to cavitation, standing wave formation and acoustic streaming.

Cavitation involves the production and vibration of micron-sized bubbles within fluids, including tissue fluid. The ultrasound beam affects small, gaseous bubbles that move within the fluids. These bubbles oscillate in the ultrasound field, alternately expanding and contracting during each cycle of the ultrasound wave. The movement and compression of the bubbles can cause changes in the cellular activities of tissues subjected to ultrasound.

- *Stable cavitation* occurs at intensities low enough for the bubbles to change little in size during each cycle. The effect of stable cavitation can result in diffusional changes across the membranes of cells located close to these bubbles. They can also distort the cell membranes causing, for example, reversible increase in membrane permeability to calcium ions, thus affecting cell activity. Stable cavitation is potentially beneficial and can stimulate healing.
- *Unstable or transient cavitation* refers to collapse of the bubbles mentioned above. Transient bubbles implode, causing local mechanical damage and free radical formation. This is potentially very hazardous. It occurs at high intensities, particularly when the sound head is not moved during treatment and standing waves develop (Sussman & Dyson, 2001).

Standing waves occur if the applicator is kept still during treatment. The ultrasound is then reflected backwards and forwards between the applicator and any reflective surface, e.g. that between soft tissue and bone, producing a standing wave in which energy can accumulate to damaging levels. There is evidence that the intravascular flow of blood cells can be stopped temporarily and that endothelial cells can be damaged (Dyson & Pond 1973). Moving the transducer disrupts the standing waves.

Acoustic streaming is the unidirectional movement of fluids along acoustic boundaries (e.g. bubbles or cell membranes) as a result of the mechanical pressure wave associated with the ultrasound beam (Ziskin & Michelovitz, 1990). Outcomes attributable to this effect include reversible increase in cell membrane permeability and increased protein synthesis.

It has been proposed that stable cavitation and microstreaming are responsible for the stimulatory effects of low intensity ultrasound (Dyson 1995).

How ultrasound stimulates wound healing

Mechanism

Wound healing can only occur if the cells involved in the process are activated. The entry of calcium ions into cells can activate them. Increase in the permeability of the plasma membranes of cells to calcium ions follows exposure to non-thermal levels of ultrasound (Dyson 1995). The physical mechanisms producing this are stable cavitation and acoustic streaming of the fluid around the cells.

Cells in the path of the beam of ultrasound migrate, divide, differentiate, grow, phagocytose and synthesize growth factors and matrix materials such as collagen according to their capabilities. Collectively these activities heal the wound, provided that they occur in an organized fashion. Therapeutic ultrasound acts as a stimulus that the cells transduce. In each affected cell an amplified response occurs, the type of which depends upon the type of cell involved: for example, polymorphs phagocytose debris, fibroblasts synthesis collagen and other matrix materials, endothelial cells migrate and divide forming new capillaries.

Effect of ultrasound on acute wounds

When wounds begin to heal they enter a phase of temporary acute inflammation. Treatment with therapeutic ultrasound during acute inflammation can shorten it. The wound therefore progresses into the subsequent proliferative phase more rapidly (Dyson 1995). Ideally, ultrasound should therefore be applied as soon as possible after an injury. During acute inflammation the growth factors necessary to progress healing are produced and secreted; this is stimulated by therapeutic ultrasound. What ultrasound therapy does is to assist the body to heal itself. It is of value if healing is suboptimal, as is generally the situation. In such circumstances healing can be accelerated. There is also evidence that acute skin injuries treated with ultrasound in the acute inflammatory phase develop stronger reparative tissue than do control wounds (Hart 1993).

Effect of ultrasound on chronic wounds

To assist the healing of chronic wounds, they must first be activated so that at least part of each wound is in the acute inflammatory phase of repair. This can be achieved by debriding the wound. Treatment with either kilohertz ultrasound via a water bath or one application of megahertz ultrasound at an intensity high enough to produce thermal effects can also activate chronic wounds. Once acute inflammation has commenced, the application of lower intensity, predominantly non-thermal, ultrasound has been shown to accelerate healing of venous leg ulcers (Dyson et al 1976).

The following treatment regime has been shown to be effective:

- Frequency = 3 MHz
- Duration of treatment = 5–10 min, three times per week
- Pulsed
- Pulse duration = 2 ms; space duration = 8 ms
- $I_{SATA} = 0.2$ W/cm^2
- $I_{SAPA} = I_{SATP} = 1.0$ W/cm^2.

The treatment was applied to the periwound area following the initiation of acute inflammation. It can also be applied to the open wound through an appropriate dressing as described above.

An alternative method using long-wave (i.e. kilohertz) ultrasound has also been shown to be effective as an adjunctive treatment for venous leg ulcers (Peschen et al 1997). Here the treatment is applied via a water bath similar to the podiatry bath shown in Figure 26.6. The acoustic streaming produced in the bath removes superficial necrotic tissue and occasionally produces a tingling sensation and pinhead-sized points of bleeding. Further treatments with kilohertz ultrasound were shown by Peschen et al (1997) to accelerate healing in comparison with a control group. The following treatment regime was used:

- Frequency = 30 kHz
- Duration of treatment = 10 min, three times per week
- Continuous
- $I_{SATA} = 0.1$ W/cm^2.

Both the ultrasound treated and the control wounds were covered with hydrocolloid dressings and compression therapy was applied. After 12 weeks, the ultrasound-treated group of wounds showed an average decrease in surface area of 55.4% compared with only 16.5% in the control wounds ($p < 0.007$; $n = 24$).

Expected outcomes

Ultrasound is most effective when applied during the acute inflammatory phase of healing. During this phase, expect an acceleration of inflammation and early progression to the proliferative phase of healing. In chronic wounds the first outcomes to treatment will be increased perfusion, observed as warmth, oedema and darkening of tissue colour

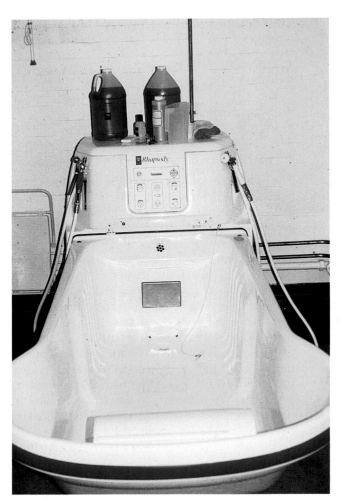

Figure 26.6 Podiatry bath incorporating a rectangular kilohertz ultrasound therapy transducer (Arjo Inc.)

compared to adjacent skin colour tones. In necrotic wounds, expect to see autolysis of the necrotic tissue; the outcome will be a clean wound bed. Wounds in two clinical trials of megahertz ultrasound progressed to closure in a mean time of 4–6 weeks (McDiarmid et al 1985, Nussbaum et al 1994). However, these times could be longer for patients with intrinsic and extrinsic factors that limit healing. Published research is a valuable guide in prediction of outcomes (Sussman & Bates-Jensen 2001) and the progress of repair should be compared with this. It is therefore necessary, as with any therapy, for the progress of repair of each wound to be monitored throughout the course of treatment.

If the wound does not change phase and/or become reduced in size (surface area and depth) within 2–4 weeks, the clinical status of the patient should be reassessed. If this has deteriorated, clinical or surgical intervention may be necessary. If it has not deteriorated, then the treatment regimen should be reviewed and, if necessary, revised. It may, for example, be necessary to re-initiate acute inflammation.

The use of high-resolution ultrasound imaging to monitor wound healing

In addition to its therapeutic role, ultrasound is also of value in wound care as a diagnostic technique

(Dyson et al 2003). In these days of evidence-based clinical practice it is essential that the effectiveness of treatment be monitored objectively. Ultrasound imaging permits this to be done non-invasively, rapidly and painlessly. Unlike surface photography, it allows tissue changes within, throughout and around the leg ulcer to be visualized in the manner of a biopsy, but without any damage to the patient. Magnified, high-resolution images of living tissue akin to low-power micrographs are produced by using 20 MHz ultrasound; the technique is therefore often referred to as *ultrasound biomicroscopy*. The images obtained are digital, can be archived and can be e-mailed to remote sites for analysis if this is required, an example of telemedicine in action.

Portable, user- and patient-friendly high-resolution scanners such as that shown in Figure 26.7 are now commercially available. It is recommended that the surface appearance of the leg ulcer be recorded with a digital camera and the tissue changes within and around with a high-resolution ultrasound scanner every time the wound is treated. These photographs and scans can be taken by the nurse or other clinician treating and/or dressing the wound and only add a few minutes to the time spent with each patient. The scanner shown here (see www.longportinc.com for further information) operates at a frequency of 2 MHz, providing a vertical resolution of the order of 65 μm and clear discrimination between acoustically dif-

ferent materials such as tissue fluid, debris, granulation tissue, scar tissue and the various layers of the epidermis, dermis and hypodermis. The software incorporated into the scanner allows linear and area measurements to be made. These are then stored, together with the scans, digital photographs and the patient's notes, in a secure, retrievable fashion. Examples of scans of intact skin and of a leg ulcer 1 and 27 days following grafting are illustrated in Figures 26.8, 26.9 and 26.10 respectively.

Digital photographs and high-resolution ultrasound scans should be taken before treatment is commenced and throughout the course of any treatment so that its effectiveness can be monitored and changes made if the response of the patient indicates this.

LOW-INTENSITY LASER THERAPY

Electromagnetic radiation in the form of photons, delivered in either laser or non-laser form, has been applied to wounds as a means of stimulating healing for over 30 years. The technique is now often referred to as *photobiomodulation*, the use of photons to modulate biological activity (Dyson et al 2002). Light consists of those wavelengths of the electromagnetic spectrum that are visible to the human eye. This part of the spectrum extends from violet (the shortest visible wavelength) to red (the longest visible wavelength). Infrared is just beyond the visible range. The perceived colour depends on the wavelength. White light is a mixture of all the visible wavelengths. For photons to reach a wound all that is required is that the wound be either exposed to air or sterile saline or covered by a transparent dressing. Exposure to red light and/or infrared radiation can stimulate the healing of both chronic wounds (Mester et al 1985) and acute wounds (Dyson & Young 1986).

Laser is an acronym for 'light amplification by the stimulated emission of radiation'. The stimulated emission of radiation occurs when a photon interacts with an energized atom. When an atom is energized, for example by electricity, one of its electrons is excited, i.e. raised to a higher-energy orbit than its orbit when in the resting state. If the energy of the incident photon is equal to the energy difference between the electron's excited and resting states, the stimulated emission of a photon

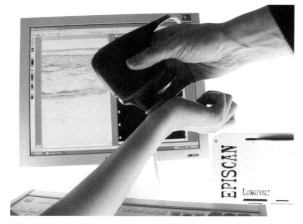

Figure 26.7 Portable high-resolution, high-frequency diagnostic ultrasound scanner (Longport Inc.)

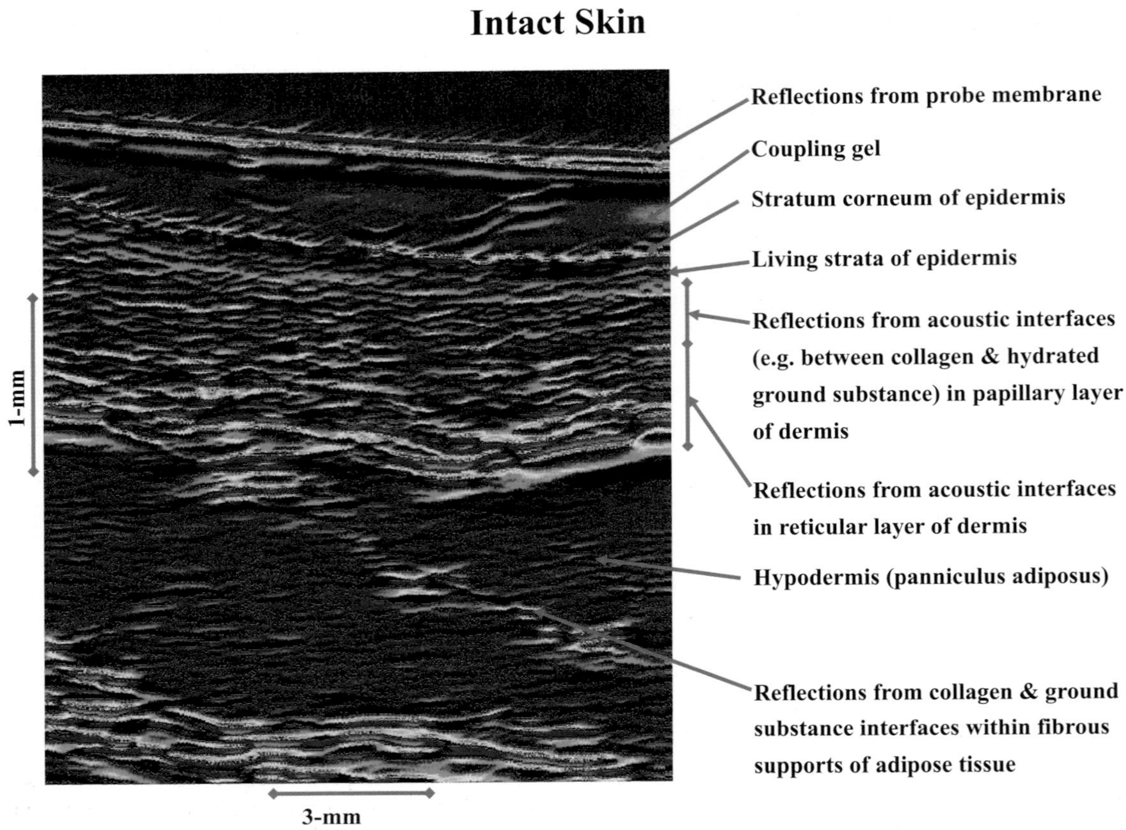

Intact Skin

Reflections from probe membrane

Coupling gel

Stratum corneum of epidermis

Living strata of epidermis

Reflections from acoustic interfaces (e.g. between collagen & hydrated ground substance) in papillary layer of dermis

Reflections from acoustic interfaces in reticular layer of dermis

Hypodermis (panniculus adiposus)

Reflections from collagen & ground substance interfaces within fibrous supports of adipose tissue

1-mm

3-mm

Figure 26.8 High-resolution ultrasound scan of intact skin on the inner aspect of the forearm

occurs and the excited electron returns to its resting state. This photon has the same properties as the incident photon, which is also emitted. This process is repeated in the adjacent energized atoms, producing a laser beam. Unlike light from non-laser sources, this light is:

- Monochromatic, i.e. of a single wavelength
- Collimated, i.e. its light rays are non-divergent
- Coherent, i.e. in phase, the troughs and peaks of the waves coinciding in time and space.

With regard to laser therapy, monochromaticity is its most important characteristic. To produce an effect, the light must be absorbed, and absorption is wavelength-specific. Different substances absorb light of different wavelengths. Mitochondria, present in all cells, contain cytochromes that absorb red light. Some cells absorb some wavelengths of infrared radiation, while other cell types absorb other infrared wavelengths.

LILT is an acronym for low-intensity laser therapy (Baxter 1994). Other names include LLLT (low-level laser therapy) and LEPT (low-energy photon therapy). Unlike the high-intensity medical lasers used to thermally cut and coagulate tissues, LILT involves the use of medical lasers that operate at intensities too low to damage living tissues. Their action is photobiomodulation: they can stimulate inactivated tissue components and inhibit some activated components (Agaiby et al 1998).

Equipment

This has three essential components:

- *Lasing medium*, which is capable of being energized sufficiently for lasing to occur
- *Resonating cavity* containing the lasing medium
- *Power source* that transmits energy into the lasing medium.

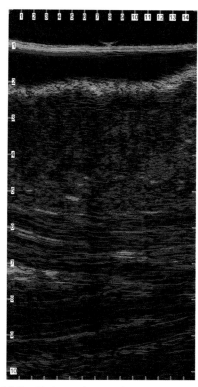

Figure 26.9 High-resolution ultrasound scan of a leg ulcer 1 day after application of a bioengineered graft (Courtesy of Dr Paul Qintavalle)

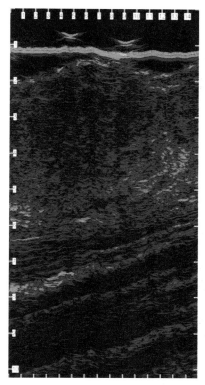

Figure 26.10 High-resolution ultrasound scan of a leg ulcer 27 days after application of a bioengineered graft (Courtesy of Dr Paul Qintavalle)

The type of lasing medium used determines the wavelength, and therefore the colour, of the laser beam. For example, a HeNe laser, in which the lasing medium is a mixture of helium and neon gases, produces red light with a wavelength of 632.8 nm. Gallium, aluminium and arsenide, the lasing medium of GaAlAs semiconductor diodes, also produces monochromatic radiation, but the wavelength of this depends on the ratio of these three materials and is in the red–infrared range of the electromagnetic spectrum, typically 630–950 nm.

The resonating cavity containing the lasing medium has two parallel surfaces, one being totally reflecting, the other being partially reflecting. Photons emitted from the lasing medium are reflected between these surfaces, some of them leaving through the partially reflecting surface as the laser beam. The cavity of a HeNe laser is many centimetres long, whereas that of a GaAlAs semiconductor diode is tiny, the diode being the lasing medium and its polished ends the reflecting surfaces. Most LILT devices are currently of the GaAlAs type. Their treatment heads may contain either one or several diodes. Those with one diode resemble laser pointers and are designed to treat acupuncture and trigger points; they can also be used to treat points in and around wounds. Those with many diodes are generally called cluster probes and allow large areas to be treated rapidly. The diodes may be housed in a rigid head (Fig. 26.11) or in a flexible material. The latter can be applied around curved surfaces such as the shoulder. Cluster probes housing up to 50 diodes are available; groups of these diodes emit different wavelengths in the red and infrared range. The red light targets all cells, whereas different wavelengths in the infrared range appear to target specific cell types. In cluster probes usually only some of the diodes produce coherent radiation but all produce monochromatic radiation.

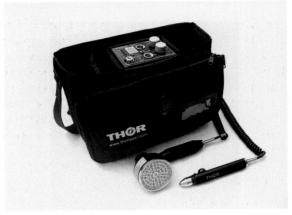

Figure 26.11 A LILT device showing a single diode probe and a multidiode cluster probe (Courtesy of Thor International Ltd)

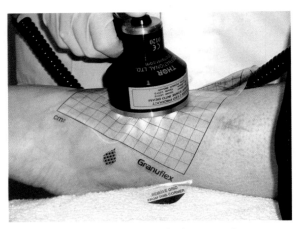

Figure 26.12 LILT cluster probe being used to treat a leg ulcer. (Courtesy of James Carroll.)

The power source for a LILT device may be either a battery or mains electricity. Many LILT devices are portable. The main function of the power source is to energize the lasing medium.

Application of LILT to a leg ulcer

When treating an open wound LILT is usually applied through a transparent dressing via a cluster probe (Fig. 26.12). This can either be placed in contact with the dressing or held just above it if the wound is painful. Mester et al (1985) recommended the use of an energy density of $4\,J/cm^2$, joules being calculated by multiplying the power density (in W/cm^2) by the irradiation time in seconds. In addition to treating the wound bed, Baxter (1996) recommends treating the intact skin around the wound with a single diode probe at points about 1–2 cm from the wound margin and about 2–3 cm apart. The probe should be pressed firmly on to the intact skin. This reduces attenuation by temporarily displacing erythrocytes that would absorb some of the incident energy. It is usually recommended that the energy density applied be no more that $10\,J/cm^2$.

When LILT is used to treat a patient the following treatment parameters should be recorded:

- Wavelength (nm)
- Treatment duration (min)
- Power output (W)
- Power density (W/cm^2): this is calculated by dividing the power output by the irradiating area (or spot size) of the laser. The spot of a semiconductor diode is typically 0.1–$0.125\,cm^2$. This value is multiplied by the number of diodes when a cluster probe is used
- Energy density (J/cm^2): this is calculated by multiplying the power density by the irradiation time in seconds
- If LILT is used in pulsed mode then the pulse repetition rate in hertz (i.e. number of pulses per second) should also be recorded.

LILT bioeffects

For LILT to be effective, the tissue targeted must absorb photons. Absorption is wavelength-dependent. Red light is absorbed by cytochromes in the mitochondria of all living cells, whereas infrared is thought to be absorbed by specific proteins of the cell membrane; these proteins vary according to the type of cell. Provided that appropriate wavelengths and energy densities are used, cell activity can be stimulated if it is suboptimal. Cells in which this has been investigated include mammalian keratinocytes, lymphocytes, macrophages, fibroblasts and endothelial cells, all cells of significance in tissue repair. Much of the research on this has been reviewed by Baxter (1994) and by Tuner & Hode (2002). Cells affected by LILT show a temporary increase in permeability of their cell membranes to calcium ions (Young et al 1990). This may be the mechanism by which LILT modulates cell activity, as has been shown to occur following ultrasound treatment. Other electrotherapeutic modalities may act in a similar fashion.

How LILT stimulates wound healing

Mechanism

The triggering of cell activity by reversible changes in membrane permeability when photons are absorbed could be responsible for the stimulation of tissue repair (Young & Dyson 1993). Increase in calcium uptake by macrophages exposed to red light and infrared *in vitro* has been shown to be wavelength- and energy-density-dependent. Of the wavelengths tested, 660, 820 and 870 nm were effective; 880 nm was ineffective. These same wavelengths also affected growth factor production by the macrophages, 660, 820 and 870 nm being stimulatory whereas 880 nm was not. Energy densities of 4 and 8 J/cm^2 were found to be effective; 2 and 19 J/cm^2 were not (Young et al 1990). Red light of 660 nm wavelength is absorbed by the cytochromes of mitochondria, where it stimulates adenosine triphosphate (ATP) production and increases cytoplasmic H^+ concentration, which can affect cell membrane permeability (Karu 1988). Infrared radiation of 820 and 870 nm may be absorbed by components of the cell membrane. Some of these components vary in different cell types, which may be why the infrared wavelengths absorbed by cells differ according to the cell type. For example, 870 nm affects macrophages (Young et al 1990) but not mast cells (El Sayed & Dyson 1990). It may be possible to selectively stimulate macrophages but not mast cells *in vivo* by exposure to an 870 nm probe; this remains to be investigated.

Following a reversible change in membrane permeability to calcium ions, the cell responds by doing what it is designed to do. In the case of macrophages, this is to produce growth factors and to phagocytose debris; mast cells degranulate, releasing histamine and other substances.

The molecular mechanisms by which LILT affects cell activity begin with photoreception, when the photons are absorbed. This is followed by signal transduction, amplification and a photoresponse, e.g. cell proliferation, protein synthesis and growth factor production, all of which may assist in tissue repair. Membrane structure differs according to the cell type, which, if infrared is absorbed by parts of the membrane, may explain why different cell types absorb different wavelengths of infrared. Theoretically, it should be possible by the judicious selection of infrared wavelengths to affect some cell types while leaving others unaffected. Red light lacks this sensitivity, being absorbed by the mitochondrial cytochromes present in all living cells.

The cellular effects of LILT relevant to tissue repair include the stimulation of:

- ATP production
- Mast cell recruitment and degranulation
- Growth factor release by macrophages
- Keratinocyte proliferation
- Collagen synthesis
- Angiogenesis
- Vasodilatation mediated by increased synthesis of nitric oxide.

At the tissue level there is an acceleration of the resolution of acute inflammation, resulting in the more rapid formation of granulation tissue and re-epithelialization than in sham-irradiated control tissue. Any or all of these effects could help to explain why wound healing can be stimulated by LILT.

Effect of LILT on acute wounds

As with any other technique, the healing of acute wounds can only be stimulated by LILT if they are healing suboptimally, e.g. if they are in a dry environment. In such wounds granulation tissue production can be stimulated, as can wound contraction (Dyson & Young 1986). The most effective energy density reported is 4 J/cm^2.

Effect of LILT on chronic wounds

In 1985 Mester et al surveyed the LILT treatment of over 1000 patients with chronic ulcers; using an energy density of 4 J/cm^2, they showed 50–100% healing, variation being related to the type of lesion and the clinical condition of the patient. It has been suggested that the induction of acute inflammation in chronic wounds by, for example, debridement should precede treatment with LILT, since growth factors released during acute inflammation stimulate healing and it has been shown that LILT can accelerate this phase of healing (Young & Dyson 1993).

More recently Gupta et al (1998) have demonstrated a significantly greater ($p < 0.002$) reduction in the surface area of leg ulcers treated with red light and infrared than in sham irradiated controls. The leg ulcers were given three treatments per week for 10 weeks, by which time the LILT-treated ulcers showed an average reduction in surface area of 193.0 mm^2 whereas the reduction in area of the controls was only 14.7 mm^2.

ELECTRICAL STIMULATION

Electrical stimulation, often referred to as E-stim, has been used since the 1960s to promote wound healing (Assimacopoulos 1968). More recent investigations include those of Gault & Gatens (1976), Akers & Gabrielson (1984) and Feedar et al (1992).

What is E-stim?

According to Sussman & Byl (2001) it is 'the use of a capacitive coupled electric current to transfer energy to a wound'. Although there are other methods of transferring electricity to tissues, capacitive coupling is the most widely available and is non-invasive. It involves the transference of electric current through an electrode pad applied to moistened skin or to the wound bed, both of which act as a wet conductive medium. At least two electrodes are needed to complete the circuit. The electrodes can be placed either within the wound bed or on the intact skin near the wound. The polarity of the electrodes can be varied to alter their effects on the wound. Polarity determines the direction of current flow; electrons move from the negative pole (the cathode) to the positive pole (the anode). Current flow can be either unidirectional or bidirectional.

E-stim can be delivered in a variety of waveforms:

- Continuous unidirectional direct current, also known as galvanic current
- Monophasic pulsed direct current, the pulses or phases being either square wave, or containing two peaks
- Continuous alternating current, also know as biphasic or bipolar. This can be:

- either balanced or unbalanced
- either symmetrical or asymmetrical.

These wave forms are illustrated in Figure 26.13.

E-stim equipment

Electrical stimulators consist of a power source, an oscillator circuit, an output amplifier and electrodes. Portable stimulators are battery-powered. The larger devices have a mains supply. Many incorporate microprocessors, which provide the user with a choice of waveforms and treatment protocols.

The electrodes complete the circuit between the stimulator and the patient. Sussman & Byl (2001) recommend using aluminium foil as electrodes because it is non-toxic, inexpensive, disposable, conformable, a good conductor and can be cut to the size required. The surface area of the electrode affects current density – the smaller the surface area the greater the current density, the deeper the penetration of the current and the greater its effect. Increasing the distance between the electrodes increases the penetration depth, as does increasing the amplitude of the voltage. Usually, one electrode is smaller than the other. The smaller electrode is referred to as the active electrode, the larger as the dispersive electrode.

Direct current devices of both low voltage (typically 60–100 V) and high voltage (typically 100–500 V) are available commercially, as are alternating current devices, which resemble the transcutaneous neural stimulators (TENS) used to reduce pain but have a different waveform.

Application of E-stim to a wound

The dressing covering the wound and on which one of the electrodes is often placed must be a good conductor and keep the wound moist so that the current can be transmitted into the wound bed. Because of their low water content occlusive film dressings are poor conductors. In contrast, fully hydrated hydrocolloid dressings and hydrogels are good conductors and promote healing by:

- Maintaining a moist environment
- Promoting an injury current through this moisture
- Retaining growth factors which stimulate healing.

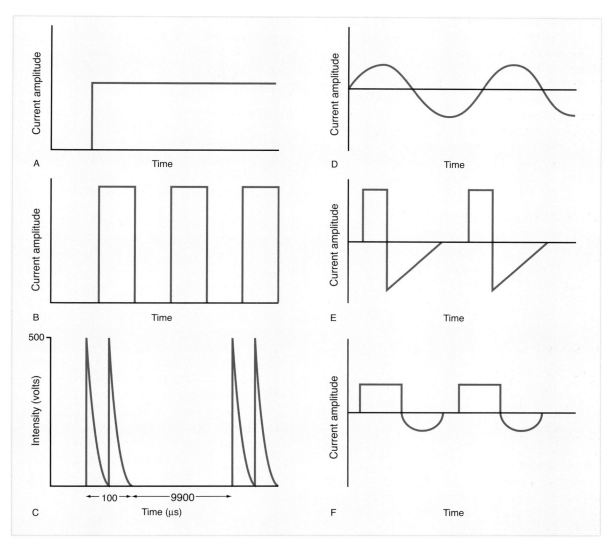

Figure 26.13 Waveforms used in electrical stimulation. (**A**) Unidirectional direct current. (**B**) Monophasic pulsed current. (**C**) High-voltage pulsed current showing twin-peaked monophasic waveform. (**D**) Balanced symmetrical alternating (b phasic) current. (**E**) Balanced asymmetrical alternating (biphasic) current. (**F**) Unbalanced asymmetrical alternating (b phasic) current. (Modified from Sussman & Byl 1998.)

Treatment parameters

Selection of treatment

The biological requirements of the wound vary as it progresses through the healing process. The biological effects of polarity, biphasic currents, frequency and voltage amplitude should all be considered before deciding on an appropriate treatment (Dyson & Lyder 2001).

- *Polarity*: The negative pole is generally used as the active pole during acute inflammation or when the wound is infected. Once this has been resolved the polarity is varied with the aim of matching polarity with changes in the polarity of the injury potential (Kloth & Feedar 1988).
- *Biphasic current*: Baker et al (1996), in their investigations into the effect of biphasic current on pressure ulcers in patients with spinal cord

injuries, found that the best results were obtained with an asymmetrical waveform biased toward the negative pole.

- *Pulsing frequency*: Varying this for high voltage pulsed currents affects blood flow, with lower pulsing frequencies producing higher blood flow velocities (Mohr et al 1987).
- *Amplitude*: This is usually kept constant throughout treatment and is reported as either voltage for high-voltage pulsed currents or as milliamperes (mA) for low-voltage direct current.

The response of the wound to treatment should be monitored non-invasively and subsequent treatments modified if necessary according to this response.

The optimum pattern of treatments using E-stim is not yet known and the treatments used have been arrived at empirically. Polarity is the main variable to have been tested. Sussman & Byl (2001) recommend that the smaller, active electrode:

- Be negative during the acute inflammatory phase and when treating oedematous regions
- Alternate between positive and negative every 3 days during granulation tissue development
- Alternate between positive and negative daily during remodelling.

Direct current

High-voltage pulsed current usually has a monophasic twin-peak waveform (Fig. 26.13C). When used to stimulate wound healing the parameters selected are usually:

- Voltage = 80–200 V
- Pulse rate = 50–120 Hz
- Peak duration = 5–20 μs
- Polarity variable.

Monophasic low voltage microcurrent: When used to stimulate soft tissue healing the parameters selected are usually:

- Voltage <100 V
- Amperage = 200–300 μA.

Alternating current

This is used without pulsing. It appears to be most effective as a wound healing stimulator when its waveform is unbalanced and asymmetrical, in con-

trast to the balanced, symmetrical waveform used in TENS devices to reduce pain (Sussman & Byl 2001).

E-stim bioeffects

Living cells interact creating a bioelectrical environment that is modified by injury. The aim of E-stim is to help normalize this environment and in doing so to accelerate healing. The intact epidermis has an electrical potential across it and acts as a battery that maintains this potential. Positively charged sodium ions are moved by the sodium pump to the deep aspect of the epidermis, leaving an excess of negatively charged chloride ions on its outer surface that develops an electronegative charge of about −23 mV. When the epidermis is injured, current can flow as ions are transmitted through the tissue fluid linking the damaged regions of the epidermis. This unidirectional flow attracts reparative cells to the wound bed by a process termed galvanotaxis. When healing is either completed or arrested, this current, referred to as the injury current, disappears. Debriding a chronic wound restores the injury current.

How electricity stimulates wound healing

Mechanism

This is unknown, but it has been suggested that E-stim may mimic the injury current and thus initiate healing in a chronic wound. This change in the bioelectric environment of a chronic wound may be sufficient to jump-start the healing process (Gentzkow et al 1991). Varying the treatment parameters may act as a stimulus that accelerate the healing process.

Effect of E-stim on acute wounds

When used correctly, E-stim accelerates the resolution of acute inflammation with the result that the proliferative phase begins more rapidly.

Effect of E-stim on chronic wounds

The restoration of an injury current by E-stim may initiate acute inflammation and thus trigger the healing process. Further treatments can accelerate healing. If healing decelerates or stops, then the treatment parameters should be changed. In such cases Kloth (1995) recommends using a high-voltage pulsed current stimulator with daily reversal of the polarity. Regular non-invasive monitoring of the healing process is essential if E-stim is to be used effectively.

HYPERBARIC OXYGEN

Hyperbaric oxygen (HBO), i.e. oxygen at a pressure greater than 1 atmosphere, has been used extensively in medicine as a therapeutic modality since the 19th century when it was used to treat bacterial infections (Irvin & Smith 1968). Among the medical uses of HBO relevant to wound healing and approved by the Undersea and Hyperbaric Medical Society (Thom 1992) are the following:

- Crush injury, the compartment syndrome and other acute traumatic ischaemias
- Enhancement of healing in selected problem wounds such as leg ulcers
- Necrotizing soft tissue infections
- Thermal burns.

The literature on HBO and the healing of diabetic wounds has been reviewed recently by Broussard (2003), the stated aim of this publication being to provide nurses with information about a technology that 'promises to increase the healing potential of foot wounds in patients with diabetes and subsequently reduce amputations in this population'. The literature has also been reviewed recently by Wang et al (2003), the conclusions of this publication being that 'the overall study quality is poor' and that although 'HBO may be helpful for some wounds' more high-quality randomized clinical trials are needed to better inform clinical decision making.

What is hyperbaric oxygen therapy?

Hyperbaric oxygen therapy is the administration of oxygen at pressures greater than 1 atmosphere. It has properties more akin to a drug than to a physical therapy (Kindwall 1993). Its actions include the following:

- It reduces oedema by about 50% in postischaemic muscle through preserving adenosine triphosphate (Nylander et al 1987)

- In acute burns it reduces fluid requirements by 35% in the first 24 hours, thus reducing oedema (Ciani et al 1989)
- It stimulates angiogenesis in ischaemic wounds (Heng 1993).

It can be administered either systemically or topically. The advantages of the topical approach include low cost and lack of systemic oxygen toxicity.

Hyperbaric oxygen therapy equipment

Systemic

Hyperbaric oxygen chambers used for systemic HBO therapy are effectively small rooms in which the patient spends several hours breathing oxygen at 2–3 atmospheres pressure. This increases the amount of dissolved oxygen in the blood and enhances oxygen delivery to hypoxic tissues, provided that the tissues have an adequate blood supply. The chambers can be *monoplace*, accommodating one patient, or *multiplace*, accommodating several patients.

Topical

Hyperbaric oxygen chambers used topically are generally engineered to fit around an injured limb, although disposable polyethylene bags in which oxygen is kept at 1.04 atmospheres have also been used (Heng et al 1984). They enclose the injury and adjacent intact skin. The chamber is sealed on to the intact skin to stop oxygen loss from the chamber. The hyperbaric oxygen is applied directly to the open wound, where it dissolves in tissue fluid, improving the oxygen content of the fluid bathing the cells without necessarily entering the blood capillaries.

This extravascular route for oxygenation is of particular importance in ischaemic wounds 'where some prior oxygenation of the ischaemic tissue is necessary before endothelial proliferation and neovascularization can take place' (Heng 1993). With topical hyperbaric oxygen delivery, the oxygen is only a few microns from the cells. Since diffusion kinetics of gases such as oxygen depend largely on diffusion distances, and with topical administration to an open wound these are minute, the topical HBO devices are very efficient and require lower pressures to stimulate angiogenesis than the

2–3 atmospheres necessary with systemic HBO chambers.

There is a reduced risk of systemic oxygen toxicity with topical HBO chambers because there is little increase in systemic absorption of oxygen. Ways in which systemic oxygen toxicity can manifest itself include grand mal seizures and pulmonary haemorrhage (Morgan et al 1963). However local oxygen toxicity can occur and particular care must be taken with diabetic leg ulcers which are prone to develop oxygen toxicity, probably due to increased levels of glutathione peroxidase induced by HBO (Morykwas & Argenta 1997).

Application of hyperbaric oxygen to a leg ulcer

For an open wound such as a leg ulcer, topical HBO is recommended. All dressings should be removed so that the oxygen can reach the tissue fluid bathing the wound unimpeded. Topical HBO is unsuitable for treating closed injuries, where the only effective method of delivering HBO is systemic. Necrotizing soft tissue infections, myonecrosis, crush injuries, compartment syndrome, refractory osteomyelitis, osteoradionecrosis and compromised skin grafts and flaps all respond well to HBO delivered systemically (Kindwall 1993).

Treatment parameters

Systemic hyperbaric oxygen
The usual regime consists:

- Duration = 90–120 min
- Pressure = 2.0–2.5 atmospheres
- Treatment spacing = 1 per day or 2 per day
- Number of treatments = 10–60, depending on the condition being treated.

Topical hyperbaric oxygen
- Duration: This is variable, for example: 20 minutes twice daily, or 4–6 hours daily
- Pressure = 1.04–2 atmospheres
- Treatment spacing = 1 per day or 2 per day, with a rest period of 2–3 days per week to decrease local endothelial cell toxicity
- Number of treatments: variable.

The above treatment schedules are cited by Morykwas & Argenta (1997). They are empirical.

With open wounds there should be frequent monitoring of response and modification of the treatment regime when indicated by this response.

Hyperbaric oxygen bioeffects

Soft tissue oxygen levels are in normal conditions approximately 40 mmHg. If the levels drop to less than 30 mmHg, metabolic activity is significantly impaired (Grim et al 1990). Local oxygen levels are frequently less than 30 mmHg in injured or infected tissue. Bacterial infection reduces local tissue perfusion and therefore oxygenation. Neutrophils use a significant amount of oxygen when they phagocytose bacteria. Oxygen has been described as an antibiotic (Knighton et al 1984). If the level of oxygen can be increased, this assists in healing and in the fight against infection. HBO is a means of achieving this objective.

Mechanism
The use of hyperbaric oxygen in treating open wounds is based on the increased solubility of oxygen in blood and tissue fluids under hyperbaric conditions (Illingworth et al 1961). The extra dissolved oxygen carried in the blood of a patient breathing oxygen at an elevated pressure of 2–3 atmospheres enhances delivery to hypoxic tissues, provided that these tissues are adequately vascularized. However, the problem in wound healing is not so much the level of oxygenation of the blood but rather inadequate vascularization of the wound. When hyperbaric oxygen is supplied topically it reaches the tissue fluid bathing the cells of the wound bed directly, bypassing the blood vessels supplying the wound. The cells involved in the healing process are therefore better oxygenated for the period that the oxygen is supplied. This temporary oxygenation of the wound bed is necessary for many of the processes involved in wound healing, including:

- Phagocytosis of bacteria by neutrophils
- Endothelial cell proliferation and thus for vascularization of the wound bed
- Collagen synthesis.

It should be appreciated that even with topical hyperbaric oxygen there is a risk of oxygen toxicity, but this is purely local. It includes the destruction of newly formed blood vessels but can be avoided by allowing several days of rest from HBO therapy each week (Heng 1993). Furthermore, the relative hypoxia occurring during the rest periods is a stimulus to growth factor release and capillary formation. When cells are hypoxic they are unable to generate reduced glutathione, which protects them against free radical attack (Andreoli et al 1986). When oxygen is reintroduced into ischaemic tissues during reperfusion, lipid peroxidation and damage of the cell membranes can occur from an excess of free radicals. However, hyperbaric oxygen inhibits lipid peroxidation, thus protecting cell membranes from damage (Raskin et al 1971). It is important to realize that the effects on injured tissues of the presence and absence of oxygen are complex. The beneficial aspects of hyperbaric oxygen on wound healing may be negated by failure to identify and react to signs of oxygen toxicity. Tissue responses should therefore be monitored non-invasively throughout the healing process and treatments should be amended where appropriate.

Effect of hyperbaric oxygen on acute wounds

Minor burns and scalds show accelerated healing when treated with topical HBO. Reported effects cited by Heng (1993) include:

- Oedema reduction
- Increased collagen synthesis
- Increased angiogenesis
- Accelerated re-epithialization.

Effect of hyperbaric oxygen on chronic wounds

Chronic ischaemic leg ulcers benefit from HBO. It can initiate healing and within about 3 weeks the wound bed is usually well vascularized. Healing generally continues after the HBO therapy has been discontinued (Heng et al 1984).

VACUUM-ASSISTED CLOSURE THERAPY

Also known as *negative pressure therapy*, and *subatmospheric therapy*, vacuum-assisted closure (VAC) therapy is a non-invasive technique entailing exposure of a wound to pressure of less than one atmosphere (Morykwas & Argenta 1997, Clare

et al 2002, Egington et al 2003). The effects of this include:

- Dilation of the arterioles, improving the blood supply to the wound
- Removal of excess fluid thus reducing oedema
- Reduction in bacterial colonization of a wound by drawing off many of the bacteria with this fluid
- Improved granulation tissue formation, resulting in progressive wound closure.

What is vacuum-assisted closure therapy?

VAC therapy is the application of subatmospheric pressure, either continuously or intermittently, to an open wound such as a leg ulcer. A VAC device to do this has been manufactured for clinical use by Kinetic Concepts, Inc. It delivers negative pressure (vacuum) uniformly to the wound bed and to the tissue adjacent to it. Case studies have documented its effectiveness (Morykwas & Argenta 1997) in the treatment of acute and chronic wounds.

Vacuum-assisted closure equipment

The VAC negative-pressure equipment consists of:

- VAC negative-pressure unit (Fig. 26.14)
- VAC PAC dressing pack, containing sterile foam dressing, suction tubing, occlusive transparent drapes
- Canister to collect the exudate and tubing for connection between the VAC unit and the foam dressing.

Application of vacuum-assisted closure to a wound

- The foam dressing is cut to the shape of the wound and applied to the wound, which has been irrigated with normal saline
- The foam dressing and at least 3.5 cm of surrounding intact skin is covered with the occlusive transparent drapes to ensure an occlusive seal and convert the open wound into a controlled closed wound; the drape is also sealed to the tube leaving the dressing
- The free end of the tubing from the foam dressing is connected to the tubing on the unit

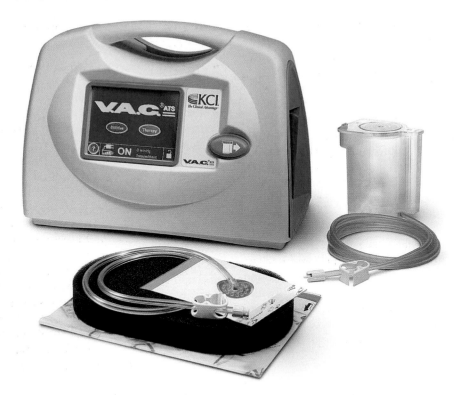

Figure 26.14 VAC unit (Courtesy of KCI Medical Ltd.)

- The unit is set to deliver the type of negative pressure required, continuous or intermittent, and the device is switched on.

Treatment parameters (supplied by Kinetic Concepts, Inc.)

These vary according to the type of wound being treated. The following example is for venous stasis, arterial insufficiency and diabetic ulcers:

- Cycle: continuous for 5 days
- Duration: ideally 24 hours a day. The dressing should be removed if therapy has to be discontinued for more than 2 hours a day
- Target pressure: 50–75 mmHg
- Dressing change: every 48 hours or every 12 hours if the wound is infected.

Bioeffects of vacuum-assisted closure therapy

The continuous subatmospheric pressure used at the commencement of treatment draws fluid from the wound bed and surrounding tissue, decreasing local interstitial pressure and allowing vessels previously compressed or collapsed to dilate, restoring blood flow. The intermittent negative pressure applied later assists the proliferative phase of repair when granulation tissue forms.

Mechanism

The use of negative pressure therapy to remove tissue fluid from the wound bed and its oedematous surroundings is based on the supposition that the removal of this fluid will enhance the healing process. Certainly reduction in oedema and therefore of pressure on the microcirculatory system is advantageous in that the reduced pressure allows the vessels to dilate, with the result that perfusion of the wound is improved. Also the fluid from chronic wounds contains factors that, when applied to cells *in vitro*, suppress cell division and protein synthesis. However later in the healing process the fluid contains beneficial growth factors secreted by macrophages and other cells, factors that can enhance the development of granulation tissue. Analysis of the fluid withdrawn from chronic and healing wounds has demonstrated this change (Morykwas & Argenta 1997). It should therefore, ideally, only be used until this change occurs.

Another mechanism of action of the VAC is the mechanical stimulation of cells by tensile forces placed on the surrounding tissue when the applied vacuum collapses the foam dressing. This results in deformation of the cells anchored in the tissues. Integrins act as transmembrane bridges between the applied extracellular forces and the cytoskeleton. Perturbation of the integrin bridges distorts the cell membrane and results in the release of second messengers that trigger changes in gene expression with subsequent increases in cell proliferation and protein synthesis.

Effect of vacuum-assisted closure therapy on acute wounds

The treatment parameters recommended by Kinetic Concepts are as follows:

- Cycle: continuous for the first 48 h to evacuate excess fluid from the wound; intermittent thereafter (standard: 5 min on, 2 min off) to promote granulation tissue formation
- Duration: ideally 24 h a day
- Target pressure: 125 mmHg
- Dressing change: every 48 h or every 12 h if the wound is infected.

This produces a rapid reduction in oedema followed by an acceleration of granulation tissue formation.

Effect of vacuum-assisted closure on chronic wounds

VAC has been used successfully to treat venous ulcers, arterial insufficiency and neuropathic (diabetic) ulcers. The recommended treatment parameters are:

- Cycle: continuous treatment for the duration of the therapy
- Duration: ideally 24 h a day
- Target pressure: 50–75 mmHg
- Dressing change: every 48 h or every 12 h if the wound is infected.

CONCLUSIONS

All the adjunctive therapies described can assist in wound healing if used in an appropriate manner. Most act by assisting in the resolution of inflammation so that the proliferative phase of healing begins earlier, leading to speedier wound closure. Cell activity is jump-started by changes in membrane permeability, with the result that healing is accelerated. The clinician responsible for treating an injured patient is better equipped to select the most beneficial treatment for the patient if armed with an understanding of each therapy and of its mode of action.

The ultimate test of any therapy is the way in which the patient responds to it. Systemic changes in the patient should be documented and their wounds should be imaged non-invasively throughout healing by, for example, digital photography and high-resolution diagnostic ultrasound. Changes in wound structure and physiology should be quantified where possible so that valid comparisons can be made. The sharing of findings via peer-reviewed journals and conference presentations will add to our understanding of these therapies and improve the lot of injured patients.

Patients heal their wounds themselves; a major role of the nurse is to help them do so.

References

Agaiby A, Ghali L, Dyson M 1998 Laser modulation of T-lymphocyte proliferation in vitro. Laser Therapy 10: 153–158

Akers T K, Gabrielson A L 1984 The effect of high voltage galvanic stimulation on the rate of healing of decubitus ulcers. Biomedical Sciences Instrumentation 20: 99–100

Andreoli S P, Mallet C P, Bergstein J M 1986 Role of glutathione in protecting cells against hydrogen peroxide oxidant injury. Journal of Laboratory and Clinical Medicine 108: 190–198

Assimacopoulos D 1968 Wound healing promotion by the use of negative electric current. American Surgeon 34: 423–442

Baker L L, Rubayi S et al 1996 Effect of electrical stimulation on healing of ulcers in human beings with spinal cord injury. Wound Repair and Regeneration 4: 21–28

Baxter D 1994 Therapeutic lasers: theory and practice. Churchill Livingstone, Edinburgh

Baxter D 1996 Low intensity laser therapy. In: Kitchen S, Bazin S (eds) Clayton's electrotherapy, 10th edn. W B Saunders, London, pp 197–217

Broussard C L 2003 Hyperbaric oxygen and wound healing. Journal of Wound, Ostomy and Continence Nursing 30: 210–216

Ciani P, Lueders H M et al 1989 Adjunctive hyperbaric oxygen therapy reduced length of hospitalization in thermal burns. Journal of Burn Care and Rehabilitation 19: 432–435

Clare M P, Fitzgibbons T C, McMullen S T et al 2002 Experience with the vacuum assisted closure negative pressure technique in the treatment of non-healing diabetic and dysvascular wounds. Foot and Ankle International 23: 896–901

Dyson M 1995 Role of ultrasound in wound healing. In: McCulloch J M, Kloth L C, Fudar J A (eds) Wound healing: alternatives in management, 2nd edn. F A Davis, Philadelphia, PA, pp 318–346

Dyson M 1997 Advances in wound healing physiology: the comparative perspective. Veterinary Dermatology 8: 227–233

Dyson M, Lyder C 2001 Wound management: physical modalities. In: Morison M J (ed.) The prevention and treatment of pressure ulcers. Mosby, Edinburgh, pp 177–193

Dyson M, Pond J 1973 The effects of ultrasound on circulation. Physiotherapy 59: 284–287

Dyson M, Young S R 1986 The effects of laser therapy on wound contraction and cellularity. Lasers in Medical Science 1: 125–130

Dyson M, Franks C, Suckling J 1976 Stimulation of healing of varicose ulcers by ultrasound. Ultrasonics 14: 232–236

Dyson M, Agaiby A, Ghali L 2002 Photobiomodulation of human T-lymphocyte proliferation in vitro. Lasers in Medical Science 17(4): A22

Dyson M, Moodley S, Verjee L et al 2003 Wound healing assessment using 20 MHz ultrasound and macrophotography. Skin Research and Technology 9: 116–121

Egington M T, Brown K R, Seabrook G R et al 2003 A prospective randomized evaluation of negative-pressure wound dressings for diabetic foot wounds. Annals of Vascular Surgery 17: 645–649

El Sayed S, Dyson M 1990 A comparison of the effect of multiwave-length light produced by a cluster of semiconductor diodes and each individual diode on mast cell number and degranulation in intact and injured skin. Lasers in Surgery and Medicine 10: 559–568

Feedar J F, Kloth L C, Gentzkow G D 1992 Chronic dermal ulcer healing enhanced with monophasic pulsed electrical stimulation. Physical Therapy 72: 539.

Gault W R, Gatens P F Jr 1976 Use of low intensity direct current in management of ischemic skin ulcers. Physical Therapy 56: 265–269

Gentzkow G D, Pollack S V et al 1991 Improved healing of pressure ulcers using Dermapulse, a new electrical stimulation device. Wounds 3: 158–160

Grim O, Gottlieb L, Boddie A 1990 Hyperbaric oxygen therapy. Journal of the American Medical Association 263: 2216–2220

Gupta A K, Filonenko N, Salansky N, Sauder D N 1998 The use of low energy photon therapy (LEPT) in venous leg ulcers: a double-blind, placebo-controlled study. Dermatologic Surgery 24: 1383–1386

Hart J 1993 The effect of therapeutic ultrasound on dermal repair with emphasis on fibroblast activity. PhD Thesis, University of London

Heng M C Y 1993 Topical hyperbaric therapy for problem skin wounds. Journal of Dermatologic Surgery and Oncology 19: 784–793

Heng M C Y, Pilgrim J P, Beck F W J 1984 A simplified hyperbaric oxygen technique for leg ulcers. Archives of Dermatology 120: 640–645

Hoogland R 1986 Ultrasound therapy. Enraf-Nonius, Delft, pp 12–13

Illingworth C F, Smith G, Lawson D D et al 1961 Surgical and physiological observations in experimental pressure chambers. British Journal of Surgery 49: 111–117

Irvin T, Smith G 1968 Treatment of bacterial infections with hyperbaric oxygen. Surgery 63: 362–376

Karu T I 1988 Molecular mechanisms of the therapeutic effect of low-intensity laser irradiation. Lasers in the Life Sciences 2: 53–74

Kindwall E P 1993 Hyperbaric oxygen. More indications than many doctors realize. British Medical Journal 307: 515–516

Kloth L C 1995 Electrical stimulation in tissue repair. In: McCulloch J M, Kloth L C, Feedar J A (eds) Wound healing: alternatives in management, 2nd edn. F A Davis, Philadelphia, PA, pp.275–310

Kloth LC, Feedar J 1988 Acceleration of wound healing with high voltage, monophasic, pulsed current. Physical Therapy 68: 503–508

Knighton D, Halliday B, Hunt T K 1984 Oxygen as an antibiotic. Archives of Surgery 119: 199–204

McDiarmid T, Burns P N, Lewith G T, Machin D 1985, Ultrasound and the treatment of pressure sores. Physiotherapy 71: 66–70

Mester E, Mester A F, Mester A 1985 The biomedical effects of laser application. Lasers in Surgery and Medicine 5: 31–39

Mohr T, Akers T, Wessman H C 1987 Effect of high voltage stimulation on blood flow in the rat hind leg. Physical Therapy 67: 526–533

Morgan T E Jr, et al 1963 Effects on man of prolonged exposure at a total pressure of 190 mmHg. Aerospace Medicine 34: 589–592

Morykwas M J, Argenta L C 1997 Nonsurgical modalities to enhance healing and care of soft tissue injuries. Journal of the Southern Orthopaedic Association 6: 279–288

Nussbaum E L, Biemann I, Mustard B 1994 Comparison of ultrasound, ultraviolet C and laser for treatment of pressure ulcers in patients with spinal cord injury. Physical Therapy 74: 812–825

Nylander G, Norstrom H, Eriksson E 1984 Effects of hyperbaric oxygen on oedema formation after a scald burn. Burns Including Thermal Injury 10: 193–196

Peschen M, Weichenthal M, Schopf E, Vanscheidt W 1997 Low-frequency ultrasound treatment of chronic venous ulcers in an outpatient therapy. Acta Dermato-Venereologica (Stockholm) 77: 311–314

Raskin P, Lipman R L, Oloff C M 1971 Effect of hyperbaric oxygen on lipid peroxidation in the lung. Aerospace Medicine 42: 28–30

Sussman C, Bates-Jensen M 2001 Wound care a collaborative practice manual for physical therapists and nurses, 2nd edn. Aspen, Gaithersburg, MD

Sussman C, Byl N 2001 Electrical stimulation for wound healing. In: Sussman C, Bates-Jensen M (eds) Wound care a collaborative practice manual for physical therapists and nurses, 2nd edn. Aspen, Gaithersburg, MD, pp 497–545

Sussman C, Dyson M 2001 Therapeutic and diagnostic ultrasound. In: Sussman C, Bates-Jensen M (eds) Wound care a collaborative practice manual for physical therapists and nurses, 2nd edn. Aspen, Gaithersburg, MD, pp pp.596–620

Thom S R 1992 Hyperbaric oxygen therapy: a committee report. Undersea and Hyperbaric Medical Society, Bethesda, MD

Tuner J, Hode L 2002 Laser therapy: clinical practice and scientific background. Prima Books, Grangesberg, Sweden

Wang C, Schwaitzberg S, Berliner E et al 2003 Hyperbaric oxygen for treating wounds: a systematic review of the literature. Archives of Surgery 138: 272–279

Ward A R 1986 Electricity, fields and waves in therapy. Science Press, Marrickville, Australia

Young S R, Dyson M 1993 The effect of ultrasound and light therapy on tissue repair. In: Macleod D A D, Maughan C, Williams C R et al (eds) Intermittent high intensity exercise. Chapman & Hall, London, pp 321–328

Young S R, Dyson M, Bolton P 1990 Effect of light on calcium uptake by macrophages. Laser Therapy 2: 53–57

Ziskin M C, Michlovitz S L 1990 Therapeutic ultrasound. In: Michlovitz S L (ed.) Thermal agents in rehabilitation. F A Davis, Philadelphia, PA, pp 141–176

Dermatological aspects of leg ulcers

Marco Romanelli, Paolo Romanelli

INTRODUCTION

The skin surrounding a chronic leg ulcer can manifest different clinical signs associated with the underlying pathology. In our experience, patients with leg ulcers are usually more concerned about the signs and symptoms of surrounding skin than about wound bed aspects. In addition, the surrounding skin often indicates the positive or negative effects of a given therapy. We can therefore classify the dermatological aspects of leg ulcers into two different groups according to their presentation:

1. Related to ulcer aetiology:
   - Lipodermatosclerosis
   - Skin hyperpigmentation
   - Atrophie blanche
2. Related to ulcer complications:
   - Eczema
   - Allergic contact dermatitis
   - Irritant contact dermatitis
   - Infection
   - Vasculitis
   - Neoplastic proliferation.

Knowledge of skin anatomy and physiology is essential in order to better understand the pathophysiological mechanisms underlying the dermatological aspects associated with leg ulcers.

AETIOLOGY

Venous leg ulcers represent the most common problem among patients suffering from peripheral vascular disease. About 1.5% of the adult population of the Western world will be affected by chronic leg ulcers at some point during their lifetimes and skin aspects have recently been considered an essential component of the CEAP classification (Beebe et al 1995). (The classification has been proposed as a uniform system for chronic venous dysfunction.) Skin changes associated with venous insufficiency of the lower leg are predominantly due to venous hypertension, which is followed by the interstitial accumulation of haemosiderin.

Lipodermatosclerosis

Lipodermatosclerosis (LDS) is a clinical condition often associated with venous insufficiency and characterized by skin induration and hyperpigmentation (Kirsner et al 1993). Prolonged venous hypertension is responsible for an increase in the size and permeability of dermal skin capillaries in the area affected and subsequently for the leaking of blood macromolecules into the dermis. Acute and chronic stages of LDS have been described: the former involves erythematous (tender and painful skin), while in the chronic stage the leg becomes shaped like an inverted bottle of champagne with a scaly, brown hyperpigmented and indurated area (Fig. 27.1), which is localized predominantly at the gaiter site. The acute phase may be misdiagnosed as a form of cellulitis, which is usually followed by an inappropriate use of antibiotics and the removal of bandages. The chronic stage is not necessarily a result of the acute stage. LDS is associated with an

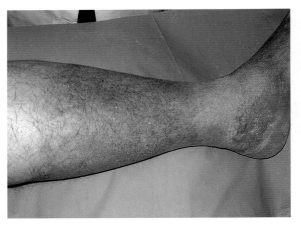

Figure 27.1 Lipodermatosclerosis in a patient with venous insufficiency of lower leg.

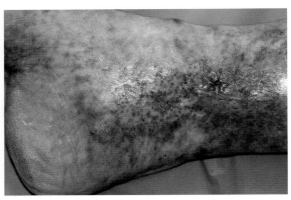

Figure 27.2 Atrophie blanche on medial area of the leg.

increased risk of leg ulceration and patients with venous leg ulcers as part of their LDS have shown a correlation between the degree of skin induration and time to healing (Nemeth et al 1989). Skin induration in LDS can be measured objectively using a durometer, thereby providing a useful prognostic tool (Romanelli & Falanga 1995). The treatment of LDS consists of graded compression stockings, which have been shown to reduce the level of pain and the mean area of induration and thickening (Browse et al 1977). The anabolic steroid stanozolol has been used to enhance fibrinolysis in several reported cases of patients with LDS. The main result of this treatment was a rapid and consistent reduction of induration and pain, which were correlating to a decrease in pericapillary fibrin (Burnand et al 1980).

Hyperpigmentation

A brown staining around the gaiter area of the lower leg is a common sign in patients with venous insufficiency and this is due to the accumulation of haemosiderin in the interstitial space. Other vasculitic processes may leave a residual post-inflammatory hyperpigmentation, which is less persistent than venous stasis. Recurrent superficial infection of the skin, such as erysipelas, can also be frequent in patients with a lymphedematous leg and may lead to a browning discoloration of the area involved.

Atrophie blanche

The term atrophie blanche is used to describe an ivory-white patch (Fig. 27.2), usually located on the medial aspect of the lower limbs, filled with telangiectasias and surrounded by hyperpigmentation (Maessen-Visch et al 1999). The area affected may be different in size, with an irregular shape. The early lesion signs may be crusting and blister formation, after which it becomes atrophic and coalesces with other lesions. In the early stage, lesions are usually without symptoms. The area is extremely fragile and prone to ulceration, which occurs in about 30% of cases (Milstone et al 1983). Such ulcers are small in size and consistently hard to heal. The aetiology of atrophie blanche is not clear, but most cases have been associated with non-inflammatory, usually thrombophilic, disorders such as venous stasis. An obliteration of capillaries from the middle and deep dermis has been hypothesized as the underlying cause of atrophie blanche. The area must be protected from further trauma; elastic compression with rest has been shown to improve the progression of this aspect. Topical treatment of atrophie blanche include the use of mild emollients and skin protectants. Use of topical steroids in this area can cause further damage, including ulceration, due to the very fragile skin, and therefore must be avoided. Pharmacological treatment that stimulates fibrinolytic activity and inhibits platelet thrombosis has also been shown to be effective in controlling the progression of atrophie blanche (Pizzo et al 1986).

ULCER COMPLICATIONS

Eczema

Eczema is a pruritic, epidermal and dermal inflammatory reaction of the skin, which is caused or complicated by a variety of external or constitutional factors (Box 27.1).

Skin changes of the lower leg associated with venous disease often manifest as stasis eczema. About two-thirds of patients suffering from chronic leg ulcers display signs of contact sensitization to

---

Box 27.1   Types of eczema

Exogenous eczema
- Irritant contact dermatitis
- Allergic contact dermatitis
- Phototoxic contact dermatitis
- Photoallergic contact dermatitis

Endogenous eczema
- Atopic eczema
- Seborrhoeic eczema
- Pompholyx
- Eczematous psoriasis
- Venous stasis dermatitis

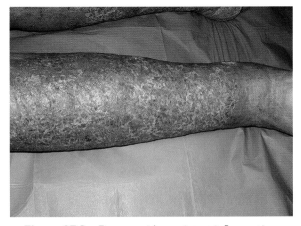

Figure 27.3 Eczema with persistent inflammation.

topical treatment (Machet et al 2004). The exact mechanism involved in the eczematous skin changes of lower legs is unclear, but an underlying hypoxic state, due to the presence of pericapillary fibrin cuffs or arteriovenous shunts, leading to poor tissue nutrition, has been postulated.

Clinical features

The typical appearance of this condition, secondary to venous hypertension, consists of a combination of erythema, oedema, scaling and weeping, accompanied by intense itching (Fig. 27.3). The onset of symptoms may be extremely rapid and in this case is frequently associated with deep vein thrombosis. The lower leg swells with an erythematous, warm and eczematous state. The superficial venous system presents many varicosities, with oedema, purpuric lesions, brown hyperpigmentation and small areas of atrophie blanche (which can lead to ulceration). The area affected by venous stasis eczema reflects the perforating veins area and is mainly located on the medial and lateral aspects of the leg above the malleoli. The progression of skin changes proximally involves the entire leg; occasionally the foot may also be affected. At this stage the frequent application of topical products can exacerbate the situation and cause recurrent flares of acute dermatitis, leading to contact dermatitis. The perpetuation of the inflammatory stage in the dermis and subcutaneous tissue causes repeated red blood cell extravasation due to venous hypertension, and results in fat necrosis due to tissue hypoxia. These two conditions create the lipodermatosclerotic status of the lower leg, which is the result of a sclerotic involvement of the interstitial spaces and replaces the oedema from the earlier stage.

Histology

Histologic examination shows either an acute, subacute or chronic dermatitis pattern. Spongiotic microvesicles or macrovesicles with oozing are present in acute dermatitis, while a combination of acanthosis and parakeratosis is the histologic picture of the chronic stage. Subacute dermatitis is a combination of the two reaction patterns and is difficult to distinguish from the other forms of dermatitis. Chronic lesions show numerous dilated capillaries embedded in a fibrotic dermis. Secondary changes can also occur in the arterioles and venules consisting of intimal proliferation and medial hyperplasia.

Differential diagnosis

The clinical picture of stasis eczema is characteristic and generally associated with positive instrumental assessment for venous insufficiency. The involvement of leg swelling could be unilateral in the presence of venous thrombosis or lymphatic obstruction, but also bilateral if caused by congestive heart failure or congenital lymphedema other than venous obstruction. If an ulcer is located in the area of dermatitis, it is necessary to make proper assessment to identify ulcer aetiology and to follow up with an appropriate treatment. There are several eczematous changes that must be differentiated before starting a therapeutic regimen.

Asteatotic eczema   This problem is commonly found in the elderly and is secondary to systemic diseases, environmental aspects, and drug treatment. The condition is clinically characterized by fine scaling with a very dry itching skin, which then fissures with a cracked appearance. The legs do not present any erythematous appearance or swelling. Use of topical emollients is recommended in these patients and products with an ointment as a vehicle are the most appropriate to avoid skin irritation.

Psoriasis   Lesions are well-circumscribed plaques with an erythematous, scaly aspect (Fig. 27.4). Other sites are involved, such as the knees, elbows and scalp.

Fungal infection   A direct mycological test must be carried out on any scaling of the foot or leg. Fungal lesions may appear as coin-shaped patches with an erythematous scaly border. The groin area is commonly involved. Fungal infection involving the intertriginous area can easily spread to the dorsum of the foot, but it is difficult and unusual that the lower leg is affected and chronic wounds management influenced by this problem. Treatment of fungal infection on the lower leg and foot must give particular attention to drying the affected area, which is frequently under a compression system because of venous insufficiency. Antifungal powders are used for this purpose together with systemic

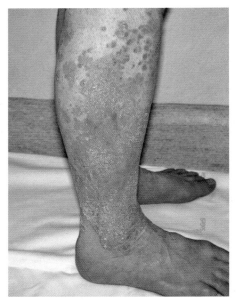

Figure 27.4   Psoriasis involving the leg.

treatment, which is today prescribed most of the time as a pulse therapy to minimize side effects.

Contact dermatitis   The development of contact dermatitis is a common complication in patients with stasis eczema and can be classified either as allergic contact dermatitis or irritant contact dermatitis. Because of the chronic nature of leg ulcers, patients are exposed to different topical treatments and sensitization therefore occurs over the course of their lives. The prevalence of contact dermatitis among patients with leg ulcers ranges from 37% to 85% (Angelini et al 1975). More than 50% of these patients tested positive for two or more allergens (Tavadia et al 2003). In the case of stasis eczema in patients with venous insufficiency, there is damage to the stratum corneum, which is normally the first barrier against the external environment. The skin becomes dry and cracked because of the loss of water, allowing the irritants to penetrate the epidermis and dermis easily. A clear distinction between allergic and irritant contact dermatitis is very difficult to make from a clinical and histological point of view; this is mainly because the inflammatory reaction that follows hapten sensitization is very similar.

Allergic contact dermatitis This is a delayed, type IV hypersensitivity, starting from a specific sensitization in a low-molecular-weight hapten. After the first contact with the skin, the sensitization occurs in the regional lymph node. During a second sensitization to the same hapten, the sensitized T lymphocytes are recruited via chemoattractants, and cytokines are released with an inflammatory reaction similar to the one that occurs in irritant contact dermatitis. The risk of developing sensitization is dependent upon several factors, ranging from the allergenic properties of the substance to the duration and type of exposure, bearing in mind the fact that in chronic wound management medications are applied frequently under occlusion, a situation that can turn a mild sensitizer into a major problem (Fig. 27.5).

Irritant contact dermatitis This is caused by external agents topically applied to legs with stasis eczema. Because the epidermal barrier is disrupted, there is an inflammatory reaction to penetration of irritants with an increase in transepidermal water loss. Symptoms and clinical appearance may be moderate to severe, according to the degree of exposure. Patients affected by irritant contact dermatitis on the legs present early symptoms such as itching, burning and stinging sensations, and pain.

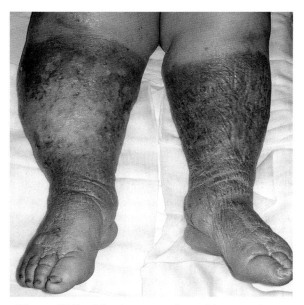

Figure 27.5 Allergic contact dermatitis to parabens.

> **Box 27.2 *Groups of leg ulcer allergens***
>
> - Lanolin and derivatives
> - Rubber
> - Topical antibiotics
> - Preservatives
> - Balsam of Peru
> - Adhesives
> - Fragrances

Because of the wide range of topical medications available today for wound management, there is an increased risk that patients may be sensitized as a result of different allergens being applied to the open wound and surrounding eczematous skin. Patch testing is the best way to identify potential allergens and must be performed on any patient attending a leg ulcer clinic with a history of contact dermatitis. The test is simple to administer but may require special expertise for its interpretation. The patient and caregivers must receive written information about the results of the tests. Patch testing must be performed as often as necessary over the years. The list of allergens to be tested is increasing every year and must include advanced wound dressing materials, although we have noted less sensitivity to dressings such as hydrocolloids, hydrogels, hydrofibres and polyurethane foams. The most common allergens in chronic venous leg ulcers are listed in Box 27.2.

Treatment of contact dermatitis is based on identification and avoidance of the allergen involved. In our experience, bed rest and systemic treatment is the most effective care for such patients. As dermatologists we prefer to avoid the use of topical corticosteroids, even for short periods, because they too may sensitize over the course of long-term application.

Infection

Most primary chronic wounds are characterized by an increased susceptibility to infection, and

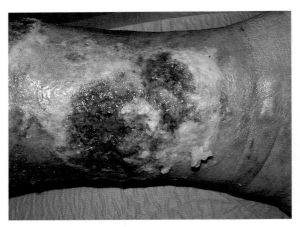

Figure 27.6 Critical colonization in a venous leg ulcer.

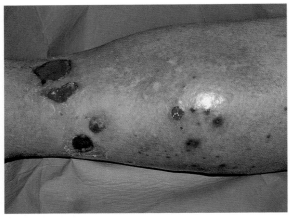

Figure 27.7 Cutaneous leukocytoclastic vasculitis.

in many the symptoms are prominent clinical features. In general, the kind of cutaneous infection that occurs reflects to some degree the role of the deficient component in the host defence. Bacterial infections due to the common pathogens *Staphylococcus aureus* and *Streptococcus pyogenes* are the most common cutaneous bacterial infections associated with chronic wounds. Treatment consists of the use of systemic antibiotics that cover penicillinase-producing organisms. If the infection is recurrent or does not respond to the usual therapies, it is very helpful to obtain a culture from the wound bed and to perform appropriate antibiotic sensitivity testing. Treatment of frequent recurrences may require prolonged courses of systemic antibiotics, associated with topical antimicrobial dressings. The response to treatment can also be different in various chronic wounds (Fig. 27.6). For this reason, biopsies should be performed on any wound bed that presents with an unusual clinical course or an unusual response to therapy, and the tissue should be sent for multiple cultures, including special media if there is a clinical indication.

Vasculitis

Vasculitis refers to disease processes involving inflammation of the blood vessel wall together with necrosis, which are the result of the deposition of circulating immune complexes. Aetiological agents in vasculitis include infection, drugs, autoimmune diseases, malignant diseases and other unknown factors. Vasculitis presents many challenges to the physician, including classification and diagnosis. A classification system for vasculitis is difficult to obtain and may be based on several issues, such as the clinical features of the disease, issues of whether the disease is systemic or cutaneous, and vessel size. In our opinion, this latter aspect is one of the most acceptable and useful working criteria, since it divides vasculitis into three types by vessel size: small-, medium- and large-vessel involvement. A histopathological confirmation of the clinical diagnosis can be obtained with a punch biopsy specimen of a lesion at the appropriate stage. Clinical features of vasculitis include a palpable purpura as a primary lesion, which then progresses to papules, nodules, vesicles, plaques, bullae or pustules. Secondary changes include ulceration, necrosis and postinflammatory hyperpigmentation (Fig. 27.7).

Because vasculitis is generally self-limiting, treatment is often unnecessary. Vasculitic ulcers are treated according to the moist wound healing concept, paying greater attention to pain control and prevention. Topical treatment includes debridement of necrotic tissue and use of occlusive dressings, which are going to protect the skin from further trauma. Systemic treatment is directed toward prevention of visceral involvement and alleviation of symptoms. Steroids are often prescribed as a systemic treatment together with immunosuppressive agents. Topical steroid creams are sometimes used on the surrounding skin to reduce the inflammatory aspect. Caution should be used with these preparations because of the risk of atrophy and skin sensitization. A mild steroid such as hydrocortisone cream 1% is usually essential for skin management.

Neoplastic proliferation

Malignant transformation in a chronic ulcer is a rare event and was first described by Marjolin in 1828 with regard to areas of ulceration in chronic burns scars. The most common type of skin cancer observed in chronic ulcers is squamous cell carcinoma; this is in comparison with basal cell carcinoma, which has also been frequently reported as a malignant degeneration in chronic wounds (Blank & Schnyder 1990). The main topic for debate is whether the malignancy originates as a primary skin cancer or manifests as a secondary transformation in a pre-existing chronic tissue. There have been several hypotheses concerning the development of skin cancer in chronic wounds, mainly reflecting the role of venous stasis as the main reason for degeneration.

Squamous cell carcinoma and basal cell carcinoma in leg ulcers have been found to be difficult to diagnose because of the absence of a clear clinical picture of malignancy. The wound bed most of the time presents with fully granulating, shiny tissue with a typical red colour and evidence of hypergranulation. The wound edge may give some indications in order to rule out skin cancer. Because the clinical aspects of malignant transformation in chronic wounds are not very well defined, the main criteria for identification are a non-healing progression (despite optimal standard care) and a positive biopsy. A wound biopsy must be taken for any suspected wound or at least after 3 months of non-progression and tissue sample has been obtained from the wound bed and the edge including surrounding skin. A proportional increase of squamous cell carcinoma on legs in females compared to males in the Swedish population (12% vs 7%) represents an interesting aspect that was connected to different clothing habits and patterns of actinic radiation (Cancer Registry 1981–1990).

Patients with chronic leg ulcers should be carefully instructed by their physicians about clinical features and changes in the wound bed and surrounding skin appearance in order to receive early and appropriate treatment.

SKIN CARE

The care of the skin surrounding leg ulcers is an essential aspect in wound management. Dry skin is a factor affecting 70% of the elderly population and is a very common feature of patients with chronic wounds. Attention to improving the dryness every day is critical. There are many emollients commercially available and patients vary in their acceptance of them. Products based on an ointment vehicle have been considered to be more effective and have fewer side effects than creams, which in general are not satisfactory emollients because they tend to have a drying effect. There is a group of substances, including paraffin, white petrolatum and some silicones, which form an occlusive and continuous film on the area to be treated, causing a reduction of transepidermal water loss and producing an effect similar to that of a polyethylene film. Other substances, such as urea, lactic acid, sodium lactate and ceramides, favour the union of water with membrane proteins through chemical interactions and are able to retain water intracellularly in the stratum corneum. Bandages that contain zinc oxide and coal tar, or zinc paste in combination with calamine, changed once or twice a week, have been shown to be helpful, especially if there is concomitant eczema. Topical and systemic use of steroids can delay healing so care should be taken to avoid any side effects in leg ulcer management.

It is important to show concern about the use of steroids and it is helpful to instruct the patients to apply a very thin smear of class II or class III steroid to the affected area only and not to normal skin. It is clear that skin care is a difficult challenge in chronic wound management. The complexity of the physiological mechanisms responsible for skin hydration leads to a lack of knowledge about the real possibilities for proper skin care.

References

Angelini G, Rantuccio F, Meneghini C L 1975 Contact dermatitis in patients with leg ulcers. Contact Dermatitis 1: 81–87

Beebe H G, Bergan J J, Bergqvist D et al 1995 Classification and grading of chronic venous disease in the lower limbs – a consensus statement. Phlebology 10: 42–45

Blank A, Schnyder U W 1990 Squamous cell carcinoma and basal cell carcinoma within the clinical picture of a chronic venous insufficiency in the third stage. Dermatologica 181: 248–250

Browse N L, Jarrett P E M, Morland M et al 1977 Treatment of liposclerosis of the leg by fibrinolytic enhancement: a preliminary report. British Medical Journal 2: 434–435

Burnand K, Clemenson G, Morland M et al 1980 Venous lipodermatosclerosis : treatment by fibrinolytic enhancement and elastic compression. British Medical Journal 280: 7–11

Cancer Registry 1981–1990 Cancer Incidence in Sweden 1977–87. Annual Publication. National Board of Health and Welfare, Stockholm

Kirsner R S, Pardes J B, Eaglstein W H et al 1993 The clinical spectrum of lipodermatosclerosis. Journal of the American Academy of Dermatology 28: 623–627

Machet L, Couhe C, Perrinaud A et al 2004 A high prevalence of sensitization still persists in leg ulcer patients : a retrospective series of 106 patients tested between 2001 and 2002 and a meta-analysis of 1975–2003 data. British Journal of Dermatology 150: 929–935

Maessen-Visch M B, Koedam M I, Hamulyak K et al 1999 Atrophie blanche. International Journal of Dermatology 38: 161–172

Marjolin J N 1828 Ulcers. Dictionnaire de medecine. Bèchet Jeune, Paris, vol 21, pp 31–50

Milstone L M, Braverman I M, Lucky P et al 1983 Classification and therapy of atrophie blanche. Archives of Dermatology 119: 963–969

Nemeth A J, Eaglstein W H, Falanga V 1989 Clinical parameters and transcutaneous oxygen measurements for the prognosis of venous ulcers. Journal of the American Academy of Dermatology 20: 186–190

Pizzo S V, Murray J C, Gonias S L 1986 Atrophie blanche. A disorder associated with defective release of tissue plasminogen activator. Archives of Pathology and Laboratory Medicine 110: 517–519

Romanelli M, Falanga V 1995 Use of a durometer to measure the degree of skin induration in lipodermatosclerosis. Journal of the American Academy of Dermatology 32: 188–191

Tavadia S, Bianchi J, Dawe R S et al 2003 Allergic contact dermatitis in venous leg ulcer patients. Contact Dermatitis 48: 261–265

Nutritional assessment and support

Susan M. McLaren

INTRODUCTION

A considerable body of evidence derived from both animal and clinical studies is now available to substantiate the vital role that nutrients play in wound healing and other patient outcomes. The role of nutrients relates to diverse aspects of healing at cellular and subcellular levels; these encompass the provision of the essential components of new cell structures, nucleic acids and extracellular matrix; formation of metabolic substrates for the cellular infiltrate and enhancement of the functions of immunocompetent cells that promote healing and prevent sepsis. In addition, nutrients play a vital role in antioxidant defence, preventing lipid peroxidation and tissue damage by oxygen free radicals.

The presence of undernutrition has been associated with a number of adverse outcomes in hospitalized patients; these include increased risks of morbidity and mortality, increased sepsis and length of hospital stay (Green 1999, Allison 2002). Overnutrition manifest in obesity also carries health risks associated with vascular disease and diabetes mellitus. From the perspective of leg ulcer development and healing, both undernutrition and obesity are important in terms of the risks they pose, and the fact that leg ulcers are most prevalent in older adults, a known risk group for malnutrition, suggests that nutritional aspects of management are vital. This chapter focuses on the risks associated with malnutrition, approaches to screening for nutritional risk and its subsequent management, with an emphasis on the older person. Wherever possible, research evidence has been included that is drawn from studies in leg ulcer populations; where these are unavailable, relevant studies in older adults have been included.

LEG ULCERS AND NUTRITIONAL STATUS

The prevalence of leg ulcers is highest in the elderly population, an age group designated as vulnerable in relation to nutritional status. In attempting to explore the potential relationships between nutritional factors, leg ulcer aetiology and healing, it is vital to define, identify and compare the sources of nutritional risk in the population of older adults and those with leg ulcers. It is on the basis of such information that intervention strategies to modify risk can be formulated.

Malnutrition

Malnutrition is a state in which a deficiency, excess or imbalance of energy, protein and other nutrients causes measurable adverse effects on tissue or body form (shape, size, composition), function and clinical outcome (Stratton et al 2003a). It can arise from a number of medical conditions that differ in both severity and cause (disease-related malnutrition) and is also influenced by social, economic, and institutional factors operating in community, hospital and nursing home settings (Green 1999). A range of terms are used to describe malnourished states; these include 'overnutrition', due to an excessive food consumption relative to requirements, and the converse, 'undernutrition', where intakes are inadequate.

Obesity

More specifically, overnutrition can result in obesity, defined as an excess of adipose tissue for a given weight; body mass indices of 26–30 are indicative of overweight and more than 30 of severe obesity. In terms of health risks, obesity has been associated with cardiovascular disease, diabetes mellitus, arthritis and specific types of cancer. Furthermore, in obese older adults, reduced functional status and decreased quality of life in the presence of vascular disease and diabetes have been identified (Defay et al 2001, Kennedy et al 2004). The prevalence of obesity and its associated medical complications is rising in Western and westernized populations, giving rise to concerns about 'obesity epidemics' (Contaldo & Pasanini 2005). A survey of older adults over 65 years old in the UK found that approximately 65% of those who were free-living and just under half of those in institutions could be identified as either overweight or obese on the basis of a body mass index (BMI) of more than 25 (Finch et al 1998).

Obesity: leg ulcer aetiology

Recent reviews research relating to the aetiology and management of venous leg ulcers have noted that the incidence is greatest in the elderly and is rising (Leach 2004, Simon et al 2004). Obesity has been identified as an important cause of venous hypertension, which contributes to some of the pathophysiological events leading to ulceration, i.e. local oedema increasing diffusion distances for nutrients and metabolites, ultimately resulting in an ischaemia–reperfusion injury during dependency and periods of walking or elevation (Simon et al 2004). Leg ulcer populations can exhibit multiple pathologies resulting from underlying medical conditions that are also associated with obesity, notably vascular disease (arterial and venous), arthritis and endocrine disease (Schofield et al 2003). Diabetes mellitus is another important neuropathic cause of venous ulceration.

Undernutrition

In contrast, 'undernutrition' has been defined as 'a state of energy, protein or other nutrient deficiency which produces a measurable change in body function and is associated with worse outcome from illness, as well as being specifically reversed by nutritional support' (Allison 2000). The prevalence of undernutrition in older populations living in the community and institutionalized settings has given cause for concern. Reported statistics vary, but surveys of nutritional status and risk conducted in nursing homes suggest that 10–85% of residents are undernourished (Green 1999, Saletti et al 2000), while in hospital settings a high prevalence of undernutrition has been found in older people admitted to hospital, with further deterioration occurring in some during their stay (Allison 2002). Among the free-living elderly, 3–5% have a BMI indicative of underweight (Finch et al 1998). Causes of undernutrition include diseases leading to reduced nutrient intake, decreased digestion/absorption and increased metabolic utilization of nutrients, together with social, economic, psychological and drug-related factors (Table 28.1).

Chronic undernutrition can lead to the deterioration of vital organ systems, resulting in impaired wound healing in the cascade of events summarized in Table 28.2. In addition, weight loss, anxiety, depression, apathy and diminished work and functional capacity can result from undernutrition. An increased risk of complications, length of hospitalization and mortality have also been reported in a number of studies in medical and surgical populations (Green 1999, Allison 2002).

Undernutrition: leg ulcer healing

Comparatively few investigations into the adequacy of the dietary intake of older adults with leg ulcers have been conducted, but the available evidence suggests that they do not differ significantly from those of elderly people without ulceration. Lewis & Harding (1997) used dietary histories, 7-day food diaries, food frequency questionnaires and measurements of BMI to investigate dietary adequacy in elderly people with leg ulcers. Key findings were that both overweight and underweight existed in the population and, in comparison with reference values, intakes of energy, protein and zinc were inadequate in some individuals. Comparisons made with age- and gender-matched controls found that the dietary intakes of older people with ulcers did not significantly differ from the control group. However, the implications of obesity and undernutrition on leg ulcer healing in the individuals affected were a cause for concern.

Table 28.1 Factors that alone or in combination can lead to undernutrition in older adults

Causes and contributory factors leading to undernutrition	Impact on diet, digestion, absorption, metabolism	Rationale for impact on older person
Disease-related causes		
Stroke, Parkinson's disease, dementia, cardiac failure, pulmonary disease, arthritis, musculoskeletal trauma	Decreased intakes	Inability to purchase or prepare food because of impairment of mobility or cognition Eating dependency
Liver, cancer, renal disease	Decreased intakes	Anorexia, nausea, vomiting
Oral, pharyngeal, oesophageal cancer, stroke, dementia	Decreased intakes	Obstructive dysphagia Neurogenic dysphagia
Ulcerative colitis, Crohn's disease, gut infection, gut cancer, enteropathies	Decreased nutrient digestion and absorption	Gut inflammation
Burns, sepsis, trauma, severe chronic wounds, cachexia, hyperthyroidism	Increased metabolic utilization and/or disposal of nutrients	Metabolic injury response, cancer cachexia syndrome, hyperthyroidism, increased energy requirements
Effects of ageing		
Altered appetite regulation	Reduced food intake	Anorexia, early satiety
Loss of taste and olfactory acuity	Consumption of monotonous diet	Sensory specific satiety
Reduced muscle mass, thyroid hormones, responsiveness to noradrenaline (norepinephrine)	Gradual reduction in food intake	Reduced basal metabolic rate Reduced energy expenditure Reduced energy requirements
Tooth loss, reduced mass of tongue and masseter muscles of jaw, reduced salivary volume, viscosity	Impaired oral food ingestion and transport Potential for reduced food intake	Reduced ability to form food bolus prior to swallowing
Socioeconomic status		
Social isolation, poverty, poor levels of education, bereavement	Reduced food intake	Restricted food purchase, facilities for storage and preparation Reduced quality and variety of nutrients consumed Irregular eating habits
Psychological status		
Anxiety, depression	Reduced food intake	Anorexia, weight loss

A later study by Wissing et al (2001) investigated ulcer healing and recurrence in relation to nutritional risk profile in a small number of elderly patients. Key findings were that those with open ulcers (unhealed or recurrent) had higher mean nutritional risk scores and lower mean activity of daily living/mobility scores than those whose ulcers had healed. Other interesting findings were that patients with healed ulcers had significantly higher mean social interaction scores than those with open ulcers. The implication of this study was that increased nutritional risk and broader social variables could affect the healing of leg ulcers; however, the small sample sizes in this and the study by Lewis & Harding (1997) limit wider generalizability of the findings.

In contrast, an investigation into the potential influence of micronutrient deficiency on chronic leg ulcer healing utilizing biochemical tests revealed that ulcer patients had significantly lower serum levels of vitamin A, zinc, carotenes and, in men, vitamin E than a control group (Rojas & Phillips

Table 28.2 The potential impact of chronic undernutrition on body systems and wound healing

Body system	Effect of undernutrition	Impact on wound healing
Gastrointestinal system	Reduced gastric acid secretion Reduced gut motility Mucosal atrophy Pancreatic acinar cell atrophy Impaired digestion Impaired nutrient absorption	Reduced nutrient digestion and absorption leads to nutrient deficits in organs and tissues Reduced nutrient availability for healing
Respiratory system	Reduced vital capacity Reduced tidal/minute volume Atrophy of respiratory muscles Risk of pulmonary sepsis	Hypoxaemia Impaired oxygen delivery Reduced tissue oxygen availability impairs healing
Haemopoietic system	Anaemia, leukopenia Marrow necrosis	Decreased tissue oxygen delivery impairs healing
Immune system	Decreased cellular immunity Decreased humoral immunity Decreased lymphocyte count Decreased serum complement except C4	Increased vulnerability to sepsis impairs wound healing Increased risk of sepsis in wound and other sites can increase morbidity, mortality
Skin and integumental tissues at wound site	Decreased neoangiogenesis Decreased fibroblast proliferation and collagen synthesis Tissue oedema (low plasma proteins due to undernutrition and exudate losses) Increased skin fragility, friability	Impaired proliferative phase Impaired remodelling phase Decreased wound tensile strength Delayed closure Risk of wound dehiscence Oedema impairs nutrient diffusion
Circulatory system	Decreased stroke volume Decreased cardiac output Decreased blood pressure	Reduced tissue perfusion Reduced oxygen and nutrient delivery

1999). Although these micronutrients are known to play an important role in wound healing generally, it is important to bear in mind that disease states can affect the concentrations of serum carrier proteins for trace elements and some vitamins. Therefore, serum levels may not reflect the tissue levels of these nutrients. For these reasons, combining biochemical test data with dietary information and other clinical features, including ulcer assessment, may be more conclusive.

In conclusion, obesity can impact negatively on leg ulcer aetiology and healing; undernutrition also has the potential to adversely affect healing. Preliminary findings suggest that further research is needed in this area, ideally combining a range of nutritional assessment techniques with leg ulcer assessments, within a controlled, longitudinal

study design. Studies that have evaluated the role of nutritional supplementation in undernourished populations of older adults and those with leg ulceration are discussed below.

MACRONUTRIENTS AND MICRONUTRIENTS: INFLUENCES ON HEALING

During the process of wound healing an array of nutrients meet the needs of tissue metabolism and also provide for the synthesis of its new structural components. These nutrients can be considered in two major categories: macronutrients, which include glucose, fatty acids and protein, and micronutrients, which can be subdivided into vitamins, trace elements and minerals. In this section most of the effects of nutrients on healing relate generally to wounds; only in relation to micronutrients is there evidence specific to leg ulcer healing.

Glucose

During the early stages of healing the cellular infiltrate containing leukocytes and macrophages releases cytokines and growth factors, which stimulate fibroblast production and collagen synthesis (Edwards & Moldawer 1998). In the performance of these vital functions both leukocytes and macrophages utilize glucose as an energy substrate; the efficiency of energy production from glucose is optimized by the factors that support aerobic metabolism, notably angiogenesis, haematocrit and local tissue perfusion. Other cells use glucose in the synthesis of new tissue components, notably fibroblasts, which synthesize hexosamines, components of the new extracellular matrix. In lymphocytes, arginine activates cells by increasing glucose uptake (Efron & Barbul 1998).

Polyunsaturated fatty acids

Polyunsaturated fatty acids (PUFA) are vital components of cell membranes, where they play a vital role in cellular signal transduction and in the production of eicosanoids, which have wide ranging effects on immune function, inflammatory and vascular responses. Macrophages, lymphocytes and monocytes can synthesize eicosanoids from PUFA in their cell membranes. For some time, interest has focused on two particular types of fatty acid, the omega-3 fatty acids found in fish oils and omega-6 fatty acids, found in specific vegetable oils such as sunflower and safflower. These two fatty acids give rise to different species of eicosanoid; in the case of omega-3 fatty acids, these include prostaglandin E_3 and leukotrienes, which can exert vasodilatory and anti-inflammatory effects, the latter by inhibition of cytokine production. In the case of omega-6 fatty acids, the eicosanoids produced are prostaglandins I_2 and E_2, which appear to be vasoconstrictive and immunosuppressive.

Clearly, the production of prostaglandin E_3 and leukotrienes have important implications for healing, in terms of local tissue perfusion and reduction of chronic inflammation. More specifically, the possibility that it might be possible to manipulate the production of the eicosanoids beneficial to healing by increasing dietary intakes of omega-3 fatty acids, which subsequently become incorporated in the macrophage membrane, was an interesting line of investigation. A number of clinical studies have been conducted to test the immune-enhancing and wound-healing benefits of omega-3 fatty acids, frequently in combination with other nutrients. Yaqoob (2003) has critically evaluated recent research relating to dietary fatty acids (omega-3 fatty acids) and immune responses and concluded that results are inconsistent in human studies for three reasons. First, the doses used in human studies do not compare with those used in earlier animal models; the preparations of fish oils used have varied in their content of two critical fatty acid components, eicosapentaenoic and docosahexanoic acids, which may exert different effects on immune function, and finally, many studies lacked statistical power. Calder & Deckelbaum (2003) have also drawn attention to the evidence that there may be genotypic factors that modify sensitivity to the anti-inflammatory effects of omega-3 fatty acids at the individual level. This raises the possibility that the effects of omega-3 fatty acids may need to be more efficiently targeted. Readers are referred to these publications for more information relating to this exciting area of research.

Protein

Dietary protein provides the amino acids necessary for the synthesis of functional body components. The proteins derived from these amino acids provide elements of cell structure and are essential for growth, immunological responses, enzyme activity and neuromuscular function. Given their vital role in cellular structure and function, it is not surprising that early animal studies demonstrated a crucial role for protein in wound healing, where it is needed to increase fibroblast proliferation, angiogenesis and collagen production (Ruberg 1984). In severe protein deficiency states, the synthesis of visceral proteins can be reduced, leading to hypoalbuminaemia and oedema. The latter can impair the local diffusion of oxygen and nutrients, resulting in adverse effects on healing. The possibility that plasma proteins can also be lost in exudate from leg ulceration, also resulting in hypoalbuminaemia, should be borne in mind here. Considerable interest has focused on the role of protein and energy supplements in the promotion of healing in malnourished states (see below). The protein recommended dietary allowance in healthy adults is 0.8 g per kg body weight per day; this is the amount of protein necessary to meet physiological needs and maintain health. A dietetic assessment is necessary to determine any additional protein requirements for healing in conjunction with other factors in any individual (see below). In order for protein to be utilized effectively in tissue repair, it is vital that the total dietary energy intake is adequate, or the protein ingested will be metabolized as an energy source.

Amino acids

Amino acids are categorized as essential or non-essential. The former cannot be synthesized by mammals and must be provided in the diet; these are leucine, isoleucine, lysine, methionine, phenylalanine, tryptophan, valine, histidine and threonine. Non-essential amino acids can be synthesized within the body from nitrogen-containing precursors; they include alanine, glutamine, arginine, aspartic acid, asparagine, cystine, glycine, proline, serine and tyrosine. During injury and healing some non-essential amino acids become vital: arginine and glutamine are exemplars of these. In a healing wound, amino acids are necessary for the synthesis of structural proteins within cytoskeletons, the components of nucleic acids, notably purines and pyrimidines; the synthesis of procollagen, components of new tissue extracellular matrix and the provision of a metabolic fuel for the cellular infiltrate. Amino acids are also utilized by the liver in the metabolic response to injury, to synthesize acute phase proteins, which are systemic mediators of the inflammatory response. In animal models dietary deficiency–repletion studies have shown that certain amino acids play prominent roles in healing: for example, methionine and cysteine are essential for collagen synthesis and fibroblast proliferation.

Glutamine

Glutamine is the most abundant amino acid in the body. It is synthesized extensively in skeletal muscle and fulfils a major transport function in the delivery of nitrogen to vital organs such as the liver, gut and kidney (Melis et al 2004). The physiological role of glutamine is of interest in wound healing and metabolism for the following reasons.

- It is the preferred metabolic fuel for macrophages, neutrophils and lymphocytes within the cellular infiltrate
- Glutamine is involved in the synthesis of antioxidants glutathione and taurine; antioxidant defence against free radical damage is vital in chronic wound healing
- Glutamine provides nitrogen for the synthesis of purine and pyrimidine nucleotides; these are essential for RNA and DNA production
- Fibroblasts convert glutamine to glutamate, a precursor of proline and, thereby, collagen.

Other important effects of glutamine include benefits on the gut barrier where it is a fuel for enterocytes and colonocytes, enhancing the function of gut-associated lymphatic tissue; beneficial therapeutic effects on tissue damage and survival in animal models of ischaemia–reperfusion injury and, when administered parenterally in clinical studies, reductions in the loss of lean body tissue in catabolic states (Melis et al 2004). Overwhelming evidence suggests that all rapidly proliferating cells, particularly those of the immune system, depend on glutamine as an energy source (Furst et al 2004). Clinical evidence suggests that provision of parenteral glutamine to critically ill patients is associated with reduced mortality, infectious morbidity and length of hospital stay (Griffiths 2004). Significantly shorter wound healing times have been reported in one clinical study (Zhou et al 2004).

Arginine

Arginine is a dibasic amino acid that has effects on wound healing that appear to change along the time-course of healing (Efron & Barbul 1998). The mechanisms whereby arginine can influence wound healing (in pharmacological doses), include those mediated by increased secretion of growth hormone, insulin and glucagon, which lead to increased protein synthesis. A number of experimental animal studies have suggested that arginine is converted by both fibroblasts and macrophages to nitric oxide and citrulline in wounds. Subsequently, in fibroblasts, the citrulline is converted to proline for incorporation into collagen. However, the fact that arginine is a substrate for the production of nitric oxide suggests that its most important role in healing is via angiogenesis. Nitric oxide is a potent vasodilator, a mediator of macrophage-induced bacterial killing and a stimulator of fibroblast activities (Schaffer et al 1997). The macrophage appears to be the most prominent producer of nitric oxide from arginine in the inflammatory environment. Other functions of arginine include its impact on immune cell populations, where in polymorphonuclear leukocytes it facilitates phagocytosis and in lymphocytes, mitogenesis. Recent clinical evidence derived from arginine supplementation in artificial nutrition, suggest benefits in terms of healing in the non-critically ill, but potentially serious side effects due to nitric oxide production in the critically ill (McFie 2004).

Micronutrients

The roles of key micronutrients in healing are summarized in Tables 28.3 and 28.4. The impact of oral zinc supplementation on leg ulcer healing is discussed in the section on nutrition support below.

NUTRITIONAL SCREENING AND ASSESSMENT

Nutritional screening has a crucial purpose: to identify individuals who either are already or are likely to become undernourished, in order that they can be referred for further in-depth assessment and where appropriate, nutritional intervention (Weekes et al 2004). The European Society for Parenteral and Enteral Nutrition Guidelines for Nutritional Screening (Kondrup et al 2003) also define the purpose of nutritional screening to be the prediction of better or worse outcomes due to nutritional factors and whether nutritional interventions are likely to influence this. Outcomes of interventions can be measured in various ways, for example changes in mental and physical functions, number and severity of morbid complications, length of hospital stay, duration of convalescence and economic costs of treatment.

Screening in community leg ulcer clinics and hospital settings

It has been recommended that all patients are routinely screened on admission to hospital or other health-care settings and that screening may be repeated periodically thereafter to monitor changes (Kondrup et al 2003). Community leg ulcer clinics have been largely responsible for the assessment and management of patients in recent years, although some patients may be admitted to hospital for treatment of the ulcer or underlying health problem. It is not clear to what extent specialist nurses and medical staff working in community leg ulcer clinics incorporate nutritional screening as part of routine assessment. As an essential preliminary step in patient management, Simon et al (2004) emphasize the need to conduct a full assessment to identify risk factors that contribute to leg ulceration and identify BMI as an important component of the assessment. While this measurement is helpful in the identification of obesity, it does not alone constitute an adequate method of screening for undernutrition; adopting one of the tools discussed below could provide more useful information relating to nutritional risk and provide useful information for dietetic referral.

A number of screening tools have been developed to assist health professionals to evaluate nutritional risk routinely in both acute and community settings, thus they should meet certain criteria for utility, i.e. be easy and quick to complete, offer clear interpretation, in addition to being acceptable to patients and clients. It is vital that they aid but do not replace professional judgement (Weekes et al 2004). Training in the use of screening instruments should be offered that incorporates measures of consistency in use (Green & McLaren 1998). Both acute and primary care organizations should develop protocols for screening and assessment linked to care plans, which contain explicit intervention monitoring and outcome information appropriate to level of risk. It is important that the care plans are in a format readily communicable to other care settings where the patient may be transferred.

Screening tools

In terms of content, screening tools vary, but a common approach is to attribute ordinal scores to

Table 28.3 Influences of selected trace elements on wound healing and features of deficiency

Trace element/reference nutrient intakes	Effects on wound healing	Signs and symptoms of deficiency
Zinc Reference nutrient intake: 7 mg/day in women >50 years and 9.5 mg/day in males >50 years	Metal cofactor for >200 enzyme systems involved in biological oxidation Essential for enzyme activity supporting the reconstruction of the wound matrix, DNA/RNA synthesis Regulation of activity of macrophages and polymorphonuclear leukocytes	Eczematous dermatitis, alopecia, ocular lesions, testicular atrophy, altered taste and smell, mouth ulceration, ataxia
Copper Reference nutrient intake in adults >50 years 1.2 mg/day	Synthesis and polymerization of collagen via action as cofactor for lysyl oxidase Plays a role in antioxidant defence via action as cofactor for superoxide dismutase	Copper-depleted individuals lose the ability to utilize stored iron (impaired ferroxidase activity) Iron deficiency anaemia and neutropenia
Iron Reference nutrient intakes in adults >50 years 8.7 mg/day	Cofactor for lysyl and prolyl hydroxylases in collagen synthesis Crucial component of haemoglobin and thereby determinant of tissue oxygen delivery	Hypochromic, microcytic iron deficiency anaemia Glossitis, cheilosis, dysphagia, gastric atrophy
Manganese Reference nutrient intake values not available, but safe intakes are above 1.4 mg/day in adults	A cofactor for many enzymes influencing healing, e.g. arginase, superoxide dismutase, hydrolases, prolinases Influential in antioxidant defence Via functions as a cofactor, production of glycoproteins and mucopolysaccharides	Manganese deficiency does not appear to develop in humans
Selenium Reference nutrient intake values in adults set at 75 μg/day in men >50 years and 60 μg/day in women >50 years	Integral component of the enzyme glutathione peroxidase, therefore crucial role in antioxidant defence	Unclear – cardiomyopathy, myopathy

Reference nutrient intakes: Department of Health 2001a.

variables (i.e. recent weight loss, dietary intakes, living conditions) considered to be indicative of undernutrition, with a summation of subscores providing an index of nutritional risk and extent of malnutrition. Critical appraisal of the scientific evidence supporting the use of any tool is essential to inform the development of an effective screening and assessment protocol. Issues of validity (the extent to which the tool measures what it is intended to measure) and reliability (consistency in use) should have been addressed during development. Specific aspects of validity that are important include content validity (adequate representation of factors known to be indicative of nutritional

Table 28.4 Role of vitamins influential in wound healing and features of deficiency

Vitamin/reference nutrient intakes	Role in wound healing	Signs and symptoms of deficiency
Vitamin A Reference nutrient intake: women >50 years 600 µg/day; men 700 µg/day	Differentiation and maintenance of cell membranes, epithelialization Cofactor for enzymes involved in collagen cross linkage Lymphocyte proliferation and natural killer cell activity Benefits wound breaking strength in animal studies Antagonizes steroid-induced delays in healing	Visual deterioration, night blindness Hyperkeratosis of skin, Bitot's spots Conjunctival dryness Bone pain in spine, pelvis, legs
Vitamin C Reference nutrient intake: adults >50 years 40 mg/day	Cofactor for hydroxylation of proline and lysine during collagen synthesis Essential for angiogenesis, wound tensile strength Inhibits free radical formation and, thereby, tissue damage Beneficial effects on cell-mediated immunity reduces sepsis	Scurvy, hyperkeratosis, purpura, joint haemorrhage Loss of gingival margin
Vitamin E Reference nutrient intake: none; safe daily intakes of 4 mg and 3 mg in men and women respectively	Antioxidant, protects against lipid peroxidation by free radicals	Deficiency syndromes rare Ataxic neurological syndromes; rare spinocerebellar degeneration
Vitamin K reference nutrient intake: none; ≈0.5–1.0 µg/kg body weight per day	Synthesis of prothrombin and clotting factors VII, IX, X haemostasis	Bruising, haemorrhage in deficiency states associated with biliary obstruction and malabsorption

Reference nutrient intakes. Department of Health 2001a

risk) and predictive validity (the extent to which the tool is a useful predictor of the outcomes of a nutritional intervention resulting from screening). Test–retest reliability determines how consistently the same rater scores the patient at two different points in time, while inter-rater reliability tests consistency in scoring when two or more independent raters screen the same patient at the same time. The levels of agreement obtained from both types of reliability testing can be determined either by calculating the correlation coefficient (i.e. Spearman rank order correlation coefficient) between scores or by calculating the kappa coefficient of agreement, which incorporates a correction for random agreement. For further information relating to measurement and levels of inter-rater agreement see Fleiss (1971). Other important scientific criteria include validity testing in different ethnic groups, sensitivity testing (the extent to which the tool can detect and measure small variations in nutritional risk), adequacy of sample sizes used for testing effectiveness of the tool and the appropriateness of the method used to determine weightings on ordinal scales (Waitzberg & Correa 2003).

Types of screening tools: exemplars used in adults

Leg ulcers are most prevalent in the older adult population, hence selection of screening tools that have been validated for use in this group and are appropriate to community or hospital settings is indicated.

Malnutrition Universal Screening Tool (MUST)

Originally developed for use in the community (Malnutrition Advisory Group 2000), this tool uses ordinal ratings of BMI, weight loss over the preceding 3 months and a single weighted score for acute disease effects on nutritional intake. These are added to give a final score indicative of the risk of undernutrition. Overall levels of risk are delineated as low (routine clinical care), medium (observe) and high (treat), with further specific action points recommended in community, care home and hospital settings. Content validity was ensured by using an expert multidisciplinary group during the development stages; kappa values reported for inter-rater reliability were 0.8–1.0, constituting excellent agreement. The risk of undernutrition assessed by MUST has been shown to be significantly related to mortality and length of hospital stay in elderly hospital inpatients (King et al 2003) and excellent concurrent validity with other screening tools has been established (Stratton et al 2003).

Mini-Nutritional Screening and Assessment Tool (MNA)

This instrument was developed for use in the elderly population in nursing home, hospital settings and home care programmes. It is a combination of a screening and assessment tool, within two clearly delineated sections. Within the screening section are six ordinal scaled subsections, relating to recent changes in food intake, weight loss, mobility, psychological stress/acute disease, neuropsychological problems and BMI. A screening score is obtained by adding the subscores together and two categories of risk are then identified, i.e. normal, not at risk (no need to complete the assessment section) and possible undernutrition (continue assessment section). Predictive validity of the MNA has been established in relation to the outcomes of mortality, length of hospital stay, health and social functioning; inter-rater reliability kappa values of 0.51 have been reported (Kondrup et al 2003, Vellas et al 1999, 2001).

Nutritional Risk Screening (NRS 2002)

Designed for screening use in adults within the hospital setting, the NRS-2002 has two components; one constitutes an initial screening, the second a final screening. The former asks four questions relating to BMI, weight loss within the last 3 months, reduced dietary intakes and severity of illness. If the answer is yes to any question, further (final) screening is completed; if the answer is no to all questions, rescreening at weekly intervals is recommended. The final screening process contains two components of impaired nutritional status and severity of disease. Within each component ordinal scaled scores are attributed, for example to the extent of weight loss and changes in BMI, (impaired nutritional status) and the severity of disease, scored in relation to different medical and surgical conditions. A total NRS score is obtained by adding the subscores of the final screening components together and including an adjustment for age. The final score identifies two levels of risk, one where a care plan is initiated because of the presence of nutritional risk and a second where weekly rescreening is recommended. In relation to validity testing, content validity was addressed by using an expert working group in the development stages and, following this, predictive validity tested in relation to length of hospital stay and morbidity. Inter-rater reliability kappa coefficients of agreement of 0.67 have been reported when tested using a nurse, dietitian and doctor (Kondrup et al 2002, 2003).

Nutritional assessment

Nutritional assessment constitutes a more detailed examination of nutritional, functional and metabolic variables by clinician, dietitian or specialist nutrition nurse, which leads to an appropriate plan of care (Kondrup et al 2003). According to Klein et al (1997), the specific aims of assessment are as follows.

- To identify individuals who have or are at risk of developing malnutrition or specific nutrient deficiencies

- To quantify a patient's risk of developing malnutrition-related complications
- To monitor the adequacy of nutritional therapy.

The scope of assessment considers the individual's dietary history in the context of health status and medical treatment. It can include, where appropriate, the investigation of selected anthropometric, biochemical, haematological, immunological and functional markers, together with tests of body composition. Since nutritional assessment techniques have limitations and can be affected by non-nutritional factors, it is usual to use three or more techniques in combination. A consideration of requirements for energy, macro- and micronutrients and the types of intervention that may be needed, including the use of specific diets, nutritional supplements and enteral and parenteral nutrition, follow on from assessment. Care plans that detail these essential aspects of management, together with the monitoring of intervention outcomes over time, are essential for effective decision-making by multidisciplinary teams.

Anthropometry

Traditionally, anthropometry measures body dimensions across age, sex and ethnic groups and has long been used as a method of nutritional assessment. Common anthropometric techniques indicative of changes in body composition encompass the measurement of body weight, height, BMI, circumference of limbs (e.g. mid-arm circumference, MAC), thickness of skinfolds, demispan and demiquet. Tables 28.5 and 28.6 summarize the rationale and approaches used in these techniques, together with the impact of non-nutritional variables on measurement. Extensive research has focussed on the relative merits of different anthropometric indices in terms of their ability to detect malnutrition (mainly undernutrition) and to predict outcomes such as morbidity, mortality and length of hospital stay. For example, a recent study by Campillo et al (2004) found that the sensitivity of BMI to detect severe malnutrition (undernutrition) was highest in specific hospitalized diagnostic groups, for example patients following surgery for hip fracture (100%), palliative care for cancer (80%) and certain medical conditions (100%). In contrast, BMI had lower sensitivity in detecting severe malnutrition in patients suffering from tense ascites (40%), cardiac diseases (33%) and stroke (50%). A BMI of less than 20 was highly sensitive in the diagnosis of severe malnutrition in elderly and cancer patients but not in cirrhotic patients with tense ascites, cardiovascular and neurological conditions. In hospitalized medical, surgical and orthopaedic patients, Powell-Tuck & Hennessy (2003) found that compared with BMI and MAC, weight loss of more than 10% was the most significant predictor of mortality. However, in patients for whom weight loss was not recorded, MAC was a significant predictor of mortality, either alone or after adjustment for BMI. BMI was not significant in predicting mortality. Furthermore, BMI, weight loss of more than 10% and MAC were poor predictors of hospital stay. Overall, MAC measurements were found to correlate highly with BMI, were easier to measure and predicted poor outcome better.

In general, anthropometric measurements confer the advantages of being non-invasive, relatively inexpensive and, following training of personnel, relatively easy to perform. Offsetting these are a number of limitations that need to be borne in mind when interpreting measurements in any individual. For further information on practical aspects of measurement see Perry 2003. Waitzberg & Correa (2003) have drawn attention to the caution necessary in using some reference tables of anthropometric values drawn from studies in healthy populations, which have raised questions relating to the methodologies used. Set against the background of medical condition and treatment, serial anthropometric measurements made on an individual over time may provide more valuable information than comparisons with reference values drawn from population studies, which may have limited applicability to an individual.

Biochemical markers

Biochemical markers of nutritional status include serum proteins, vitamins, trace elements and urinary urea, creatinine and ketone excretion. Many are available as routine tests conducted in clinical biochemistry laboratories, others only through specialist regional centres (Selberg & Sel 2001). In this chapter exemplars of commonly used biochemical markers will be discussed and the reader will be referred to other specialist publications for details of

Table 28.5 Anthropometric measurements using body weight that are indicative of changes in body composition in adults

Parameter	Indicative changes	Performing measurement and calculating values	Impact of extraneous variables and limitations in interpretation
Body weight	Sum of fat, protein, water and skeletal mass No information on nature of tissue loss Approximate guide to changes in energy stores and body cell mass	Use scales frequently calibrated with standard weights Scale accuracy ±0.1 kg Weigh on weekly basis, consistently at same time of day (diurnal variation) wearing same clothing	Extensive tumours and fluid balance changes can affect measurements Renal and cardiac failure Malignancy associated with ascites Diuretic and corticosteroid therapy
Percentage weight change	Recent non-intentional weight loss over 3–6 months Arr. 'MUST' screening tool: >10% clinically significant, 5–10% early indicator of risk, <5% within normal variation	Current weight as above Previous/usual weight by patient recall or reference to medical records Previous or usual body weight minus current weight ×100, divided by previous/usual weight	Memory recall of usual weight can introduce error See also above variables
Body mass index (BMI)	An index of weight in proportion to height Does not distinguish changes in body fat from muscle <19 underweight, 20–25 normal, 26–30 overweight, >30 obese	Weight measured as above Height measured using stadiometer on horizontal surface, erect posture, looking straight ahead, back of head shoulders and buttocks in contact with stadiometer Weight (kg) divided by height (m)^2	Problematic measurement if patient cannot stand for height measurement Health risks indicated by BMI may vary across age groups In older adults BMI <23 may indicate underweight (Beck & Ovesen 1998)
Demiquet	An index of body mass in relation to skeletal size based on measurement of weight and demispan	Weight (kg) divided by demispan (m)^2	Measure demispan in centimetres using non-stretchable tape measure, i.e. distance from web between middle and ring finger along outstretched arm to sternal notch Useful where height cannot be measured Range of reference values for older adult populations unavailable

Table 28.6 Anthropometric measurements using limb skinfolds and circumference that are indicative of changes in body composition

Parameter	Indicative changes	Performing measurement and calculating values	Impact of extraneous variables and limitations in interpretation
Limb skinfold thickness Triceps skinfold thickness (TSF)	Index of changes in body fat stores Usually measured weekly over months to monitor changes sensitively Not useful in detecting short-term changes TSF used in measurement of MAMC (below)	Skinfolds can be measured at subscapular, suprailiac, biceps, triceps (common), thigh and calf sites Calipers of resolution 0.1 mm with application of uniform standard pressure of 10 g/mm^2 over contact area of 30–90 mm^2 desirable Skinfolds measured at same midpoint as limb circumference (see below) Lift skin and fat clear from underlying tissue and apply calipers to middle of fold Take measurement after 2–3 s Average of readings in triplicate gives final value of TSF Average of readings from all six sites most accurate	Not exactly proportional to total body fat Variations in distribution of body fat occur with age, sex, ethnic group, which can affect thickness and compressibility of skinfolds Hydration status, oedema can modify compressibility Minimize error by training assessors, using same assessor on each occasion, marking skinfold with hypoallergenic tape Reference values available for percentile ranges of selected skinfolds but some out of date
Limb circumference (LC) Mid-arm circumference (MAC)	Index of fat, muscle and bone Mid-arm circumference (MAC) used in MAMC measurement (below)	Sites are mid-upper arm (midpoint of acromial and olecranon processes), mid-thigh (midpoint between lower gluteal fold and posterior patella crease), mid-calf (maximal circumference) Use non-stretch tape measure, avoid compressing skin in application	See above
Mid-arm muscle circumference (MAMC)	Index of changes in protein reserve in skeletal muscle Assumes that that mass of muscle group is proportional to protein content and also reflects total body muscle mass; both can be challenged.	From TSF (cm) and LC (cm) derive MAMC (cm) as follows. MAMC = MAC − (3.142×TSF) Note TSF measurement divided by 10 to convert to centimetres	Limb and layers of muscle and bone not concentric and continuous Muscle composition affected by ageing, muscular dystrophies, semistarvation Muscle mass can change with immobility, neurological disorders impairing innervation Reference values see above

Measurements usually made on the non-dominant arm.

methods used to measure some vitamins and trace elements.

Serum proteins   Albumin, transferrin, thyroxine-binding prealbumin (transthyretin) and retinol-binding protein, all of which are synthesized by the liver, have been used selectively as nutritional markers of visceral protein status, based on the assumption that undernutrition leads to a decline in hepatic protein production. The criteria for the ideal serum protein marker encompass short half-life, rapid rate of biosynthesis and small body pool size, which would ensure a high sensitivity to undernutrition. However, hepatic protein synthesis is adversely affected by several non-nutritional factors, for example hepatic diseases (cirrhosis), infection and inflammation. Contraction or expansion of extracellular fluid volume (concentrating and dilutional effects), loss of proteins from the vascular compartment in certain disease states (glomerulonephritis, nephrotic syndrome) or in wound exudate, and intravenous administration of blood products can all affect serum protein concentrations. Losses of proteins in exudate from extensive leg ulceration could limit the usefulness of serum proteins as nutritional markers.

The role of visceral proteins in the nutritional assessment of critically ill patients who have a metabolic injury response as a result of trauma, injury or sepsis has recently been evaluated, drawing on a number of research papers (Raguso et al 2003). Conclusions were that thyroxine-binding prealbumin and C-reactive protein (an inflammatory marker), measured twice weekly in the early stages of metabolic injury responses, were valuable, as they provided a view on the metabolic picture of anabolism versus catabolism. As the injury response and inflammatory markers gradually subside, the continued monitoring of thyroxine-binding prealbumin provides an index of the adequacy of nutritional status and support. It is not clear whether or not patients with severely inflamed and infected leg ulcers have a metabolic injury response but, since evidence exists to support the idea that this occurs in severe pressure ulceration, the possibility cannot be excluded.

Albumin   The body pool size of albumin is substantial, estimated to be 5000 mg/kg body weight in an adult, of which one third is distributed in the intravascular and two-thirds in the extravascular compartment. The half-life is relatively long, at 21 days; hence, chronic starvation is marked by a slow fall in the serum albumin concentration; in some cases no change in the serum albumin concentration occurs because of a compensatory shift from the extravascular compartment and lower rates of albumin degradation. Serum albumin concentrations decline during conditions that trigger metabolic injury responses resulting in protein catabolism (trauma, surgery, sepsis); renal diseases that result in albuminuria (see above); and septic shock associated with increased vascular permeability, in which albumin shifts to the extravascular compartment can occur. A number of studies have indicated that albumin is an important predictor of morbidity and mortality in a range of clinical conditions (Selberg & Sel 2001); a recent report by Rapp-Kesek et al (2004) found low serum albumin predictive of an increased risk for sepsis following cardiac surgery. Normal values for the serum albumin concentration range from 35–45 g/litre; values of less than 21 g/litre have been considered to be indicative of undernutrition in the absence of the non-nutritional factors summarized above.

Transferrin   In contrast to albumin, the body pool size of this plasma protein is 100 mg/kg body weight and the half life is 8–10 days. Therefore, it is potentially more sensitive to changes in nutritional status. However, non-nutritional variables can affect the synthesis of transferrin, for example pregnancy, iron deficiency and hypoxaemia (increased synthesis), and chronic sepsis and protein-losing enteropathies (decreased synthesis). Normal concentrations are in the range 2.5–3.0 g/litre; less than 1.0 g/litre indicative of severe undernutrition.

Retinol-binding protein and thyroxine-binding prealbumin   Both proteins have short half-lives of 12 hours and 2 days respectively. Body pool sizes are small; only 2 mg/kg body weight for retinol-binding protein and 10 mg/kg body weight for thyroxine-binding prealbumin; sensitivity to undernutrition is therefore potentially high. Serum concentrations of both proteins are affected by some non-nutritional variables, notably stress, injury and trauma (both decline); iron deficiency (decrease in thyroxine-binding prealbumin); and deficiency of vitamin A, zinc and hyperthyroidism (decrease in retinol-binding protein). Retinol-binding protein is renally filtered, so serum concentrations rise in acute renal failure. In selected patient groups, serum concentrations of these proteins rise in response to refeeding (Raguso et al 2003). Normal serum concentrations are 0.16–0.30 g/litre for thyroxine-binding prealbumin (severe undernutrition <0.05 g/litre) and 0.026–0.1 g/litre for retinol-binding protein.

Other biochemical markers   A number of trace elements, notably the metals zinc, iron and copper, are thought to play a vital role in the healing of chronic wounds such as leg ulcers; information about deficiency states could therefore be helpful in planning either nutritional interventions or the application of topical treatments containing trace metals such as zinc. It is acknowledged that assessment of trace element status is complex in healthy individuals and, in the unhealthy, the presence of a number of complications can limit the ability to diagnose a deficiency state. Reasons for this are that trace metals are transported by plasma proteins; the levels of these can change in disease states, injury and trauma, so that changes in plasma proteins, and thus of trace metals, can vary without any appreciable changes in tissue stores. Levels of both may also be affected by haemodilution and haemoconcentration. With regard to zinc, the plasma reference interval is 12–18 µmol/litre and levels consistently below 8.0 µmol/litre merit further investigation. Although monitoring the plasma zinc levels can detect deficiency before the onset of physical signs, the laboratory methods for diagnosing mild deficiency are problematic (Fell & Talwar 1998). With regard to the latter, a positive clinical response to controlled zinc supplementation is probably the most reliable index in diagnosis of a deficiency state. For more detailed information on the assessment of both trace element and vitamin status see Fell & Talwar (1998), Shenkin (1998) and World Health Organization (1996).

Dietary assessments

Two broad approaches to dietary assessment can be discerned; the dietary history (qualitative) and records of dietary intake (quantitative). A number of approaches to dietary history have been developed, some encompassing both qualitative and quantitative elements. A dietary history is taken directly from the patient during an assessment interview and requires the collection of data relating to the range and varieties of foods eaten together with disease-related, social and cultural factors that could affect intakes. The following information could be included.

- A review of eating patterns, types and frequency of foods consumed and portion sizes, incorporating questions about typical daily and weekend patterns of meal consumption, snacks, beverages and condiments
- Ethnic background and its influence on eating habits
- Levels of physical mobility and activity, particularly as they relate to the ability to shop independently for food and to prepare it
- Facilities within the home for storing and preparing food; living alone or with others
- Current health status, noting the presence, duration and treatment of any acute or chronic illnesses that, either directly or as a consequence of treatment, may affect dietary intakes
- Modifications in diet due to chronic diseases such as diabetes mellitus, renal or hepatic disease
- Impact of dental status, presence of distressing symptoms associated with ill health and effects on dietary intakes, e.g. anorexia, nausea, vomiting, dysphagia, taste changes, pain, diarrhoea
- Drug treatment and any potential effects on nutritional status through side effects or drug–drug or drug–nutrient interactions, e.g. side effects of corticosteroids and antineoplastic drugs
- Financial status as affecting ability to purchase foods.

Recording dietary intakes   Approaches that can be used here to complement the above information include food diaries, food frequency questionnaires, recall and weighed food methods. Westerterp & Goris (2002) have reviewed a number of studies that have used either dietary records or recall methods (see below) to quantify food intakes and have provided an analysis of misreporting and its implications. Bias in assessment of dietary intake was analysed from studies comparing dietary intakes with doubly-labelled-water-assessed energy expenditure. Many studies showed a lower value for reported energy intake than total energy expenditure. Physical and psychological features of study participants influenced reporting bias.

- Food diaries (dietary records) can be used for variable periods of time (usually 3–7 days) to enable subjects to record all foods and beverages consumed, based on household measures or portion sizes. Variant approaches have used weight scales to record foods consumed and leftovers. Methods of cooking, brand names, condiments and environment (home, restaurant, etc.) are also recorded. It is usual to include week and weekend days in the recording period. The potential drawbacks of this approach are that it requires commitment, time and patient understanding on the part of the subject. Compliance problems can occur, as can bias and inaccuracy in recording. Monthly and seasonal variations in food intake can be missed.
- Recall methods require the subject to remember, describe and quantify the foods and beverages consumed either in the preceding 24 hours or over longer time periods. A standardized protocol is used to record information; portion sizes and food models quantify intake. Potential limitations with this method are that memory may be unreliable, recall over certain days may not cover typical dietary patterns over weeks and months and subjects may be economical with the truth. The advantages include high compliance and speed in use.
- Weighing methods, in which food is weighed before meals and any remaining is re-weighed at the end, can provide greater accuracy than recall or diary methods. Usually, weighed intakes are made over a 3-day consecutive period, including one weekend day. Disadvantages are that this method can lead to food cooling, which alters its palatability, and it may miss both weekly and seasonal variation.
- Food frequency questionnaires (self administered or by interview) provide detailed information on the frequency with which foods are consumed on a daily, weekly and monthly basis.

Information on portion sizes is also required. Various approaches have been described, including selective sampling of food areas believed to be deficient, or more global approaches to food consumption.

Interview approaches require sensitivity, good interpersonal skills and the avoidance of judgemental attitudes which could bias responses. At the end of any interview reading the information back to the subject is helpful in confirming points of accuracy. Following the collection of dietary data, information can be entered on computer software programmes and analysed for energy, macro and micronutrient content. Following this, comparisons of intakes with reference values can provide an estimate of the adequacy of dietary intakes (Department of Health 2001a).

Clinical examination
A number of physical signs can be indicative of a nutritional deficiency state, notably in the features of vitamin and trace element deficiency summarized below. A problem with their use in the diagnosis of deficiency states is that some may be features of the underlying disease.

Body composition assessment
A number of specialist methods are available to quantify different body compartments: magnetic resonance imaging, neutron activation analysis, dual energy X-ray absorptiometry (DEXA), isotope techniques (using tritiated water and labelled potassium) and hydrostatic weighing. As Waitzberg & Correia (2003) have commented, very little work has been done in applying these methods to routine monitoring of malnourished patients. Costs, impracticality, limited availability and accessibility have constrained their use, although less costly and more readily available methods such as bioelectric impedance analysis, which measures fat free mass, are under evaluation.

New approaches
A relatively new approach to body composition testing is provided by air displacement plethysmography. The fundamental principle here is use of the subtraction method to determine body volume. The

body volume is equal to the volume of the empty chamber minus the volume of the chamber when an individual sits quietly within it (Fields & Hunter 2004). Corrections are employed for the air in the lung during measurement. To date this technique is undergoing extensive reliability and validity testing. Its applications could be invaluable for precision nutritional assessment in elderly populations. It has advantages over other high-precision methods such as DEXA and hydrostatic weighing, which are uncomfortable for individuals with back pain, immobility and other medical problems.

Another promising technique is the measurement of the thickness of the adductor pollicis muscle located in the hand, between thumb and forefinger, to provide a reflection of muscle mass. This muscle is flat and located between two bony structures, and is therefore relatively easy to measure; thickness of the muscle has been found to correlate positively with other anthropometric variables that estimate muscle mass in healthy subjects. Further field testing is under way and appears hopeful (Lameu et al 2004).

ASSESSMENT OF NUTRITIONAL REQUIREMENTS

Following screening and assessment, the confirmation that an individual is either at high risk of developing malnutrition or is already malnourished is followed by further assessment of nutritional requirements for energy, protein and micronutrients. This is usually conducted by a dietitian and is a prelude to considering how nutritional support can be most effectively delivered, either orally or artificially by the enteral or parenteral routes. Patients suffering from leg ulceration may have raised energy, nitrogen and micronutrient requirements, due to the fact that the presence of an extensive area of ulceration may trigger a metabolic injury response. Unfortunately there is a paucity of research in leg ulcer patients regarding this, but biochemical investigations to establish its presence are fairly easy to conduct and could include measurement of acute phase reactants, cytokines and hormonal mediators in serum. Assessments of requirements should consider any evidence for this against the wider background of requirements for

healing, medical diagnoses, pre-existing nutritional status and any needs for nutrient repletion. The presence of ulcer sepsis accompanied by a pyrexia could also increase requirements, for example an increase in body core temperature of 1°C can increase energy requirements by 5–10% (Selberg & Sel 2001).

In chronically undernourished individuals, the risks of refeeding syndrome should be borne in mind when assessing requirements and initiating feeding. This is marked by hypophosphataemia and can progress to serious fluid and electrolyte disequilibrium, cardiac arrhythmias and cardiac failure. Correction of any electrolyte imbalances before initiating feeding, together with a slow build-up in energy provision, is necessary to avoid this, while continuing to monitor serum phosphate and other electrolytes.

Energy requirements can be determined in a number of ways, for example by indirect calorimetry, predictive equations, nomograms and reference tables. Some reference tables are suitable only for use in healthy populations, for example Department of Health (2001a), and are not relevant to unhealthy, metabolically compromised individuals. Predictive equations are commonly used in clinical practice to approximate energy requirements; a number have been published and subjected to tests of validity and reliability. Since physical characteristics such as sex, age, height and weight account for most of the variation in body cell mass, they can be used to estimate energy requirements (Selberg & Sel 2001). These are incorporated in the Harris–Benedict equations for healthy men and women, as follows, where REE is resting energy expenditure:

Men REE (kcal/d) = 66.47 + 13.75 × weight (kg) + 5.0 × height (cm) − 6.76 × age (years)

Women REE (kcal/) = 655.09 + 9.56 × weight (kg) + 1.85 × height (cm) − 4.66 × age (years)

In healthy people, total resting energy expenditure per day approximates to 1.3 times the value of the Harris–Benedict prediction in men and women. Further correction factors (e.g. for activity) must be applied to obtain total energy expenditure. In the case of the unhealthy, the Harris–Benedict equation has been used in conjunction with correction factors to reflect physical activity and the altered energy expenditure associated with clinical conditions. Correction factors have been developed by comparing indirect calorimetry measurements in hospitalized patients with the REE of normal subjects. Examples of these correction factors are 1.2 (confined to bed), 1.3 (out of bed), surgery (1.1 minor, 1.2 major), infection (1–1.2 mild, 1.2–1.4 moderate, 1.4–1.8 severe), blunt trauma (1.15–1.35), burns (1–1.95) (Long 1984). Considerable debate is evident in the literature regarding the accuracy of the Harris–Benedict equation and the various correction factors used for clinical conditions. Readers are referred to the papers by Reid & Carlson (1998) and Siervo et al (2003) for further consideration of the use of calorimetry and limitations of predictive equations.

An alternative approach is to use a combination of predictive equation to determine basal metabolic rate, apply an adjustment from a nomogram for metabolic stress, add an adjustment for activity and diet-induced thermogenesis and make a final correction dependent on whether it is intended that energy stores are increased or decreased (McAtear 1996). The nomogram used in this approach was developed by Elia (1990) to indicate metabolic rate adjustments caused by various stressors, including burns, sepsis and fractures.

Indirect calorimetry offers a means of measuring energy expenditure from information on respiratory gas exchange; these measurements can now be made at the bedside using a metabolic monitor, most commonly in critical care settings. The physiological basis of this is that, in the steady state, a constant amount of oxygen is consumed, a constant amount of carbon dioxide is produced and a constant amount of energy is released for each mole of a specific nutrient (carbohydrate, fat, protein) oxidized. Energy expenditure is determined from the respiratory quotient (RQ = ratio of volume of CO_2 produced to that of O_2 consumed) and the urinary nitrogen excretion. From this data it is possible through a sequence of steps to eventually compute total resting energy expenditure in kcal/24 h; however the value derived depends on the conditions under which measurements were obtained; in a resting patient it is usual to make several measurements over periods ranging from a few minutes up to an hour, in any 24-hour period.

The measurements do reflect any alterations in energy expenditure induced by clinical condition but they do not allow for periods of activity, episodic pyrexia or the need for nutritional repletion in an undernourished individual; correction factors are needed to make these adjustments.

It is acknowledged that many clinical units do not have access to metabolic monitors and the use of predictive equations can be unreliable in the critically ill. It has been suggested that the majority of adult hospitalized patients can be maintained on 25–35 non-protein kcal/kg body weight per day and that an upper limit of 40 kcal/kg body weight should not be exceeded in the critically ill (Pennington 1996).

Basal protein requirements in adults are approximately 0.8 g/kg ideal body weight per day (Selberg & Sel 2001). Nitrogen requirements can be determined using nitrogen balance studies or from reference tables, which provide ranges of intakes based on metabolic status and body weight. For the latter see McAtear 1996. Dietary protein values can be converted to nitrogen, based on the fact that 6.25 g protein contains approximately 1 g nitrogen. Nitrogen balance studies require three sequential 24-hour urine collections to be completed accurately; this can be problematic in clinical practice. Essentially, nitrogen balance is calculated from nitrogen input (from dietary protein) and nitrogen output (losses as urinary nitrogen, plus 2–4 g per day in hair, sweat, skin and faecal losses). To avoid cumbersome methods, urinary urea nitrogen (80% of the total nitrogen) is measured and a correction is made that considers changes in the serum urea nitrogen:

$$\text{Nitrogen balance} = \text{protein intake (g)}/6.25 - \text{urinary nitrogen} + 4 \text{ g.}$$

This does not consider losses in wound exudate, fistula outputs or severe diarrhoea, for which fluids, further collections, analyses and adjustments to overall balance are necessary. In non-catabolic individuals, nitrogen intakes are usually calculated to exceed losses by 3–5 g per day. Substantial negative nitrogen balances can occur during the peak catabolic response to injury. In this situation matching nitrogen provision to urinary nitrogen excretion is not advocated, particularly if this results in intakes of nitrogen greater than 0.3 g/kg body weight, which can be dangerous. Nitrogen balance can be achieved in most patients at 0.2 g/kg body weight per day (Pennington 1996).

Micronutrients (vitamins, trace elements and minerals)

Most commonly, reference tables are used to estimate requirements and provide information on the needs of metabolically compromised patients and those receiving artificial nutritional support. Further information is available in Shenkin (1995, 1997, 1998) and Fell & Talwar (1998). Recommendations for vitamin and trace element intakes in healthy populations can be found in Food and Nutrition Board (2001), Department of Health (2001a) and World Health Organization (1996). See also the section on Macronutrients and micronutrients: influences on healing, above.

NUTRITIONAL SUPPORT

Scope of support

As discussed earlier, patients with leg ulceration are predominately elderly, frequently have a number of underlying pathological conditions and may be free-living in the community or receiving care in acute or long-term residential settings. In its broadest sense, nutritional support aims to improve nutritional status through the maintenance of lean body mass, organ function and immunocompetence. Restoring body composition and preventing malnutrition-related complications such as delayed wound healing and sepsis are also vital aspects of nutritional support. In patients suffering from leg ulceration, this can encompass the prevention and treatment of obesity, removing a contributory factor for venous hypertension; however, there is little evidence about the influence of obesity on leg ulcer healing. In addition, nutritional interventions that aim to treat undernutrition and promote the healing of leg ulceration and other aspects of recovery can be instituted; these can encompass oral feeding, use of supplements and, when appropriate, artificial feeding, for example via the enteral route.

Healing of leg ulcers requires the delivery of a coordinated service, using evidence-based protocols involving the expertise of specialist nurses (Simon et al 2004). Leg ulcer nurse specialists are in the best position to coordinate referral to nutrition support services for expert advice in the management of obesity and undernutrition. Subsequently, the effective delivery of nutritional support requires a multidisciplinary team approach, integrating the knowledge and skills of leg ulcer specialists, clinicians, dietitians, nurses and pharmacists.

Obesity: causes in older adults

As indicated above, the prevalence of obesity is increasing among older adults in westernized cultures, where it can predispose to the development of vascular disease, diabetes mellitus and, via venous hypertension, leg ulceration. Although obesity is relatively common, in extreme old age its prevalence declines, because of the 'anorexia of ageing' (see below). Underlying the development of obesity are a number of contributory factors, notably reductions in energy expenditure due to a decline in basal metabolic rate, reduced physical activity and lower whole-body fat oxidation. Decline in muscle mass underpins both the fall in metabolic rate and reduction in physical activity. If energy intake does not decline alongside the decline in energy expenditure, the inevitable result is weight gain (Kennedy et al 2004). Other factors that can be contributory to weight gain are low-grade inflammatory processes linked to endocrine changes (integral components of ageing), which can lead to a reduction in lean body mass, immune function and insulin resistance (Grimble 2003). Hypothyroidism and treatment with drugs that have metabolic side effects (e.g. corticosteroids) can also be contributory.

PREVENTION OF OBESITY

The cornerstones of prevention are lifestyle modifications that aim to ensure dietary adequacy and prevent decline in muscle mass and accumulation of fat with increasing age. The nutritional requirements necessary to maintain the health of older people have been identified in guidelines published by the Department of Health (1992, 2001a). Exercise offers another important facet of prevention, since its benefits can increase muscle mass and raise metabolic rate, increasing energy expenditure. Gentle to moderate exercise that is taken regularly, for example walking, swimming and tai chi, can benefit weight maintenance and improve circulatory efficiency.

Established obesity

Lifestyle modifications incorporating both exercise and diet can be indicated here as part of a holistic approach to treatment. Exercise is an effective intervention in obese older adults but, since many cannot tolerate aerobic exercise, alternative approaches have been evaluated. Several studies have demonstrated benefits of moderate resistance training, some using home-based programmes (Deschenes & Kramer 2003, Irwin et al 2003). Improvements in lean body mass and feelings of wellbeing have been experienced by participants. Since maintenance of mobility and independence are important facets of leg ulcer treatment, engagement in gentle resistance exercise programmes could be beneficial. Sufficient mobility to activate the calf muscle pump is one of several indications for superficial venous surgery directed at the improvement of leg ulcer healing in venous incompetence (Simon et al 2004).

The effect of obesity on mortality appears to be less marked with age (Calle et al 1999) and evidence supporting the presence of modest overweight as a risk factor for vascular disease is lacking. At what point are dietary modifications indicated as part of a weight-reducing programme? Opinions vary but medically supervised weight reduction has been thought necessary in morbidly obese older adults (Morley & Glick 1995). Control of obesity (BMI <30) is also an indication for superficial venous surgery (Simon et al 2004). Where weight reduction is thought necessary, setting goals for slow, steady weight loss, for example 0.25–0.5 kg per week, on a diet that is nutritionally balanced, considers requirements for healing and is within financial budget, is advisable. Care should be taken when treating obesity in older age groups, since reduction in energy intakes may lead to reduced fat mass and muscle mass. For these reasons, expert advice should be sought about the initiation and choice of any dietary regime. Information about the influence of obesity on healing, which could usefully contribute to a rehabilitation programme is lacking.

UNDERNUTRITION: PREVENTION AND TREATMENT, PROMOTION OF HEALING

Causes of undernutrition are multifactorial (see above) and elderly patients with leg ulcers exhibit similar dietary risk patterns to those found in the general population of older people. Thus, some are at risk of developing nutritional deficiencies that could adversely affect healing. Strategies aimed to improve dietary intakes in older people in diverse care settings, include the use of fortified foods, supplements, flavour enhancement, food delivery systems that benefit choice and skilled feeding assistance at mealtimes.

Fortified foods

These have been used to increase energy and protein nutrient density, with or without changes in portion sizes. However, smaller-portion meals may be preferred by older people whose appetites are decreased as a result of 'the anorexia of ageing' and ill-health. Means of increasing nutrient density include the addition of cream or evaporated milk to puddings, grated cheese or cream to soups, sauces and butter to mashed potato. A number of studies have shown that use of fortified foods in elderly care units increased energy intakes significantly and reduced food wastage (Barton et al 2000).

Flavour enhancement

This can be a useful tactic to compensate for the impairment of taste and smell in older people. Increased hunger, average body weight and improvements in smell perception have been reported in one controlled nursing home study where flavour enhancers were used (Mathey et al 2001).

Food delivery systems

Food delivery systems that comprise decentralized bulk food portioning, in which food is served at the point of delivery, may be beneficial. This allows choice on the basis of visual and olfactory stimuli and can influence portion sizes. Increased average energy intakes in nursing home residents have been reported using this system (Shatenstein & Ferland 2000).

Feeding assistance

Feeding assistance is necessary to enable dependent, disabled people to maintain an adequate dietary intake. Using a protocol for assisted feeding that comprised one-to-one assistance, social interaction, attention to preferences for dining location, extended access to meal trays and verbal/physical prompts significantly improved food intakes in a residential care setting (Simmons et al 2001).

Supplements

Supplements can be used for varying lengths of time to complement dietary intakes in patients who are unable to eat enough to meet their nutritional needs. The rationale for the latter can be increased nutrient requirements, anorexia or difficulties with chewing foods. Supplements are usually fruit- or milk-based, energy- and nutrient-dense beverages that are available in the form of commercially prepared sip feeds and drinks. To be effective, it is vital that they are administered at the time prescribed and in the quantities recommended. Some patients find supplements unpalatable and there is evidence of failure to comply with the prescription, which can limit effectiveness (Bruce et al 2003). The use of supplements has been evaluated in older adults at risk of malnutrition and specifically in patients suffering from leg ulceration.

Protein and energy supplementation in older adults

This was the subject of a Cochrane Review by Milne et al in 2002, which included 31 trials with 2464 randomized patients. This review included patients with a range of medical conditions but excluded those in critical care or suffering from cancer. Principal findings were that supplementation produced a small but consistent weight gain, together with a significant beneficial effect on mortality and a shorter length of hospital stay. More evidence from multicentre studies is needed to confirm this finding. A later systematic review by Baldwin & Parsons (2004) evaluated evidence regarding the efficacy of no dietary advice, dietary advice alone, advice with the use of supplements and supplements alone in adults suffering from disease-related

malnutrition (undernutrition). Findings were that nutritional supplements may have a greater role than dietary advice in the short-term improvement of body weight. A prospective, randomized, controlled evaluation of supplement use by Edington et al (2004) found that nutritional status improved significantly over a 24-week period in an intervention group of malnourished elderly patients who had been discharged from hospital. However, no significant differences between intervention and control groups could be detected at week 24 in terms of nutritional status. Conclusions were that all elderly patients should be assessed and interventions initiated earlier before discharge from hospital.

Supplementation in leg and foot ulceration

Clinical studies investigating the impact of supplements on healing are lacking in the literature. A randomized controlled trial was conducted by Eneroth et al (2004) to determine if oral nutritional supplements improved wound healing in malnourished patients with diabetic foot ulcers, in comparison with placebo. An interesting finding was that, on the basis of anthropometric, biochemical and haematological evidence, 32% of all the patients in this study were undernourished at inclusion and 40% were malnourished 6 months later. Because of methodological problems, the fact that intervention and placebo groups were not comparable regarding measures of peripheral circulation, and lack of information regarding compliance with supplementation, the findings of this study were not able to show any benefits on wound healing.

An earlier study by Wissing et al (2002) used a case study design (six patients) to determine whether an individualized programme of nutritional support could improve healing in therapy-resistant venous leg ulcers. An individualized dietary plan was designed that included the use of a dietary supplement containing macro- and micronutrients (vitamin C and zinc) together with ordinary meals. Patients were followed up over a 9-month period, during which they received home dietetic support, and ulcer area, anthropometric, biochemical and dietary indicators of nutritional status were assessed. Outcomes were complete healing in two patients and almost complete healing in two others. Two patients stopped taking the supplements at 5 and 20 weeks respectively. Findings were that nutritional support might have assisted healing.

The potential influence of zinc, both dietary and topically applied, on the healing of venous leg ulcers has been a focus of research interest for many years. A Cochrane Review of published research was conducted by Wilkinson & Hawke (1998), which evaluated the effectiveness of oral zinc on the healing of arterial and venous ulcers. Only six trials met criteria for inclusion, four of which measured the serum zinc at baseline or later during the period of study. Although no benefits of zinc sulphate on numbers of healed ulcers could be demonstrated, in people with a low serum zinc at baseline, some evidence of a positive effect was present. This is an important area for further research in borderline and established zinc deficiency states.

Enteral nutrition

Since patients with leg ulcers can have a number of underlying conditions, situations can arise when enteral feeding is necessary. An introduction to selected aspects of use and the potential impact of feeding on clinical outcomes is included here. A considerable body of evidence is now available to guide the selection of different types of feeding regimens, equipment for administration and monitoring metabolic changes. This is well outside the scope of this text, so readers are referred to further sources at the end of the chapter.

Indications

Enteral nutrition is a mainstay of artificial nutrition support, given its benefits in preservation of gut function, integrity, immune function and cost-effectiveness. Although not risk free, it is generally regarded as safer than parenteral nutrition (Gopalan & Khanna 2003). Enteral nutrition is indicated in a number of situations where an individual is unable to meet their nutritional requirements via normal processes of food ingestion, yet has sufficient accessible, functioning bowel to allow the absorption of nutrients. Specific indications for using enteral nutrition include obstruction of the upper gastrointestinal tract (malignant disease affecting oesophagus or pharynx); trauma to the face and jaw; oropharyngeal dysphagia (stroke and other neurological diseases); and raised nutrient requirements (severe sepsis, trauma, injury). A number of contraindications for use of enteral nutrition exist; these include paralytic ileus, gastrointestinal haemorrhage, peritonitis and severe, intractable vomiting or diarrhoea. Acute pancreatitis, enterocutaneous fistula and gut ischaemia can be relative contraindications to use depending on the individual clinical situation; for example, in a proximally sited enterocutaneous fistula it may be possible to deliver enteral nutrients distal to the fistula.

Routes

Choice of enteral feeding route is determined by the precise level and adequacy of gastrointestinal function; accessibility for the insertion of an enteral catheter; practicality in the light of anticipated duration of use, comfort and safety of positioning, and patient preference. A number of enteral delivery routes exist, including nasogastric, nasoduodenal and nasojejunal techniques, gastrostomy and jejunostomy (the latter two endoscopically or surgically inserted). Nasogastric, nasoduodenal and nasojejunal fine-bore catheters are used for short-term feeding and other routes where longer-term nutritional support is needed. Radiological verification and verification through aspiration and testing of gut fluids are necessary before commencing enteral feeding.

Impact on outcomes

Of particular relevance to the healing of chronic wounds are the comparative outcomes associated with enteral feeding in groups that vary in terms of nutritional status (e.g. mild, moderately and severely undernourished versus well nourished). Also of interest are any benefits resulting from the use of feeding regimens augmented with novel nutrients, for example glutamine, arginine (see above). Although few research studies have investigated the impact of enteral feeding on chronic wound outcomes, animal and some clinical studies have shown that, in other types of wound, undernutrition is associated with 'slow' or 'delayed' healing, altered tensile strength, dehiscence, anastomotic leakage, breakdown and fistula formation (Albina 1994, Satyanarayana & Klein 1998). In many studies, the absence or lack of specifically clinical significance and visibility of wound outcomes used (frequently merged within general categories of 'infectious complications'); the lack of comparability in feeding regimens (formulation, duration, continuity), together with the impact of non-nutritional variables such as case mix and drug therapy on outcomes, renders interpretation of findings difficult.

- Reviews of randomized controlled trials by Klein et al (1997) and Satyanarayana & Klein (1998) found evidence of benefit from short-term enteral feeding with regard to reduced rates of complications. Numbers of trials demonstrating benefit were small.
- Based on a meta-analysis and consideration of up-to-date clinical trials, conclusions were that glutamine supplementation had a beneficial effect on infectious complications and reduced hospital stay. Evidence was stronger for parenteral than for enteral nutrition. In critically ill patients it may reduce morbidity and mortality (Melis et al 2004).
- Concerns have arisen that arginine may contribute to mortality in critically ill patients through excessive production of nitric oxide (Heyland et al 2001, Dent et al 2003). A recent expert view is that arginine-enriched enteral formulae should not be used in the critically ill but that weak evidence suggested benefit in other groups of surgical patients (MacFie 2004). With regard to the latter, early postoperative enteral nutrition augmented with arginine, omega-3 fatty acids and ribonucleic acid improved surgical wound healing (specific wound outcomes provided) in patients undergoing surgery for gastric cancer (Farreras et al 2005).

Complications

Enteral nutrition can cause complications, so careful monitoring is necessary to ensure prompt intervention if any problems occur. The technique should only be used in institutions where the expertise is available for general management and monitoring (McFie 2004). Complications can include the following.

- *Aspiration pneumonia*: anterograde aspiration of fluid into the respiratory tract during swallowing, or retrograde aspiration due to reflux of enteral contents; for diagnosis see Gomes et al 2004. Elevation of the head and shoulders to 30° during nasogastric or gastrostomy feeding and for 1 hour after is advocated to assist gravitational drainage (McAtear 1999).
- *Metabolic disequilibration*: fluid and electrolyte imbalances; acidosis, alkalosis; hypophosphataemia (refeeding syndrome in the chronically malnourished); routine biochemical monitoring is mandatory prior to and following feeding. Phosphate repletion is necessary if hypophosphataemia occurs.
- *Enteral catheter misplacement, obstruction*: risk factors for nasoenteral tube misplacement include endotracheal intubation, tracheostomy, altered mental status and impaired cough reflexes (Gopalan & Khanna 2003); technical expertise for insertion and maintenance and guidelines for checking safe positioning are essential.
- *Tissue damage and wound infections*: perforation of the oesophagus (nasogastric); minor maceration and infections or more serious complications of necrotizing fasciitis, bleeding, perforation and ileus have been reported (gastrostomy).
- *Diarrhoea*: can be attributed to contamination of feeds, side effects of drugs, gut infections or pre-existing bowel disorders, feed osmolality, lack of fibre in feed formulation; diagnosis and treatment of contributing factors are necessary, including microbiological screening.
- *Interactions between drugs and constituents of enteral feeds*: such interactions can either modify the effects of nutrients by the prior or concurrent administration of a drug or modify the effects of a drug by prior of concurrent administration of nutrients (Lourenco 2001). The results can include changes in the efficacy of nutrition support or modifications in the pharmacological response to a drug. Such interactions can have relevance to wound healing. For example, formation of insoluble complexes between tetracyclines, antacids and the trace metals zinc and iron can occur, reducing absorption of these micronutrients, which are vital for healing. Dietary fibre (now a component of fibre-enhanced

enteral feeds) can decrease the amount of amoxicillin absorbed from the gut, reducing therapeutic effect through adsorption of the drug on to the fibre; if the drug is prescribed for a wound infection, this could delay healing. Separating medication and enteral feeding with a specified interval is necessary to prevent these interactions. Drug nutrient interactions are not confined to enteral feeding but to ingestion of diet and drugs more broadly; expert pharmacological advice is necessary to ensure that these interactions do not compromise patient outcomes.

Ensuring the quality of nutritional support

Past reviews of the literature relating to the quality of nutritional support have shown that sometimes organizational factors can impede the delivery of a high-quality nutritional service (Green 1999, Elia 2000). These can include inadequate provision of support to individuals at high risk, lack of awareness of the problem of malnutrition because of lack of knowledge and training in nutrition of medical and nursing staff, inadequate hospital management policies and poor organization of services. Many local, national and international evidence-based standards, guidelines and protocols are now available to assist health professionals in the provision of optimal nutritional services to users, for example ESPEN (Kondrup et al 2003) and the Malnutrition Advisory Group (MAG; Elia 2000). The National Minimum Standards for Care Homes

(Department of Health 2001b) contain the key precept that older people resident in care settings should receive 'a varied, appealing, wholesome and nutritious diet that is suited to individual assessed and recorded requirements and that meals are taken in a congenial setting and at flexible times'. This has significant implications for screening, assessment and delivery in relation to quality improvement. Extremely useful information on eating well, aimed at older adults living in the community, is available within guidelines published by the Nutrition Advisory Group for Elderly People (1995) and the Caroline Walker Trust (1995).

CONCLUSIONS

Both under- and overnutrition can pose risks for individuals suffering from leg ulceration in terms of the development of ulceration (obesity) and adverse effects on healing (undernutrition). Within the context of effective multidisciplinary working, the use of valid, reliable screening and assessment procedures, rapid referral for nutrition support for those at risk and efficient management of nutritional interventions linked to routine monitoring is advocated. A number of interventions, encompassing oral and enteral artificial nutrition, can help to improve outcomes in individuals at nutritional risk. Rigorous quality mechanisms including evidence-based standards, guidelines and protocols offer a means of ensuring that the prevalence of malnutrition and its wound related complications are reduced, benefiting patients and service.

References

Albina J E 1994 Nutrition and wound healing. Journal of Parenteral and Enteral Nutrition 18: 367–376

Allison S 2000 Malnutrition and disease related outcomes. Clinical Nutrition 16: 590–593

Allison S 2002 Institutional feeding of the elderly. Current Opinion in Clinical Nutrition and Metabolic Care 5: 31–34

Baldwin C, Parsons T J 2004 Dietary advice and nutritional supplements in the management of illness-related malnutrition: a systematic review. Clinical Nutrition 6: 1267–1279

Barton A D, Beigg C L, Macdonald I A, Allison S P 2000 A recipe for improving intakes in elderly hospital patients. Clinical Nutrition 19: 451–454

Beck A M, Ovesen L 1998 At which body mass index and degree of weight loss should hospitalised elderly patients be considered at risk? Clinical Nutrition 17: 195–198

Bruce D, Laurance I, McGuiness M 2003 Nutritional supplements after hip fracture: poor compliance limits effectiveness. Clinical Nutrition 22: 497–500

Calder P C, Deckelbaum R J 2003 Fat as a physiological regulator: the news gets better. Current Opinion in Clinical Nutrition and Metabolic Care 6: 127–131

Calle E E, Thun M J, Petrelli J M 1999 Body mass index and mortality in a prospective cohort of US adults. New England Journal of Medicine 341: 1097–1105

Campillo B, Paillaud E, Uzan I et al 2004 Value of body mass index in the detection of severe malnutrition: the influence of pathology and changes in anthropometric parameters. Clinical Nutrition 23: 551–559

Caroline Walker Trust 1995 Eating well for older people: report of an expert working group. Caroline Walker Trust, London

Contaldo F, Pasanisi F 2005 Obesity epidemics: simple or simplistic answers? Clinical Nutrition 24: 1–4

Defay R, Delcourt C, Ranvier M 2001 Relationships between physical activity, obesity and diabetes mellitus in a French elderly population: the POLA study (Pathologies Oculaires Liées a l'Age). International Journal of Obesity Relating to Metabolic Disorders 25: 512–518

Dent D L, Heyland D K, Levy H 2003 Immunonutrition may increase mortality in critically ill patients with pneumonia. Critical Care Medicine 30: A17

Department of Health 1992 The nutrition of elderly people. Report on Social Subjects 43. HMSO, London

Department of Health 2001a Dietary reference values for food energy and nutrients for the United Kingdom. Department of Health Report on Health and Social Subjects 41. HMSO, London

Department of Health 2001b National minimum standards: care homes for older people. HMSO, London

Deschenes M R, Kramer W J 2003 Performance and physiologic adaptations to resistance training. American Journal of Physiology and Medical Rehabilitation 81: S3–S16

Edington J, Barnes R, Bryan F 2004 A prospective randomised controlled trial of nutritional supplementation in malnourished elderly in the community: clinical and health economic outcome. Clinical Nutrition: 23: 195–204

Edwards P D, Moldawer L L 1998 Role of cytokines in the metabolic response to stress. Current Opinion in Clinical Nutrition and Metabolic Care 1: 187–190

Efron D T, Barbul A 1998 Modulation of inflammation and immunity by arginine. Current Opinion in Clinical Nutrition and Metabolic Care 1: 531–538

Elia M 1990 Artificial nutritional support. Medical International 82: 3392–3396

Elia M 2000 Guidelines for detection and management of malnutrition. Malnutrition Advisory Group. British Association for Parenteral and Enteral Nutrition, Maidenhead

Eneroth M, Larsson J, Oscarsson C, Apelquist J 2004 Nutritional supplementation for diabetic foot ulcers: the first RCT. Journal of Wound Care 13: 230–234

Farreras N, Artigas V, Cardona D et al 2005 Effect of postoperative enteral nutrition on wound healing in patients undergoing surgery for gastric cancer. Clinical Nutrition 24: 55–65

Fell G S, Talwar D T 1998 Micronutrients: assessment of status. Current Opinion in Clinical Nutrition and Metabolic Care 1: 491–497

Fields D A, Hunter G R 2004 Monitoring body fat in the elderly: application of air displacement plethysmography. Current Opinion in Clinical Nutrition and Metabolic Care 7: 11–14

Finch S, Doyle W, Lowe, C 1998 National Diet and Nutrition Survey: people aged 65 years and over. HMSO, London

Fleiss J L 1971 The measurement of inter-rater agreement. Statistical Methods for Rates and Proportions. John Wiley, New York

Food and Nutrition Board 2001 Standing Committee on the Scientific Evaluation of Dietary Reference Intakes. National Academy Press, Washington, DC

Furst P, Alteheld B, Stehle P 2004 Why should a single nutrient – glutamine – improve outcome? The remarkable story of glutamine dipeptides. Clinical Nutrition 1(Suppl 1): 4–15

Gomes G F, Campos A C, Pisani J C et al 2004 Diagnostic methods for the detection of anterograde aspiration in enterally fed patients. Current Opinion in Clinical Nutrition and Metabolic Care 7: 285–292

Gopalan S, Khanna S 2003 Enteral nutrition delivery techniques. Current Opinion in Clinical Nutrition and Metabolic Care 6: 313–317

Green C J 1999 Existence, causes and consequences of disease related malnutrition in the hospital, and the community and clinical and financial benefits of nutritional intervention. Clinical Nutrition 183–28

Green S, McLaren S 1998 Nutritional assessment and screening: instrument selection. British Journal of Community Nursing 3: 233–242

Griffiths R D 2004 Glutamine in the critically ill patient: can it affect mortality? Clinical Nutrition 1(Suppl 1): 25–32

Grimble R F 2003 Inflammatory response in the elderly. Current Opinion in Clinical Nutrition and Metabolic Care 6: 21–29

Heyland D K, Novak F, Drover J W 2001 Should immunonutrition become routine in critically ill patients? Journal of the American Medical Association 286: 944–953

Irwin M L, Yasui Y, Ulrich C M 2003 Effect of exercise on total and intra-abdominal fat in post menopausal women: a randomized controlled trial. Journal of the American Medical Association 289: 323–330

Kennedy R L, Chokkalingham K, Srinivasan R 2004 Obesity in the elderly: who should we be treating, and why, and how. Current Opinion in Clinical Nutrition and Metabolic Care 7: 3–9

King C L 2003 Predictive validity of the malnutrition universal screening tool (MUST) with regard to mortality and length of stay in elderly in-patients. Clinical Nutrition 22(Suppl 1): S4

Klein S, Kinney J, Jeejeebhoy K 1997 Nutritional support in clinical practice: review of published data and recommendations for future research directions. Journal of Parenteral and Enteral Nutrition 21: 133–156

Kondrup J, Rasmussen H H, Hamberg O, Stanga Z 2002 Nutritional risk screening (NRS 2002): a new method based on an analysis of controlled clinical trials. Clinical Nutrition 22: 321–336

Kondrup J, Allison S, Elia M et al 2003 ESPEN guidelines for nutritional screening 2002. Clinical Nutrition 22: 415–421

Lameu E D, Gerude M F, Campos A C, Luiz R R 2004 The thickness of the adductor pollicis muscle reflects the muscle compartment and may be used as a new anthropometric measure for nutritional assessment. Current Opinion in Clinical Nutrition and Metabolic Care 7: 285–301

Leach M J 2004 Making sense of the venous leg ulcer debate: a literature review. Journal of Wound Care 13: 52–56

Lewis B K, Harding K G 1997 Nutrition in elderly people with leg ulcers. Proceedings of the 7th European Conference on Advances in Wound Management. EMAP Publishing London, pp 106–108

Long C R 1984 The energy and protein requirements of the critically ill patient. In: Wright R A, Heymsfield S (eds) Nutritional assessment. Blackwell Scientific, Oxford, ch. 8, pp 157–175

Lourenco R 2001 Enteral feeding: drug–nutrient interactions. Clinical Nutrition 20: 187–193

McAtear C 1999 Current perspectives on enteral nutrition in adults. British Association for Parenteral and Enteral Nutrition, Maidenhead

MacFie J 2004 European round table: the use of immunonutrients in the critically ill. Clinical Nutrition 23: 1426–1429

Malnutrition Advisory Group 2000 Explanatory notes for the screening tool for adults at risk of malnutrition. British Association for Parenteral and Enteral Nutrition, Maidenhead

Mathey M, Siebelink E, de Graf C, Van Staveren W A 2001 Flavour enhancement of food improves dietary intake and nutritional status of elderly nursing home residents. Journal of Gerontology 56A: M200–M205

Melis C, Wengel N, Boelens P, van Leeuwen P 2004 Glutamine: recent developments in research on the clinical significance of glutamine. Current Opinion in Clinical Nutrition and Metabolic Care 7: 59–70

Milne A C, Potter J E, Avenell A 2002 Protein and energy supplementation in elderly people at risk from malnutrition. In: Cochrane Database of Systematic Reviews, issue 2: CD003288. John Wiley, Oxford

Morley J E, Glick Z 1995 Obesity. In: Morley E, Glick Z, Rubenstein L Z (eds) Geriatric nutrition: a comprehensive review. Raven Press, New York, pp 245–256

Nutrition Advisory Group for Elderly People 1995 Dietetic standards of care for the older adult in hospital. British Dietetic Association, Birmingham

Pennington C R 1996 Current perspectives on parenteral nutrition in adults. British Association for Parenteral and Enteral Nutrition, Maidenhead

Perry L 2003 Nutritional screening tools. In: Nutrition a practical guide. EMAP Healthcare, London, pp 6–7

Powell-Tuck J, Hennessy E M 2003 A comparison of mid upper arm circumference, body mass index and weight loss as indices of undernutrition in acutely hospitalised patients. Clinical Nutrition 22: 307–312

Raguso C A, Dupertuis Y M, Pichard C 2003 The role of visceral proteins in the nutritional assessment of intensive care unit patients. Current Opinion in Clinical Nutrition and Metabolic Care 6:211–216

Rapp-Kesek D, Stahle E, Karlsson T T 2004 Body mass index and albumin in the preoperative evaluation of cardiac surgery patients. Clinical Nutrition 23: 1398–1404

Reid C L, Carlson G 1998 Indirect calorimetry: a review of recent clinical applications. Current Opinion in Clinical Nutrition and Metabolic Care 1: 281–286

Rojas A R, Phillips T J 1999 Patients with chronic leg ulcers show diminished levels of vitamins A and E, carotenes and zinc. Dermatologic Surgery 25: 601–604

Ruberg R 1984 Role of nutrition in wound healing. Surgical Clinics of North America 64: 705–714

Saletti A, Lindgren E Y, Johansson L, Cederholm T 2000 Nutritional status according to mini-nutritional assessment in an institutionalised elderly population in Sweden. Gerontology 46: 139–145

Satyanarayana R, Klein S 1998 Clinical efficacy of perioperative nutritional support. Current Opinion in Clinical Nutrition and Metabolic Care 1: 51–58

Schaffer M R, Efron P A, Thornton F J 1997 Nitric oxide: an autocrine regulator of wound fibroblast synthetic function. Journal of Immunology 158: 2375–2381

Schofield M, Aziz M, Bliss M, Bull R 2003 Medical pathology in patients with leg ulcers: a study carried out in a leg ulcer clinic in a day hospital for the elderly. Journal of Tissue Viability 13: 17–22

Selberg O, Sel S 2001 The adjunctive value of routine biochemistry in nutritional assessment of hospitalised patients. Clinical Nutrition 20: 477–485

Shatenstein B, Ferland G 2000 Absence of nutritional or clinical consequences of decentralised bulk food portioning in elderly nursing home residents with dementia in Montreal. Journal of the American Dietetic Association. 100: 1354–1360

Shenkin A 1995 Adult micronutrient requirements. In: Payne-James J, Grimble R, Silk D (eds) Artificial nutrition support in clinical practice. Edward Arnold, London, pp 151–156

Shenkin A 1997 Micronutrients. In: Rombeau J L, Rolandelli R H (eds) Clinical nutrition: enteral and tube feeding. W B Saunders London, pp 96–111

Shenkin A 1998 Micronutrients in adult nutritional support: requirements and benefits. Current Opinion in Clinical Nutrition and Metabolic Care 1: 15–19

Siervo M, Boschi V, Falconi C 2003 Which REE prediction equation should we use in normal-weight, overweight and obese women? Clinical Nutrition 22: 193–204

Simmons S F, Osterweil D, Schnelle J F 2001 Improving food intake in nursing home residents with feeding assistance: a staffing analysis. Journal of Gerontology 56A: M790–794

Simon D A, Dix F P, McCollum C N 2004 Management of venous leg ulcers. British Medical Journal 328: 1358–1362

Stratton R J, Green C J, Elia M 2003a Disease-related malnutrition: an evidence-based approach to treatment. CABI Publishing, Cambridge, pp 1–34

Stratton R J, Longmore D, Elia M 2003b Concurrent validity of a newly developed malnutrition universal screening tool. Clinical Nutrition 22(Suppl 1): S10

Vellas B, Guigoz Y, Garry P J 1999 The mini-nutritional assessment (MNA) and its use in grading the nutritional state of elderly patients. Nutrition 15: 116–122

Vellas B, Lauque S, Andrieu S et al 2001 Nutritional assessment in the elderly. Current Opinion in Clinical Nutrition and Metabolic Care 4: 5–8

Waitzberg D L, Correa T D 2003 Nutritional assessment in the hospitalised patient. Current Opinion in Clinical Nutrition and Metabolic Care 6: 531–538

Weekes C E, Elia M, Emery P 2004 The development, validation and reliability of a nutrition screening tool based on the recommendations of the British Association for Parenteral and Enteral Nutrition (BAPEN). Clinical Nutrition 23: 1104–1112

Westerterp K R, Goris A 2002 Validity of the assessment of dietary intake: problems of misreporting. Current Opinion in Clinical Nutrition and Metabolic Care 5: 489–493

Wilkinson E A J, Hawke C 1998 Oral zinc for arterial and venous leg ulcers. The Cochrane Database of Systematic Reviews, issue 4: CD 001273. Oxford, Update Software

Wissing U, Ek A C, Unosson M 2001 A follow up study of ulcer healing, nutrition and life situation in elderly patients with leg ulcers. Journal of Nutrition, Health and Ageing 5: 37–42

Wissing U E, Ek A C, Skold G, Unoson M 2002 Can individualised nutritional support improve healing in therapy resistant leg ulcers? Journal of Wound Care 11: 15–20

World Health Organization 1996 Trace elements in human nutrition and health. World Health Organization, Geneva

Yaqoob P 2003 Lipids and the immune response: from molecular mechanisms to clinical applications. Current Opinion in Clinical Nutrition and Metabolic Care 6: 133–150

Zhou Y P, Jiang Z M, Sun Y H et al 2004 The effects of supplemental glutamine dipeptide on gut integrity and clinical outcome after escharectomy in severe burns: a randomised controlled clinical trial. Clinical Nutrition 1(Suppl 1): 55–60

29

Minimizing pain at wound-dressing-related procedures: a consensus document

Medical Education Partnership Ltd

FOREWORD

Professor Keith Harding

This guide is a World Union of Wound Healing Societies' educational initiative. It has been inspired by two seminal documents: the European Wound Management Association (EWMA) position document *Pain at wound dressing changes* (2002) and a supplement to *Ostomy/Wound Management* on 'Practical treatment of wound pain and trauma: a patient-centred approach' (Reddy et al 2003). As an international educational initiative, this document is aimed at anyone involved in dressing-related procedures anywhere in the world.

The principles presented are based on statements from the two documents mentioned above and the consensus opinion of an international expert working group (Best Practice 2003). For the concept of best practice to make a real difference to patient care, clinicians should adopt these recommendations and share them with colleagues, patients and carers.

The expert working group comprised: Michelle Briggs, Leeds University (UK); Frank D Ferris, San Diego Hospice & Palliative Care (USA); Chris Glynn, Churchill Hospital, Oxford (UK); Keith Harding, University of Wales College of Medicine, Cardiff (UK); Deborah Hofman, Churchill Hospital, Oxford (UK); Helen Hollinworth, Suffolk College, Ipswich (UK); Diane L Krasner, Rest Haven, York (USA); Christina Lindholm, Karolinska University Hospital, Stockholm (Sweden); Christine Moffatt, CRICP, Thames Valley University, London (UK); Patricia Price, University of Wales College of Medicine, Cardiff (UK); Marco Romanelli, University of Pisa (Italy); Gary Sibbald, University of Toronto (Canada); Mike Stacey, University of Western Australia (Australia); and Luc Téot, University Hospital Montpellier (France).

This document was supported by an unrestricted educational grant from Molnlycke Health Care and published by Medical Education Partnership Ltd in 2004. It is reprinted here in full with permission of MEP Ltd. To cite the original source of this document please use the following: Minimising pain at wound dressing-related procedures. A consensus document. Medical Education Partnership Ltd, London, 2004.

PRINCIPLES OF BEST PRACTICE

Unresolved pain negatively affects wound healing and has an impact on quality of life. Pain at wound-dressing-related procedures can be managed by a combination of accurate assessment, suitable dressing choices, skilled wound management and individualized analgesic regimens. For therapeutic as well as humanitarian reasons it is vital that clinicians know how to assess, evaluate and manage pain.

Having a basic understanding of pain physiology will help anyone involved in a wound-dressing-related procedure to understand the patient's pain experience. It is fundamental to appreciate that pain from wounds is multidimensional, and the patient's psychosocial environment will influence and impact on the physiological experience of pain.

The International Association for the Study of Pain (www.iasp-pain.org) defines pain as 'an unpleasant sensory and emotional experience associated with actual or potential tissue damage, or described in terms of such damage'.

UNDERSTANDING TYPES OF PAIN

There are two types of pain: nociceptive pain and neuropathic pain. Nociceptive pain may be defined as an appropriate physiological response to a painful stimulus. It may involve acute or chronic inflammation. Acute nociceptive pain occurs as a result of tissue damage and is usually time-limited. Where wounds are slow to heal, the prolonged inflammatory response may cause heightened sensitivity in both the wound (primary hyperalgesia) and the surrounding skin (secondary hyperalgesia).

Neuropathic pain has been defined as an inappropriate response caused by a primary lesion or dysfunction in the nervous system. Nerve damage is the commonest cause of the primary lesion, which may be due to trauma, infection, metabolic disorder or cancer. Neuropathic pain is a major factor in the development of chronic pain. It is often associated with altered or unpleasant sensations whereby any sensory stimulus such as light touch or pressure or changes in temperature can provoke intense pain (allodynia). The clinician must recognize that this requires specific pharmacological management and referral for assessment by a specialist who is able to diagnose (and treat) neuropathic pain.

Patients with increased sensitivity who feel pain at the slightest touch, are likely to find the additional pain from a dressing-related procedure excruciating

---

Application to practice

- Assume all wounds are painful
- Over time wounds may become more painful
- Accept that the skin surrounding the wound can become sensitive and painful
- Accept that for some patients the lightest touch or simply air moving across the wound can be intensely painful
- Know when to refer for specialist assessment

CAUSES OF PAIN

Using a layered approach

The terms background, incident, procedural and operative can be used to describe the cause of pain (Fig. 29.1). Whatever the cause of pain, the patient's experience will be influenced by his/her psychosocial environment.

- *Background pain* is the pain felt at rest, when no wound manipulation is taking place. It may be continuous (e.g. like a toothache) or intermittent (e.g. like cramp or night-time pain). Background pain is related to the underlying cause of the wound, local wound factors (e.g. ischaemia, infection and maceration) and other related pathologies (e.g. diabetic neuropathy, peripheral vascular disease, rheumatoid arthritis and dermatological conditions). The patient may also have pain that is unrelated to the wound, which may impact on the background pain experience (e.g. herpes zoster (shingles), osteoarthritis and cancer)
- *Incident (breakthrough) pain* can occur during day-to-day activities such as mobilization, when coughing or following dressing slippage
- *Procedural pain* results from a routine, basic procedure such as dressing removal, cleansing or dressing application. Non-pharmacological techniques and analgesia may both be required to manage the pain
- *Operative pain* is associated with any intervention that would normally be performed by a specialist clinician and require an anaesthetic (local or general) to manage the pain.

Psychosocial/environment

Factors such as age, gender, educational level, environment and previous pain history can all influence patients' experience of pain and ability to communicate their pain. Clinicians must validate the pain experience and acknowledge the patient's beliefs about the cause of pain as well as the potential benefits of different methods of pain management.

Causes of wound pain

Understanding that there are layers of pain is central to effective assessment and management.

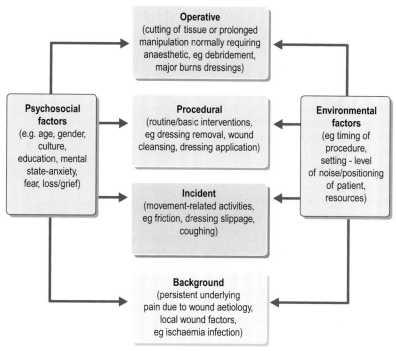

Figure 29.1 Causes of wound pain. Understanding that there are layers of pain is central to effective assessment and management. Pain from a clinical intervention may occur on top of background pain (i.e. pain at rest) and incident pain (i.e. breakthrough pain)

Pain from a clinical intervention occurs on top of background pain (i.e. pain at rest) and incident pain (i.e. breakthrough pain).

ASSESSMENT OF PAIN

Using a layered approach

Given the wide range of wounds and individual responses, it is impossible to guarantee that every patient will feel no pain and it is important to set realistic goals with each patient. Patients can expect to feel some sensation during a dressing-related procedure, but the aim should be to limit pain and discomfort to a minimum. This can only be achieved with the patient's involvement and by using an agreed pain assessment method involving a layered approach to evaluate and, if necessary, change the choice and timing of any analgesics and/or intervention.

Initial assessment

An initial assessment should be carried out by an experienced clinician. This will include a full pain history, building up a picture of background, incident, procedural and operative pain. A body map diagram may be useful to show the location/site of the pain, especially if there is more than one painful area that needs to be scored independently. This assessment provides knowledge of the wound and the patient's pain experience and places it within a patient-centred environment.

Assessment should also try to explore factors such as feelings, perceptions, expectations, meaning of pain and impact of pain on daily/family life. A clinician will need to be a good listener and build up a picture of the patient's beliefs about pain, using simple questions such as 'Where do you believe the pain comes from?' or 'What helps you cope with the pain?' Skilled clinicians may need to use tools such as a Sickness Impact Profile (SIP; Bergner et al

1981) or Quality of Life Scale (QOLS; Flanagan 1978).

On-going assessment

On-going assessment is performed each time a dressing-related procedure is carried out. Background pain in the wound and surrounding tissue, plus any new regional pain that may have developed, should be assessed and the intensity rated before the dressing-related procedure.

Pain intensity should also be rated during and after the intervention as appropriate.

Documenting this in the patient's notes should enable a later evaluation of whether the pain is increasing or decreasing over time. Events related to increased or reduced pain should also be documented.

> Ensure that each pain assessment is individualized, relevant and does not become an additional stressor

Review assessment

A review assessment should be carried out by an experienced clinician as part of a wider case review and ongoing evaluation to assess treatment strategies and progress. The triggers for pain and reducers of pain should be identified and documented. Details such as documented pain scores may be represented graphically, allowing trends to emerge over time and changes in practice, such as pre-emptive analgesia, to be evaluated. An audit review may also reveal unknown relationships, such as different levels of pain after treatment by different carers.

Pain scoring can help reveal trends

In this hypothetical graph (Fig. 29.2), pain scores are recorded before, during and after a dressing-related procedure. The pain is clearly at its worst during the procedure, and a combination of appropriate medication, 'time outs' and adjustments to technique and dressing choices result in a decline in severity. This also has an impact on the pain experience following the procedure.

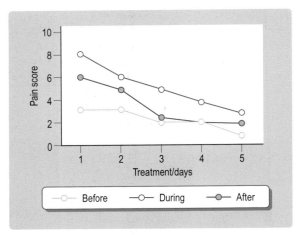

Figure 29.2 Pain scoring can help to reveal trends. In this hypothetical graph, pain scores are recorded before, during and after a dressing-related procedure. The pain is clearly at its worst during the procedure, and a combination of appropriate medication, 'time outs' and adjustments to technique and dressing choices result in a decline in severity. This also has an impact on the pain experience following the procedure

ASSESSMENT STRATEGIES

Pain is whatever the patient says it is, but sometimes the patient doesn't say

Assessment should always involve the patient. In special circumstances, such as dealing with non-communicative young children, the frail elderly or the cognitively impaired, greater patience and understanding is required. In these situations steps must be taken to ensure a comprehensive evaluation of patients' pain management requirements. It can be difficult to isolate pain from general anxiety, agitation, unhappiness or distress, but a caring approach can do much to alleviate suffering.

Age, culture and differences in the interpretation of pain or words used to describe it can make it difficult to empathize with patients, especially if the pain reported appears to be out of proportion to the perceived stimuli. At the very least, the patient's feelings should be believed, and respected.

Assessing the character of pain using questions

Clinicians should begin by listening to patients and observing their responses. Pain assessment can be as basic as asking how the patient feels, both generally and specifically in relation to background, incident and procedural pain. Clinicians should ask questions to gather information on what triggers pain or what the pain feels like, for example, and then listen to and observe the patient's behaviour, as some may modify their answers so as not to appear difficult or troublesome.

Other indicators

Dressing-related procedures provide an opportunity to observe the wound for factors that may impact on pain such as signs of inflammation and infection; these may include delayed healing, wound deterioration, erythema, purulence, heat, oedema and odour. In addition, the condition of the surrounding skin and whether there is evidence of dressing adherence (too dry) or excessive exudate (too wet), necrosis or maceration may provide useful information.

MEASURING PAIN INTENSITY

The basic principles of pain assessment should be the same for all wound types: the goal is to minimize pain and create optimal conditions for wound healing. Pain scoring is a vital sign for wound management: if the pain is getting worse, it may be indicative of healing problems such as infection, or the use of an inappropriate treatment, for example poor dressing choice.

Clinicians should not simply ask 'Do you have pain, yes or no?', but 'How would you grade your pain?' Unless extreme, the absolute figure on the pain scale is less important than the direction of travel. If the pain management is correct then the direction of travel should be downwards (i.e. reducing).

An unacceptable level of background pain or uncontrolled pain during or after dressing changes may necessitate a change in management. Individual goals can be set with each patient, but as a general guide pain rated as 'moderate' or scores above 4 (on a scale of 1–10) or above 40% of any other scoring range should prompt 'time out' breaks, top-up and/or improved maintenance analgesia, and a review of the current dressing or procedural technique used. Scores that persist above 4

can be considered to indicate uncontrolled pain (Royal College of Anaesthetists 2000). Scores below 4 (or below 40% of the range) may indicate a level of discomfort that is acceptable, with no lingering pain. However, it is vital to keep this under review.

WHICH PAIN SCALE?

The routine, systematic use of a pain scale provides a method of measuring the success of analgesic and wound care choices. No one tool is suitable for all patients and it is important that both the clinician and the patient understand the scoring system to be used and how to interpret it. The choice of scale will depend on individual patient needs and/or circumstances but, once chosen, the same scale should be used to ensure consistency in documentation (Fig. 29.3).

- *Visual scales* include the Faces scale, which uses cartoon faces ranging from a smiling face for 'no pain' to a tearful face for 'worst pain'. The visual analogue scale (VAS) is commonly drawn as a 10 cm line indicating a continuum between two extremes, for example 'no pain' to 'worst pain'. Patients are asked to point to a position on the line that best represents their level of pain. This score is then measured and recorded.
- *Numerical and verbal scales*: The numerical rating scale (NRS) presents the patient with a range of numbers (e.g. 0–10) to indicate the range from no pain to worst possible pain. The patient is asked to choose a number on the scale that best places his or her current pain on that scale. The verbal rating scale (VRS) is one of the simplest scales to use and usually consists of no more than four or five words (for example 'none', 'mild', 'moderate' and 'severe').

Pain diaries – continuous pain scoring

These provide a personalized, detailed account of the pain experience not only during dressing-related procedures, but also when patients are performing daily routines. A pain diary can combine a brief narrative with a self-assessment tool for patients to rate their pain at specific times of the day. This can build up a picture of background pain problems and help to evaluate pain at dressing-related procedures.

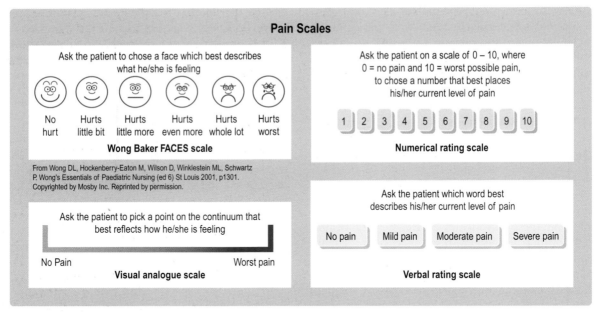

Figure 29.3 Pain scales

Assume all patients can use a pain rating scale until proven otherwise
    Routine pain scoring during dressing-related procedures can impact significantly on management

Patients' previous negative pain experience can lead to increased expectations of pain

PROFESSIONAL ISSUES

A vital element in spreading best practice is the concept of professional accountability. The patient has a right to a minimum standard of professionalism from clinicians and carers, and clinicians can be held accountable by their regulatory body. This means also that clinicians have responsibility for the quality of care of those working under their direction. Ignorance of modern knowledge and techniques is no defence.

If a patient has severe pain during a dressing-related procedure, it is negligent to repeat the procedure without adequate pain relief. Systematic and documented patient-centred pain assessments, which may result in changes in practice or appropriate referral where necessary, are evidence of a good quality of care.

MANAGEMENT OF PAIN

Every person and every wound should have an individualized management plan: uncontrolled pain should signal an immediate adjustment to that plan. Wounds differ in their origins and prospects for healing, which has potential implications for the likelihood and severity of pain experienced and should guide the choice of treatment options and strategies used in dressing-related procedures. The aim is to treat all causes of pain and the clinician will need to consider the patient's level of background and incident pain prior to any clinical intervention.

Background and incident pain

Treat underlying cause

The most important factor in reducing background pain is to treat, where possible, the underlying aetiology of the wound or associated pathologies. Correcting the underlying cause of the wound is likely to promote healing and may coincide with a reduction in background pain.

Address local factors causing wound pain

Clinicians need to consider how best to treat and manage factors that may alter the intensity or character of wound pain. The approaches available to manage local wound factors are many and varied. Clinicians must follow local wound management protocols and consider which treatment options are suitable, available, affordable and practical within their particular health-care settings.

> **Local wound factors**
> These include: ischaemia, infection, excessive dryness or excessive exudate, oedema, dermatological problems and maceration of the surrounding skin

Consider analgesic options

Clinicians should always work quickly to control background and incident pain using a combination of analgesic drugs from different classes as appropriate. The World Health Organization has developed a three-step ladder for managing cancer pain (www.who.int/cancer/palliative/painladder/en). This is also suitable for managing background pain as regular, simple analgesics (e.g. oral non-opioids), are the first step. Then, if pain is uncontrolled, weak opioids such as codeine or tramadol should be added or used alone. A third step, based on a full evaluation of the previous strategies used, is the addition of a stronger opioid (e.g. morphine).

The WHO analgesic pain ladder

Step 1: Non-opioid ± adjuvant
Step 2: Opioid for mild to moderate pain (± non-opioid/adjuvant)
Step 3: Opioid for moderate to severe pain (± non-opioid/adjuvant)
Note: Depending on the pain assessment it may be appropriate to start at a higher step

Co-analgesic medications

Some classes of non-analgesic drugs, such as tricyclic antidepressants and anticonvulsants, can be given as an additional therapy as they enhance the management of neuropathic pain. These should only be prescribed after a full assessment and due consideration of other prescribed medications and comorbidities.

> **Application to practice**
> ● Background pain and incident pain must be well controlled to minimize pain intensity at wound dressing-related procedures effectively
>
> ● The clinician must act early to relieve pain and prevent provoking pain
>
> ● If an intervention such as dressing removal or wound cleansing is causing increasing pain requiring more aggressive analgesia, then the clinician must reconsider treatment choices

Minimize risk of adverse events

The main classes of common analgesics are appropriate for both children and older people, but some adjustment to doses and timing may be necessary.

As all analgesics are associated with adverse effects, it is important to anticipate potential problems and avoid analgesics with a high risk. With older people, in particular, who may be taking other medication such as anticoagulants, caution must be exercised to prevent interactions. Impaired renal or hepatic function may delay the metabolism of analgesics, and consideration must be given to managing the side effects of opioids, which can cause more severe constipation in older people and increased nausea in the young.

Procedural pain

Most analgesics can be administered before a painful event ('preventatives'), but clinicians should ensure that other drug options are available to deal with pain that becomes uncontrollable ('fire-extinguishers'). If analgesics have been required in this way, this should lead to better planning next time the treatment intervention is performed. Analgesia may be continued post-procedure, but if wound pain persists and is poorly controlled, background medication should be reviewed.

> Local policies and protocols should be developed to ensure a safe and effective level of prescribing. These must be reviewed and improved in the light of ongoing assessment

Classes of analgesics

Opioids

Weak to strong opioids are effective for moderate to severe pain. There are long-acting and slow-release formulations available for background pain but oral, buccal or sublingual opioids are also of use as fast-acting top-up analgesics for managing the pain of more invasive or sensitive procedures.

Consideration must be given to the use of strong opioids as appropriate where pain is difficult to control and is interfering with the smooth completion or toleration of the procedure for the patient.

NSAIDs

Non-steroidal anti-inflammatory drugs dampen down peripheral sensitivity and are particularly useful in controlling the throbbing or aching pain felt after a procedure has been completed. As long as there are no contraindications, these should be given 1–2 hours in advance of the procedure to reach peak effect when most needed. However, caution must be exercised in the over-65 age group and patients with known contraindications (e.g. history of duodenal ulcer, clotting or renal problems).

Paracetamol (acetaminophen)

Paracetamol (acetaminophen) can be given alone or in combination with another analgesic (e.g. codeine or morphine) 1–2 hours prior to a dressing-related procedure.

Topical local anaesthetics

In small doses, topical local anaesthetics (e.g. lidocaine) can provide a degree of numbness for a short period of time. This may be useful during a specific procedure or operative event but should not be used as the only method of pain relief.

50% nitrous oxide and 50% oxygen gas

This mixture of gases can be used alongside other pain relief techniques, but regular use may be associated with bone marrow depression.

Note: For general pain management dosing see www.epeconline.net/EPEC/Media/ph/module4.pdf

Preparing the environment: Prepare, Plan, Prevent

In order to Prevent pain, Preparation and Planning are key to effective management:

- Choose an appropriate non-stressful environment – close windows, turn off mobile phones, etc.
- Explain to the patient in simple terms what will be done and the method to be used
- Assess the need for skilled or unskilled assistance, such as help with simple hand-holding
- Be thoughtful in positioning the patient to minimize discomfort and avoid unnecessary contact or exposure
- Avoid prolonged exposure of the wound, e.g. waiting for specialist advice
- Avoid any unnecessary stimulus to the wound – handle wounds gently, being aware that any slight touch can cause pain
- Involve the patient throughout – frequent verbal checks and use of pain tools offer real-time feedback
- Consider preventative analgesia.

In some cases, dressing-related procedures can become more painful over time and a new assessment must be undertaken each time the procedure is carried out.

The simplest outcome of listening to and involving the patient is a prompt for 'time out' breaks to allow the patient's comfort levels to recover. At this time analgesia can be supplemented and the clinician, who needs to understand what the patient recognizes as triggering the pain and what brings relief, can consider how best to proceed. Slow, rhythmic breathing is recommended to distract the patient and reduce anxiety.

PROCEDURAL INTERVENTIONS

There are a vast array of dressing-related procedures. Specific interventions will require specific management, but the following general principles should be considered:

- Be aware of current status of pain
- Know and avoid, where possible, pain triggers
- Know and use, where possible, pain reducers
- Avoid unnecessary manipulation of the wound
- Explore simple, patient-controlled techniques, such as counting up and down, focusing on the breath entering and leaving the lungs or listening to music
- Reconsider management choices if pain becomes intolerable and document as an adverse event
- Observe the wound and the surrounding skin for evidence of infection, necrosis, maceration, etc.
- Consider the temperature of the product or solution before applying to the wound
- Avoid excessive pressure from a dressing, bandage or tape
- Follow the manufacturer's instructions when using a dressing or technology
- Assess comfort of intervention and/or dressing/bandages applied after the procedure
- Ongoing evaluation and modification of the management plan and treatment intervention is essential as wounds change over time
- More advanced non-pharmacological techniques that require specialist training or skilled personnel, such as the use of hypnosis or therapeutic touch, can be considered.

Dressing removal

It is important that the clinician recognizes the potential to cause pain during dressing removal. By talking to the patient it is possible to negotiate the most appropriate removal technique – for example the patient may want to remove the dressing him/her self. Pain intensity scoring at dressing removal should be offered to evaluate practice. Dressing removal has the potential to cause damage, especially to delicate healing tissue in the wound and surrounding skin. It is therefore important to consider using dressings that promote moist wound healing (e.g. hydrogels, hydrofibres) and are

known to be atraumatic (Thomas 2003) on removal (i.e. soft silicones).

> Reconsider dressing choice if soaking is required for removal or removal is causing bleeding/trauma to the wound or surrounding tissue

Dressing selection

Correctly matching the parameters of a dressing to the state of the wound and surrounding tissues helps to manage pain. Factors affecting dressing choice must include appropriateness to the type and condition of the wound. The following dressing parameters should be considered:

- Maintenance of moist wound healing
- Atraumatic to the wound and surrounding skin
- Absorbency capacity (fluid handling/retention capacity)
- Allergy potential.

Where appropriate, clinicians should select dressings that stay in situ for a longer period to avoid frequent removal. In addition, there is a need to evaluate the dressing used when the wound conditions change, as some of the pain the patient is experiencing may be due to dressing choice: what may have been a good choice on day 1 becomes a poor choice on day 5 when the conditions have changed.

CHALLENGING MYTHS

Clinicians need to challenge the assumptions that underpin their beliefs and attitudes as there are some common misconceptions about minimizing trauma and pain. These include:

- *Myth 1*: 'Wet to dry dressings are still the gold standard for wound care'
  Adherent gauze can disrupt delicate healing tissue and provoke severe pain
- *Myth 2*: 'Transparent films are the best dressings for treating and reducing the pain of skin tears and other minor acute wounds'

The misuse of transparent films is a common cause of skin tears

- *Myth 3*: 'Using paper tape is the least painful way to secure a dressing'
  Heightened nerve sensation in a wide area around a wound can make any adhesive tape painful to remove
- *Myth 4*: 'Pulling a dressing off faster rather than slower reduces pain at dressing changes'
  This method has the potential to inflict tissue damage and traumatic pain
- *Myth 5*: 'Using a skin sealant on periwound skin reduces the risk of pain and trauma'
  Skin sealants only create a thin topical layer and do not protect deeper dermal layers
- *Myth 6*: 'People with diabetic foot wounds do not experience pain'
  There may be some loss of peripheral nerve sensation but also heightened sensitivity
- *Myth 7*: 'Pain comes from the wound. The surrounding skin tissue nerves play little role'
  Spinal cord responses to incoming pain signals can give rise to abnormal sensitivity in the surrounding area (allodynia)
- *Myth 8*: 'The only way to treat wound pain is by an oral analgesic 30–60 minutes before dressing changes'
  Oral analgesics can give some relief but should not be seen as a single solution. A full pain assessment must be used to evaluate and fine-tune any prescribed therapy.

PRINCIPLES OF BEST PRACTICE

Questions to assess character of pain

Does the patient have background and/or incident pain?

- *Quality*: Describe the pain or soreness in your wound at rest. Is the pain aching or throbbing (likely to be nociceptive pain) or sharp, burning, or tingling (likely to be neuropathic pain)?

- *Location*: Where is the pain? Is it limited to the immediate area of the wound or do you feel it in the surrounding area? Consider using body map
- *Triggers*: What makes the pain worse? Do touch, pressure, movement, positioning, interventions, day versus night trigger pain?
- *Reducers*: What makes the pain better? Do analgesia, bathing, leg elevation, etc. help to relieve pain?

Does the patient experience pain during or after dressing-related procedures?

- *Quality*: Describe the pain the last time your dressing was removed
- *Location*: Where was the pain? Was it limited to the immediate area of the wound or did you feel it in the surrounding area?
- *Triggers*: What part of the procedure was most painful, e.g. dressing removal, cleansing, dressing application, having the wound exposed?
- *Reducers*: What helped to reduce the pain, e.g. time out, slow removal of dressing, removing the dressing yourself, etc.?
- *Timing*: How long did it take for pain to resolve after the procedure?

Measure pain intensity

Pain scales can record trends in pain intensity before, during and after a procedure and, when used together with appropriate assessment strategies, provide a broad understanding of the patient's pain experience.

> The simple act of routine pain scoring during dressing-related procedures can impact significantly on management

References

Bergner M, Bobbitt R A, Carter W B, Gilson B S 1981 The Sickness Impact Profile: development and final revision of a health status measure. Medical Care 19: 787–805

Best Practice 2003 Best practice: minimising pain at wound dressing changes. Summary of the proceedings of a meeting of key opinion leaders, Amsterdam, 23–24 September 2003

European Wound Management Association 2002
  Position document: pain at wound dressing changes.
  MEP Ltd, London. Available on line at:
  www.ewma.org
Flanagan J C 1978 A research approach to improving
  our quality of life. American Psychologist 33:
  138–147
Reddy M, Kohr R, Queen D et al 2003 Practical
  treatment of wound pain and trauma: a patient-
  centred approach. Ostomy/Wound Management
  49(4A Suppl): 2–15

Royal College of Anaesthetists 2000 Raising the
  standard: a compendium of audit recipes. Royal
  College of Anaesthetists, London. Available on line
  at: www.rcoa.ac.uk
Thomas S 2003 Atraumatic dressings. Worldwide
  Wounds. Available on line at:
  www.worldwidewounds.com/2003/january/
  Thomas/Atraumatic-Dressings.html

CHAPTER 30

Health-related quality of life with chronic leg ulceration

Peter J. Franks, Christine J. Moffatt, Philip A. Morgan

INTRODUCTION

Health has become an increasingly important component of quality of life. The concept of health related quality of life (HRQoL) has become an important element of health-care evaluation over the past 30 years (Rokeach 1973). However, it is only over the past 12 years that studies have been undertaken in HRQoL assessment in patients suffering from leg ulceration (Lindholm et al 1993, Franks et al 1994). This delay in interest is partly a reflection of the general lack of development in this condition relative to other higher-priority areas of health care. The treatment of leg ulceration was considered to be intractable and labour-intensive, and professionals held stereotypical views about patients (Browse et al 1988). The literature refers to patients being described as of lower social class, unwilling to comply with treatment and uninterested in their own health prospects (Muir Gray 1983).

Quality of life assessment in leg ulceration developed following the epidemiology studies that highlighted the size and complexity of the problem, with some patients experiencing ulceration for many decades (Callam et al 1987). There was a new appreciation of the impact that this condition could have on many aspects of patients' lives. This coincided with major advances in the way care was being delivered, using evidence-based practice and the search for outcome measures that could reflect the benefits for patients of effective treatment (Moffatt et al 1992, Franks et al 1994, Simon et al 1996, Stevens et al 1997).

Most of the HRQoL literature has emerged from westernized populations, particularly the UK and Scandinavia, which have also been important centres for treatment development. Our current knowledge of the impact of leg ulceration reflects a very westernized approach to illness and its consequences. There may be many cultural factors influencing how ulceration impacts on patients that have yet to be determined. A major limitation is the lack of international consensus on the assessment of quality of life in leg ulceration or the availability of well validated disease-specific tools to facilitate this, making comparisons between populations problematic.

These developments are set against the backdrop of major international changes in health care. The traditional relationship between professional and patients is now being challenged, with increased expectations of treatment and greater availability of information (Department of Health 2001). This is creating a more informed and empowered patient who will demand more recognition of their suffering and greater access to best available treatment.

PROFESSIONAL ATTITUDES TO QUALITY OF LIFE ASSESSMENT IN LEG ULCERATION

The traditional medical model with its focus on clinical descriptors has been the most important factor in shaping the way in which care is structured and delivered. While clinical factors are of vital importance in ensuring appropriate treatment, these should not be used at the expense of understanding the wider issues that impact on a patient and their family. In the past, clinical features of ulceration have been used by health professionals as proxy measures of the quality of life impact of leg ulceration. As an example of this, the differential diagnosis between venous and arterial ulceration focused on the absence of pain in venous ulceration and the presence of severe pain in patients with peripheral vascular disease. The quality of life literature, which revolves around patient self-reporting of symptoms, has since disputed this simplistic approach, with a number of studies indicating severe pain in a high proportion of patients with uncomplicated venous ulceration (Franks et al 1994, Phillips et al 1994, Hofman et al 1997).

Professionals frequently determine suffering using clinical criteria for severity, while the literature has shown that these measures may not accurately reflect quality of life impact from the patient's perspective. As an example, some patients with a small ulcer may have significant quality of life deficits, while those with a large ulcer may not. Professional interactions with patients may also affect their judgements on the quality of life of their patients. Patients who are viewed as difficult or non-compliant with treatment may be unpopular (Moffatt et al 2002). The sociology literature would suggest that this may lead to a reduction in the ability of professionals to determine suffering, caused by a blunting of their responses (Duxbury 2000, Moffatt 2004). This may also change their own professional behaviour, to induce more confrontational behaviour, thus perpetuating the cycle (English & Morse 1988). Patients with severe deteriorating ulceration may cause high levels of anxiety in staff who feel unable to control the deterioration they observe. This may lead to the development of social defensive behaviour such as avoiding continuity of care, distancing from patients' emotional reactions and ultimately the denial of significant suffering (Moffatt et al 2002).

There is evidence that health professionals are poor at determining the quality of life impact of disease, consistently either over- or underestimating it (Wigton 1988). Professionals tend to underestimate psychological aspects and empha-size more obvious symptoms (Bowling 2001). Of particular relevance to leg ulcer patients is the underestimation of the importance to patients of pain. It is questionable whether patients always feel able to express exactly how they feel during quality of life assessment if this is carried out by professionals, particularly when they are dependent on them for care. There is evidence from other conditions that staff only report severe events, with professionals basing their quality of life assessments on the severity of obvious clinical symptoms (Bowling 2001). Staff who are used to relying on clinical information to inform their decisions may consider quality of life issues less important or relevant to them.

It is difficult to know how often quality of life is used in clinical decision-making. It may be that, in more severe or critical situations, such as the need for amputation, these factors are taken into consideration, although how often quality of life is used in less acute situations is debatable. While in many countries there is a great deal of rhetoric on the use of quality of life indicators to influence health service planning, there is little evidence of quality of life being a main driver to develop services that meet the needs of patients in this way.

PHILOSOPHY OF QUALITY OF LIFE AND ITS ASSESSMENT

Over the past 50 years there has been a shift in emphasis away from regarding health as the absence of disease towards a multidimensional approach that focuses on the patients' own sense of well being and ability to contribute to their own social environment. As early as 1947 the World Health Organization (WHO) began to appreciate the multidimensional nature of health with their definition as 'a state of complete physical, mental and social well being and not merely the absence of disease or infirmity' (World Health Organization 1947).

This has been criticized as utopian, but reflected a shift away from reliance on clinical diagnosis to determine the impact of ill-health on a patient. The WHO added the term 'autonomy' in 1984 in recognition of the need for people to be independent and to contribute to their social environment. Quality of life has been recognized as an important issue in its own right, with a WHO working party specifically charged with the development of concepts and tools. Their definition of quality of life is defined as:

> an individual's perception of their position in life in the context of the culture and value systems in which they live, and in relation to their goals, expectations, standards and concerns. It is a broad ranging concept affected in a complex way by the person's physical health, psychological state, level of independence, social relationships, and their relationships to salient features of their environment.
>
> WHOQoL Group 1993

Chronic leg ulceration is immersed in a medical model of health, and this has influenced the way that quality of life has been assessed. Few studies have attempted to examine leg ulceration in a broader model of health, although those studies so far undertaken have indicated that there are areas of great importance to be explored (Callam et al 1987, Franks et al 1995). Two examples of this are that younger men experience the greatest deficits in measured quality of life, although the reasons for this have yet to be explored (Franks & Moffatt 1998). Similarly, little is known of the potential role that social support may play in both ulcer healing and quality of life (Morgan et al 2004).

Because of the clinical nature of the disease and the prominent role of medical professionals in shaping leg ulcer care, little or no attention has been given to other views of health and quality of life. A sociological approach to leg ulceration would focus on the ability of patients to have acceptable levels of physical and social functioning in society, whereas a humanistic approach would focus on patients as autonomous individuals and their ability to positively influence their lives and develop self mastery over their condition.

In questioning why quality of life in leg ulceration has been so poorly valued by health professionals, a number of issues can be considered. The age of the patients may have influenced both professional and patient attitudes, with low expectations of health and little appreciation of the true impact of the condition on the patient. The relative impact of leg ulceration must be placed in the context of concurrent conditions. We know little about the relative contribution of ulceration compared with these other conditions and the contextual issues that will influence this. The field of gerontology has addressed the issues of illness in a more elderly population with their focus on cognitive efficacy, personal control, motivation, social competence and productivity (Baltes & Baltes 1990, Day 1991). Quality of life has not been assessed in this way for patients suffering from leg ulceration. In addition to the general lack of understanding of the impact, little is known about how different professional groups rate the impact of ulceration on patients. However, studies on other patient groups have shown low levels of agreement between professionals (Wigton 1988). In addition, there are discrepancies between the way in which the professional and the patient assess the HRQoL issues that require addressing. An example of this was shown in a patient with sickle-cell disease who reported that professionals were only concerned with the clinical issues of her illness and failed to appreciate the significant psychological and social issues that she was facing in her day-to-day life (Anionwu 2002). It also highlighted the value she placed in identifying a professional group who also addressed these issues.

Leg ulceration is described as a chronic condition, yet little is known about the patients' perception of their illness. It may be that they consider their ulcer episodes as acute events rather than as part of a chronic illness paradigm. Perceptions of leg ulceration as an acute or chronic condition may affect the way that it impacts on HRQoL and its effect on care delivery. Thus, the patient who perceives their ulcer to be an acute problem will consider that healing should return them to a normal health state, whereas those that consider it to be a chronic condition for which they are at permanent risk may not return to their pre-ulcer health state. This also has to be explored within the context of patients who may be suffering from other conditions and who may be facing other social and psychological issues in their daily lives.

The primary goal of ulcer care has been complete healing, and many studies have evaluated quality of life within the context of this. The results which show improved quality of life in patients who heal have reinforced this association, despite patients who fail to heal also experiencing improvements (though less dramatic) in quality of life (Franks et al 1999a, b). There is a new recognition that, despite appropriate treatment, there may be a small but important group of patients who have delayed healing or who fail to heal completely (Moffatt et al 1992). We know little of the long-term consequences for these patients. Ebbs et al (1989) have argued that in chronic conditions a comprehensive evaluation of quality of life may be critical in making treatment decisions. The emphasis in this patient group may shift towards improving comfort and assisting them in being as socially and functionally able as possible.

Traditionally, patients with leg ulceration have not been encouraged to exercise choice in their treatment. A heavy emphasis has been placed on the development and use of international standards of practice, which have been based on trials and studies that rely on clinical outcomes as measures of effectiveness. There is a dearth of information on how these treatments affect the HRQoL of patients and little information on patient satisfaction or patient experience. There has been a reliance on the reporting of adverse events with different treatments as indicators of safety, rather than criteria that patients might use in deciding which treatment is best for them as an individual. Patient choice may conflict with professional opinion over a treatment; however, quality of life issues should be more important in these instances. The use of patient satisfaction as an outcome of care is poorly developed because of problems with definition and measurement in the literature (Fitzpatrick 1990, Davies & Ware 1991, Wilkin et al 1992). Little attempt has been made to evaluate satisfaction in the area of leg ulcer care with outcomes such as improved healing and quality of life acting as proxy measures. The literature has recently begun to examine the issues of satisfaction with illness, with the development of tools such as the Oxford Happiness Scale (Argyle et al 1995) and the Satisfaction with Illness Scale (Hyland & Kenyon 1992). We know little of whether patients feel satisfied about living with an ulcer. However, it can be postulated that poor control of symptoms such as pain and exudate associated with ulceration may intrude on people's lives and influence the satisfaction they feel in living with their condition.

MEASUREMENT ISSUES IN LEG ULCERATION

In considering the measurement of quality of life in patients with ulceration several issues must be considered. There are a number of approaches to assessment of quality of life, the choice of which will be determined by factors such as the type of information that is required, access to patients and the context in which the patient is seen. We would argue that quality of life assessment should be integral to every assessment of patients with ulceration, and should be used to plan and evaluate care. The tools that have been developed to assess quality of life are frequently complex and used in the context of research rather than for routine clinical practice. However, clinicians should be encouraged to explore the impact of the condition on all patients in order to plan care that is sensitive to their needs.

Traditional approaches to quality of life assessment have encouraged the use of well validated generic tools such as the SF-36 (Ware & Sherbourne 1992) and the Nottingham Health Profile (Hunt et al 1986), and more recently the application of tools specifically related to the underlying condition. The generic tools are valuable in their validation across cultures, languages and diseases but may be limited in their sensitivity to areas of life that are implicated in the individual disease process. The disease specific tools that are discussed in detail later in this chapter are often limited in their development. While they may be sensitive to disease-related issues, they have generally not been extensively validated across different patient groups and cultures.

The qualitative approach, which has been used particularly by nurses, has allowed for a deeper understanding of the impact of ulceration on patients. The nature of this approach requires small numbers of patients, which limits the ability to generalize these findings across ulcer populations. Phenomenologists have recognized the value of capturing the individual perceptions of patients rather than the simple listing of quality of life issues (Cohen 1982). Recently developed tools have taken into account the individual's perception of the impact of their illness rather than the use of a tool that looks at limited predetermined areas of life that may not be relevant to the patient (Ruta et al 1994, Garratt & Ruta 1999). In this design, patients are asked to identify the areas of their life that they judge to be the most important. The aim of this approach is to quantify the difference between their expectations and the reality of their lives, with treatment aiming to narrow the gap between them (Garratt & Ruta 1999). To date, little attempt has been made to link the qualitative and quantitative paradigms.

When considering an approach to quality of life assessment, it is important to consider the patient profile that is being examined. A key limitation to certain tools is the so called ceiling and floor effects. The ceiling effect occurs when patients achieve the maximum score for the scale, which usually indicates best possible health or complete absence of a particular problem. An example might be patients who have complete mobility. In studies that aim to improve quality of life this ceiling effect prevents any improvement being detected. Conversely, the floor effect occurs when patients have the poorest possible health or worst possible manifestation of a problem. In this situation the patient cannot report a deterioration within the scale being used. Thus, important effects (either positive or negative) may be lost.

In the leg ulcer literature there has been a reliance on cross-sectional data in the assessment of quality of life. While this may give some indication of the impact of the disease on patients, it presents a static view of the condition, which may be liable to change over time. Follow-up studies have used clinical time points for evaluation, and this has determined when quality of life assessments have been made. Often patients are assessed at 3-monthly intervals, which may not capture the early changes that occur with new treatments. Similarly, there is a dearth of longitudinal data, which limits the interpretation of the long-term consequences of this chronic disease. Cross-sectional studies may be limited in that they select patients at a particular time period rather than at a particular point in their disease trajectory. Patients with long-term ulceration may have undergone considerable adaptation to their illness, which will affect their reported HRQoL. In addition, patients with new ulceration may focus on stressors that may be different at later time points. Practical

issues may arise in lengthy interviews in elderly patients, who may suffer from impaired cognition, failing eyesight or poor hearing.

LITERATURE REVIEW

Information for this review was gathered from articles published and referenced through the medical literature (MEDLINE, EMBASE) and nursing (CINAHL) systems. Research evidence was categorized into four broad areas of evidence

- Qualitative research
- Development and validation of disease-specific tools
- Cross-sectional quantitative studies
- Longitudinal and outcome studies.

The criterion for inclusion was investigation of quality of life for patients with leg ulceration. Specific exclusions were for individual case studies and studies that refer to quality of life but which give no results for its evaluation or measurement. Tool development studies that evaluated chronic venous insufficiency were included provided that the questionnaire was appropriate to patients with chronic venous leg ulceration. A further search was undertaken to examine the literature on diabetic foot ulceration, which is presented separately.

Qualitative research in chronic leg ulcers

The majority of qualitative research studies into the HRQoL of patients with venous ulcers has been undertaken by nurses and highlights the importance of the 'lived experience' of the patient for this professional group. This perspective is in keeping with the holistic philosophy that underpins nursing practice and stresses the importance of understanding the patient's total experience of their venous ulcer (Hayes 1997) so that care may be given more effectively (Walshe 1995) and sensitively (Chase et al 1997). Twelve qualitative studies were reviewed and spanned the years 1994–2003. Six were conducted in the UK, three in the USA and one in Sweden, New Zealand and Australia respectively (Table 30.1).

A number of themes can be identified that are common across these studies and that describe features and consequences of chronic venous

Table 30.1 Qualitative analysis

Reference	Research question/aim	Study design	Participants	Methods	Conclusions
Hyland & Thomson 1994 UK	Development of a disease-specific quality of life tool	Stage 1 of a three stage project. Qualitative phase to identify issues relevant to HRQoL deficit in leg ulcer patients	22 patients recruited opportunistically through district nurses and for whom leg ulcer was main morbid condition.	Focus groups ×6. Patients asked to discuss the effect leg ulcers had on their lives	Four main categories: Pain Restriction of activities Mood and feelings Ulcer preoccupation and treatment
Walshe 1995 UK	To explore and describe the experience of living with venous leg ulcers	Phenomenology	13 participants from a purposeful sample of 26 (women $n = 12$, men $n = 1$). 11 received care from district nurses. All were elderly with half >85 years. Ulcer duration 4 months to 10 years	Single unstructured tape-recorded interview in patients own home. Phenomenological analysis using ETHNOGRAPH software to organise data.	Four main themes: Description of symptoms Description of treatment Restrictions caused by ulceration Perceptions of and coping with ulceration
Bland 1996 NZ	To examine the experience of living with a leg ulcer and how it impacts on quality of life	Heideggerian hermeneutic phenomenology	9 participants in one health district in New Zealand (women $n = 4$, men $n = 5$)	Single semi-structured interviews	Ulcers impact on virtually every aspect of daily life Patients work hard to heal ulcers Differences created by ulcers become part of a taken-for-granted way of being in the world Some treatment-regimes cause major disruption to quality of life Need to move away from focus on wound management to individual needs based care
Chase et al 1997 US	What is the lived experience of healing a venous ulcer for patients treated in an ambulatory surgical clinic?	Phenomenology	37 patients whose wounds were managed with weekly dressing changes (54 invited to take part)	Review of patient notes Activity and pain log Participant observation over one year Semi-structured interviews with 7 patients Van Manen's thematic analysis	Four major themes: A forever healing process Limits and accommodation Powerlessness Who cares?

Table 30.1 Qualitative analysis, cont'd

Reference	Research question/aim	Study design	Participants	Methods	Conclusions
Krasner 1998a,b US	To describe, understand and interpret the meaning of the lived experience of people who have painful venous ulcers	Heideggerian hermeneutic phenomenology	Purposeful sampling. 14 patients and six staff members. Wide range of ages and socioeconomic backgrounds sought. Women $n = 7$, men $n = 7$. Age range = 30–86 years. Ulcer present 2–84 months	Semistructured interviews at OPD at Baltimore Hospital. Phenomenological analysis (reflexive, reflexive and circular). MARTIN software for text analysis	Eight key themes: Expecting pain with the ulcer; Feeling frustrated; Swelling = pain; Not standing; Interfering with the job; Starting the pain all over again; Having to make significant life changes; Finding satisfaction in new activities
Hyde et al 1999 Australia	To give a voice to women with leg ulcers and to focus on the experience of living with leg ulcers	Descriptive study	Purposive sampling. 12 English speaking women aged >70 years who had experienced leg ulcers for 3 years or more and were being treated by the Sidney Home Nursing Service	Two interviews per participant: one in-depth semi-structured; one follow-up 30 minute interview to verify subthemes	Two overarching themes: Gaining and maintaining control over vulnerable limbs. Lifestyle consequences. Subthemes: Nagging pain; Self-expertise and infection; Leakage, smell and embarrassment; Fighting for skin integrity; Wearing non-preferred clothes; Loneliness; Coping, determination and hope
Neil & Munjas 2000 US	What is it like to live with a wound that does not heal	Heideggerian hermeneutic Phenomenology	Purposive sampling: 10 English speaking men ($n = 4$) and women ($n = 6$) from diverse cultural backgrounds. Recruited from outpatient wound healing clinics, in-patient hospital units, and referrals from home healthcare nurses and physical therapists	In-depth semi-structured interviews, eight in participant's own home, two in hospital wards. Analysis: Diekelmann's framework of Heideggerian hermeneutical analysis. MARTIN software used to organise themes	Two patterns with six themes. Contending with the wound: • Noticing • Oozing & smelling • Losing sleep • Being in pain Staying home, staying back: • Trouble walking • Being isolated

table continued on following page

Table 30.1 Qualitative analysis, cont'd

Reference	Research question/aim	Study design	Participants	Methods	Conclusions
Ebbeskog & Ekman 2001 Sweden	To illuminate elderly people's experience of living with a venous ulcer	Hermeneutic phenomenology	15 elderly people with venous leg ulcers (women n = 12, men n = 3). Mean age: 79.4 years. Ulcer present for 4 months to 2 years; 11 participants had recurrent ulcers	Semi-structured interview using the 'trigger' 'what is it like to live with a leg ulcer?' Analysis used a three step phenomenological hermeneutical method: Naive reading Structural analysis Comprehensive understanding	Four main themes: Emotional consequences of altered body image Living a restricted life Achievement of wellbeing in connection with a painful wound and bandage Struggle between hope and despair with regard to a lengthy healing process
Husband 2001 UK	To explore the patient's experience of venous ulceration and how it is shaped with primary care	Grounded theory	Self electing sample of 14 GPs and 33 nurses asked patients on their caseloads to participate. 39 patients (women n = 35, men n = 4), average age of men = 67 years; average age of women = 74 years. Ulcer experience = 5 months to 28 years. 20 district nurses, 14 GPs in a major health district in England	Semi-structured interviews with all participants Field notes and memos Ongoing and simultaneous analysis and continuous hypothesis testing 2-year process until saturation was achieved	Patients take decision to consult professional seriously Patients do not want to lose control over their ulcer Pain usually dominant factor leading to GP visit, followed by wound deterioration GPs usually leave leg ulcer care to nurses This leads to symptom control and a focus on ulcer not on the whole patient Reciprocal impact Feelings of dissatisfaction in nurses and conditions of poor quality of life for the patient Guarded alliance Patients need supportive assistance to navigate their health trajectory

Table 30.1 Qualitative analysis, cont'd

Reference	Research question/aim	Study design	Participants	Methods	Conclusions
Douglas 2001 UK	To explore and describe the feelings and experiences of patients with chronic venous ulcers.	Descriptive grounded theory.	Purposeful sampling: • Leg ulcer for more than one year • Diagnosis of venous leg ulcer • Under care of a district nurse • Able to give informed consent Eight participants (women $n = 6$, men $n = 2$); age range = 65–94 years	Initial unstructured interviews followed by semi-structured to progressively focus on specific areas identified in previous interview. Grounded theory analysis	Five major categories: 1. The physical experience 2. Vision of the future 3. Health-care professional and patient relationship 4. Loss of control 5. Carer perspective *Category 3 selected as core category on the basis that all others relate to it*
Rich & McLachlan 2003 UK	To explore the patient's experience of living with leg ulcers	Phenomenology	First eight 'willing' consecutive new patients attending a secondary-care-based leg ulcer clinic	Semi-structured interviews about their experiences of living with a leg ulcer; its effects on lifestyle, physical implications and what they thought of their care	Five main themes: Pain Lack of consistent care Social and physical restrictions Self-consciousness about odour and appearance of the limb Fear of further injury

HRQoL, health-related quality of life.

ulcers that affect HRQoL. These include, pain, a restricted lifestyle, loss of mobility, powerlessness and major life changes. Hyland & Thomson (1994) carried out a three-stage study to develop a disease-specific quality of life tool. The first stage was qualitative and used six focus group interviews with a total of 22 opportunistically sampled patients with leg ulcers. Pain was found to be an important factor affecting quality of life, as were sleep disturbance and impairment of mobility, and was a major contributor to the restriction of activities reported by patients. These restricted activities influenced the patient's mood, with sadness, depression, loss of willpower and feelings of helplessness commonly described. Quality of life was also affected by a preoccupation with the ulcer and its treatment, as well as avoidance strategies adopted to protect the integrity of the skin and prevent ulcer recurrence.

A descriptive study by Walshe (1995) using phenomenological analysis explored the lived experiences of 13 elderly patients with leg ulcers (12 female and one male, half being over 85 years), and reported similar conclusions. Pain emerged as the most profound and unremitting experience of this patient group. Ulcer leakage, smell, impaired mobility and a pessimistic view of the potential of their ulcer to heal affected the quality of life of these patients and their ability to cope with everyday activities. It is worth noting that this study identified a lack of appropriate help to enable these patients to cope with their chronic illness and recommended a more holistic approach to assessment and care.

A phenomenological study conducted in the USA by Chase et al (1997) involved 37 patients and used a range of methods to construct a picture of the experience of living with chronic venous ulcers. Methods included a review of patient notes, participant observation over a 1-year period, weekly pain and activity logs and semi-structured interviews with seven of the patients. Four major themes were identified: a forever healing experience; limits and accommodations; powerlessness and a sense of 'who cares?' This study focused on the lengthy healing time associated with venous ulcers. An important finding was that, whereas healing usually has positive connotations, for the patient with venous ulcers this is not always the case. The chronicity of the healing process changes the nature of the healing experience, in which pain is a dominant feature. Again, venous ulcers appeared to limit mobility and normal activities, including work, through the effects of pain, treatment and changes to body image. The patients in this study also described a lack of information and understanding about their venous ulcers that negatively affected not only their 'ownership' of the ulcer but also their ability to take control and contribute to their care.

The conclusions of other phenomenological studies echo the negative effects on HRQoL of pain, restricted lifestyle, sleeplessness and social isolation (Charles 1995, Bland 1996, Krasner 1998a, 1998b, Ebbeskog & Ekman 2001, Rich & McLachlan 2003, Neil & Munjas 2000). In addition, these studies found a number of physical, psychological and social consequences that might not be immediately obvious. As an example of this, Charles (1995) found feelings of hopelessness to be the most significant theme, while Bland (1996) reported how venous ulcers impacted on virtually every aspect of daily life. Patients in her study worked hard to minimize these effects and desperately wanted their ulcers to heal. Krasner (1998a, 1998b) identified eight key themes, four of which were concerned with pain, and listed 20 descriptors of pain used by patients in her study that indicate the diversity of individual pain experience. The remaining four themes were feeling frustrated, disruption to work, having to make significant life changes and satisfaction with new activities.

Ebbeskog & Ekman (2001) conducted semi-structured interviews with 15 elderly patients with chronic venous leg ulcers. They concluded that elderly people were greatly influenced by the illness experience. They describe it as a dialectical ongoing process between two opposite poles. On the one hand is a sense of altered body image and of being imprisoned in a disrupted body, the consequences of which are major life changes. On the other hand there is hope of a positive outcome through healing, and indeed an end to the ulcers. Hope has its basis in a desire for freedom from a burdensome body, from having to cope with a painful wound, and from the restrictions to everyday life that a venous ulcer imposes.

Three of the studies reviewed use grounded theory to explore the patient's feelings and experiences of living with venous ulcers. A study by Hyde et al (1999) in Australia used gender-specific data collection methods (allowing women respondents to express their views in their own way) to 'give voice' to women suffering from venous leg ulcers. The findings confirm the importance of pain, leakage, smell and social isolation as major determinants of HRQoL. Equally important, however, was the fact that, while the community nurse addressed the everyday wound-related problems, other more subtle aspects were often overlooked. These included patient concern about ongoing use of analgesics, changes to preferred modes of dress and the frustration felt at the failure by professionals to acknowledge the expertise of patients in their own ulcer, in particular, their ability to recognize the early stages of infection. Equally significant were the personal qualities developed by the women to cope with the 'myriad' practical, physical, social and emotional consequences of venous ulceration. These qualities included willpower, determination, perseverance and a realistic sense of hope.

A small study by Douglas (2001), in which eight patients with venous leg ulcers (aged 65–94 years) under the care of the district nurse were interviewed using an unstructured approach followed by progressively focused semi-structured interviews, developed five major categories. These were: the physical experience; vision of the future; health-care professional and patient relationships; loss of control and the carer's perspective. Particularly interesting is that the category 'health-care professionals and patient relationships' was identified as the core category because all other categories were heavily influenced by their relationship to it. Central to this core category were issues around conflicting advice; lack of information; patient loss of control; inconsistency of treatment and care; and patient non-adherence to treatment. The author concluded that a greater awareness of the consequences of venous ulceration by the professional, and a more collaborative relationship with the patient would enhance their perceptions of control over their lives, boost self-esteem and improve active coping strategies.

The relationship between health-care professionals and patients with venous ulcers and the effect this can have on HRQoL has been examined by Husband (2001) in a grounded theory study in a major health district in the UK. 39 patients, 33 nurses and 14 GPs were interviewed over a 2-year period. The findings indicate that, because of the way venous ulcer patients are initially diagnosed by the GP, the 'trajectory projections' for the patient are based on a symptom-specific diagnosis rather than a medically defined condition-specific diagnosis. This led to a serious but unrecognized conflict of focus between the nurse and the patient. Nurses in this study set priorities related to the ulcer and to the underlying pathology, whereas the patients wanted help with pain management and in normalizing their lives. The outcome was that the professionals 'usurped' the self-care potential of the patients, prompting them to adopt a position of 'guarded alliance' with the nurse. This study describes a situation that resulted in frustration for the nurses, who were failing to achieve the outcomes they wanted, and provided the conditions for ongoing poor quality of life for the patients. Recommendations from this study argue for nurses having and practising skills not simply in ulcer-focused direct care but also in helping patients to meet their biographical needs and to perform the everyday activities that affect quality of life.

Development and validation of disease specific tools in chronic leg ulceration

The development of disease specific tools to evaluate HRQoL for patients suffering from chronic leg ulceration has been undertaken by a number of groups (Table 30.2). In 1994 Hyland & Thomson (1994) published information on the development of a tool to assess HRQoL for patients suffering from chronic leg ulceration. Using factor analysis they reduced a 54-item questionnaire down to 34 items. Among these, four main areas were identified: pain from the ulcer; sleep disturbance; time spent trying to heal the ulcer; time spent thinking about the ulcer. In addition, 29 questions examined the impact of the ulcer on functional limitations, dysphoric mood and treatment. Although this was a preliminary investigation, no further validation studies have yet been published.

In the same year, Phillips et al (1994) published the results of a semi-structured interview for 62 patients suffering from chronic leg ulceration. Of

Table 30.2 Development of disease-specific tools

Reference	Subjects	Methods	Measures	Results	Conclusions
Hyland & Thomson 1994 UK	50 patients with chronic leg ulceration	Single interview	Validation of a 54-item questionnaire produced through patient interviews	Questionnaire reduced to 34 items. Four key domains: ulcer pain, sleep quality, helping heal ulcer and thinking about ulcer, with 29 factors related to life impact of ulcer	Nurses' perceptions of ulcer healing similar to patients. Self care behaviour unrelated to level of pain or HRQoL.
Phillips et al 1994 US	62 patients with chronic leg ulceration	Single interview to determine impact of ulceration on patient	Author-devised questionnaire with physical, functional, financial and psychological domains	81% believed mobility related to ulcer, associated with leg swelling ($p < 0.001$). Leg ulcer related to time lost from work, job loss and adverse effect on finances. 58% caring for the ulcer burdensome. 68% negative emotional impact	Leg ulcers pose a substantial threat to a variety of dimensions of patients' HRQoL
Launois et al 1996 France	2001 patients, 1001 with CVI, and 1000 non-venous patients	Cross-sectional study and follow up after 2 months	Scale validation producing 20 questions in four domains, psychological, physical, social and pain	$\alpha > 0.82$ for three of four domains. Reproducibility confirmed in 60 patients, and good responsiveness to change (ES >0.8)	Questionnaire can be used to assess HRQoL in clinical trials of CVI
Augustin et al 1997 Germany	246 patients with CVI including 64 with venous ulcer	Validation study using cross-sectional and follow-up information	FLQA comprising of 83 questions in seven scales	Small floor and ceiling effects, $\alpha > 0.7$. Good discriminant validity, change sensitivity good. High acceptance by patients	FLQA suitable in reliably recording HRQoL in patients with CVI
Klysz et al 1998 Germany	142 patients with CVI, 41 with venous ulceration	Validation study using cross-sectional data	TLQ-CVI questionnaire comprising 108 questions in nine scales	$\alpha > 0.7$ for all scales. Good discrimination among disease severity	TLQ-CVI suitable tool for HRQoL in CVI. Provides practical target criteria for clinical research

Table 30.2 Development of disease-specific tools, cont'd

Reference	Subjects	Methods	Measures	Results	Conclusions
Smith et al 2000 UK	98 patients with venous ulceration confirmed by duplex	Validation of a newly developed tool using cross-sectional and follow up information	Charing Cross Venous Ulcer Questionnaire, comprising 32 questions	Factor analysis reduced the questions to 20, within four domains: social interaction, domestic activities, cosmesis and emotional status	Good evidence of a clinically derived measure for patients with venous ulcer; has validity to measure quality of life
Lamping et al 2003 International	1672 patients suffering from chronic venous disorders of the leg	Cross-sectional validation of the tool	VEINES-QOL/Sym., a 26-item questionnaire	Questionnaire acceptable, reliable, valid and responsive to change	Practical and scientific outcome measure that is quick and easy to administer
Price & Harding 2000 UK	49 patients (17 pilonidal sinus, 32 venous leg ulcers)	Cross-sectional comparative study with repeatability assessment	CWIS (Cardiff Wound Impact Schedule)	Significantly higher HRQoL in the domains of physical symptoms and wellbeing in patients with venous ulcers compared with patients with pilonidal sinus	Patients with chronic wounds may have adjusted their lives to cope with chronic wounds compared with patients with acute wounds

α, Cronbach's alpha coefficient; CVI, chronic venous insufficiency; ES, effect size; FLQA, Freiburger Questionnaire of quality of life in venous diseases (Augustin et al 1997); HRQoL, health-related quality of life; TLQ-CVI, Tübingen questionnaire for measuring quality of life of CVI patients (Klysz et al 1998); VEINES-QOL/sym, Venous Insufficiency Epidemiological and Economic Study for Symptoms and Quality of Life (Lamping et al 2003).

these, 81% believed that the ulceration had a direct affect on their mobility, which was associated with leg swelling. Ulceration was related to time lost from work, and attributed to job loss and adverse effects on finances. 58% believed the ulcer to be burdensome, with 68% believing it had a negative emotional impact. In all, 65% stated that the pain from their ulcer was severe.

More recent studies have developed and validated disease specific tools in greater detail. The Charing Cross venous ulcer questionnaire was developed specifically to address issues in relation to venous ulceration (Smith et al 2000). Factor analysis reduced the 32-item questionnaire down to 20 questions. The themes of the four domains were social interaction, domestic activities, cosmesis and emotional status. All domains were highly negatively correlated with the SF-36 questionnaire, which was administered at the same time (direction of worst and best being reversed in the two questionnaires). As expected, the highest correlation for emotional status was with mental health ($r = -0.561$). However social interaction was most closely correlated with physical functioning ($r = -0.698$), whereas domestic activities and cosmesis were best correlated with social functioning ($r = -0.593$ and -0.493 respectively), rather than domains that purport to measure similar things. It would appear that some of the characteristics of this tool may be less than ideal.

While leg ulceration is the focus of this chapter, a number of tools have been developed to measure HRQoL in patients suffering from the range of chronic venous insufficiency (CVI). The CIVIQ questionnaire was developed and validated in France using a sample of 1001 patients suffering from CVI and 1000 patients without signs and symptoms of the disease (Launois et al 1999). Factor analysis of the 1001 patients identified 20 items that reduced to four domains: psychological, physical, pain and social repercussions. These domains discriminated well between patients with and without CVI and with the presence and absence of associated symptoms. There were also substantial changes in all domains for patients whose clinical status improved over a two month follow up.

The Freiburger Questionnaire on Quality of Life in Venous Diseases (FLQA) was developed in Germany and validated in a sample of 246 patients with varying stages of CVI including 64 (26%) patients with chronic venous ulceration (Augustin et al 1997). This 83-item tool differentiates between limitations in HRQoL in seven domains: physical complaints, everyday life, social life, emotional status, therapy, satisfaction and occupation. The results showed good internal consistency for the domains (all α >0.7), with small floor and ceiling effects. The tool provided good convergence with the NHP, and was capable of good discrimination between the clinical stages of CVI. Sensitivity to changes in the patients' clinical status was also good. While the characteristics of this tool appear to be good, the large numbers of items and completion time (≈21 minutes), may make it less useful in situations where time with patients is limited, or where other questionnaires may be required for completion at the same visit.

The Tubingen Questionnaire for Measuring Quality of Life of CVI patients (TLQ-CVI) was also developed in Germany for patients over the whole range of CVI, to understand the patients' perception of their disease and how they cope (Klysz et al 1998). While the original questionnaire had some 108 items divided into eight domains this has since been reduced to 60 items (Klysz T, personal communication). The domains identified are: disease-specific leg symptoms, consequences of CVI symptoms, other symptoms, functional status, state of health and satisfaction with life, everyday fears and worries, hopes with respect to treatment and living with others. The questionnaire was validated in a sample of 142 patients with a range of CVI, including 41 (29%) patients with venous ulceration. Again, the questionnaire was able to discriminate between the different stages of CVI, with high levels of internal consistency within domains (all α >0.74). No evidence on sensitivity to change has yet been published.

Most recently, a large multiprofessional group has collaborated on an international study of CVI (Lamping et al 2003). The Venous Insufficiency Epidemiological and Economic Study (VEINES) was established to examine the clinical outcomes, quality of life, costs and use of health services in French-speaking Belgium, France, Italy and Canada and has since been extended to the English-speaking areas of Canada. The VEINES-QOL/Sym is a new 26-item patient-reported tool to evaluate symptoms and quality of life for patients with CVI. Standard psychometric properties appear to be good, with small ceiling/floor effects, good validity and some evidence of sensitivity to change. The authors state that it is the only fully validated measure of quality of life and symptoms that is appropriate across the range of CVI conditions.

While most developed tools have concentrated on the underlying aetiology of the ulceration, one condition-specific tool has been developed for investigating patients with wounds (Price & Harding 2000). The Cardiff Wound Impact Schedule is a 28-question tool that gives scores in four domains (physical symptoms and daily living, social life, wellbeing and overall HRQoL). It has been used in a study to compare responses in patients with an acute wound (pilonidal sinus) with those with a chronic wound (venous ulcer). The results indicated that patients with a venous ulcer rated themselves more highly with respect to symptoms and daily living and overall wellbeing than the group with acute pilonidal sinus. This may indicate a degree of adjustment to the chronic problem compared with the effects of an acute wound.

While there has been a lot of activity in the development of these tools, as yet there is little evidence that groups outside those who developed the tools are using them. As these are all relatively new it remains to be seen whether one will dominate the evaluation of ulcer-specific quality of life in the future.

Cross-sectional studies in chronic leg ulceration

The first attempt to use generic tools to assess the impact of chronic leg ulceration on patients with chronic leg ulceration was undertaken by Lindholm et al in 1993 using the Nottingham Health Profile. Since then, other studies have used this tool in evaluations of chronic leg ulceration (Franks & Moffatt 1998) and a randomized trial of therapy in patients with venous ulceration (Franks et al 1999a). Other studies have examined the use of the MOS SF-36 questionnaire in relation to normative data in chronic leg ulceration (Price & Harding 1996, Franks et al 2003). Details of the studies identified in the literature are given in Table

30.3. Comparisons with normative data have been made in different ways and different tools have been used, making interpretation between studies difficult; however, some general themes have emerged. Bodily pain and physical mobility are consistently poorer in patients with ulceration compared with normative controls (Lindholm et al 1993, Price & Harding 1996, Franks & Moffatt 1998, Franks et al 1999a, Franks et al 2003), with mean differences reaching around 20 units on either NHP or SF-36 scales. While other areas of HRQoL (social, emotional, mental) are substantially poorer in patients with leg ulceration, the magnitude of the effect is usually somewhat less. When adjusted for social class the differences were smaller, but this may be a consequence of patient selection within the RCT design (Franks et al 1999a). It appears that, while overall HRQoL is poorest in elderly women, it is younger men who may experience the greatest impact from their ulceration, particularly in the areas of bodily pain, mobility and sleep quality (Lindholm et al 1993, Franks & Moffatt 1998).

Longitudinal and outcome studies in venous ulceration

As with the cross-sectional analysis, the emphasis of research has fallen on the use of generic tools, in particular the NHP (Franks et al 1999a, 1999b, 2001) and SF-36 (Walters et al 1999, Franks et al 2003) and Euroqol (EQ-5D) (Walters et al 1999, Mathias et al 2000, Loftus 2001) (Table 30.4). Studies that have used the NHP have found large changes over time with treatment, particularly with respect to bodily pain and sleep (Franks et al 1999a, 1999b, 2001). These differences were greatest for patients whose ulcers healed over the period of follow-up. In general, the changes observed using the SF-36 have been less dramatic, with some evidence of improvement in patients with healed ulceration over those patients who failed to heal, particularly in the areas of bodily pain and mental health (Walters et al 1999, Franks et al 2003). The difference in magnitude of the effect may be due in part to the sensitivity of the tools in this patient population or a consequence of methodological differences in the studies undertaken, in particular patient selection, treatments

Table 30.3 Cross-sectional studies

Reference	Subjects	Methods	Measures	Results	Conclusions
Lindholm et al 1993 Sweden	125 patients with chronic vascular ulcers	Cross-sectional study examining patient scores in relation to expected normal score	NHP administered at one time point	Generally poorer energy, pain, emotion, sleep, socialisation and mobility scores in men compared with population data. Higher scores in women for pain, and mobility. Difference in sexes for pain and mobility	Male ulcer patients should be observed for symptoms of emotional stress, pain, social isolation and poor mobility. More efforts should be made to alleviate pain. Need to consider the whole patient
Price & Harding 1996 UK	63 patients treated in a specialist wound clinic for chronic leg ulceration	Cross-sectional study comparing patients with normative data (aged 70–74 years)	SF-36 administered at one time point	Significant differences in seven of eight subscores of the SF-36 (except mental health)	Indications of poorer HRQoL in patients with leg ulceration compared with normative controls
Franks & Moffatt 1998 UK	758 patients with chronic leg ulceration treated in six health trusts	Cross-sectional study comparing patients with age and gender matched normative controls	NHP administered at one time point	Significantly poorer scores for all domain of the NHP in patients vs normative data. Greatest deficits in HRQoL observed in younger patients and in men	While HRQoL assessed by NHP poorest in elderly women, the impact of chronic leg ulceration is greatest on young men
Franks et al 1999a UK	200 patients with chronic venous ulceration	Cross-sectional study comparing patients with age/ gender/social class normative data	NHP administered at one time point	Significantly poorer HRQoL for bodily pain and physical mobility than controls. Socialization significantly better in patients than controls	Adjustment for social class produced generally less difference between patients and controls than in previous studies
Franks et al 2003 UK	118 patients with chronic leg ulceration	Cross-sectional study comparing patients with age/ gender matched normative controls	SF-36 administered at one time point	Significantly poorer HRQoL in patients vs normative controls for physical, bodily pain, social functioning, role emotional and mental health ($p < 0.05$)	Patients with chronic leg ulcers experience significantly poorer HRQoL than expected from normative data

HRQoL, health-related quality of life; NHP, Nottingham health profile (Hunt et al 1986); SF-36, Medical Outcomes Short Form 36 questionnaire (Ware & Sherbourne 1992)

Table 30.4 Longitudinal and outcome studies

Reference	Subjects	Methods	Measures	Results	Conclusions
Franks et al 1994 UK	188 patients with ABPI >0.8 in community leg ulcer clinics	Cohort evaluated pre- versus post-treatment using 4LB (12 weeks)	SRT and questions designed by author	Significant reduction in anxiety, depression, hostility and improved cognition (p <0.05) after treatment. Greatest improvements in patients whose ulcers healed vs unhealed for depression (p = 0.006) and hostility (p = 0.013). Significant improvements in ulcer pain and going out to socialize	Clear changes in HRQoL following 12 weeks of treatment. Greatest improvements in patients whose ulcers healed
Walters et al 1999 UK	233 patients with venous leg ulcers	Cohort evaluated during an RCT of compression treatment in community clinics	SF-36, EQ-5D, SF-MPQ, FAI at baseline, 3 and 12 months	At 3 months SF-MPQ more responsive to changes in HRQoL. At 12 months SF-MPQ, SF-36 and EQ-5D all responsive	In the absence of disease specific tool, recommended that SF-MPQ used for short follow up whereas the SF-36 and/or SF-MPQ in longer follow up studies
Franks et al 1999b UK	231 patients newly presenting with venous ulceration (ABPI >0.8)	RCT of original four layer vs Profore bandage systems	NHP at baseline, 12 and 24 weeks in trial	Significantly greater improvements in sleep (d = 10.5) and pain (d = 8.9) in healed vs unhealed. No difference between treatments	Improved HRQoL following effective leg ulcer treatment, with greatest improvements in healed ulcers. No difference between treatments
Franks et al 1999a UK	200 patients with chronic (>2 months) ulceration of venous origin	RCT (factorial) of bandages (4LB vs single), dressings (NA vs HCD) and drug (oxpentifylline vs placebo)	NHP at baseline and 24 weeks	Significant improvement in all scores following treatment except for social isolation. Improvements in energy, pain, emotion, sleep and mobility greater in healed vs unhealed. Significantly greater improvement in energy and pain in 4LB vs single	Greater improvements in patients whose ulcers healed. Difference in HRQoL for bandage trial could be explained by improved healing in 4LB group

table continued on following page

Table 30.4 Longitudinal and outcome studies. cont'd

Reference	Subjects	Methods	Measures	Results	Conclusions
Mathias et al 2000 Canada	14 patients with venous leg ulcers	Pre vs post series of patients treated with Apligraf	EQ-5D, SF-12 and parts of other validated pain tools	Significant improvements in pain interference, average leg pain, worse leg pain and days with leg pain (all $p <0.01$)	Greatest improvements noted in pain and other health dimensions
Loftus S 2001 UK	24 patients with venous ulceration	Non-random study comparing patients treated with 4LB and those who underwent venous surgery	EQ-5D plus questionnaire devised by author	HRQoL significantly improved for both groups following treatment ($p <0.05$). No difference between treatments	Improvement in HRQoL after treatment. Improvements greater in 4LB group (NS)
Franks & Moffatt 2001 UK	383 patients suffering from chronic leg ulceration in four health trusts	Cohort of patients followed up after 12 weeks	NHP administered at baseline and after 12 weeks of usual care	Significant improvements in all domains of the NHP after 12 weeks ($p <0.01$). Bodily pain improved significantly more in healed vs unhealed patients ($p = 0.004$)	NHP has limitations in terms of large floor effect, but is sensitive to change in patients' ulcer status
Franks et al 2003 UK	118 patients suffering from chronic leg ulceration in a single health trust	Cohort of patients followed up after 12 weeks	SF-36 administered at baseline and after 12 weeks of usual care	SF-36 scores hardly changed between baseline and 12 weeks but bodily pain improved in the 31 patients who healed ($p = 0.006$) whereas it did not change in those who did not heal. Significantly greater improvements (healed vs unhealed) for bodily pain and mental health	SF-36 may be able to detect changes in health status, with largest differences observed in patients whose ulcers heal

4LB, four-layer bandage; ABPI, ankle to brachial pressure index; EQ-5D, Euroqol version 5D (Euroqol Group 1990); FAI, Frenchay Activities Index (Holbrook & Skilbeck 1983); HCD, hydrocolloid dressing; HRQoL, health-related quality of life; NA, non-adherent dressing; NHP, Nottingham health profile (Hunt et al 1986); NS, not significant; RCT, randomized controlled trial; SF-12, Medical Outcomes Short Form 12 questionnaire (Ware et al 1995); SF-36, Medical Outcomes Short Form 36 questionnaire (Ware & Sherbourne 1992); SF-MPQ, Short Form McGill Pain Questionnaire (Melzack 1987); SRT, Symptom Rating Test (Kellner 1982)

available and duration of follow-up. The Euroqol showed improvements in two studies over 12 weeks (Mathias et al 2000, Loftus 2001) and deterioration in one study, with later improvement after 1 year (Walters et al 1999). Despite little evidence of difference in total bodily pain between patients with healed and unhealed ulceration, the McGill Pain Questionnaire did provide evidence of greater improvement in healed patients, particularly with respect to current sensory pain and visual analogue scales (Walters et al 1999). A similar pattern was observed with visual analogue scores used in a study of skin equivalents (Mathias et al 2000).

At present only one RCT has demonstrated greater improvements in HRQoL for patients randomized to one treatment compared with an alternative. A factorial design randomizing patients to a dressings, bandages and drug/placebo found significant improvements in pain and mobility in patients randomized to a four-layer compression bandage compared with a single-layer compression system (Franks et al 1999a). This greater improvement was probably a consequence of the greater healing achieved in this group (69% vs 49%). A positive effect of healing on the patients' psychological status was observed in an early study (Franks et al 1994), which showed significantly greater improvements in depression and hostility in patients whose ulcers healed. This supports the evidence previously discussed from the SF-36 on mental health.

Quality of life and diabetic foot ulceration

There is a substantial literature base in quality of life for patients suffering from diabetes, although only a few of these are devoted to the specific issues around foot care and diabetic foot ulceration. These results are presented in Table 30.5. Foot ulcers are a serious complication of diabetes and may have a significant impact on quality of life of patients affecting their mobility, socialization and ability to undertake simple everyday tasks (Vileikyte 2001).

A qualitative study using focus groups was undertaken by Brod (1998) in 14 patients with lower limb ulceration associated with diabetes, and 11 caregivers. A semi-structured discussion was undertaken related to four quality of life issues:

social (daily, leisure, family and social life); economic (employment and finances); psychological (emotional health and positive consequences); and physical (physical health and treatment impact). Both patients and carers reported an impact on all these aspects due to the loss of mobility, which required both patient and family to adopt a new lifestyle. A reduction in social activities was reported to increase tension within the family and had a negative impact on general health experienced by both patients and carers. The authors point out the necessity to separate out the impact of the ulcer from the general condition of the diabetes to target appropriate interventions.

Two studies have undertaken to develop and validate a tool to measure patients' perception of the impact of foot ulcers on diabetic patients (Abetz et al 2002, Vileikyte et al 2003). The first of these used semi-structured interviews and focus groups to develop a tool that was then validated in 173 diabetic patients. Of these, 48 had current foot ulcers, 54 healed ulcers and the remainder had no history of foot ulceration. The developed tool of 58 items and 11 domains was then tested in a further group of 288 patients. The authors concluded that the properties of internal consistency, test–retest reliability and sensitivity to change make it appropriate for use in clinical trials. The second tool (NeuroQol) was developed to examine the impact of peripheral neuropathy and ulceration on diabetic patients. It was developed following 57 interviews with patients with peripheral neuropathy and 15 without, and was then administered to 418 patients (290 in the UK, 128 in the USA) with peripheral neuropathy, 35% of whom had a history of foot ulceration. All patients were being treated within diabetic centres. The psychometric properties were assessed, and results were compared using the SF-12 measure of health-related functioning. Factor analysis revealed three physical symptom measurements and two psychosocial function measures, all of which had good internal consistency. The NeuroQol was strongly associated with the severity of the neuropathy and the authors stated that it provided a reliable measure to capture the patients' experience of their peripheral neuropathy.

Cross-sectional studies have been undertaken using a number of generic tools. In one study,

Table 30.5 Studies relating to the diabetic foot

Reference	Subjects	Methods	Measures	Results	Conclusions
Brod 1998 US	14 patients with diabetes and lower limb ulcers, 11 caregivers	Semi-structured focus group	Four domains of social, psychological, physical and economic	Negative impact on all domains assessed by both patients and carers, due to limitation of mobility, required adaptation of lifestyle. Reduced social activity, increased family tension and time off work	Need to separate out the impact of the ulcer from the general condition of diabetes
Abetz L et al 2002 UK	Two studies, 173 patients with foot ulcers (48), healed ulcers (54) or no ulcers (71). Tested in 288 patients		New tool developed (Diabetic Foot Ulcer Scale-DFS). Compared with SF-36	58 items grouped into 11 domains. Good internal consistency. Significant difference between healed and current ulcers for leisure, emotions, financial (p <0.05). Adequate test–retest reliability and sensitivity to change in ulcer status	DFS scale is suitable for HRQoL assessment in clinical trials
Vileikyte 2003 UK & US	418 patients with diabetic peripheral neuropathy (35% with foot ulcer history)	Cross-sectional study	New tool developed (Neuroqol) from responses and compared with the SF-12	Factor analysis gave three physical measures and two psychosocial measures, all with good reliability (α >0.86). More strongly associated with neuropathic severity than SF-12	Neuroqol reliably captures key dimensions of diabetic neuropathy and is a valid tool for examining impact of neuropathy and foot ulceration on HRQoL
Meijer et al 2001 Netherlands	14 patients with clinically stable foot ulcers compared with 24 diabetic patients without ulcers	Case control study	SF-36, Barthel score and questionnaire on walking and walking up stairs (WSQ).	Significant differences in physical functioning, social functioning, role-physical, and general health, and all four sub scales of the WSQ between groups ($p<0.05$)	Presence or history of foot ulcers has a large impact on HRQoL, particularly with respect to patient mobility. Need to target care to improve mobility to improve HRQoL

Table 30.5 Studies relating to the diabetic foot, cont'd

Reference	Subjects	Methods	Measures	Results	Conclusions
Carrington et al 1996 UK	13 diabetic amputees (DA), 13 diabetic foot ulceration (DU) and 26 diabetic controls with no foot problems	Case-control study matched for age and gender	PAIS, HAD and specially designed foot questionnaire	Compared with controls, poorer psychosocial adjustments to illness found with both DA and DU patients ($p <0.05$). DU more depressed than controls ($p <0.05$). DU more dissatisfied with personal lives than controls. DU had more negative attitudes to feet than controls or DA ($p <0.05$)	Psychosocial status of mobile amputees better than patients with current foot ulcers but poorer than diabetic controls
Ragnarson Tennvall & Apelqvist 2000 Sweden	457 patients treated for diabetes	Cross-sectional study comparing patients with no history of ulcer, current ulcer, previous ulcer and amputation	Euroqol	Patients with current ulcers rated their HRQoL lower than healed patients. Major amputation led to lower HRQoL, as did other diabetic complications, but improved in patients who lived with a healthy partner	Patients with current ulcer value their health lower than healed patients, with HRQoL reduced after major amputation

Barthel, Barthel (ADL) Index (Mahoney & Barthel 1965); Euroqol, Euroqol version 5D (Euroqol Group 1990); HAD, Hospital Anxiety & Depression Scale (Zigmond & Snaith 1983); HRQoL, health-related quality of life; PAIS, Psychosocial Adjustment to Illness scale (Derogatis 1977); SF-12, Medical Outcomes Short Form 12 questionnaire (Ware et al 1995); SF-36, Medical Outcomes Short Form 36 questionnaire (Ware & Sherbourne 1992).

diabetic patients either with a previous or former foot ulcer were compared with those who had not suffered an episode of foot ulceration (Meijer et al 2001). Patients were comparable for age, sex, duration and type of diabetes. 14 patients with previous or present stable foot ulceration were compared to 24 patients without a history of foot ulceration. Neither group suffered from complications of diabetes that would be considered to affect their HRQoL. The SF-36, Barthel scale and Walking and Walking Stairs Questionnaire (WSQ) were used, together with a diabetic foot risk score. There were significant differences in physical functioning, health experience, social functioning and role-physical between the two groups, patients with foot ulceration experiencing the greatest deficits in these scores. Significantly poorer walking was also observed in this groups using the subscores of the WSQ. Associations were found between physical functioning and role-physical dimensions of the SF-36 compared with the diabetic risk score. The authors concluded that diabetic foot ulceration has a major impact on physical functioning and mobility and the physical role of patients. It would appear that impairments in mobility have a great impact on quality of life in these patients.

A further case control study investigated the impact of HRQoL in patients with diabetic foot ulceration and lower limb amputation (Carrington et al 1996). Controls for this study were diabetic patients with no evidence of foot problems. Patients were interviewed using the Psycho-Social Adjustment to Illness Scale, the Hospital Anxiety and Depression Scale, the Quality of Life Ladder and a foot questionnaire. 13 unilateral lower limb amputees were matched for age and sex with 13 unilateral patients with diabetic foot ulceration. These patient groups were matched by age and sex to 26 diabetic patients with no history of foot complications. Patients with ulceration were significantly more depressed than the controls. The ulcer patients were more dissatisfied with their lives than the control patients according to the Quality of Life Ladder. Both amputees and ulcer patients experienced poorer psychosocial adjustment to illness than the controls. The foot questionnaire showed that the ulcer group had more negative attitudes to their feet than either amputees or controls. The authors concluded that the psychological status of

the mobile amputees was better than patients with ulceration but not as good as the control group.

A Swedish study undertook to evaluate the Euroqol in patients with healed or unhealed diabetic foot ulcers and those who had undergone a minor or major amputation (Ragnarson Tennvall & Apelqvist 2000). A postal survey was sent to 457 patients who were being treated for foot ulcers by a multidisciplinary team over a 3-year period. Patients were classified according to whether they had never had a lower extremity amputation, whether ulceration was present at the time of the survey or whether it had healed. Those with amputations were classified according to the level of amputation. A response rate of 70% was obtained. Patients with current foot ulcers rated their quality of life significantly lower than those who had healed without amputation. A major amputation led to a reduced Euroqol index, while the presence of another diabetic complication reduced the visual analogue score (VAS) of the Euroqol. Living with a healthy partner increased the VAS score, but both values were reduced by a current foot ulcer. The authors concluded that patients with a current foot ulcer had a greater quality of life deficit than those with healed ulceration, and that quality of life was substantially reduced after major amputation.

Discussion

Evaluations of HRQoL in patients with chronic leg ulceration have come largely from the nursing profession, where qualitative methods have been used to evaluate the lived experience of patients. These have highlighted the impact that this condition has on patients, and add an important dimension to our understanding of the physical, psychological and social impact that a chronic ulcer has on patients. Such studies provide the patient's perspective of 'being in the world' with an ulcer. Even though many of the qualitative studies cannot be generalized with confidence and many of those reviewed here are small, they should not be ignored. It is the patient's perspective of the experience of this condition, rather than simply the outcome of treatment, that is increasingly bringing to the fore differences in priorities that can affect the HRQoL of patients. On one hand are the ulcer-focused priorities of the health-care professional that emphasize healing, symptom control and adherence to treatment. On the other hand are the life-focused priorities of patients, who speak of healing but also of wanting to retain control of their lives and to be included in the management of their ulcer.

The evidence is that chronic leg ulceration can be excruciatingly painful irrespective of the ulcer aetiology, with relatively few patients achieving complete pain relief. Mobility appears to be directly affected by the ulceration, which is also manifested as a reluctance to socialize. This is further compounded by patients avoiding situations with a high risk of further ulceration and embarrassment about the odour associated with many ulcers. Other areas affecting HRQoL include psychological disturbance, including depression, anxiety and a negative body image.

The use of generic tools in cross-sectional studies has highlighted the fact that, while it is elderly women who appear to have the poorest general quality of life, it is younger men who experience the greatest impact in relation to their leg ulceration. The benefits of appropriate treatment have been demonstrated in a number of studies, with the greatest improvement seen in the areas of pain reduction, increased mobility and psychological status. To date, HRQoL data have only been published in two trials of therapy, only one of which achieved statistically greater improvements in one treatment (four layer) over another (single layer) compression system in relation to pain and mobility.

The literature on the diabetic foot has indicated the complex issues around ulceration versus amputation. It has been shown that patients with active ulceration may have a poorer quality of life than those who have undergone minor amputation, although there is evidence that major amputation leads to an even greater deficit. The patients with healed ulceration showed a better quality of life than those with current ulceration, indicating the profound effect of this ulceration on the patient. The literature has concentrated on patients with neuropathic ulceration, and the issues for patients with neuro-ischaemic ulceration may be quite different, particularly since their perception of pain will be greater. The role of peripheral arterial disease would also require examination in these patients.

KEY ISSUES IN FUTURE RESEARCH

The studies so far undertaken have demonstrated a clear deficit in assessed HRQoL compared with normative populations. However, many of the studies that developed normative data were carried out up to 20 years ago, and it is reasonable to suggest that changes in the population may have occurred. Moreover, it is questionable whether data collected in one environment may be appropriately applied in another. For example, do patients who live in the country experience similar quality of life deficits to those in urban areas? It is also questionable how the individual's personal situation may affect their assessment of quality of life and the impact of ulceration on it. Little is known on the impact of social deprivation on HRQoL in patients with leg ulceration, although there is some evidence to suggest that these factors are associated with poor healing (Franks et al 1995).

Most studies in this field have focused on white patients. Clearly there may be strong ethnic and cultural differences that may influence the patient's perception of quality of life and attitudes to illness. As an example of this, there may be different levels of family support in other cultures that may influence the social interaction of patients and may affect daily functioning in other ways.

Little is known about how other clinical and sociological factors impact on HRQoL in these patients. While it has been demonstrated that psychological status is affected by the presence of ulceration, how do depression and mood state affect social functioning and relationships? Does depression develop as a consequence of ulceration or is it a factor in the delayed healing of ulceration, or both?

Little is known of the impact of ulceration on the ability of patients to work and the corresponding economic consequences, and how that affects quality of life. Moreover, little attempt has been made to evaluate the impact on families and significant others. While leg ulceration is associated with a negative impact there may be situations where the ulceration provides a benefit in terms of increased social interaction and support.

As patients are faced with living with an ulcer there may be many things they miss doing, but there may also be new hobbies and activities that they develop and enjoy as a consequence of the ulceration.

Professionals may play a key role in the care of these patients, yet little is known about how the relationship between patient and professional may impact either positively or negatively on the patients quality of life.

One question that has puzzled researchers is why social isolation doesn't improve following ulcer healing. Possible reasons for this may be that when ulcer healing occurs there is a withdrawal of professional care, which perpetuates the sense of isolation. It may also be that other factors might influence the patient's ability to go out, such as their poor mobility. A further observation is that younger men appear to suffer the greatest deficit in quality of life due to their ulceration. We can speculate that this may be because of greater health expectations in this group, or the consequences of ulceration on their work.

While there is some evidence on the clinical effectiveness of products used in the treatment of patients with leg ulceration, relatively little is known on the impact of particular treatments on quality of life. It may be that some treatments that are clinically highly effective reduce quality of life in some patients to an unacceptable level. Conversely, some products that are less effective may provide greater benefits to patients in improving quality of life. At present the emphasis is on clinical effectiveness, which may be at the expense of quality of life. With the greater involvement of patients in choice of their care in the future, this balance may change.

In this chapter we have outlined the present state of knowledge on the impact of ulceration on patients. Present knowledge has indicated the deficits in quality of life experienced by patients with ulceration and the potential improvements following effective treatment. We acknowledge that there are deficits in a number of related issues. We need to understand within the patient group differences in perceived quality of life so that these may be addressed on an individual basis. Most importantly the assessment of quality of life must not be considered as a research tool but must be integrated into improving clinical practice. Future challenges must include the use of sociological and humanistic-based approaches to quality of life, which will provide a richer picture of the true impact of this condition on the patient and their families.

Acknowledgement

Part of this chapter has been published previously as a research article in *Expert Review of Pharmacoeconomics & Outcomes Research*. We thank the publishers, Future Drugs Ltd,. for permission to reproduce these extracts.

References

Abetz L, Sutton M, Brady L et al 2002 The diabetic foot ulcer scale (DFS): a quality of life instrument for use in clinical trials. Practical Diabetes International 19: 167–175

Anionwu E N 2002 Leg ulcers and sickle cell disorders. Nursing Times 98(25): 56–57

Argyle M, Martin M, Luo L 1995 Testing for stress and happiness: the role of social and cognitive factors. In: Speilberger C D, Sarason I G (eds) Stress and emotion, vol 15. Taylor & Francis, Washington, DC

Augustin M, Dieterle W, Zschocke I et al 1997 Development and validation of a disease specific questionnaire on the quality of life of patients with chronic venous insufficiency. Vasa 26: 291–301

Baltes P B, Baltes M M 1990 Successful aging: perspectives from the behavioural sciences. Cambridge University Press, New York

Bland M 1996 More than just a bit of a nark: living with chronic leg ulcers. Primary Intention 4: 17–19

Bowling A 2001 Measuring disease, 2nd edn. Open University, Buckingham

Brod M 1998 Quality of life issues in patients with diabetes and lower extremity ulcers: patients and caregivers. Quality of Life Research 7: 365–372

Browse N L, Burnand K, G Lea-Thomas M 1988 Diseases in the veins: pathology, diagnosis and treatment. Edward Arnold, London

Callam M J, Harper D R, Dale J J, Ruckley C V 1987 Chronic ulcer of the leg: clinical history. British Medical Journal 294: 1389–1391

Carrington A L, Mawdsley S K, Morley M et al 1996 Psychological status of diabetic people with or without lower limb disability. Diabetes Research and Clinical Practice 32: 19–25

Charles H 1995 The impact of leg ulcers on patient's quality of life. Professional Nurse 10: 571–572

Chase S K, Melloni M, Savage A 1997 A forever healing: the lived experience of venous ulcer disease. Journal of Vascular Nursing 15: 73–78

Cohen C 1982 On the quality of life: some philosophical reflections. Circulation 66(Suppl III): 29–33

Davies A R, Ware J E 1991 GHAA's consumer satisfaction survey and user's manual. Group Health Association of America, Washington, DC

Day A T 1991 Remarkable survivors: insights into successful aging among women. Urban Institute Press, Washington

Department of Health 2001 The expert patient: a new approach to chronic disease management for the 21st Century. Department of Health, London

Derogatis L R 1977 Psychosocial Adjustment to Illness Scale (PAIS and PAIS-SR: scoring, procedures and administration. MD. Clinical Psychometric Research

Douglas V 2001 Living with a chronic leg ulcer: an insight into patients' experiences and feelings. Journal of Wound Care 10: 355–360

Duxbury J 2000 Difficult patients. Butterworth-Heinemann, Oxford

Ebbeskog B, Ekman S-L 2001 Elderly people's experiences: the meaning of living with venous leg ulcers. EWMA Journal 1: 21–23

Ebbs S R, Fallowfield L J, Fraser S C A, Baum M 1989 Treatment outcomes and quality of life. International Journal of Technology Assessment in Health Care 5: 391–400

English J, Morse J M 1988 The 'difficult' elderly patient: adjustment or maladjustment? Journal of Nursing Studies 25: 23–29

Euroqol Group 1990 Euroqol- a facility for the measurement of health related quality of life. Health Policy 16: 199–207

Fitzpatrick R 1990 Measurement of patient satisfaction: measuring the outcomes of care. In Hopkins A, Costain D (eds) Measuring the outcomes of medical care. Royal College of Physicians, London

Franks P J, Moffatt C J 1998 Who suffers most from leg ulceration? Journal of Wound Care 7: 383–385

Franks P J, Moffatt C J 2001 Health related quality of life in patients with venous ulceration: use of the Nottingham health profile. Quality of Life Research 10: 693–700

Franks P J, Moffatt C J, Connolly M et al 1994 Community leg ulcer clinics: effect on quality of life. Phlebology 9: 83–86

Franks P J, Bosanquet N, Connolly M et al 1995 Venous ulcer healing: effect of socio-economic factors in London. Journal of Epidemiology and Community Health 49: 385–388

Franks P J, Bosanquet N, Brown D et al 1999a Perceived health in a randomised trial of treatment for chronic venous ulceration. European Journal of Vascular and Endovascular Surgery 13: 3–17

Franks P J, Moffatt C J, Connolly M et al 1999b Quality of life in a randomised trial in venous leg ulceration. Phlebology 14: 95–99

Franks P J, McCullagh L, Moffatt C J 2003 Assessing quality of life in patients with chronic leg ulceration using the Medical Outcomes Short Form 36 questionnaire. Ostomy/Wound Management 49: 26–37

Garratt A M, Ruta D A 1999 The patient generated index. In: Joyce C R B, McGee H M, O'Boyle C A (eds) Individual quality of life: approaches to conceptualisation and assessment. Harwood Academic Publishers, Amsterdam

Hayes M 1997 Quality of life in patients with chronic leg ulceration. Journal of Wound Care 6: 348–349

Hofman D, Ryan T J, Arnold F et al 1997 Pain in venous leg ulcers. Journal of Wound Care 6: 222–224

Holbrook M, Skilbeck C 1983 An activities index for use with stroke patients. Age and Ageing 12: 166–170

Hunt S M, McEwan J, McKenna J 1986 Measuring health status. Croom Helm, London

Husband L L 2001 Shaping the trajectory of patients with venous ulceration in primary care. Health Expectations 4: 189–198

Hyde C, Ward B, Horsfall J, Winder G 1999 Older women's experience of living with chronic leg ulcers. International Journal of Nursing Practice 5: 189–198

Hyland M E, Kenyon C A P 1992 A measure of positive health related quality of life: the satisfaction with illness scale. Psychological Reports 71: 1137–1138

Hyland M E, Thomson B 1994 Quality of life of leg ulcer patients: questionnaire and preliminary findings. Journal of Wound Care 3: 294–298

Kellner R 1982. Abridged version of the Symptom Rating Test – seven scale version (SRT).: University of New Mexico, Albuquerque, NM

Klysz T, Junger M, Schanz S et al 1998 Quality of life with chronic venous insufficiency (CVI). Hautartzt 49: 372–381

Krasner D 1998a Painful venous ulcers: themes and stories about living with pain and suffering. Journal of Wound, Ostomy and Continence Nursing 25: 158–168

Krasner D 1998b Painful venous ulcer: themes and stories about their impact on quality of life. Ostomy/Wound Management 44: 38–50

Lamping D L, Schroter S, Kurz X et al 2003 Evaluation of outcomes in chronic venous disorders of the leg: development of a scientifically rigorous, patient reported measure of symptoms and quality of life. Journal of Vascular Surgery 37: 410–419

Launois R, Reboul-Marty J, Henry B 1996 Construction and validation of a quality of life questionnaire in chronic lower limb venous insufficiency (CIVIQ). Quality of Life Research 5: 539–554

Lindholm C, Bjellerup M, Christensen O B, Zederfeld B 1993 Quality of life in chronic leg ulcers. Acta Dermato-Venereologica (Stockholm) 73: 440–443

Loftus S 2001 A longitudinal, quality of life study comparing four layer bandaging and superficial venous surgery for the treatment of venous leg ulcers. Journal of Tissue Viability 11: 14–19

Mahoney F I, Barthel D W 1965 Functional evaluation: the Barthel Index. Maryland State Medical Journal 14: 61–65

Mathias S D, Prebil L A, Boyko W L, Fastenau J 2000 Health related quality of life in venous leg ulcer patients successfully treated with Apligraf: a pilot study. Advances in Skin and Wound Care 13: 76–78

Meijer J W, Trip J, Jaegers S M et al 2001 Quality of life in patients with diabetic foot ulcers. Disability and Rehabilitation 23: 336–340

Melzack R 1987 The short form McGill Pain Questionnaire. Pain 30: 191–197

Moffatt C J 2004 Perspectives on concordance in leg ulcer management. Journal of Wound Care 13: 243–248

Moffatt C J, Franks P J, Oldroyd M et al 1992 Community leg ulcer clinics and impact on ulcer healing. British Medical Journal 305: 1389–1392

Moffatt C J, Doherty D C, Franks P J 2002 Professional dilemmas of non-healing. Ostomy/ Wound Management 48: 77

Morgan P A, Franks P J, Moffatt C J et al 2004 Illness behaviour and social support in patients with chronic venous ulcers. Ostomy/Wound Management 50: 25–32

Muir Gray J A 1983 Social aspects of peripheral vascular disease in the elderly. In: McCarthy S (ed.) Peripheral vascular disease in the elderly. Churchill Livingstone, Edinburgh, pp 191–199

Neil J A, Munjas B H 2000 Living with a chronic wound: the voice of sufferers. Ostomy/Wound Management 46: 28–38

Phillips T, Stanton B, Provan A, Lew R 1994 A study of the impact of leg ulcers on quality of life: financial, social and psychologic implications. Journal of the American Academy of Dermatology 31: 49–53

Price P, Harding K 1996 Measuring health-related quality of life in patients with chronic ulcers. Wounds 8: 91–94

Price P E, Harding K G 2000 Acute and chronic wounds: differences in self reported health related quality of life. Journal of Wound Care 9: 93–95

Ragnarson Tennvall G, Apelqvist J 2000 Health related quality of life in patients with diabetes mellitus and foot ulcers. Journal of Diabetes and its Complications 14: 235–241

Rich A, McLachlan L 2003 How living with a leg ulcer affects people's daily life: a nurse-led study. Journal of Wound Care 12: 51–54

Rokeach M 1973 The nature of human values. Free Press, New York

Ruta D A, Garratt A M, Leng M et al 1994 A new approach to the measurement of quality of life: The patient generated index (PGI). Medical Care 32: 1109–1126

Simon D A, Freak L, Kinsella A et al 1996 Community leg ulcer clinics: a comparative study in two health authorities. British Medical Journal 312: 1648–1651

Smith J J, Guest M G, Greenhalgh R M, Davies A H 2000 Measuring the quality of life in patients with venous ulcers. Journal of Vascular Surgery 31: 642–649

Stevens J, Harrington M, Franks P J 1997 Audit: a community/hospital leg ulcer service. Journal of Wound Care 6: 62–68

Vileikyte L 2001 Diabetic foot ulcers: a quality of life issue. Diabetes/Metabolism Research and Reviews 17: 246–249

Vileikyte L, Peyrot M, Bundy C et al 2003 The development and validation of a neuropathy and foot ulcer-specific quality of life instrument. Diabetes Care 26: 2549–2555

Walshe C 1995 Living with a venous leg ulcer: a descriptive study of patient's experiences. Journal of Advanced Nursing 22: 1092–1100

Walters S J, Morrell C J, Dixon S 1999 Measuring health-related quality of life in patients with venous ulcers. Quality of Life Research 8: 327–336

Ware J E, Sherbourne C D 1992 The MOS 36 item short form health survey (SF-36). Medical Care 30: 473–483

Ware J E, Kosinski M, Keller S D 1995 SF-12: how to score the SF-12 physical and mental health summary scores, 2nd edn. Health Institute, New England Medical Center, Boston, MA

WHOQoL Group 1993 Study protocol for the World Health Organization project to develop a quality of life assessment instrument (WHOQOL). Quality of Life Research 2: 153–159

Wigton R S 1988 Medical applications. In: Brehmer B, Joyce C R B (eds) Human judgment: the SJT view. Advances in psychology 54. North-Holland, Amsterdam

Wilkin D, Hallam L, Doggett A M 1992 Measures of need and outcome of for primary health care. Oxford University Press, Oxford

World Health Organization 1947 Constitution of the World Health Organization.. World Health Organization, Geneva

Zigmond A S, Snaith R P 1983 The hospital anxiety and depression scale. Acta Psychiatrica Scandinavica 67: 361–370

Psychological aspects of wound healing

Patricia Price, Christine Moffatt

INTRODUCTION

This chapter is designed to introduce you to the area of psychosocial aspects of health, in particular the application of some psychological and sociological concepts to the process of wound healing. This is a very substantial area of study: books have been written on many of the concepts, which can only be discussed briefly within this chapter.

What will the chapter cover?

'Health psychology' encompasses all areas of behaviour related to health, illness and health care. Little empirical work has been conducted that is specific to the application of the principles of health psychology to wound care and healing, but the work conducted in other areas is sufficiently sophisticated to warrant application to this exciting area. The main focus will be on models of health behaviour, adaptation to illness and the psychosocial sequelae of chronic illness. The effect of stress on health and the role of social support and coping strategies used by individuals will also be discussed. Some wounds have a devastating effect both physically and psychologically; the chapter outlines the development of body image and how wounds may cause unique problems. Finally, the ways in which we, as health professionals, communicate to those in our care plays a crucial role in achieving a successful outcome will be covered.

HEALTH AND ILLNESS BELIEFS

There has been a growing interest in the nature of beliefs about health and illness, and in health-related behaviours due to the rise in 'twentieth century' illnesses which are, in part, determined by behaviours such as smoking, eating and exercise (McKeown 1979). There are numerous models which have now been proposed to explain and/or predict the performance of health-related behaviours, these include:

- Attribution theory
- Health locus of control
- Unrealistic optimism
- Transtheoretical model of behaviour change
- Health Belief Model
- Protective motivation theory
- Theory of reasoned action/planned behaviour
- The health action process approach
- Self-efficacy.

It is beyond the scope of this chapter to describe and evaluate each of these approaches, so two have been chosen to represent the range of approaches that have been adopted.

The Health Belief Model

Developed in the early 1950s, the Health Belief Model has been extended by Becker (e.g. 1977) to investigate the predictors of health behaviours likely to prevent illness.

According to this model, health behaviour is based on several fundamental aspects of how individuals view health. The work of Becker and colleagues has resulted in a development of the model to include the influence of demographic factors and the role of an individual's general health motivation (i.e. a readiness, or susceptibility, to be concerned about health issues).

The Health Belief Model has received a great deal of research attention, probably more than any of the other social cognition models; Harrison et al (1992) in a meta-analysis found 234 published empirical tests of the model. It has been used for a variety of health situations, including health screening behaviour, risk behaviours (e.g. smoking, taking exercise), adherence to treatment regimens and attendance at clinics. Not all findings have been consistent, which could reflect the fact that there is no set conceptualization of the elements in the model so researchers often develop research specific assessments, making comparison between studies very difficult, e.g. combining the severity and susceptibility elements to form a 'threat index' or combining the benefits and barriers elements into an 'evaluation index'.

In evaluating this model you should consider the following points:

- Are we always rational about making changes to our behaviour? Do we really weigh up the pros and cons in a clear, level-headed manner?
- What about our emotional reaction to a given condition? Although 'severity' is included in the model, this doesn't encompass feelings of fear or denial?
- What about the wider social and economic factors? The feelings of those close to us are often very important in performing and maintaining health behaviours
- Do the elements of the model exist independently or are they related? If they are related, in what way are they related?
- What about the amount of control we may have over a given situation?
- Other models (e.g. the theory of planned behaviour, Ajzen 1991) have demonstrated that the intention to behave is the best predictor of behaviour, but this element is not included in the model. Studies using this model have now focused on those who intend to comply and then carry through that intention, compared with those who intend to comply and fail to carry out the behaviour (Gollwitzer 1993), or the relative importance of beliefs in predicting behaviour (Steadman & Rutter 2004)
- Is the model static or is it dynamic? Our thinking about a health situation may change dependent on mood or circumstances.

Health locus of control

The area of social psychology that relates to the ways in which we attribute causation for events in our lives is known as 'attribution theory', an element of social learning theory. One part of this theory has identified individuals who, based on their previous experiences, have an internal locus of control (i.e. they believe that events in their lives are directly under their control) and those who have an external locus of control (i.e. individuals who believe that what happens to them is governed by external forces, such as luck). Steadman et al (1976) applied this concept to health and developed the Multidimensional Health Locus of Control Scale, which evaluates perceptions of health related to three key dimensions:

- Health is controlled by the individual (internality)
- Health is controlled by chance (externality)
- Health is controlled by powerful others (e.g. health professionals).

Using examples from individuals with chronic leg ulceration, this would represent views such as:

- 'If I take care of myself, I can avoid getting an ulcer' (*internality*)
- 'No matter what I do, if I'm going to get an ulcer, I will get an ulcer' (*externality*)
- 'It's nothing to do with me, I can only do what the doctor/nurse tells me' (*powerful others*).

The main proposition of this model is that those with an internal health-related locus of control should be more likely to engage in health behaviours, although a strong belief in the role of powerful others can be a useful strategy when adapting to chronic conditions. There have been numerous studies conducted on preventative behaviours such as taking exercise, dietary choices and reducing alcohol intake. Studies on breast examination have indicated that there is a positive relationship between beliefs that health is controlled by powerful others and *physician* examination, while high scores on internality are associated with *self*-examination (Bundek et al 1993).

The health locus of control has also been shown to be related to the type of communication style individuals require from health professionals and their ability to adhere to medical advice. For example, those with an external locus of control may have difficulty in changing a lifestyle behaviour that they believe is outside their control. However, many of the studies using this model have been criticized as very few investigate the *value* placed on health, which reflects either a lack of appreciation of the complexity of social learning theory or an assumption that everyone values their health (Conner & Norman 1996). In spite of being intuitively appealing this theory also has a few unresolved questions:

- Are individuals always 'internal' or 'external'?
- Could this be a temporary state of mind dependent on health status, or are the concepts of 'internal' and 'external' representative of stable personality traits? For instance a patient with leg ulceration may feel that the ability to get a good night's sleep is within their control (e.g. by using whichever relaxation techniques they find are useful), but the choice of a comfortable dressing is often solely the choice of the health professional
- When seeking medical advice, are individuals using external representations by using a 'powerful other' to sort out the problem or are they using internal representations by taking the initiative and seeking out information? For instance, if a patient with leg ulceration asks for additional/stronger medication to cope with pain, are they depending on the 'powerful other' to solve the problem or are they asserting their internality by seeking appropriate help?

Lay theories about health and illness

An alternative approach to using a formal theoretical model has been adopted by social anthropologists and medical sociologists, which involves in-depth qualitative interviews to examine beliefs about health and illness. Based on this work, Radley (1994) concludes that:

- Health and illness are not seen solely as opposite terms (we have a clearer idea about the nature of illness): the experience of one will help to understand the other (e.g. health is the absence of disease)
- Not every one has a clear idea of what health is, nor is it important to everyone

- Individuals may differ in the accounts of their health they give in private and in public
- Beliefs about health are not always part of a logically organized system of beliefs.

Sociologists have also looked at the differences between disease and illness. Whereas disease can be attributed to a pathological condition, illness may be viewed as a subjective concept, i.e. it is possible to be diseased without feeling ill and to feel ill without having a disease. Prevailing beliefs and knowledge may influence the way in which a patient perceives their illness and the relative significance they attribute to the physical signs of disease. Even in a westernized science-based culture, a great deal of non-scientific thinking exists about causes and remedies of disease.

Lay explanations of health and illness often go beyond common-sense meaning and biomedical dysfunction. Health and illness can emerge as the outcome of a struggle between an individual and their way of life or purely as a matter of fate (Pill & Stott 1985). The focus of work using this approach is to make sense of the experience of health and illness, and the influence of society on these experiences.

This more qualitative, structured approach has been used to investigate the nature of communication between doctors and patients, the experience of stress, gender issues and health, and the meaning of health promotion, while interviews have been conducted with those who are chronically ill to understand the patient perspective (e.g. Ebbeskog and Eckman, 2001).

PSYCHO-SOCIAL EFFECTS OF CHRONIC ILLNESS

This section attempts to cover the main themes that emerge from this work, and is closely related to the section on stress, where the experience of the condition acts as a stressful life event that requires the patient to appraise and then cope with the situation.

Some of the common themes which emerge from work in this area focus on:

- The loss of self-identity
- Changes to the physical self
- The interruption to 'normal' life, including medicalization of life

- Dealing with uncertainty and unpredictability, especially in terms of outcome
- Trying to understand 'why'
- Changes in relationships with significant others.

Given that there is a high value put on being 'fully functioning' in our society, there is pressure to find meaningfulness in our lives and be able to manage our own existence.

Concerns about chronic illness include:

- Identifying the illness (e.g. wanting a diagnosis following the experience of symptoms)
- The consequences of the illness (e.g. wanting to know about the ultimate effects of the illness)
- Time elements (e.g. how long will the illness last? how long before my condition starts to deteriorate? how long before I will be unable to care for myself?)
- Causes (e.g. have I contributed to this illness? what happened to trigger it off?)
- Outcomes (e.g. is there a cure? can the symptoms be controlled?).

Illness as a crisis

Moos & Schaefer (1984) have applied crisis theory to the experience of illness. Crisis theory postulates that psychological systems are geared towards maintaining equilibrium in life so, when experiencing a 'crisis' (such as illness), individuals wish to return to a stable state and attempt to achieve this through a series of coping strategies. Illness is seen as a 'crisis' in terms of the number of changes that can occur in a person's life:

- Changes in location, e.g. move to a hospital/new area to get the appropriate treatment
- Changes in role, e.g. from main carer of young children to a 'sick' person who needs care
- Changes in identity, e.g. not knowing who you are any longer, often following a change in role
- Changes in the future, e.g. plans now become uncertain.

These changes, together with the unpredictability and uncertainty of illness and the speed at which certain treatment-related decisions have to be made, means that illness can be categorized as a turning point in life, which calls for a major reappraisal of many features of everyday living that may have been taken for granted.

Adaptation to chronic illness

Chronic disorders may last for a very long time, during which time the aim is to adapt to the new situation. Adaptation refers to the process of making changes (both cognitive and behavioural) in order to adjust constructively to the new set of circumstances. People who are chronically ill have to make a range of decisions about how they will live their lives, about domestic arrangements to care for others and possibly about career changes: those individuals who continuously use avoidance strategies to cope with the situation avoid making informed and realistic assessments about their lives. Successful adaptation will depend on the personality of the individual, the physical and social resources available to them, and the nature of the health problem. Not everyone can always endure the process of adapting to illness: there will be times when the whole experience becomes overwhelming – these are often the result of a relatively trivial incident that means that the total burden is unbearable (Dewar & Morse 1995).

Although not a new paper, the autobiographical account by Kelly (1985) graphically highlights many phases that an individual can go through in coming to terms with a chronic illness (in this case ulcerative colitis), in particular the experience of life-changing surgery.

Impact on significant others

Adaptation to chronic illness is a process that involves the patient, the family and the carers (both formal and informal). Chronic illness can place an enormous strain on a family unit, particularly if that family is going through a transitional life change. As health professionals often visit the chronically ill within their own homes, it is important to be cognisant of the impact and strain that such circumstances can have on families.

The impact of chronic illness on health professionals must also be borne in mind, as it has been reported that some professionals caring for cancer patients experience high levels of distress, the death of a patient being the most stressful event. In addition, many of those caring for the dying feel that they are inadequately trained to help dying patients. One of the biggest concerns expressed in a survey was that staff felt that patients were unaware that psychological care could help them (Schoberberger et al 1996); in an environment of limited numbers of psychologists available within the health care system, much of the psychological support has to be provided by other health professionals. Schoberberger also outlines the usefulness of running psychological training programmes in health-care settings to aid in the reduction of work-related stress, often by improving communication with patients. This view is reinforced by Clarke & Cooper (2001) who concluded that nurses can take on the role of delivering psychosocial support to patients provided they are given training and appropriate resources. The delicate balance between frustrations with care and trust in their health-care profession is outlined in a qualitative study by Haram & Dagfinn (2003). The coping strategies used by health professionals when working in palliative care (in particular working with patients with malignant, often malodorous wounds) are sometimes negative, with staff coping in silence (Wilkes et al 2003).

STRESS, SOCIAL SUPPORT AND COPING STRATEGIES RELATED TO HEALTH

Ways of looking at stress

One of the first people working in the area of stress defined this concept in terms of the response of the individual to a wide variety of events and/or conditions. Selye (1956) called this response 'the general adaptation syndrome', which he felt consisted of three phases – alarm, resistance and exhaustion. This pioneering work set the path for an explosion of research into the various physiological responses to stressful situations.

More recent approaches to this area focus on the life events that may trigger a stress response. Holmes & Rahe (1967) developed the Social Readjustment Rating Scale to identify the major events that have taken place during the past months; each event has an agreed stress rating, such that death of a spouse has a rating of a maximum 100 while moving house scores 20. The scale includes positive and negative events, although negative events are better predictors of the stress response, which suggests that 'change' in itself is not a major causal factor.

Kanner et al (1981) felt that there should be a distinction between major life events and everyday difficulties. The Daily Hassles Scale focuses on everyday difficulties, which may be relatively short term. The work in this area has suggested that the onset of depression can be attributed separately to events and difficulties.

The final approach to investigating stress is to look at the interaction between the individual and the environment. Lazarus (1966) focused on the interaction of the individual and the demands of the environment, while Cox (1978) investigated the imbalance between perceived demands from the environment and an individual's perceived coping resources.

Measurement of stress

There are a number of ways to measure stress, each reflecting the theoretical framework used during the investigation:

- Physiologically, e.g. palmar sweating, peripheral blood flow, neuroendocrine secretion, electro-myelogram, immune function
- Task performance, e.g. speed of task completion, number of errors
- Paper and pencil tests/interview method:
  - Those reflecting the effects of the stressful experience, e.g. the State-Trait Anxiety Inventory (STAI; Spielberger 1983)
  - Those focusing on life events or daily hassles, e.g. Life Events and Difficulties Schedule (LEDS; Brown & Harris 1989).

Effects of stress on health

A simplified version of a model to explain how stress impacts on health has been proposed by Crosby (1988) in her study on the relationship between stress and health in patients with rheumatoid arthritis (Fig. 31.1). This study proposed that there is a psychophysiological feedback loop in which emotional stress levels and disease activity each serve as a cause and a consequence of this relationship (i.e. disease activity increases so does emotional stress, also as emotional stress increases so does disease activity).

The second model is one proposed by Gottlieb in 1983 (Fig. 31.2), which suggests that social

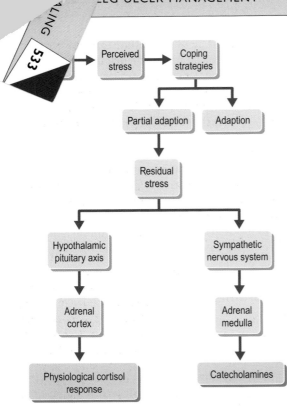

Figure 31.1 Physiological response to stress (after Crosby 1988)

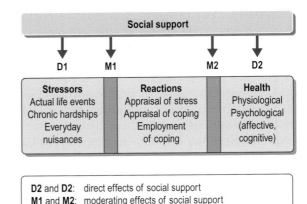

Figure 31.2 The relationship between social support, stress and health outcomes (Gottlieb 1983)

support may play a key role in the effects of stress on health. Social support can directly help by mediating the everyday stressors and the stresses related to the disease/disorder, and by providing beneficial effects on health by creating a sense of stability and self-worth. Social support can also help indirectly by assisting in the process of appraisal and employment of coping strategies.

Stress and wounds

There has been a limited amount of work relating presurgical anxiety to postsurgical recovery, which suggests that preoperative measures of fear and anxiety are linearly related to postoperative states, such that the more anxious a patient is preoperatively the worse the recovery outcome is likely to be (Johnson & Carpenter 1980, Mitchell 2000).

Research into the relationship between stress and health in patients with non-healing wounds has been limited (Olshansky 1992). Some researchers have tried to investigate the aspects of living with a wound that are most stressful, i.e. to identify the stressors associated with the condition.

There have been a number of qualitative studies that have investigated the key concerns/problems/stressors associated with different wound types. For example, Walshe (1995) identified that key symptoms such as lack of mobility, pain, leakage and odour can be particularly problematic. Other authors have proposed a similar situation for their patients with leg ulcers (e.g. Charles 1995, Hopkins 2001, 2002, Rich & McLachlan 2003), while Husband (2001) and Briggs et al (2002) have highlighted the importance of pain as a potential stressor. Studies investigating the impact of ulceration on patients with diabetic foot complications have also identified mobility and restrictions on daily living as potential stressors (e.g. Brod 1998, Sutton et al 2000, Kimmond et al 2003).

These stressors may in themselves interfere with the healing process. A paper published in *The Lancet* in 1995 represents one of the first attempts to link stress to delays in wound healing using both psychological and physiological measures, proposing that psychological stress adversely affects the immune system. Kiecolt-Glaser et al (1995) studied 13 women caring for demented relatives and 13 matched controls, and found that healing took significantly longer in caregivers. This paper has important clinical implications and highlights the impact on carers of living with long-term chronic stress. More recent studies (Kiecolt-Glaser et al 1998, Marucha et al 1998, Glaser et al 1999,

Cole-King & Harding 2001) have reinforced the view that the role of stress in wound healing is a potentially exciting area of investigation that is currently under-researched.

Social support

Models of social support

Authors such as Cohen & Wills (1985) have classified the function of social support into:

- Emotional support (including the expression of empathy, caring and concern, providing companionship, a shoulder to cry on, etc.)
- Practical support (including financial assistance, providing information, advice, suggestions, etc.).

Social support may come from a variety of sources, e.g. personal (e.g. friends, relatives), formal (e.g. work, hobby groups) and professional (e.g. counselling, support groups). There will be considerable overlap between these groups, depending on the needs of the individual.

It is also important to distinguish between actual support received and perceived support (ratings of the adequacy of support provided). Perceived support has been found to be more useful: an individual who is ill may change their feelings about the adequacy of the support they receive depending on their need for support, which changes over the course of a chronic condition (Keeling et al 1996).

There are two main hypotheses, related to how social support relates to health, both of which have received empirical support:

- *The buffering hypothesis*: Social support affects health by protecting the person against the negative effects of high stress. This protective function is most effective when the person experiences a strong stressor
- *The direct effects hypothesis*: Social support is beneficial to health and wellbeing regardless of the amount of stress people experience, i.e. the beneficial effects are similar regardless of stress level. This approach argues that social support is not only helpful after a stressful event but can also help to avert problems.

Cohen (1988) has argued that the effects of social support can be twofold:

- *Direct effect*: The direct effect of social support is that it reduces stress responses, usually by changing the cognitive appraisal of that stressor (i.e. changing how a person looks at the situation) or alternatively by changing physiological processes (e.g. getting a person to calm down and relax)
- *Indirect effects*: The indirect effects of social support are related to changing general behaviour related to health, e.g. helping to cut down the number of cigarettes smoked or encouraging someone to lose weight.

It must be borne in mind that individuals do not always get social support, and not just because they are living alone. People are unlikely to receive support if they are unsociable, don't help others or don't let others know that they need help – this could be because they aren't assertive enough, don't know who to ask or don't want to lose their independence or become a burden to others. In addition, people may ask for help but not get it because others don't have the resources needed to provide support, are stressed themselves and in need of help or are insensitive to the needs of others.

Some segments of society are more at risk of not getting support. Men tend to have larger social networks than women, but women use their networks more efficiently. Many elderly people live in isolated conditions. The lower an individual's social prestige, income and education the smaller the social network is likely to be and the more it is likely to be grouped around kin (Sarafino 1994).

There is a substantial body of evidence (e.g. Blazer 1982) that suggests that social support is beneficial; however, there are situations in which social support can be negative, such that the individual becomes overly dependent on the support, or the support prevents the individual from regaining independence following a chronic condition (Schwarzer & Leppin 1989).

Coping strategies

The strategies that people use to cope with demanding situations include a range of thought processes (e.g. thinking positively) and actions (e.g. seeking information). The strategies are often grouped into 'approach' (e.g. trying to deal with the problem head on) or 'avoidance' (e.g. distracting attention) strategies. They may also be either problem-focused (e.g. dealing with the situation in a practical way) or 'emotion-focused (e.g. dealing with the feelings associated with a situation). Miller (1987) used an avoid/approach distinction and classified coping into 'monitoring' (actively seeking and processing information relevant to the condition/illness) and 'blunting' (=avoiding or distracting oneself from the stressor).

The coping process

Crisis theory proposes that the process of coping starts with the cognitive appraisal of the situation (e.g. how serious is this illness? what changes will it make to my life?). The individual then develops a range of adaptive tasks; the first three relate to the illness, the final four to general wellbeing:

- Dealing with the symptoms of the condition
- Adjusting to the medical procedures and hospital environment
- Developing a good relationship with the relevant health professionals
- Retaining an emotional balance, controlling negative feelings and focusing on positive thinking
- Maintaining feelings of good self-image and feelings of competence
- Maintaining positive relationships with family and friends
- Preparing for an uncertain future.

Achieving all these goals can be very difficult, particularly if the condition results in visible deformity, disfigurement or death. An individual's ability to work on these tasks is related to a whole range of individual differences and the type of illness experienced.

Coping skills or strategies

Moos & Schaefer (1984) have described a series of strategies that can be used to deal with physical illness. They have grouped these skills into:

- *Appraisal-focused coping*: i.e. trying to understand the illness
- *Problem-focused coping*: i.e. tackling the problem and trying to view the problem as manageable
- *Emotion-focused coping*: i.e. dealing with the feelings associated with the illness.

Many professionals refer to 'good' or 'poor' coping strategies, but recent evidence suggests that a wide range of strategies are associated with good health outcomes, and that individuals may use different coping strategies to deal with different parts of the stressful experience. There is no linear relationship between the seriousness of the illness and the ability to cope or the strategies used; but individuals tend to differ in their perception of the stressful situation and in the way they cope. In addition, coping strategies may change over the course of an illness, depending on the nature of the illness and resources of the individual. We should be aware of the changing nature of coping strategies, as these are related to the individual's desire for information and willingness to seek advice or support. There has been little research into the coping strategies used by patients with chronic wounds but Walshe (1995) suggests that patients cope via normalization, a process advocated by Husband (2001). Barrett & Teare (2000) suggest that taking account of coping strategies should be part of a holistic assessment approach for patients with leg ulceration.

A study by Keeling et al (1996) used the Coping Response Inventory to investigate the coping strategies used by patients with chronic leg wounds and diabetic foot wounds. They found that the whole range of strategies was used at around the expected levels; however, the strategies did not change over a 4-month period, which would be expected as part of the adaptation process.

Walshe (1995) suggested that four main strategies were used by patients with venous ulceration: coping by comparison (e.g. 'there are thousands like me'), coping by feeling healthy (e.g. 'my general health is all right, there is nothing wrong with me'), coping by altered expectation (e.g. 'given my age, I'm not too bad'), and coping by being positive (e.g. 'I'm very lucky at the moment'). The strategies suggested by Hyland et al (1994) focus on more practical ideas including avoiding crowds, children and pets to prevent damage to the wound, avoiding public places and engaging in distracting activities.

BODY IMAGE AND THE EFFECTS OF WOUNDING

Today's society places great importance on physical beauty. Physical characteristics and their value in the eyes of society are part of an individual's overall body image. The mass media bombards society with images of healthy, slim, intact individuals. Great attention is now focused on health farms, fitness centres and beauty clinics.

Lacey & Cumming (1988), Birchnell (1986), Brown et al (1990) and Newell (1999), have all argued that one of the main problems in the literature associated with body image is that the construct has been used in a loose and ill-defined way. Body image was described first in the 1920s by Head as the unity in the sensory cortex developed from past and current body sensations. It was not until the writings of Goin & Goin (1981) that body image incorporated the emotional significance that we attach to various physical parts of our bodies. However, it is the definition of body image by Price (1990) that is most familiar to nurses: 'Body image is the totality of how one feels and thinks about one's own body and its appearance'. This definition is summative of the work that has gone before but is also ground-breaking, as for the first time three elements of body image are incorporated: body reality, body ideal and body presentation. The model is important as it is one of the few that goes beyond mere description of the construct; it has gained a high profile among British nurses, not least because it is closely tied to clinical practice. However, many of the assumptions behind the model have not been tested empirically (Gournay et al 1997).

The list of factors affecting the development of body image are numerous but include genetics, socialization, fashion, peer groups, cultural influences and messages delivered through health education. We enter adulthood with a relatively static perception of our own body and its image. However, while age may not be associated with negative body image, there can be little doubt that any 'significant alteration to body image occurring outside the realms of expected human development' (Price 1990) will lead to a range of psychological reactions. The work in relation to 'altered body image' has focused on the impact of trauma, acute wounds and disfigurement (Magnan 1996, Papadopoulos & Bor 1999).

Body image is closely related both to self-concept and self-esteem (Price 2001). Certainly self-concept and body image are both influenced by how positively or negatively others appraise us in both our social and cultural environment. Rogers (1961) defined self-esteem as 'the extent to which our real self measures up to ideal self, and the way we are perceived by others', a definition not dissimilar to that proposed by Price (1990) for body image. Self-esteem is a personal resource that may moderate the effects of disfigurement, incapacitating illness and injury or threatening life events.

Hospitalization, illness and surgery can all affect the perception an individual has of themselves. Procedures that invade and disrupt body privacy can incur alarming effects. The patient with an altered body image may attempt to deny the changes by refusing to look at or touch the affected part (Royle & Walsh 1992).

Very few studies have focused on the relationship between body image and chronic ulceration, even though many practitioners may intuitively feel that this is an important area. Reference to body image is often reported incidentally to health-related quality of life data (Phillips et al 1994, Walshe 1995, Ebbeskog & Eckman 2001). In such studies the anxiety or depression that is reported following leg ulceration may be due to any number of symptoms or related to the overall impact of the experience.

Two papers related to body image and leg ulceration have indicated that this is an important area for these patients. In a small study Flett et al (1994) showed that those with ulceration experienced significantly more pain in the previous 3 months ($p < 0.01$), significantly more health worries ($p < 0.05$) and were significantly less mobile ($p = 0.02$) than age-matched controls. There were also significant differences in terms of self-esteem ($p < 0.01$) and negative affect ($p < 0.05$). In 1998 Neil & Barrell concluded that people with chronic wounds face significant transitions in their lives. They experience a period of disrupted reality when their wounds do not heal and this is followed by a period of uncertainty when the individual must face a range of interventions that lead to frustration with lack of healing. During this period of uncertainty individuals may experience denial, anxiety, pain, immobility and altered body image. Neil & Barrell conclude that changes in body image can be part of this process.

Both studies have a number of limitations, including small sample sizes, non-random methods of recruitment and lack of homogeneity in wound types used. However, the studies are important in terms of the specific focus on self-esteem and body image. For those patients who lose a limb the role of the health professional in helping them takes on an additional dimension (Flannery & Faria 1999), although the relationship between limb loss and body image is often conceptual rather than empirical, as not all individuals with an amputation experience body image disruption (Fisher & Hanspal 1998).

In summary the findings are very limited, so care must be taken not to come to conclusions about the experiences of chronic wounds until more data are available.

Self-inflicted injury (factitious wounds)

Factitious means not real, genuine, or natural. Factitious disorders are therefore characterized by physical or psychological symptoms that are intentionally produced or feigned. The sense of intentionally producing a symptom is subjective and can only be inferred by an outside observer. Patients with a factitious disorder consciously induce or simulate illness but they are not conscious of their underlying motivation. This is a potentially fatal disorder and has a high cost to both the patient and the NHS. DSM-IIIR subclassifies factitious disorders into the following:

- Factitious disorder with psychological symptoms
- Factitious disorder with physical symptoms
- Factitious disorder not otherwise specified.

Münchhausen's syndrome is a term coined by Asher to describe wandering patients with dramatic medical presentations and pseudologia fantasia (i.e. pathological lying), and is a particular form of factitious disorder with physical symptoms. Self-inflicted illness is far from uncommon, although there is little detailed research into self-inflicted wounds (with the exceptions of gunshot wounds).

Reports of self-mutilation include:

- Self-cutting
- Orificial insertion
- Self-induced lymphoedema
- Ingestion of dangerous objects
- Autonucleation of the eye
- Autocastration.

The more bizarre acts usually present no problem in diagnosis. Factitious skin ulcers may constitute a greater diagnostic challenge because of several factors:

- Cutaneous ulceration can be perpetuated by a variety of metabolic, infectious, immunological, vascular and other causes
- A factitious ulcer frequently appears subsequent to the treatment of a skin wound or performance of a surgical procedure
- Patients with factitious disease may be intelligent and cunning, disguising the self-inflicted trauma and fabricating ingenious tales to distract the team, in a manner reminiscent of Münchhausen's syndrome.

Very few studies have focused on research evidence to look at the incidence of factitious wounds in patients with chronic ulceration. However, the studies described below give an indication of the sorts of cases which can be encountered.

A case study of a patient who was thought to be interfering with her wound to prevent healing was outlined by Baragwanath et al (1994), and suggests ways in which the management of such patients could be structured, promoting the idea that avoiding direct confrontation may be beneficial. Rates of self-harm appear to be on the increase: self-cutting is the second most common form of self-harm after drug overdose (Schmidtke et al 1996). Excellent reviews of many of the key issues can be found in Hawton et al 1998, Moffatt 1999 and Corser & Ebanks 2004. The problems underlying many of these conditions are outside the scope of this chapter and will involve the specialized multidisciplinary wound care team as well as specialist professional psychiatric support.

CONCORDANCE AND COMMUNICATION

Extent of patient concordance

It is very difficult to accurately estimate the extent to which patients adhere to medical advice; studies have covered a range of behaviours from non-attendance at clinic appointment, through 'cheating a little' on restrained dietary advice to not taking medication (or amending the dosage/

frequency of medication). DiMatteo (1985) reported an average rate of non-concordance at about 40%, although there are variations depending on the type of illness and the treatment regimen which has been suggested. Sarafino (1994) summarizes the work in the area as:

- There is a difference in adherence rates between acute and chronic conditions: short-term regimens may have an adherence rate of 78% but this falls to 54% for chronic conditions
- Adherence for taking medicine for preventative purposes is around 60%
- Clinic attendance is higher if the appointment is organized by the patient.

If health professionals are asked why patients do not comply with their advice, they tend to attribute non-compliance to the 'uncooperative' personality of the patient (DiMatteo 1985) but research has shown that personality traits do not influence concordance, although there may be combinations of characteristics of the patient (e.g. demographic features such as age, sex or social class), the practitioner and the illness that may contribute to this complex area.

- *Patient characteristics*: The age of a patient may influence concordance, e.g. adolescents are less likely to comply with advice if they feel that they will be singled out as being different; many of the elderly have failing eyesight and/or hearing, which may interfere with concordance behaviour
- *The nature of the advice*: Advice that requires changes to life-long habits is more difficult to adhere to; the complexity of the advice can also affect concordance rates, such that the more complex the advice the greater the chance that the patient will make an error (e.g. advice such as 'take one of these pills three times a day after meals and two of the big ones four times a day before meals; and three of these at equal intervals over a 24-hour period' can be confusing)
- *The duration of the illness*: Studies have confirmed that the longer an illness lasts the more likely it is that concordance will fall over time.
- *The seriousness of the illness*: Concordance rates for an illness that is considered by the *physician* to be serious are no higher than for any other ill-

ness – however, if the illness is rated as serious by the *patient*, then concordance is likely to be higher than for other disorders
- *The health beliefs of the patient and professional*: The models discussed earlier in the chapter outline the complex nature of the beliefs that we all have about health, and this includes health-professionals, who may influence the behaviour of the patient through their interactions with the patient
- *Rational non-adherence*: Much of the literature in this area refers to non-adherence in a tone that suggests 'wicked' or 'naughty' behaviour that must be corrected; however, some patients deliberately do not adhere to advice for very rational reasons:
  - They do not believe the treatment is working
  - They are genuinely confused about the instructions
  - They feel that the side-effects are too unpleasant, and seriously reducing their quality of life
  - They lack the financial or practical resources to continue with the treatment
  - They want to know if the illness is still there when they stop adhering to advice, or whether the condition will go away if they 'leave things alone'.
- *Communication between professionals and patients*: The clarity of the information given to patients and the manner in which it is given to patients can greatly influence concordance, as does the quality of the relationship between patient and professional. Edwards et al (2002) have shown that the level of understanding about the disease process and expectations of outcome are often poor in patients with leg ulceration, leading to misunderstandings and a desire for more information.

These suggestions are all geared towards involving the patient in their own treatment and empowering the patient to take a responsible role in their own health care. Most of the suggestions have a financial cost (either in terms of further training for professionals or time taken by professionals for the additional work involved) but if reports are accurate then in one year alone US$792 million is lost on 'wasted' drugs through non-adherence.

The work on adherence in wound care is closely related to research into the evaluation of different educational interventions, especially in terms of adherence to compression systems (e.g. Taylor 1996, Edwards 2001) or maintaining diabetic control (Bloise et al 1997). Factors influencing adherence to compression treatment have been outlined by Harker (2000), Jull et al (2004) and Moffatt (2004), and include gender motivation and health beliefs. The role of the practitioner in 'shared responsibility' for adherence in venous disease includes holistic assessment and negotiated care plans (Furlong 2001).

SUMMARY

The full range of psychologically important variables relevant to patients with chronic wounds is outside the scope of this chapter; however, several of the key concepts have been outlined. With increasing demands on the time of health-care professionals and the complexity of the treatment interventions available, it is important we do not lose sight of the human aspects of delivering care. Both patients and carers have psychological needs that must be addressed if we are to provide high-quality care in the economically competitive context of health care in the 21st century.

References

Ajzen I 1991 Theory of planned behaviour. Organisational Behaviour and Human Decision Processes 50: 179–211

Baragwanath P, Shutler S, Harding KG 1994 The Management of a patient with a factitious wound. Journal of Wound Care 3: 286–287

Barrett C, Teare J A 2000 Quality of life in leg ulcer assessment: patients' coping mechanisms. British Journal of Community Nursing 5: 530–540

Becker M H, Maiman L A, Kircht J P et al 1977 The health belief model and prediction of dietary compliance. A field experiment. Journal of Health and Social Behaviour 18: 348–366

Birchnell S A 1986 Body image and its disturbance. Journal of Psychosomatic Research 30: 623–631

Blazer D G 1982 Social support and mortality in an elderly community population. American Journal of Epidemiology 115: 684–694

Bloise D, Maldonato A, Assal J 1997 Education of the diabetic patient. In: Pickup J, Williams G (eds) Textbook of diabetes, vol 2. Blackwell, Oxford

Briggs M, Torra I, Bou J E 2002 Pain at wound dressing changes: a guide to management. EWMA Position Document. London, MEP

Brod M 1998 Quality of life issues in patients with diabetes and lower extremity ulcers: patients and caregivers. Quality of Life Research 7: 365–372

Brown G W, Harris T 1989 Life events and illness. Unwin Hyman, London

Brown T A, Cash T F, Milulka P J 1990 Attitudinal body-image assessment: factor-analysis of the Body-Self relations questionnaire. Journal of Personality Assessment 55: 135–144

Bundek N I, Marks G, Richardson J L 1993 Role of health locus of control beliefs in cancer screening of elderly Hispanic women. Health Psychology 12: 193–199

Charles H 1995 The impact of leg ulcers on patients' quality of life. Professional Nurse 10: 571–574

Clarke A, Cooper C 2001 Psychosocial rehabilitation after disfiguring injury or disease: investigating the training needs of specialist nurses. Journal of Advanced Nursing 34: 18–26

Cohen S 1988 Psychosocial models of the role of social support in the aetiology of physical disease. Health Psychology 7: 269–297

Cohen S, Wills T A 1985 Stress, social support and the buffering hypothesis. Psychological Bulletin 98: 310–357

Cole-King A, Harding K G 2001 Psychological factors and delayed healing in chronic wounds. Psychosomatic Medicine 63: 216–220

Conner M, Norman P 1996 Predicting health behaviour. Open University Press, Buckingham

Corser R, Ebanks L 2004 Introducing a nurse-led clinic for patients who self-harm. Journal of Wound Care 13: 167–170

Cox T 1978 Stress. Macmillan Press, London

Crosby L J 1988 Stress factors, emotional stress and rheumatoid arthritis disease activity. Journal of Advanced Nursing 13: 452–461

Dewar A L, Morse J M 1995 Unbearable incidents: failure to endure the experience of illness. Journal of Advanced Nursing 22: 957–964

DiMatteo M R 1985 Physician-patient communication: promoting a positive health care setting. In: Rosen J C, Solomon L J (eds) Prevention in health psychology. University Press of New England, Hanover, NH

Ebbeskog B, Eckman S L 2001 Elderly persons' experiences of living with venous leg ulcers: living in a dialectal relationship between freedom and imprisonment. Scandinavian Journal of Caring Sciences 15: 253–243

Edwards L M 2001 Views of patients deemed non-compliant. Leg Ulcer Forum Spring: 11

Edwards L M, Moffatt C, Franks P 2002 An exploration of patients' understanding of leg ulceration. Journal of Wound Care 11: 35–39

Fisher K, Hanspal R 1998 Body Image and patients with amputations: does the prosthesis maintain the balance? International Journal of Rehabilitation Research 21: 355–363

Flannery J C, Faria S H 1999 Limb Loss: alterations in body image. Journal of Vascular Nursing 17: 100–106

Flett R, Harcourt B, Alpass F 1994 Psychosocial aspects of chronic lower leg ulceration in the elderly. Western Journal of Nursing Research 16: 183–192

Furlong W 2001 Venous disease treatment and compliance: the nursing role. British Journal of Nursing 10(Suppl): S18 –S35

Glaser R, Kiecolt-Glaser J K, Marucha P T et al 1999 Stress-related changes in proinflammatory cytokine production in wounds. Archives of General Psychiatry 56: 450–456

Goin J, Goin M. 1981 Changing the body: psychological effects of plastic surgery. Williams & Wilkins, Baltimore, MD

Gollwitzer PM 1993 Goal achievement: the role of intentions. European Review of Social Psychology 4: 142–185

Gottlieb B H 1983 Social support strategies: guidelines for mental health practice. Sage, Thousand Oaks, CA

Gournay K, Veale D, Walburn J 1997 Body dysmorphic disorder: pilot randomised controlled trial of treatment: implications for nurse therapy and practice. Clinical Effectiveness in Nursing 1: 38–43

Haram R B, Dagfinn N 2003 Errors and discrepancies: a patient perspective on leg ulcer treatment at home. Journal of Wound Care 12: 195–199

Harker J 2000 Influences on patient adherence with compression hosiery. Journal of Wound Care 9: 379–381

Harrison J A, Mullen P D, Green L W 1992 A meta-analysis of studies of the health belief model with adults. Health Education Research 7: 107–116

Hawton K, Arensman E, Townsend E et al 1998 Deliberate self-harm: systematic review of efficacy of psychosocial and pharmacological treatments in preventing repetition. British Medical Journal 317: 441–447

Head H 1920 Studies in neurology, vol 2. Oxford University Press, London

Holmes T H, Rahe R H 1967 The social readjustment rating scale. Journal of Psychosomatic Research 11: 213–218

Hopkins S 2001 Psychological aspects of wound healing. NT Plus 97: 57–58

Hopkins A 2002 A disrupted life: living with non-healing venous leg ulcers. Conference of the European Wound Management Association, Granada, Spain

Husband L 2001 Shaping the trajectory of patients with venous ulceration in primary care. Health Expectations 4: 189–198

Hyland M, Ley A, Thompson B 1994 Quality of life of leg ulcers patients: questionnaire and preliminary findings. Journal of Wound Care 3: 294–298

Johnson M, Carpenter L 1980 Relationship between pre-operative anxiety and post-operative state. Psychological Medicine 10: 361–367

Jull A B, Mitchell N, Arroll J et al 2004 factors influencing concordance with compression stockings after venous ulcer leg healing. Journal of Wound Care 13: 90–93

Kanner A D, Coyne J C, Scaefer C, Lazarus R S 1981 Comparison of two modes of stress measurement: daily hassles and uplifts versus major life events. Journal of Behavioural Medicine 4: 1–39

Keeling D, Price P E, Jones E, Harding K G 1996 Social support: some pragmatic implications for health care professionals. Journal of Advanced Nursing 23: 76–81

Kelly M P 1985 Loss and grief, reactions as responses to surgery. Journal of Advanced Nursing 10: 517–525

Kiecolt-Glaser J K, Marucha P T, Malarkey W B et al 1995 Slowing of wound healing by psychological stress. Lancet 346: 1194–1196

Kiecolt-Glaser J K, Page G G, Marucha P T et al 1998 Psychological influences on surgical recovery, perspectives from psychoneuroimmunology. American Psychologist 53: 1209–1218

Lacey J H, Cumming W J K 1988 The neurobiology of the body schema. British Journal of Psychiatry 153(Suppl 2): 7–11

Lazarus S 1966 Psychological stress and the coping process. McGraw-Hill, New York

McKeown T 1979 The role of medicine. Blackwell, Oxford

Magnan M A 1996 Psychological considerations for patients with acute wounds. Critical Care Nursing Clinics of North America 8: 183–193

Marucha P T, Kiecolt-Glaser J K, Favagehi M 1998 Mucosal wound healing is impaired by examination stress. Psychosomatic Medicine 60: 362–365

Miller S M 1987 Monitoring and blunting: validation of a questionnaire to assess styles of information seeking under threat. Journal of Personality and Social Psychology 52: 345–353

Mitchell M 2000 Nursing intervention for pre-operative anxiety. Nursing Standard 14(37): 40–43

Moffatt C 1999 Self-inflicted wounding 1: psychosomatic concepts and physical conditions British Journal of Community Nursing 4: 502–514

Moffatt C J 2004 Perspectives on concordance in leg ulcer management. Journal of Wound Care 13: 243–248.

Moos R, Shaefer J A 1984 The crisis of physical illness: an overview and conceptual approach. In: Moos R H (ed.) Coping with physical illness: new perspectives. Plenum Press, New York, pp 3–25

Neil J A, Barrell M 1998 Transition theory and its relevance to patients with chronic wounds. Rehabilitation Nursing 23: 295–299

Newell R J 1999 Altered body-image: a fear-avoidance model of psycho-social difficulties following disfigurement. Journal of Advanced Nursing 30: 1230–1238

Olshansky K 1992 Psychological factors in recurrent pressure sores. Plastic and Reconstructive Surgery 90:5; 930

Papadopoulos L, Bor R 1999 Psychological approaches to dermatology. BPS Books, Leicester

Phillips T, Stanton B, Provan A, Lew R 1994 A study of impact of leg ulcers on quality of life: Financial, social and physiologic implications. Journal of the American Academy of Dermatology 31:49–153

Pill R, Stott N C H 1985 Choice of chance: further evidence on ideas of illness and responsibility for health. Social Science and Medicine 20: 981–991

Price B 1990 Body image: nursing concepts and care. Prentice Hall, Hemel Hempstead

Price P 2001 Body image and self-esteem. Leg Ulcer Forum 14: 15–17

Radley A 1994 Making sense of illness: the social psychology of health and disease. Sage, London

Rich A, McLachlan L 2003 How living with a leg ulcer affects people's daily life: a nurse-led study. Journal of Wound Care 12: 51–54

Rogers C R 1959 A theory of therapy, personality and interpersonal relationships as developed in the client-centred framework. In: Koch S (ed.) Psychology: a study of science, vol 3: Formulations of the person and the social context. McGraw-Hill, New York

Royle J A, Walsh M 1992 Watson's medical–surgical nursing and related physiology, 4th edn. Baillière Tindall, London

Sarafino E P 1994 Health psychology: biopsychosocial interactions, 2nd edn. John Wiley, New York

Schmidtke A, Bille-Brhe U, de Leo D 1996 Attempted suicide in Europe: rates, trends and sociodemographic characteristics of suicide attempts during the period 1989–1992. Results of the EHO/EURO multicentre study on parasuicide. Acta Psychiatrica Scandinavica 93: 327–338

Schoberberger R, Schmeiser-Reider A, Kunze M 1996 Problems in treatment and nursing of cancer patients. Journal of Health Psychology 1: 241–250

Schwarzer R, Leppin A 1989 Social support and health: a meta-analysis. Psychology and Health 3: 1–15

Selye H 1956 The stress of life. McGraw Hill, New York

Spielberger C D 1983 Manual for the state-trait personality inventory. Consulting Psychologists Press, Palo Alto, CA

Steadman L, Rutter D R 2004 Belief importance and the theory of planned behaviour: comparing modal and ranked modal beliefs in predicting attendance at breast screening. British Journal of Health Psychology 9: 447–463

Steadman B S, Wallston K A, Kaplan G D, Maides S A 1976 Development and validation of the health locus of control (HLC) scale. Journal of Consulting and Clinical Psychology 44: 580–585

Sutton M, McGrath C, Brady L, Ward J 2000 Diabetic foot care: assessing the impact of care on the whole patient. Practical Diabetes International 17: 147–151

Taylor P 1996 Assisting patients to comply with leg ulcer treatments. British Journal of Nursing 5: 1355–1360

Walshe C 1995 Living with a venous leg ulcer: a descriptive study of patients' experiences. Journal of Advanced Nursing 22: 1092–1100

Wilkes L M, Boxer E, White K 2003 The hidden side of nursing: why caring for patients with malignant malodorous wounds is so difficult. Journal of Wound Care 12: 76–80

32

Health promotion and patient education

Janice M. Beitz

INTRODUCTION

Any contemporary discussion of leg ulcer care will eventually focus on the critical nature of quality education within the context of patient health promotion. However, improving the knowledge base of patients does not necessarily guarantee successful treatment and health maintenance.

Health promotion and patient education have to be approached from a comprehensive perspective. Any programmatic initiative or individual interaction must be based on the recognition that these activities include cognitive, affective, developmental and sociocultural components, and that barriers and facilitators for effective health promotion and patient education exist. After these critical considerations are systematically addressed, health-care clinicians need to select evidence-based teaching–learning strategies for use in enacted care activities. If these structures and processes are ignored, patients' leg ulcers may not heal or recidivism rates may be excessive. Case study 1 exemplifies some of these issues:

Case study I   *Poorly controlled diabetes mellitus*

Eileen is a 60-year-old obese white woman with insulin-dependent diabetes mellitus and a chemically recurring plantar ulcer on the right foot. She has severe neuropathy in both feet with significant loss of protective sensation, has a Charcot's foot on the right extremity and a developing one in the left ankle joint.

Eileen is a high school graduate, is very well read and can 'talk a good story', revealing her excellent knowledge base regarding diabetes self-care. Despite this understanding, she constantly violates her recommended diet, takes more insulin so she can 'eat strawberry shortcake' and only sporadically applies the bilateral leg braces and special shoes she is supposed to wear. Consequently, her Charcot's joints are not supported and the foot ulcer is not consistently offloaded.

In addition, Eileen has bipolar disorder, for which she takes lithium. In general, her mental health episodes tend towards depression rather than excitement. She lost her part-time secretarial job 6 months ago because she was chronically late or absent. Consequently, she is currently unemployed, although she is receiving unemployment benefit.

Eileen's live-in boyfriend is angered by her job loss and constant mental and/or physical health problems. He berates her for her 'gluttony'. Eileen comes to her primary care health-care provider's office, where the diabetes specialist advanced practice nurse notes an enlarged plantar ulcer and surrounding erythema. Eileen's fasting blood sugar is high.

Issues for reflection include the following:

- What are possible barriers to Eileen's optimal self-care of the diabetic ulcer and diabetic extremities?
- What are some short-term goals appropriate to her care? What are some longer-term health promotion and patient education goals pertinent to Eileen's case?
- What teaching–learning approaches may be helpful in altering Eileen's suboptimal lifestyle?

ISSUES DICTATING QUALITY HEALTH PROMOTION AND PATIENT EDUCATION

In the world community, and especially in westernized developed countries where chronic illnesses are expanding at an explosive rate, health promotion and disease prevention have assumed a 'centre-stage' position in the international health-care agenda. No country, no society, no community can ignore the need for optimal health promotion based in large part on efficient and effective, strategy-based patient education. The serious, complex issues driving this focus are significant and pervasive.

Forces mandating scrutiny and/or activity include the surge in chronic illness, the cost control crisis and projected future financial burden, litigation, social pathologies, poor lifestyles with mediocre public health outreach, and the demands of modern patients. Contemporary patients want to be seen as partners in their health care, they want meaningful, clear communication and they demand understanding of their health-care challenges, and personal circumstances.

Chronic illnesses are diseases that are usually prolonged, do not resolve spontaneously and are rarely cured. No modern nation that seeks to control health-care costs can ignore the consequence of poor prevention in the situation of chronic illness.

In the USA, the statistics regarding chronic illness are sobering. A recent survey demonstrated that chronic illness is the immediate cause of death for three out of four Americans (Borenstein 2000). Currently 125 million Americans (45% of the population) have one or more chronic illnesses with direct medical costs of over $510 million. 30% have accompanying disabilities sufficient to limit daily activities (Funk & Tornquist 2001). It is noteworthy that chronic illness disproportionately affects women and minorities. Black men have twice as high a death rate for prostate cancer as white men; black women have significantly higher breast and cervical cancer death rates than white women (Centers for Disease Control 2000). The American population's statistics and trends mirror those of other industrialized nations of the western hemisphere (Nolan & Nolan 1999). The disparity in health is partially explained by access to health care (employment, job status, marital status) but a larger less controllable segment is affected by culture, risk attitudes, etc. (Zuvekas & Taliaferro 2003).

The most prominent contributors to chronic illness and mortality/morbidity are factors that are amenable to health promotion, disease prevention and good patient management. For lower extremity ulcers, tobacco use, diet, activity level and alcohol usage really affect whether they improve or deteriorate. Although there may be a genetic predisposition, the development of leg ulcers of various aetiologies can have strong behavioural components. Therefore, many may be preventable or at least amenable to alteration and amelioration, especially if found early in the disease process (Funk & Tornquist 2001).

With the surge in the elderly and chronically ill populations, the slowing of disease process and prolongation of healthy years is absolutely crucial financially. Effective health promotion, chronic illness prevention, and disease management can slow disease progression and maximize normality creating a 'compression of morbidity' (Fries 1987, 2003, Kart & Kinney 2001). The USA, the UK and other affected nations will simply be unable to afford the same level of financial burden as the prevalence of chronic illness rises in the coming decades unless the time period of morbidity is 'compressed' (Fries 2003).

Social pathologies and poor lifestyles have greatly contributed to chronic illness mortality and morbidity. Morbid obesity, substance abuse, social isolation, mental health challenges and the disintegration of traditional family structures have created groups of 'high-risk' individuals for chronic illness development and/or deterioration. Some authors suggest that the medical model and traditional public health approaches are, and will continue to be, ineffective with the chronic illness phenomenon. Lorig (2001) suggests that nurses and other health-care clinicians must be ready to help patients enact a 'self-management model' (p. 36). For persons with leg ulcers, nurses and other health clinicians must teach people who have already fallen into the 'chronic illness river' to learn to swim quickly and efficiently. Patient education can be both the life and the quality of life preserver.

Litigation is another force compelling health-care professionals, professional organizations and local, regional and national governments to scrutinize the human and financial burdens of chronic illness and the quality of care rendered. The movement for national benchmarks in pressure ulcer wound care and other areas of chronic health problems (e.g. the Agency for Health Care Policy and Research (now the Agency for Health Care Research and Quality) national guidelines) is emblematic of this scrutiny. Unfortunately, lawsuits, legal revisions and judicial decisions have exerted a stronger wake-up call to health-care clinicians than internal initiatives. Historical events have supported the belief that litigation acts as an impetus for increased emphasis on prevention, better family communication and wound care protocols. Ironically, the consequences of poor care can stimulate the move towards improving the quality of care (Beitz 2001).

A final force centrally positioning health promotion and disease prevention through patient education is the demand of today's patients for a different relationship with their health-care professionals. Informed patients are more likely to cooperate with treatment regimens and demonstrate better management of their health problems and chronic illnesses (Oermann et al 2001).

However, knowledge itself is insufficient to change patient behaviour. Patients want health-care professionals to engage with them, to understand the realities of living with their chronic illnesses and to acknowledge the personal circumstances that help or hinder patients' adapting to a particular lifestyle, healthy or unhealthy. This new relationship is demanding and longer-term (Anderson 2000, Saarmann et al 2000, Whitehead 2001).

HEALTH PROMOTION AND PATIENT EDUCATION: DEFINITIONS, MODELS AND THEIR APPLICATIONS

Health promotion has been explained by many authors and theorists and can be focused on the wellness behaviours of individuals, families, and/or communities (Pender 1996). For the purpose of the current discussion, health promotion is defined as the encouragement of healthy lifestyles, the creation of environments supportive of health and the focusing of health services on promoting healthy communities supported by appropriate public policy.

A number of models of health promotion and behaviour have been proposed. They include the Health Belief Model, the Health Promotion Model, the Precede-Proceed Model and the theory of reasoned action (Pender 1996, Rankin & Stallings 2001). The full description of these models or theories is beyond the scope of this chapter. However, it is noteworthy that these propositions have commonalities. In these models there is a major emphasis on cognitive components such as knowledge and beliefs, a focus on affective aspects (feelings, emotions), a consideration of biological factors that people bring to their lifestyles (genetic predisposition), interpersonal relationships and realities, and situational influences such as society and culture (e.g. dietary practices, self-care practices). These core components offer critical insights and implications for where and when patient education is enacted for optimal health promotion, and are discussed later in this chapter.

Patient education has also been scrutinized and defined in several ways. Within the context of health promotion, patient education can be defined as the process of influencing behaviour and producing changes in knowledge, attitudes and skills in order to maintain and/or improve health (Rankin & Stallings 2001). Based on a set of theories and research findings, patient education involves the imputing, interpretation and integration of information to bring about behavioural changes. Patient education is central to the practice of all health-care professionals. The process involves needs assessment, diagnosis of requisite goals, targeted interventions and evaluation of the efficacy of the activity (Babcock & Miller 1994, Redman

2001). Needs assessment plays a leading role in effective patient education. Whatever strategies are selected or evaluation methodologies are enacted, they can be off target if the critical needs of patient learners are not clearly and thoroughly identified by patients who are integrally involved in goal setting, progress monitoring and compliance facilitation (Davis & Chesbro 2003).

Notably, health promotion and patient (health) education are different constructs, with the former construct subsuming the latter. Both activities need to be evaluated separately. Whitehead (2003) has written an excellent article targeting the challenges of meaningful evaluation because the two areas are frequently confused. Biomedical individualized foci used in evaluating patient education (blood sugar levels, skin integrity, etc.) may not be pertinent for health promotion. The latter should likely include broader indices such as client social well-being, social programming, etc.

The link between health promotion and patient education is strong and models can provide valuable guiding principles. Some of the models and theories' postulates are tantamount to basic tenets of quality patient education. They include wise advice such as the following:

- It is important to ascertain people's perceived susceptibility to health problems
- The educator must consider critical variables when attempting patient education, including perceived benefits and barriers/costs to treatment from the patient's perspective
- It is critical to consider and ascertain the patient's commitment to a plan of action and any immediate competing demands
- A target group for patient education should help in determining health promotion needs and desired outcomes
- Psychosocial variables play a profound role in influencing care-seeking behaviour, including patients' feelings, affect, expectations, values, norms and personal habits; all these variables must be examined and addressed
- Information-related health data are processed both cognitively and emotionally. If both segments are not considered, negative emotions can interfere with optimal cognitive processing (Rankin & Stallings 2001).

Generic strategies that evolve from these tenets may be helpful when selecting specific teaching approaches. Patient educators should be certain to:

- Frame patient teaching to respect patients' perceptions and cultural perspectives
- Educate patients about purposes and expected effects of interventions and inform them about illness trajectory and susceptibility
- Begin by suggesting small changes rather than major alterations in order to gain success
- Add new behaviours rather than eradicating old ones, and make the new behaviours achievable in terms of both behaviour and cost
- Link new behaviours to healthy old ones
- Obtain explicit commitments from patients to behavioural change
- Be flexible with educational strategies; combining strategies is likely to be more effective
- Involve staff by creating health promotion and patient education efforts that are a 'team sport'
- Monitor progress addressing both cognitive and emotional components.

BARRIERS AND FACILITATORS TO QUALITY HEALTH PROMOTION AND PATIENT EDUCATION

Barriers

Many barriers exist to effective health promotion and patient education. Any effective patient education initiative should be premised on a comprehensive, realistic acknowledgement of the barriers that may hinder and the facilitators that may be helpful in pertinent situations. Specific examples are given below.

Barriers include poor client or caregiver knowledge base, literacy issues, dissonant cultural belief systems, lack of self-care habits or passivity, financial obstacles, poor lifestyle habits and lack of research-based approaches (Beitz 2001).

Patient and caregiver knowledge
Patient and caregiver knowledge can have enormous impact on leg ulcer care for good or ill. Patients who do not understand that venous hypertension is a life-long problem will be unlikely to be faithful users of compression therapy. Mental illness can impact approaches to patient education. MacHaffie's

(2002) research suggests that those with persistent mental health challenges are most likely to receive health promotion information from physicians, psychiatrists, nurses and pharmacists. They are much less likely to use print and media sources. Public service announcements may be less effective with this population.

Literacy issues

Literacy issues can have a major impact on quality patient education for health promotion. More than half of the entire American population cannot read beyond fifth-grade level. Illiteracy is especially rampant in the elderly and in urban dwellers (Doak et al 1995, Weiss 2002). If diabetics with neuropathic ulcers cannot read simple directions, the problems for self-care are evident. The situation is compounded by the fact that most patient education materials are written at least 5 years above patients' comprehension levels (Davis et al 1990).

Cultural belief systems

Cultural belief systems can be a major hindrance or they can be harnessed to strongly support patient education for health promotion. It is critical that the key cultural health beliefs of the target audience (patient or group) are understood. Is health promotion (e.g. preventing illness) understandable to that culture? What family structures and values affect health-care choices (Weiss 2002)? In my experience, women in traditional cultures may find great difficulty in adhering to leg elevation suggestions for their venous stasis ulcers if they interfere with cooking, childcare or care of very elderly parents. In many cultures, women are expected to be self-sacrificing.

Financial obstacles

Financial obstacles hinder quality patient education and health promotion the world over. The barriers can become especially acute as persons with chronic illness age. Venous ulcer patients, for example, are encouraged to wear compression therapy for life to prevent ulcer recurrence. However, some of the most effective compression systems that are easier to apply and wear are significantly more expensive. Effects of the climate and environment can play a part too. I have encountered female venous stasis patients who chose not to wear their full-length compression stockings because they developed vaginal yeast infections in the summer heat and could not afford the medicine to treat their bodies' natural responses.

Poor lifetime/lifestyle habits

Poor lifetime/lifestyle habits are an enormous barrier to quality health promotion and patient education. For many patients, healthy living activities are simply less attractive than poor lifestyle habits. Arterial ulcer patients, for example, may undergo bypass surgery to re-establish blood supply to an extremity but continue to smoke. Even when an individual understands their susceptibility to further problems this may be over-ridden by the gains supplied by an addictive action such as smoking or poor diet.

Passivity in self-care

Passivity in self-care or lack of self-care can be highly detrimental to vascular ulcer healing. Mental health challenges can certainly interfere but gender and health professional relationships can also act as blocks. In some situations affected clients will be less concerned with learning self-care techniques because they expect their spouse, partner, children, etc. to provide the care. Some patients, especially older ones, defer to caregiver (e.g. physician) mandates blindly without researching the 'why' behind the self-care interventions that have been ordered.

Lack of research-based approaches

Lack of research-based approaches is also a great hindrance to successful patient education and health promotion. The health-care literature is replete with suggestions for patient education activities for health promotion, but most of the articles are simply theoretical or, if research-based, are descriptive of small time-limited projects with small sample sizes. Only recently has this situation started to alter.

Facilitators

Facilitators to health promotion and patient education are also available and are becoming increasingly understood. These include newer perspectives on health, innovative electronic communication in various forms, innovations in cognitive educational approaches, a collective sense of concern about cost control, a focus on evidence-based clinical interventions, and clinical practice guidelines (Beitz 2001, Rycroft-Malone et al 2002).

Newer perspective on health

A newer perspective on health has emerged in increasing groups of people across the world. Healthy living and healthy eating are becoming valued by larger segments of the population. Although there are still 'hard core' high risk takers, many younger and older patients are working to improve and/or maintain their health status. The proliferation and success of health clubs is testimony to this activity. Even in continuing care/residential care facilities for the aged and ageing, architectural development includes exercise and recreational facilities for the elderly. Longman (2003) appropriately suggests that the health of nations depends not on 'forcing seniors into HMOs' but expecting and facilitating them to exercise.

Innovative electronic communication processes

These are becoming increasingly available. The Internet has profoundly changed methods of communication and its fullest potential for education has not even been discovered yet let alone tapped. Telemedicine and telehealthcare are currently being used to improve the care of patients with leg ulcers (Samad et al 2002). Future health-care providers and patients will probably have access to national care standards based on research evidence via hand-held computers, television interfaces and virtual educational experiences. 'Just in time' education approaches will allow continuing education. The prospect is exciting for improving future patient education and health promotion (Sullivan 2002).

New educational approaches

New educational approaches have undergone scrutiny in recent decades and innovations have emerged. Acceptance of traditional teaching techniques is no longer accepted without question. Newer research in neurophysiology and learning has suggested that alternative approaches may be more effective for long-term learning. Teaching/learning approaches targeted at the natural underlying structures of brain functioning by recognizing metacognition, active learning, cognitive arousal and memory limitations are increasingly evidence-based for appropriate use. Schenk & Hartley (2002) suggest that educational interventions (e.g. patient education) based on behavioural, affective and especially cognitive enhancements produce better outcomes. They suggest that a nurse or health educator's role is more appropriately one of 'coach' rather than teacher, and client-focused rather than illness-focused.

Collective concern and increased public awareness of health issues

This has affected enlarging segments of the population. For example, increased public awareness has helped with decreasing cardiovascular disease and some forms of cancer, but that has not occurred across the board. For example, smoking cessation programmes have worked well in some groups but have failed in others. AIDS/HIV education efforts are another example of where worry and concern has peaked and backsliding has been observed. For over a decade, nationwide HIV education efforts decreased significantly the spread of the virus among gay men. However, recent reports suggest that the virus is spreading again more quickly among young gay men and heterosexuals (Haverkos et al 2003, Moore 2003).

An emerging focus on evidence-based health care

A focus on evidence-based health care and evidence-based teaching/learning has emerged. Health care and educational practitioners (and consumers) are learning to ask questions like 'What is the evidence for …?' and 'How strong is the evidence for …?' Two international organizations have greatly aided the use of techniques and approaches that are research-based – the Cochrane Collaboration (www.cochrane.org) (for health care) and the Campbell Collaboration (www.campbellcollaboration.org) (for humanities, including the social, behavioural and educational arenas).

The recently constituted Cochrane Developmental, Psychosocial and Learning Problems Group has been established to bring the Cochrane methodology of systematic review to social, educational and sociolegal research issues (www.bris.ac.uk/depts/cochranebehav/).

In addition, research-based algorithms, critical pathways and special software have been developed related to chronic wound care. Their use will increasingly improve wound care on a national and international basis (Beitz et al 2001).

HEALTH PROMOTION AND PATIENT EDUCATION INITIATIVES: SOME PRACTICAL CONSIDERATIONS

Up to this point, the focus of the discussion has targeted general topics of health promotion and patient education and a discussion of specific learning guidelines from their theoretical perspectives. This section addresses more clearly defined topics pertinent to the care of adults with lower extremity ulcers.

Any health-care professional teaching adults, especially those with a chronic health problem, must consider the following health promotion and educational components: motivation and learning, adult learning principles, cultural competence and cultural sensitivity and personal empowerment for self-management of chronic illness (Rankin & Stallings 2001).

Motivation

In the context of patient education, motivation refers to the willingness of the learner to embrace learning (Redman 2001). Multiple theories of motivation exist, and are touched upon in Chapter 7 (see, for example Figure 7.4, which explores some of the psychological factors that can determine the extent to which individuals may engage in self-help activities). While a full description of them is beyond the scope of the current discussion, the principles of motivation that derive from these theories can be articulated and applied to multiple learning situations. These principles include the following:

- Internal motivation is longer-lasting and more self-directive than external pressure
- Learning 'works' better when people are ready to learn
- The environment can be used to focus patients' attention on learning needs

- Motivation can be enhanced by the organization of teaching materials
- Motivation is augmented by realistic goals
- Mild anxiety is helpful to increase motivation
- Affiliation and approval are good motivators.

In general, a positive learning atmosphere with adults who are internally motivated and who are ready to and want to learn will generate positive outcomes. Patients value the accolades and acknowledgements of health teachers (Redman 2001). A health educator can use select strategies to create this milieu.

Good organization of instruction makes learning meaningful and motivational. Involving learners in ascertaining goals will promote success. Health educators can create both these situations and work with learners to decrease anxiety.

Adult learning principles

Adult learning principles are also critical considerations for effective patient educators. Although Thorndike and Lindemann wrote well known monographs about adult learning, it was the work of Malcolm Knowles on andragogy (adult learning) that transformed modern education (Knowles 1990, Babcock & Miller 1994). A successful health educator will strategically structure health promotion and patient education activities to:

- Relate learning to the learner's need to know
- Recognize adults need for self-direction
- Relate learning to learner's previous experience
- Determine the adult's readiness to learn and how it relates to social roles
- Show how learning will add to problem-solving abilities
- Relate learning to adults' internal motivation and long-term life goals.

In summary, adult learners see themselves as producers or doers and derive self-esteem from their contributions. They like to be self-directed and respond well to informal, friendly learning environments where new learning helps to solve problems in daily life (Rankin & Stallings 2001).

Cultural competence

Given the increasing diversity of the industrialized world, cultural competence is essential in any patient educator's approach to teaching and health promotion. In the USA, for example, the percentage of the population who are ethnically diverse will approach 50% by the year 2050 (Rankin & Stallings 2001, p. 52).

What does cultural competence entail for a nurse or health educator who has to teach persons with chronic leg ulcers? It means that the person is not just the venous leg ulcer but the sociocultural patient with a venous leg ulcer. Examination of associated societal and ethnic community expectations is crucial before any discussion of any therapy. Lack of recognition of the critical nature of ethnic or cultural processes may doom any patient education to failure. A real-life example from my experience exemplifies its prominence. A patient with a venous stasis ulcer was a member of a religious group that proscribed the use of pork products. The patient perceived (wrongly) that the enzymatic debriding agent that was ordered for her ulcer smelled like pork, and consequently she failed to apply it as ordered. Only after several weeks of non-progress did careful questioning of the patient, along with discussion of the ingredients with her and a member of the clergy, did she agree that the ordered topical therapy was not 'forbidden'.

Personal empowerment

Personal empowerment for self-management of chronic illness is now seen as an imperative. Schenk & Hartley (2002) provide a compelling argument for the role of the 'nurse coach'. Using Bandura's (1997) social cognitive perspective and his idea of self-efficacy, nurses and other health educators need to build and maintain the client's sense of personal empowerment (self-efficacy). Using active listening, the nurse engages the client in the process of identifying problems related to their leg ulcer and its sequelae. The process of finding solutions to these self-generated questions provides the person with a sense of personal power and control. To promote meaningful lifestyle change, the nurse must know the patient's 'story'. By helping patients reach truthful self-reflection, nurses can generate the self-understanding along with knowledge and cognisance of their illness that truly contributes to self-confidence and success.

SPECIFIC TEACHING/LEARNING TECHNIQUES

Whatever the teaching/learning situation, and especially in the case of chronic leg ulcers, active teaching learning activities and techniques are preferable to passive approaches for patient education. Techniques targeting the learner and not the teacher and those that enact active cognitive processes in patients are almost guaranteed to be more effective than teacher-oriented, passive 'traditional' approaches.

Traditional approaches such as lecture, discussion and 'handouts' can be effective if they are used strategically, sparingly and teamed up with newer cognitive–behavioural approaches. One example of newer thinking is the concept of social marketing. Thackeray & Neiger (2002) note that diabetics (who are high risk for leg ulcers) are in contact with the formal health-care system less than 1% of their time. They suggest that social marketing techniques are appropriate for persons with chronic illness. This includes audience segmentation and channel analysis, i.e. identification of various constituents and the best ways to reach them. Persons with neuropathic ulcers might be in their fourth decade of life or, conversely, in their 80s. An approach designed for the elderly audience will likely be less effective for the younger group.

What strategies are available that generate active learner engagement? Many choices are available including role modelling, simulations, gaming, collaborative learning and programmed self-instruction (Babcock & Miller 1994, Rankin & Stallings 2001). It is beyond the scope of this chapter to discuss each strategy in depth. However, any clinician who is involved in patient education for health promotion has to understand the strengths and limitations of these active approaches. Many helpful resources are available. Table 32.1 lists the advantages and disadvantages of selected strategies.

Lecture and discussion can be combined with visually stimulating accessories such as audiovisuals, overheads, lifelike models, pamphlets and posters. Humorous strategies such as cartoons or gag photographs can be used to activate higher cognitive arousal for better learning and can be teamed up with many teaching/learning approaches. The body of literature supporting the cognitive efficacy of

Table 32.1 Teaching/learning strategies: advantages and disadvantages

Strategy	Primary type of learning	Advantages	Disadvantages
Lecture/discussion	Cognitive	Excellent for organizing and delivering larger amounts of content Makes focusing on critical content easier Highly efficient if supported by audience discussion	Lacks patient feedback Possible information overload Potential loss of interest (if without discussion) Less effective for affective and psychomotor learning Very passive if no group input
Demonstration/ return demonstration	Psychomotor	Multifactorial approach Involves multiple learning senses Commands interest Higher participation and cognitive arousal Teacher can diagnose performance problems Learner gets practice opportunities	Time consuming Focuses on 'how' and less on 'why'
Simulations	Affective	Promotes greatest transfer of knowledge Allows for realistic practice Permits anticipatory questioning Develops coping strategies Facilitates management of unpredictability	Time consuming Uncomfortable for some participants May evoke negative emotional responses
Programmed instruction	Cognitive	Learner sets own pace Learning divided into segments (modules) Frees teacher time Allows mastery of content before progressing to new content	Decreases teacher-learner personal contact Decreases motivation in some learners Requires development of materials Requires good visual and hearing ability
Group activities: Collaborative learning Problem-based learning	Cognitive	Allows greater teacher and learner interaction Teachers and learners learn from one another Allows divergent points of view Requires active learner participation Higher cognitive arousal Permits affective issues discussion	Time consuming Requires development of learning situations and expected activities Can be hampered by poor group process Teacher must understand theory and applications of group teaching
Testing	Cognitive	Analyses current knowledge level Stimulus for learners to remediate deficits Can be used to guide learning and give feedback	Test anxiety may interfere with true 'reading' Language may be a barrier Not appropriate for affective issues

table continued on following page

Table 32.1 Teaching/learning strategies: advantages and disadvantages, cont'd

Strategy	Primary type of learning	Advantages	Disadvantages
Role play	Affective	Promotes greater transfer of knowledge Permits acknowledgement of feelings Develops coping strategies	Time consuming Potential for negative emotional response
Gaming	Cognitive	Promotes greater transfer of knowledge Increased novelty promotes increased learning Develops coping strategies	May threaten some learners Time consuming May appear frivolous to some learners
Independent study	Cognitive	Permits learners to pace themselves Can incorporate various educational media Responsibility to learn rests on learner	Some learners do not learn efficiently without social contact Literacy issues may affect outcomes Outcomes dependent on quality of media used

humour and laughter is substantial and can be applied to many health-related issues (Beitz 1999).

Newer metacognitive approaches are also exceptionally helpful in imparting clinical information. This includes the use of problem-based learning wherein patients are asked to solve real-life dilemmas in advance (see Ch. 1), care or clinical maps (where patients see the planned steps in their own care) and mnemonics that address care issues. These can be complex memory aids or as simple as 'ACE' – the usual treatments for venous leg ulcers (ambulation, compression and elevation; Beitz 1997). The novelty of the mnemonic devices helps with long-term retention.

The easiest approach for a health educator to organize the 'big picture' of the teaching/learning experience is to develop a teaching plan. Multiple resources are available to health educators to learn how to develop a teaching plan and how to formulate behavioural objectives (Babcock & Miller 1994, Rankin & Stallings 2001). Teaching plans can be applied to a variety of health-care topics and settings (Beitz 1996). The first step in the process is to conduct a needs assessment of the participants' learning deficits. What patients perceive as their needs is of course valuable. However, pretesting of baseline knowledge may prove helpful in delineating the real knowledge gaps existent in a group. Once the missing components in knowledge, skills, and attitudes are revealed, the health educator can develop a helpful 'learning scaffold', the teaching plan.

Development of behavioural objectives is the next step. Generally the objectives address three foci: cognitive (knowledge), affective (emotions, feelings) and psychomotor (skills and actions) and are focused on the learner, not the teacher (Babcock & Miller 1994, Rankin & Stallings 2001, Redman 2001). Each objective consists of a specific action and an area of content. Sometimes educators include the expected evaluation method and its level of performance. For example, an objective may be stated as follows:

The learner will:

- Describe the epidemiology of and risk factors for arterial ulcers
- Describe the epidemiology of and risk factors for arterial ulcers with 90% proficiency on an essay question.

The health educator then lists the critical content in a bulleted list. For arterial ulcers, for example, content might include non-alterable risk factors (gender, age, heredity) vs alterable risk factors (hypercholesterolaemia, high blood pressure and smoking).

Teaching strategies that will actively engage learners can be preselected and matched to content. In general, educators should vary teaching strategies, tap into multiple learning senses (auditory, visual, musical and kinaesthetic) and generally respect adult learners by involving them in the learning experience. Educators can plan the allotted time in advance and how they will measure learning outcomes. A special caveat is in order. Evaluation methods should be matched to the nature of the objective. Namely, teaching wound care clinicians about the role of taking an ankle-brachial pressure index (ABPI) involves cognitive and psychomotor aspects. Learners could be tested via objective test questions for the theoretical content but they should also have to demonstrate actual performance of the test itself with proficiency.

The enormous benefits created by the generation of a teaching plan is that health educators are required to examine the teaching/learning process related to specific areas. Over time, the process becomes assimilated within experienced teachers and the plan becomes a form of cognitive scaffolding that expert educators use almost unconsciously to structure learning opportunities.

A newer approach is the development of behavioural objectives that address the complexities of learning, including the metacognitive level (Anderson & Krathwohl 2001). The objectives and associated content and evaluation are matched for not only cognitive domain (cognitive, affective, etc.) but the level of thinking that is involved (knowledge, comprehension, metacognition, synthesis). A sample teaching plan for a venous leg ulcer patient is given in Table 32.2.

HEALTH PROMOTION AND PATIENT EDUCATION: PUBLIC POLICY ISSUES

It is a simple truth that politics and policy-making influence health promotion and, less directly, patient education. Special interest groups and other policy-makers can alter the health promotion

Table 32.2 Sample teaching plan

Behavioural objectives	Content	Teaching/learning activities	Time	Evaluation methods
• Cognitive ♦ Affective ♦ Psychomotor	Bulleted list of major topics	Selected strategies listed	Timeframe per objective	Measurement method selected by educator
Sample plan for venous leg ulcer patients initiating compression				
The patient will: Describe the aetiology and pathophysiology of venous leg ulceration (cognitive)	**Aetiologies** • DVT • Immobilization • Trauma **Pathophysiology** • Normal venous flow • Damage to veins and valves or blood flow • Reversal of blood flow	Problem-based activity: Case study Discussion Handouts – guided questions	20 minutes	Objective exam – 100% correct answers to multiple choice questions
Value adherence to lifelong treatment therapies (affective)	• Purpose of compression therapy in self-care • Benefits of staying healthy • Barriers to staying healthy	Group discussion Role-playing	10 minutes	Role play with essay response – positive answers regarding value of self-care
Demonstrate correct application of compression stockings (psychomotor)	• Purpose of stockings • Variety of compression hose available • Actual demonstration of compression stocking application	Video demonstration of therapy Hands-on practice	30 minutes	Return demonstration with 100% efficacy

process by withholding health promotion programmes from various segments of society. The poor, the elderly, ethnic minorities and other disenfranchised groups (e.g. substance abusers) have been under-represented in research studies, and consequently programmes targeting their special needs have been lacking.

Patient education is also susceptible to political influence. For most major disorders (with diabetes as a significant exception), patient education and aspects of problem prevention are not a reimbursed activity in the USA. By way of example, for elderly persons at high risk for pressure ulcers, Medicare does not pay for prevention interventions like air mattresses, although the sequelae of skin breakdown and increased costs are virtually predictable.

Health educators of all disciplines need to recognize their ability to influence health policy by developing their knowledge of public policy and the political process. It is critical that health professionals know how to implement change and can teach political decision-makers about the efficacy and timelines of educational interventions (Rankin & Stallings 2001).

A major way in which to promote quality health promotion and patient education is to tap into the power of health partnerships. Community organizations, health-care facilities, colleges and universities, and other educational entities, can link together to share the wealth. For example academic health clinicians with grant writing expertise can partner with clinical practitioners to obtain funding for needed patient education initiatives (Pender 1996).

CONCLUSION

Health promotion and patient education are imperatives, both for care givers and for the patients actually experiencing leg ulcers. Whereever possible, patient education should be focused on preventing lower extremity ulceration. In Greek mythology, the emphasis was clear. The god of medicine, Asclepios, had two daughters, Hygeia and Panacea, who were responsible for prevention and cure respectively. To the detriment of the health of many Western nations, the focus has been on medical care producing a panacea. However, a philosophy of prevention requires health-care professionals and consumers to pay more attention to the immense benefits that can result from an active policy of health promotion, aided by sound educational principles.

References

Anderson I 2000 Quality of life and leg ulcers: will NHS reform address patient need? British Journal of Nursing 9: 830–834

Anderson L W, Krathwohl D R 2001 A taxonomy for learning, teaching, and assessing. A revision of Bloom's taxonomy of educational objectives. Longman, New York

Babcock D E, Miller M A 1994 Client education theory and practice. C V Mosby, St Louis, MO

Bandura A 1997 Self-efficacy: The exercise of control. Freeman, New York

Beitz J 1996 Developing behavioral objectives for perioperative staff development. AORN Journal 64: 87–95

Beitz J 1997 Unleashing the power of memory: the mighty mnemonic. Nurse Educator 22: 25–29

Beitz J 1999 Keeping them in stitches: humor in perioperative education. Seminars in Perioperative Nursing 8: 71–79

Beitz J 2001 Overcoming barriers to quality wound care: a systems perspective. Ostomy/Wound Management 47: 56–64

Beitz J, Bates-Jensen B 2001 Algorithms, critical pathways, and computer software for wound care: contemporary status and future potential. Ostomy/Wound Management 47: 33–40

Borenstein S 2000 Citing chronic diseases financial, human toll, doctors stress prevention. Philadelphia Inquirer, 30 November, p 1

Centers for Disease Control 2000 National Center for Chronic Disease Preventions and Health Promotion – Agency on Aging. Available on line at: www.cdc.gov/nccdphp/aag-aging.html

Davis L A, Chesbro S B 2003 Integrating health promotion, patient education, and adult education principles with the older adult. Journal of Allied Health 32: 106–109

Davis T C, Crouch M A, Willis G 1990 The gap between patient reading comprehension and readability of patient education materials. Journal of Family Practice 31: 533–538

Doak C, Doak L, Root J 1995 Teaching patients with low literacy skills, 2nd edn. J B Lippincott, Philadelphia, PA

Fries J 1987 An introduction to the 'compression of morbidity'. Gerontologica Perspecta 1: 5–7

Fries J 2003 Measuring and monitoring success in compressing morbidity. Annals of Internal Medicine 139: 455–460

Funk S G, Tornquist E M 2001 Chronic illness improving nursing practice through research. In: Funk S G, Tornquist E M, Leeman J et al (eds) Key aspects of preventing and managing chronic illness. Springer, New York, pp 3–11

Haverkos H, Chung R C, Norville Perez L C 2003 Is there an epidemic of HIV/AIDS among heterosexuals in the USA? Postgraduate Medical Journal 79: 444–448

Kart C S, Kinney J M 2001 The realities of aging: An introduction to gerontology. Allyn & Bacon, Boston, MA

Knowles M 1990 The adult learner: a neglected species. Gulf, Houston, TX

Longman P J 2003 The health of nations. Washington Monthly April: 16–23

Lorig K 2001 Self-management in chronic illness. In: Funk S G, Tornquist E M, Leeman J et al (eds) Key aspects of preventing and managing chronic illness. Springer, New York, pp 35–53

MacHaffie S 2002 Health promotion information: sources and significance for those with serious and persistent mental illness. Archives of Psychiatric Nursing 16: 263–274

Moore N 2003 Black women urged to be wary of AIDS. Detroit News 20 June, p 1 sec 3

Nolan M, Nolan J 1999 Rehabilitation, chronic illness, and disability: the missing elements in nurse education. Journal of Advanced Nursing 29: 958–966

Oermann M H, Harris C H, Dammeyer J A 2001 Teaching by the nurse: how important is it to patients? Applied Nursing Research 14: 11–17

Pender N J 1996 Health promotion in nursing practice, 3rd edn. Appleton & Lange, Stamford, CT

Rankin S H, Stallings K D 2001 Patient education: principles and practice, 4th edn. Lippincott Williams & Wilkins, Philadelphia, PA

Redman B K 2001 The practice of patient education, 9th edn. C V Mosby, St Louis, MO

Rycroft-Malone J, Gill H, Kitson A et al 2002 Getting evidence into practice. Nursing Standard 16(37): 38–43

Saarmann L, Daugherty J, Riegel B 2000 Patient teaching to promote behavioral change. Nursing Outlook 48: 281–287

Samad A, Hayes S, Dodds T 2002 Telemedicine: an innovative way of managing patients with leg ulcers. British Journal of Nursing 11(Suppl): S38–S52

Schenk S, Hartley K 2002 Nurse coach: healthcare resource for this millennium. Nursing Forum 37: 14–19

Sullivan E J 2002 Are we ready for the future? Journal of Professional Nursing 18: 305–307

Thackeray R, Neiger B C 2002 Using social marketing to develop diabetes self-management education interventions. Diabetes Educator 28: 536–543

Weiss R 2002 Literacy issues in patient care. Health Progress 83: 10–11

Whitehead D 2001 A social cognitive model for health education/health promotion practice. Journal of Advanced Nursing 36: 417–425

Whitehead D 2003 Evaluating health promotion: a model for nursing practice. Journal of Advanced Nursing 41: 490–498

Zuvekas S H, Taliaferro G S 2003 Pathways to access: health insurance, the healthcare delivery system, and racial/ethnic disparities, 1996–1999. Health Affairs 22: 139–153

Further reading

Banks N, Razor B 2000 Preoperative stoma site assessment and marking: Trained RNs can improve ostomy outcomes. American Journal of Nursing 103: 64A–B, 64E

Bennett R G 2001 Pressure ulcers. Clinical Geriatrics 9: 70–75

Best J T 2001 Effective teaching for the elderly: Back to basics. Orthopedic Nursing 20: 46–52

Bolton L L, Monte K, Pirone L A 2000 Moisture and healing: Beyond the jargon. Ostomy/Wound Management 46 (Suppl IA): 51S–62S

Cannuscio C, Block J, Kawachi I 2003 Social capital and successful aging: the role of senior housing. Annals of Internal Medicine 139: 395–400

Dailey M, Jasper A, Regan S 2000 PPS & wound care: how product formularies help to achieve cost efficiencies in the home care setting. Remington Report 8(14): 16–18

Daugherty J, Saarman L, Riegel B et al 2002 Can we talk? Developing a social support nursing intervention for couples. Clinical Nurse Specialist 16: 211–218

Davison B J 2003 Utilizing research to guide clinical practice in prostate cancer education. Oncology Nursing Forum 30: 377–379

Dolynchuk K, Keast D, Campbell K et al 2000 Best practices for the prevention and treatment of pressure ulcers. Ostomy/Wound Management 46: 38–52

Dowd T, Kolcaba K, Steiner R 2003 The addition of coaching to cognitive strategies: Interventions for persons with compromised urinary bladder syndrome. Journal of Wound, Ostomy, and Continence Nursing 30: 90–99

Dreger V, Tremback T 2002 Optimize patient health by treating literacy and language barriers. AORN Journal 75: 278–304

Healy M L 2001 Management strategies for an aging workforce. AAOHN Journal 49: 523–529

Hilton B A, Thompson R, Moore-Dempsey L, Hutchinson K 2001 Urban outpost nursing: the nature of the nurses' work in the AIDS prevention street nurse program. Public Health Nursing 18: 273–280

Jordan S 2000 Educational input and patient outcomes: exploring the gap. Journal of Advanced Nursing 31: 461–471

Landefeld C S 2003 Improving health care for older persons. Annals of Internal Medicine 139: 421–424

Liimatainen L, Poskiparta M, Sjogren A et al 2001 Investigating student nurses' constructions of health promotion in nursing education. Health Education Research 16: 33–48

Maloy J P, Gute R 2000 Overcoming the challenges of wound care education with PPS. The Remington Report 8: 24–27

Massaro E, Claiborne N 2001 Effective strategies for reaching high-risk minorities with diabetes. Diabetes Educator 27: 820–828

McCullough J, Knight C A 2002 Noncontact normothermic wound therapy and offloading in the treatment of neuropathic foot ulcers in patients with diabetes. Ostomy/Wound Management 48: 38–44

Mills A C, McSweeney M 2002 Nurse practitioners and physician assistants revisited: do their practice patterns differ in ambulatory care? Journal of Professional Nursing 18: 36–46

Milne J 2000 The impact of information on health behaviors of older adults with urinary incontinence. Clinical Nursing Research 9: 161–176

Moore Z 2001 Improving pressure ulcer prevention through education. Nursing Standard 16(6): 64–70

Oermann M H, Webb S A, Ashare J 2003 Outcomes of videotape instruction in clinic waiting area. Orthopedic Nursing 22: 102–105

Perls T, Terry D 2003 Understanding the determinants of exceptional longevity. Annals of Internal Medicine 139: 445–449

Resnick B 2003 Health promotion practices of older adults: Model testing. Public Health Nursing 20: 2–12

Resnick B 2001 Promoting health in older adults: a four-year analysis. Journal of the American Academic of Nurse Practitioners 13: 23–33

Rew L, Chambers K B, Kulkarni S 2002 Planning a sexual health promotion intervention with homeless adolescents. Nursing Research 51: 168–174

Russell L 2000 Understanding physiology of wound healing and how dressings help. British Journal of Nursing 9: 11–18

Saarmann L, Daugherty J, Riegel B 2002 Teaching staff a brief cognitive–behavioral intervention. MEDSURG Nursing 11: 144–151

Salcido R 2001 The point of education in wound care. Advances in Skin and Wound Care 14: 6

Sharp C, Burr G, Broadbent M et al 2000 Pressure ulcer prevention and care: a survey of current practice. Journal of Quality Clinical Practice 20: 150–157

Snowdon D 2003 Healthy aging and dementia: findings from the non-study. Annals of Internal Medicine 139: 450–454

Turnbull G 2001 The role and source of power. Ostomy/Wound Management 47: 11–12

Weiner M, Callahan C, Tierney W et al 2003 Using information technology to improve the health care of older adults. Annals of Internal Medicine 139: 430–436

Whitehead D 2001 Applying collaborative practice to health promotion. Nursing Standard 15(20): 33–37

Whitehead D 2001 Health education. Behavioral change and social psychology: nursing's contribution to health promotion? Journal of Advanced Nursing 34: 822–832

Yetzer E A 2002 Causes and prevention of diabetic foot skin breakdown. Rehabilitation Nursing 27: 52–58

INDEX